HEALTH LITERACY

Studies in Health Technology and Informatics

This book series was started in 1990 to promote research conducted under the auspices of the EC programmes' Advanced Informatics in Medicine (AIM) and Biomedical and Health Research (BHR) bioengineering branch. A driving aspect of international health informatics is that telecommunication technology, rehabilitative technology, intelligent home technology and many other components are moving together and form one integrated world of information and communication media. The series has been accepted by MEDLINE/PubMed, SciVerse Scopus, EMCare, Book Citation Index – Science and Thomson Reuters' Conference Proceedings Citation Index.

Series Editors:
B. Blobel, O. Bodenreider, E. Borycki, M. Braunstein, C. Bühler, J.P. Christensen, R. Cooper, R. Cornet, J. Dewen, O. Le Dour, P.C. Dykes, A. Famili, M. González-Sancho, E.J.S. Hovenga, J.W. Jutai, Z. Kolitsi, C.U. Lehmann, J. Mantas, V. Maojo, A. Moen, J.F.M. Molenbroek, G. de Moor, M.A. Musen, P.F. Niederer, C. Nøhr, A. Pedotti, O. Rienhoff, G. Riva, W. Rouse, K. Saranto, M.J. Scherer, S. Schürer, E.R. Siegel, C. Safran, N. Sarkar, T. Solomonides, E. Tam, J. Tenenbaum, B. Wiederhold and L.H.W. van der Woude

Volume 240

Recently published in this series

ISSN 0926-9630 (print)
ISSN 1879-8365 (online)

Health Literacy

New Directions in Research, Theory and Practice

Edited by

Robert A. Logan

U.S. National Library of Medicine, Bethesda, MD, USA

and

Elliot R. Siegel

U.S. National Library of Medicine (Retired), Bethesda, MD, USA

Amsterdam • Berlin • Washington, DC

ISBN 978-1-61499-789-4 (print)
ISBN 978-1-61499-790-0 (online)
Library of Congress Control Number: 2017955590

Publisher
IOS Press BV
Nieuwe Hemweg 6B
1013 BG Amsterdam
Netherlands
fax: +31 20 687 0019
e-mail: order@iospress.nl

For book sales in the USA and Canada:
IOS Press, Inc.
6751 Tepper Drive
Clifton, VA 20124
USA
Tel.: +1 703 830 6300
Fax: +1 703 830 2300
sales@iospress.com

Foreword

Richard H. CARMONA[1]

M.D, M.P.H., FACS

In 2002 I had the privilege to be nominated by the President of the United States and unanimously confirmed by the U. S. Senate as the United States Surgeon General. Little did I know that health literacy and cultural competence would not only become a significant portion of my portfolio, both would at times dominate every topic in the Surgeon General's portfolio! This is because the Surgeon General has to communicate with the largest medical practice in the nation, at that time more than 300 million fellow citizens as well as a global population of more than seven billion—who are equally interested in what and how America approaches health and disease.

The job description for the Surgeon General is to protect, promote, and advance the health, safety, and security of the United States. As the Surgeon General, I was the commander of the United States Public Health Service Commissioned Corp. But equally, if not more important, I was the chief health communicator for our nation and often the world.

As a result, it became rapidly apparent that health literacy and cultural competence were essential tools as I addressed a wide array of national health, safety, and security issues of relevance to the most linguistically and culturally diverse nation on earth.

The challenge then and today remains how do I summarize, reduce, explain, translate, and deliver the most complex science the world has ever known to the most diverse population in history? How should one impact sustainable individual and population behavioral change that results in improved health, decreased morbidity, mortality, and health costs while improving the quality and quantity of life?

While simply articulated, the aforementioned challenges are extraordinarily difficult to execute even with health literacy and cultural competence expertise. However, these challenges are *impossible* to address *without* the contributions of health literacy and cultural competence practitioners and researchers.

Many disciplines have contributed to the young multidisciplinary field of health literacy. The field of health literacy rightfully morphed into assessing daily health and medical jargon mostly because this essential element enables us to successfully engage each other and our fellow citizens who we have the privilege to serve.

Nevertheless, as the disease and economic burden of the nation continue to increase and politicians stake out their positions based on partisan ideology, the major contributor to the rising disease and economic burden is being overlooked. It is aberrant actions, such as smoking and sedentary behaviors, that often lead to preventable chronic diseases. Currently, from the U.S. federal government budget of about $3 trillion, approximately one in five dollars is spent on 'health care.' More precisely, most of the money is spent on 'sick care'—about 75¢ to 80¢ of each dollar is disbursed for preventable chronic disease.

---

[1] 17th Surgeon General of the United States, Distinguished Professor, University of Arizona

Consequently, unless we can successfully use health literate and culturally competent resonant messaging to engage, educate, and inspire our patients to pursue optimal health and wellness, the disease and economic burden will continue to rise irrespective of who is the nation's leader or which party is in power. While challenging enough, the latter tasks become even more daunting when most of a nation's population is health illiterate, as evidenced internationally by 21st century health literacy research.

To address these and other overwhelming challenges, the peer reviewed health literacy literature continues to grow as it appropriately defines the direct relationship between health literacy skills and ultimate health outcomes. Recent research additionally suggests individuals and communities with reasonable levels of health literacy are able to understand and integrate health messaging into their own lives to stay healthy, prevent disease, and recover from illness.

While the health literacy field began with extrapolating data from general literacy programs and lessons from teaching English as a second language as well as the basic seminal work of Len and Ceci Doak almost a half century ago, the evolution of the understanding of health literacy's complexity is now a legitimate science, which is exemplified by this textbook entitled, *"New Directions in Research, Theory and Practice."*

The science of health literacy is robust as it simultaneously evolves and challenges us. While health literacy is the lowest common denominator for all health related communication, its complexity and multidisciplinary nature defies a single equation or explanation.

The chapters in this text begin the journey of dissecting the variables of health literacy to a granular level where more questions are generated and some answers provided.

A future agenda for health literacy is emerging and includes, but is not limited to, leadership, policy, research, and practice—all topics covered in this textbook.

The commitment to become a health literate organization facilitates the education of staff and simplifies navigation through the health care system for our patients. Health organizations must pursue this goal so a culture of health literacy is promulgated. In addition, in certain communities where there is very low health literacy, shared decision making may be needed to meet the unique needs of vulnerable populations.

As much as the understanding and practice of health literacy has progressed, the book identifies an array of gaps that require further research. These areas include, but are not limited to, assessing how to measure the contributions of health literacy, how to best "activate" our patients and populations to effect sustainable positive behavioral change, as well as collaboration with other disciplines such as educational learning scientists and possibly neuroscientists to learn how to maximize the neuroplasticity associated with learning. I dare say that genomics will one day also be a variable we assess to better understand the genetic contributions of learning and behavior!

For those who master health literacy as practitioners or patients, the world of public health and all its aspirations become possible. For in the end, no matter how simple or complex the science, it is translation within a culturally competent, health literate manner that fosters desired, sustainable behavioral changes. The authors have provided us with a provocative and thoughtful next iteration in health literacy science as well as potential applications. This is essential reading for all health practitioners.

Preface

Robert A. LOGAN

Ph.D. U.S. National Library of Medicine

Overview

'New directions in health literacy research, theory, and practice' provides an introduction to health literacy research and practice and highlights similar scholarship in related disciplines. Although the book is intended primarily for health literacy researchers, practitioners and students, the editors suggest the book's diverse topics and approaches are of interest to health care and public health researchers, practitioners, and students in addition to scholars in related fields, such as health communication, science communication, consumer health informatics, library science, health disparities, and mass communication.

Some of the book's chapters on related fields (e.g. shared decision-making, patient engagement, patient activation, health prevention, design science, and mHealth) and related areas (e.g. the U.S. National Cancer Institute's Health Information National Trends Survey) also summarize some current research within each area. The book's editors and authors hope readers will mine individual chapters to write backgrounds for literature reviews well as to plan health literacy (and related) research and practice initiatives as well as interventions.

Organization and Chapter Contents

The book is organized as such: the initial chapter explains the still-evolving definition of health literacy; three chapters discuss developments and new directions in health literacy research; two chapters are devoted to developments and new directions in health literacy theory; two chapters detail health literacy interventions for vulnerable populations; four chapters cover health literacy leadership efforts; six chapters describe developments and new directions in disciplines that are similar to health literacy; and six chapters portray diverse health literacy practices. A preface from Richard Carmona, the former U.S. Surgeon General, is included in addition to this forward.

More specifically, in the book's first chapter Sorensen and Pleasant outline some conceptual differences in health literacy definitions and suggest current disagreements provide a foundation for the evolution of a more comprehensive health literacy definition. Sorensen and Pleasant explain that how health literacy is defined remains a foundational issue for health literacy researchers and practitioners.

The chapters devoted to developments and new directions in health literacy research feature three different themes. The chapter by Nguyen, Paasche-Orlow, and McCormack notes the recent progress and challenges to provide more empirical rigor within existing health literacy measures. The authors also discuss the Health Literacy Tool Shed (that they helped develop) which critiques health literacy tools and enables researchers to assess diverse health literacy measures. The chapter is especially recommended for health literacy scholars who are writing the methods section within a research paper. The chapter by Pelkian and Ganahl summarizes the development, psychometric properties, and results from recent health literacy population surveys within some European Union (EU) nations. Pelikan and Ganahl note the EU survey is integrative and based on 12 published models and 17 definitions of health literacy. The authors provide some specific suggestions to future researchers to measure health literacy in general populations. They report the survey's findings suggest low but varying health literacy levels among the participating nations. In this section's third chapter, Rudd identifies some gaps within the health literacy research literature as well as in health literacy practice. In an environmental scan of current research and practice, Rudd furnishes important issues for future health literacy researchers to consider including increased attention to the institutional and system wide norms, policies, and regulations that facilitate or impede access to health information, services, and care. The chapter is especially recommended for health literacy scholars who are writing the literature review section within a research paper.

The chapters devoted to developments and new directions in health literacy theory cover health literacy and the arts, and the conceptual crossroads between health literacy and health disparities research. Ike, Parker, and Logan describe research that suggests the arts are associated with better health outcomes and explain how this correlation has important implications for health literacy research and practice. The chapter additionally provides a theoretical framework that suggests why the arts may be therapeutic. In the second chapter within this section, Logan argues while health disparities and health literacy research are different disciplines, they share common conceptual foundations. The chapter suggests there are vacuums in current research knowledge that need attention – especially regarding the integration of health literacy and health disparities research to assess the social and structural determinants of health.

The two chapters devoted to health literacy interventions for vulnerable populations discuss initiatives within diverse community settings. A chapter by Smith and Carroll summarizes findings from U.S. social work interventions to improve maternal health within vulnerable populations where health literacy (in conjunction with other variables) is associated with improved health outcomes. Smith and Carroll's comprehensive findings yield an intricate web of interactions that occur among health literacy with other social, structural, cultural, family, and individual determinants of health. In this section's second chapter, Pleasant describes the Canyon Ranch Institute's (CRI) health literacy/integrative health interventions, which serve vulnerable populations in the U.S. and internationally. While Pleasant covers several CRI projects, he highlights a health literacy/theater for health intervention (utilizing community participation) within a low-income area of Lima, Peru that fostered favorable health outcomes.

Four chapters describe an array of health literacy leadership efforts. Hernandez, French, and Parker outline some of the initiatives launched by the U.S. National Academies of Sciences, Engineering, and Medicine's Roundtable on Health Literacy since its inception in 2004. The authors provide an overview of the Roundtable's contributions to health literacy. Hernandez, French, and Parker note the Roundtable has focused on evidence-based health literacy approaches that foster high-quality, patient centered care. Baur, Harris, and Squire explain the developments that prompted the 2010 U.S. National Action Plan to improve health literacy and note how the planning and activities associated with the effort became a model for positive organizational change. Brach describes the advancement of now-widely used criteria to assess and implement health literacy initiatives and perspectives within health care organizations. Brach explains the progress of health care organizations as they journey from implementing discrete health literacy initiatives to adopting a systems perspective focused on becoming health literate organizations. Besides providing some background about the criteria's development, Brach profiles some implementation efforts within three U.S. health care organizations (Carolinas Healthcare System, Intermountain Health, and Northwell Health). In this section's last chapter, Aldoory tracks health literacy higher education and related professional training efforts in the U.S. Aldoory's overview is one of the first efforts to describe health literacy higher education activities; she provides a case example that notes how policy developments in one U.S. state (Maryland) impacted the role of health literacy in professional higher education.

The six chapters devoted to developments and new directions in disciplines similar to health literacy describe six separate fields that provide collaborative opportunities for health literacy researchers and practitioners. Hibbard describes some similarities and differences between patient activation and health literacy research. Hibbard also provides a helpful summary of patient activation research in the U.S. and other nations. Stacey, Hill, McCaffery, Boland, Lewis, and Horvat review shared decision making's theoretical and empirical underpinnings and note the research's implications for health literacy scholarship. Stacey, Hill, McCaffery, Boland, Lewis, and Horvat provide international examples and suggest the integration of health literacy principles is important to develop interventions that facilitate shared decision making and essential to overcome the inequalities among patients with varying health literacy levels. Krist, Tong, Aycock, and Longo describe recent research efforts to engage patients in decision-making and behavior change to promote health care prevention. The authors note the theoretical underpinnings of engagement, the systems required to better support patient engagement, how social determinants of health influence patient engagement, and practical examples to demonstrate approaches to better engage patients in their health and wellbeing.

In one of the other three chapters within this section, Neuhauser provides an introduction to participatory design theory and endorses more collaboration between participatory design and health literacy researchers. Neuhauser supplies some research tips and case examples for researchers, practitioners, and policymakers. Hesse, Greenberg, Peterson, and Chou explain that the U.S. National Cancer Institute's Health Information National Trends Survey (HINTS) provides a downloadable, generalizable data set about how consumers utilize cancer health information resources. Hesse, Greenberg, Peterson, and Chou provide some HINTS-derived research that addresses consumer health engagement, consumer health informatics, consumer health awareness, and media utilization. In the last chapter in this section, Kreps describes the interactions between mHealth, health communication, consumer health informatics, and health literacy research. Kreps also addresses the use of mHealth in successful consumer health interventions and notes its potential for future use in health literacy initiatives.

The book's remaining six chapters provide a range of innovative health literacy practices. In the first of two chapters (by a team of international authors from diverse nations), Rowlands, Dodson, Leung, Levin-Zamir et. al. discuss how diverse global health systems and policy development provide opportunities for health literacy research, theory, and practice. The authors suggest a health literacy framework provides a pragmatic way to address health inequities and monitor progress across policy domains. In their second chapter, Levin-Zamir, Leung, Dodson and Rowlands et. al. note how individual, family, community, and cultural health challenges within diverse international settings impact health literacy initiatives as well as provide opportunities for health literacy researchers and practitioners. Among other issues, the authors note current cultural competence gaps among international health care providers exemplify how capacity building in health literacy is critical to improve a nation's health care delivery system. In the third chapter within this section, Whitney, Keselman, and Humphreys provide an overview of how libraries and librarians have contributed to health literacy practice and research. Whitney, Keselman, and Humphreys explain libraries often provide advantageous settings for health literacy initiatives and the authors encourage the collaborative participation of libraries and librarians in future health literacy research.

In the three remaining chapters within this section, Villaire, Gonzalez, and Johnson describe how health literacy initiatives contribute to innovative approaches in chronic disease management. Villaire, Gonzalez, and Johnson add the inclusion of health literacy assessment tools optimizes validation efforts within chronic disease management research. Kurtz-Rossi, Rikard, and McKinney describe how the U.S.-based Health Literacy Discussion List (which is an interactive listserv) yields ongoing data about contemporary topics of interest to health literacy practitioners. The authors' findings suggest the Health Literacy Discussion List provides a platform to share information and resources, announcements and calls for action, technical assistance, and professional discourse. In the book's final chapter Roberts, Callahan, and O'Leary describe the U.S.-based, Health Literacy Media's efforts to elevate health literacy via the use of social media. Roberts, Callahan, and O'Leary find social media are an effective mass communication tool for health promotion and health literacy initiatives. The authors provide tips for practitioners to use in future social media/health literacy efforts intended for vulnerable populations as well as other audiences.

Diversity of Nations, Institutions, and Universities Among the Book's Authors

The book's authors represent diverse nations including: Australia; Brazil; Canada; China; Denmark; India; The Netherlands; United Kingdom; and the United States.

Represented international colleges and universities include: Boston College; Boston University; Emory University; George Mason University; Harvard University; Michigan State University; Tufts University; Virginia Commonwealth University; University of California-Berkeley; University of Maryland, University of Oregon; University of Washington; Mayo Clinic College of Medicine; University of Ottawa; University of Vienna, University of Newcastle; La Trobe University; Aarhaus University; Hong Kong Polytechnic University; University of Haifa; Manipal University; Brazilian National School of Public Health; and Deakin University.

Represented international health care institutions and organizations include: the Global Health Literacy Academy; International Health Literacy Association; Canyon Ranch Institute/Health Literacy Media; RTI International; U.S. National Library of Medicine; U.S. National Cancer Institute; U.S. Office of the Surgeon General; Office of Disease Prevention and Health Promotion, U.S. Department of Health and Human Services; U.S. Agency for Healthcare Research Quality; U.S. National Academies of Sciences, Engineering, and Medicine; Mayo Clinic; Clalit Health; Institute for Healthcare Advancement; Victoria State Department of Health and Human Services; Fred Hollows Foundation; Bundesministerium fur Gesundheit und Frauen; and the Community Health and Learning Foundation.

Background

Overall, 'New directions in health literacy research, theory, and practice' took about 26 busy months from start to finish. It began during Elliot Siegel's consultation visit to the

U.S. National Library of Medicine (NLM) in spring 2015 when he told Rob Logan about a publishing initiative from IOS Press called 'Studies in Health Technology and Informatics.' Logan responded by preparing an outline of 26 chapters designed to cover contemporary health literacy theory and research as well as some developments in related disciplines in the U.S. and around the world. In the outline, Logan suggested the book's eventual title and recommended that he co-edit the volume with Siegel, NLM's emeritus Associate Director of Health Information Programs and Outreach.

To Logan's delight, IOS Press quickly embraced the outline's plans and initial invitations were sent to selected authors in summer 2015. Twenty-two months later, Logan and Siegel are pleased to report that 23 of the 24 of the current book's chapters are authored or co-authored by the originally invited contributors – and 23 of the 24 topics are either identical or highly similar to the ideas suggested within the initial invitations. The book's editors note the impressive participation by the original authors suggests the interest and pent-up demand to write a book about diverse aspects of health literacy research and practice. To put this another way, Logan and Siegel benefitted from an unprecedented rate of contributor acceptance, perseverance, cooperation, and occasional enthusiasm.

Most of the book's chapters were written and current as of late fall and winter 2016-17. The book was edited to foster some consistency in the quality of writing among and between chapters, which befits the book's health literacy focus. Yet, as explained in the first paragraph, the book was edited for health literacy researchers and practitioners rather than the general public.

Full disclosure: some of the book's chapters have been published in *Information Services and Use* with the consent of IOS Press (which is the publisher of the latter journal, this book, and the 'Studies in Health Technology and Informatics' initiative). Previous NLM contracts helped support the research presented in the chapter by Sandra Smith and Lauren Carroll and the development of the Health Literacy Tool Shed (described by Nguyen, Paasche-Orlow, and McCormack in their chapter).

Appreciation

Logan and Siegel are proud to have been associated with this book's development. We especially thank Betsy Humphreys MLS, who was NLM's acting director at the time of the book's inception (and co-authored a chapter) as well as Patricia Flatley Brennan Ph.D., who became NLM's director in September 2016. Brennan and Humphreys graciously supported Logan's time commitment to provide original contributions and serve as the book's co-editor.

The editors also gratefully acknowledge the interest in this book's development from diverse members of the U.S. National Academies of Sciences, Engineering, and Medicine's Roundtable on Health Literacy and the new International Health Literacy Association. Some of the ideas for the book's topics (as well as some authors) came from members of these organizations. In addition to our kudos to all of the book's authors and Kairi Look, Paul Weij, Kim Willems, and Arnoud de Kemp @ IOS Press, the editors thank Rachel Fudge (a free lance editor in San Francisco, CA.), for her assistance in the conversion of some manuscripts to meet IOS Press' technical publication requirements.

We hope 'New directions in health literacy research, theory, and practice' attains the 2015 request to the initial invitees to 'create a gem.'

Contents

Health Literacy Leadership

Developments and New Directions in Disciplines Similar to Health Literacy

Developments and New Directions in Health Literacy Practice

Defining Health Literacy

Health Literacy
R.A. Logan and E.R. Siegel (Eds.)
IOS Press, 2017
doi:10.3233/978-1-61499-790-0-3

Understanding the Conceptual Importance of the Differences Among Health Literacy Definitions

Kristine SØRENSEN[1]
Director, Global Health Literacy Academy, the Netherlands

Andrew PLEASANT
Director of Health Literacy and Research, Canyon Ranch Institute, Arizona, US

Abstract. This chapter aims to provide an overview of health literacy definitions, how the definitional work on health literacy has developed, and why it is important to understand the conceptual differences among diverse definitions. Since the introduction of the term 'health literacy' in the 1970s, research interest has grown exponentially.

Keywords. Health literacy, definitions, concepts

1. Introduction

Health literacy concerns the ability to manage health and navigate the health system. It is relevant for making informed health decisions, patient health outcomes, and resulting healthcare costs. Because of its importance across many areas of health, significant attention has been given to studying and measuring health literacy in recent years.

Conversely, the field lacks a consensus on how health literacy should be defined and measured, which fosters diverse definitions and assessments. The resulting fragmentation and inconsistencies create a barrier to conceptualizing, measuring, and understanding health literacy across health domains and fields. In addition, various studies operationalize health literacy within diverse health domains, populations, contexts, and languages, which can undermine comparative research [1].

This chapter aims to provide an overview of health literacy definitions, how the definitional work on health literacy has developed, and why it is important to understand the conceptual differences among diverse definitions. Whilst the blame of a lack of one commonly accepted definition has been an occasional barrier to action, recent research suggests health literacy's definitions may be more overlapping and similar than they initially appear. Although disputes about definitional-derived uncertainties dominate contemporary health literacy discourse, a common ground is being established that emphasizes more unifying than divisional approaches. Indeed, the latter discrepancies may occur because researchers are busy studying the differences among trees rather than agreeing to be in the same forest [1]. Notably, this

---

[1] Corresponding author: Director, Global Health Literacy Academy, Spilstraat 2, 6129JE Urmond, the Netherlands. E-mail: contact@globahealthliteracyacademy.org.

chapter argues the definitions that suggest health literacy is a multi-dimensional, complex, and heterogeneous phenomenon may themselves describe different aspects of the same phenomenon.

The chapter is written for researchers, policy-makers and practitioners to help them understand how their interpretation and perspectives on health literacy – based on their choice of definition (or lack of choice) – influence their work and outcomes.

The chapter is divided into four parts that include: an overview of health literacy definitions and their origin; a description of the evolution of health literacy definitions and their conceptual underpinnings; a discussion of the implications with regards to the application of health literacy definitions in policy, research, and practice; followed by concluding remarks.

At the outset, it is important to address how health literacy is defined because in the Oxford dictionary the definition of 'Definition' refers to 'an exact statement or description of the nature, scope, or meaning of something' [2]. As an emerging term, that was first cited in 1974 by Simonds as part of social policy with regards to health education in schools, health literacy has been of interest for stakeholders to understand and study as well as describe its meaning [3].

PubMed suggests the rate that scientific articles focusing on health literacy are published has increased with exponential speed. The first article was published in 1985; the second in 1992; and then only a handful of papers per year until 1999, when 15 articles were published. 2006 was the first year when more than 100 articles were issued and in 2016 almost a thousand articles focused on the topic. To date, 6129 articles are indexed in PubMed that address 'health literacy' [4]. Whereas many publications mention one definition, only a few of the indexed articles specifically address the analysis of health literacy definitions [5–10].

2. Health Literacy Definitions – an Overview

Three studies provide in-depth overviews of health literacy definitions. The first systematic literature review on health literacy definitions and models was conducted by Sørensen et al. in 2012 [9]. A second review focuses on health literacy definitions, their interpretations, and implications for policy initiatives [7]; and a more recent study provides an analysis of health literacy definitions with relevance for children and adolescents [5].

While not exhaustive, Table 1 provides commonly used health literacy definitions. Among the definitions included in Table 1, health literacy often is identified as part of the possession of knowledge about health among individuals. Contextually, health literacy is perceived as a skill-based process that individuals use to identify and transform information into knowledge. This translation process, then, inherently involves decoding a symbol system, such as printed words, spoken language, or visual elements, coupled with the placement of information within a useful context [11].

However, recent discussions about the role of health literacy (and subsequent definitions) emphasize the importance moving beyond an individual focus – and perceive health literacy as the interaction between the demands of health systems and the skills of individuals [9].

Table 1: Definitions of health literacy

1	WHO (1998)	"The cognitive and social skills which determine the motivation and ability of individuals to gain access to understand and use information in ways which promote and maintain good health" (12)
2	American Medical Association's (1999)	"The constellation of skills, including the ability to perform basic reading and numeral tasks required to function in the healthcare environment" (13)
3	Nutbeam (2000)	"The personal, cognitive and social skills which determine the ability of individuals to gain access to, understand, and use information to promote and maintain good health" (14)
4	USDHHS, 2000	"The degree to which individuals have the capacity to obtain, process and understand basic health information and services needed to make appropriate health decisions"
	Fok & Wong	"To understand and act upon physical and psycho-social activities with appropriate standards, being able to interact with people and cope with necessary changes and; demands reasonable autonomy so as to achieve complete physical, mental and social well-being" (15)
4	Institute of Medicine (2004)	"The individuals' capacity to obtain, process and understand basic health information and services needed to make appropriate health decisions" (16)
5	Kickbusch, Wait & Maag (2005)	"The ability to make sound health decision(s) in the context of everyday life--at home, in the community, at the workplace, the healthcare system, the market place and the political arena. It is a critical empowerment strategy to increase people's control over their health, their ability to seek out information and their ability to take responsibility" (17)
6	Zarcadoolas, Pleasant & Greer (2003, 2005, 2006)	"The wide range of skills, and competencies that people develop to seek out, comprehend, evaluate and use health information and concepts to make informed choices, reduce health risks ad increase quality of life" (10,18)
7	Paasche-Orlow & Wolf (2006)	"An individual's possession of requisite skills for making health-related decisions, which means that health literacy must always be examined in the context of the specific tasks that need to be accomplished. The importance of a contextual appreciation of health literacy must be underscored" (19)
	(Kwan et al., 2006)	'people's ability to find, understand, appraise and communicate information to engage with the demands of different health contexts to promote health across the lifecourse' (20)
8	EU (2007)	"The ability to read, filter and understand health information in order to form sound judgments" (21)
9	Pavlekovic (2008)	"The capacity to obtain, interpret and understand basic health information and services and the competence to use such information to enhance health" (22)
10	Rootman & Gordon-Elbihbety (2008)	"The ability to access, understand, evaluate and communicate information as a way to promote, maintain and improve health in a variety of settings across the life course" (23)
11	Ishikawa & Yano (2008)	"The knowledge, skills and abilities that pertain to interactions with the healthcare system" (24)
12	Mancuso (2008)	"A process that evolves over one's lifetime and encompasses the attributes of capacity, comprehension, and communication. The attributes of health literacy are integrated within and preceded by the skills, strategies, and abilities embedded within the competencies needed to attain health literacy" (25)
13	Australian Bureau of Statistics (2008)	"The knowledge and skills required to understand and use information relating to health issues such as drugs and alcohol, disease prevention and treatment, safety and accident prevention, first aid, emergencies, and staying healthy" (26)
14	Yost et al. (2009)	"The degree to which individuals have the capacity to read and comprehend health-related print material, identify and interpret information presented in graphical format (charts, graphs and tables), and perform arithmetic operations in order to make appropriate health and care decisions" (27)
15	Adams et al. (2009)	"The ability to understand and interpret the meaning of health information in written, spoken or digital form and how this motivates people to embrace or disregard actions relating to health" (28)
16	Adkins et al. (2009)	"The ability to derive meaning from different forms of communication by using a variety of skills to accomplish health-related objectives" (29)
17	Freedman et al. (2009)	"The degree to which individuals and groups can obtain process, understand, evaluate, and act upon information needed to make public health decisions that benefit the community" (30)
18	Massey et al.	"A set of skills used to organize and apply health knowledge, attitudes and practices relevant when managing one's health environment" (8)
19	Paakkari & Paakkari	"Health literacy comprises a broad range of knowledge and competencies that people seek to encompass, evaluate, construct and use. Through health literacy competencies people become able to understand themselves, others and the world in a way that will enable them to make sound health decisions, and to work on and change the factors that constitute their own and others' health chances" (31)

20	Wu et al.	"Health literate individuals are able to understand and apply health information in ways that allow them to take more control over their health through, for example, appraising the credibility, accuracy, and relevance of information and action on that information to change their health behaviours or living conditions" (32)
21	Gordon et al.	"The degree to which individuals have the capacity to obtain, access, process, and understand basic health information and services needed to take appropriate health decisions and involves an ongoing process of building individual and community capacity to understand the components of health"
22	Calgary Charter on Health Literacy (2011)	"Health literacy allows the public and personnel working in all health-related contexts to find, understand, evaluate, communicate, and use information. Health literacy is the use of a wide range of skills that improve the ability of people to act on information in order to live healthier lives. These skills include reading, writing, listening, speaking, numeracy, and critical analysis, as well as communication and interaction skills."
23	Sørensen et al. (2012)	"Health literacy is linked to literacy and entails people's knowledge, motivation and competencies to access, understand, appraise and apply information to make judgements and take decisions in everyday life concerning healthcare, disease prevention and health promotion to maintain or improve quality of life during the life course" (9)
24	Osborne et al. (2015)	"The personal characteristics and social resources needed for individuals and communities to access, understand, appraise and use information and services to make decisions about health. Health literacy includes the capacity to communicate, assert and enact these decisions" (33)

3. The Evolution of Health Literacy Definitions

In 1998, the World Health Organization (WHO) defined health literacy as "the cognitive and social skills which determine the motivation and ability of individuals to gain access to, understand and use information in ways which promote and maintain good health" in the Health Promotion Glossary [12]. In contrast, since 1999 the American Medical Association's Committee on Health Literacy has defined health literacy as a constellation of skills, including the ability to perform basic reading and numerical tasks required to function in the health-care environment [13]. Healthy People 2010 in the United States also defined health literacy as the degree to which individuals have the capacity to obtain, process and understand basic health information, and services needed to make appropriate health decisions [14].

In 2002, Fok and Wong emphasized the importance of individual autonomy in their definition and noted health literacy is "to understand and act upon physical and psycho-social activities with appropriate standards, being able to interact with people and cope with necessary changes and; demands reasonable autonomy so as to achieve complete physical, mental and social well-being" [15].

The U.S. Institute of Medicine suggests "health literacy is a shared function of social and individual factors, which emerges from the interaction of the skills of individuals and the demands of social systems" [16]. Similarly, Kickbusch and Maag [17] propose a context-driven definition of health literacy as: 'the ability to make sound health decision[s] in the context of every day life – at home, in the community, at the workplace, the health-care system, the market place and the political arena. It is a critical empowerment strategy to increase people's control over their health, their ability to seek out information and their ability to take responsibility.'

Kwam et al. provide a similar definition and suggest that health literacy refers to: 'people's ability to find, understand, appraise and communicate information to engage with the demands of different health contexts to promote health across the lifecourse' [20]. Kwan et al. further highlight the importance of engaging and equipping *all* parties involved in communication and decisions about health, including patients, providers, health educators, and lay persons [20]. This broader view also is found in Zarcadoolas, Pleasant and Greer's definition, which supplements that a health literate person can apply health concepts and information to novel situations, and participate in ongoing public and private dialogues about health, medicine, scientific knowledge, and cultural beliefs. Hence, Zarcadoolas, Pleasant and Greer define health literacy as 'the wide range of skills and competencies that people develop to seek out, comprehend, evaluate, and use health information and concepts to make informed choices, reduce health risks, and increase quality of life' [18].

The Calgary Charter on Health Literacy also was among the first to embrace an emerging 'two-sided' nature of health literacy that health literacy exists both within individuals as well as the demands created by health systems and health professionals.

Similarly, Freedman et al. argue that health literacy should reflect a broader social perspective than an individual orientation. Freedman et al. suggest public health literacy occurs when the conceptual foundations of health literacy also impact a larger group or a community [30].

3.1. Health Literacy – a Heterogeneous Phenomenon

The aforementioned definitions suggest health literacy is a heterogeneous phenomenon that has significance for both individuals and society [34]. For example, Mårtensson and Hensing identify two different approaches to health literacy. In the first, health literacy is characterized as a polarized phenomenon that focuses on the differences among adults with low versus high health literacy. In this approach, health literacy definitions are associated with a functional understanding as well as highlighting the individual basic skills that are needed to understand health information. Yet Mårtensson and Hensing's second approach advances a complex understanding of health literacy that acknowledges a wide range of interactive skills within social and cultural contexts. They suggest an individual's health literacy may fluctuate from situation to situation depending on content and context. In turn, the latter approach addresses the interactive and critical skills needed to use information and knowledge as a foundation for appropriate health decisions [34].

Pleasant and Kuruvilla explain the aforementioned approaches represent two conceptual dimensions that are grounded in differing clinical versus public health perspectives about health literacy. For example, Pleasant and Kuruvilla explain clinical encounters focus on obtaining information about and from the patient, whereas public health work focuses on delivering information such as knowledge of safe sex practices, abstinence to prevent HIV/AIDS, or the use of oral rehydration solution to prevent dehydration from diarrhea [11].

Similarly, a public health approach to health literacy often regards the acquisition of health knowledge as an integral part of health literacy rather than a separate outcome [14,35–36]. For instance, Nutbeam explains health literacy is an outcome of health promotion and explicitly places knowledge within a model of health literacy by defining functional health literacy as the basic understanding of factual health information [14]. Inspired by educational theory, Nutbeam identifies two additional levels of health literacy: interactive health literacy and critical health literacy. Respectively, these reflect individual cognitive, literacy, and social skills as well as the ability to critically analyze and apply health information to enhance personal control [14]. In addition, Abel conceptualizes knowledge as undergirding health literacy by describing health literacy as a 'knowledge-based competency for health promoting behaviors' [37]. Zarcadoolas et al. widen the latter approach to health literacy by noting health literacy's scientific, civic and cultural domains and defining the acquisition, understanding, evaluation, and use of knowledge as an integral component of health literacy.

In contrast, Baker provides a clinical perspective that notes knowledge is a resource within individuals that 'facilitates health literacy but does not in itself constitute health literacy' [38].

Although the concept of health literacy features diverse definitions and conceptual approaches, definitions grounded in clinical and public health tend to find a common ground because each tends to focus on peoples' ability to find, understand, evaluate and put information to use to improve decision making and, ultimately, improve health and quality of life and/or reduce inequities in health during one's life course [11]. Some definitions also contextualize health literacy by including a focus on interaction and participation within surrounding communities and society [9].

3.2. Lost in Translation?

The fact that 'health literacy' is neither included in the *Encyclopaedia Britannica* nor other American and British dictionaries suggests that 'health literacy' has yet to attain mainstream English use. Of course, its derivation (from the words 'health' and 'literacy') is included as separate terms.

While there is consistency in defining 'health' among dictionaries, the explanations concerning the meaning of 'literacy' within English dictionaries are somewhat polarized. One perspective emphasizes functional aspects and defines 'literacy' as, literally, the ability to read and write. A second perspective suggests 'literacy' is obtaining individual knowledge or competence, which links literacy with educational attainment [39].

The differences in how 'literacy' is defined somewhat parallel the heterogeneous range of health literacy definitions, which suggests an acceptance of functional health literacy within clinical settings parallels a wider, more comprehensive interpretation within public health and health promotion (that includes interactive and critical health dimensions).

Otherwise, an analysis of health literacy term translations made by Sørensen and Brand suggests the polarization of the term health literacy sometimes mirrors its translation from English into other languages [39]. Sørensen and Brand's analysis also suggests that 'health literacy' frequently is translated into related words such as 'health competencies', 'abilities', 'capabilities', 'skills', 'capacities', 'knowledge' and 'awareness.' The latter finding suggests a thesaurus of related health terms often suggests how health literacy is defined and interpreted in non-English languages. The translations of health literacy sometimes represent nuances of the same term, and different translations even overlap at times, such as [39]:

- Competence can be understood as 'the ability to do something successfully or efficiently' or as 'the scope of a person's or group's knowledge or ability', thus it can also mean 'skill or ability'.
- Skill means 'the ability to do something well; expertise' and has its origin in late Old English scele, knowledge.
- Ability means 'the capacity to do something' and 'talent that enables someone to achieve a great deal'.

- Capacity means 'the ability or power to do, experience, or understand something'.
- Knowledge means 'facts, information and skills acquired by a person through experience and education; the theoretical or practical understanding of a subject as well as awareness or familiarity gained by experience of a fact or a situation'.
- Awareness refers 'to having knowledge or perception of a situation or a fact'.

In a systematic review of health literacy definitions, Sørensen et al. suggest while there is no unanimous definition of health literacy within an array of languages, many of the current definitions of related terms overlap significantly [9].

3.3. Risk of Fragmentation?

Given the breadth of research on health literacy, the variance in definitions is sometimes suggested to foster a risk of fragmentation within the field. Indeed, Mackert et al. identify four domains of health literacy research that suggests some fragmentation is operant. For example, Mackert et al. note the field of health literacy is divided into research about health domains (e.g., various conditions and diseases), populations (e.g., by role or age), specific channels and contexts (e.g., e-health), and languages [1].

Regarding health domains, health literacy is frequently associated with specific illnesses and conditions, such as AIDS [40], diabetes [41], cancer [42], and mental health [43]. Regarding populations, health literacy research focuses on specific patient populations [44] as well as specific individual roles, such as caregivers [45], mothers [46], and parents [47]. Herein, a life course perspective also is often used, e.g., in terms of children [48], adolescents [49], adults [50], and elderly [51]. The potential gender-issues associated with health literacy also are explored among and between men [52] and women [53].

Regarding specific channels and contexts, a third stream of research focuses on the various channels by which people receive health information, such as media health literacy [54]. Finally regarding languages, health literacy research about languages other than English often includes a focus on translations and the adaptation of health literacy instruments and tools within Asian and European cultural and linguistic contexts [55–56].

While Mackert et al., explain the proliferation of research spurs more specialized approaches to health literacy assessment, they counter the field's diversity may be a testament to the range of scholars interested in the topic, as well as their creativity and interest in advancing evidence [1]. Mackert et al. add the effort to study health literacy in different contexts and develop new tools and measurements to be used in research also are crucial elements that advance the health literacy field. They explain the development of more focused research domains can advance rather than undermine a broader conceptual understanding of health literacy [1].

4. The Implications of Application of Health Literacy in Policy, Research and Practice

While new definitions of health literacy continue to be published, it is important to be mindful of how definition(s) of health literacy are adopted in practice as well as the differing, and potentially problematic, ways in which definitions may be interpreted, which impacts health literacy-derived policy initiatives [7].

The existence of many definitions of health literacy and the various interpretations that are derived from commonly used definitions sometimes may be problematic for policymakers, practitioners, and researchers. For example, it may unclear which definition of health literacy is best in any given context. Similarly, the criteria to assess the merits of diverse definitions can be nebulous. In addition, vague definitions open the possibility of misunderstandings because unclear definitions can generate false assumptions and research operationalizations, which undermine the reliability and validity of research methods [7]. In addition, it is difficult to compare research with different conceptual underpinnings, which limits the advancement of systematic reviews and comparative effectiveness research in the health literacy field. Since systematic reviews and comparative effectiveness research represent the most rigorous research approaches, implicit and explicit constraints inhibit the development of health literacy as an evidence-based discipline.

It also should be recognized that an imprecise meaning of a translated literacy component might foster one-dimensional research approaches that potentially impact health literacy research, policy, and practice. For instance if health literacy is translated narrowly to reflect a functional focus, subsequent research and implementation may be relegated to functional issues without assessing health literacy's other, diverse dimensions. Similarly, if the focus of a translated definition of health literacy is the competences related to abilities to evaluate and act on information, assessments may only address decision-making and critical thinking in terms of applying information to a personal situations and actions. Basically, the consequences of the choice of translation additionally have the potential to influence the discourse and agenda setting concerning health literacy among and between diverse nations [39].

Unsurprisingly, some countries opt to use the term 'health literacy' in English due to the challenge to find an appropriate term to explain 'literacy.' For similar reasons, some health researchers and practitioners in non-English speaking nations do not translate the term 'empowerment,' which is becoming a well-accepted, self-contained term internationally.

4.1. Missing the Forest through the Trees?

Given diverse definitions and different conceptual underpinnings, Mackert et al. find it is crucial that scholars separate the "forest" of health literacy through the "trees" associated with their specific research interests [1]. Mackert et al. suggest there are more similarities than differences in health literacy definitions. Hence, they encourage health literacy scholars to pay more attention to their research methods and goals than become immersed in the subtle differences among and between health literacy definitions [1].

5. Concluding Remarks

Health literacy arises from a convergence of education, health services, social and cultural factors and advances research and practice from diverse fields [16]. Linguistically, the term implies multiple interpretations that build on the separate understanding of 'health' and 'literacy.' Still, it is clear health literacy's 'whole' is more than the sum of its linguistic parts, and 'health literacy' is an emerging field in its own right. The exponential developments within health literacy research, policy, and practice keep adding new details and insights about health literacy's impact as a social and structural determinant of health. In turn, each of health literacy's multidimensional aspects provides a piece of a puzzle that helps us define what health literacy is and why it is important.

Overall, health literacy's definitions conceptually support making health and other information more accessible, understandable, evaluable, applicable, and actionable so health improves for individuals, families, communities, and society. The discussions about the strengths and weaknesses of various definitions should not be a barrier to address health literacy's challenges in health systems worldwide, such as how to overcome limited health literacy and the strong social gradient within health that challenges health policies and practices. Health literacy deficits and associated social inequalities need to be addressed by health planners and policymakers, who also must attend to the social determinants of health as well as foster appropriate public health and health promotion strategies that strengthen citizens, patients, and the health care delivery system's capacities to meet peoples' needs [57].

Ultimately, health literacy is a socially constructed concept. The idea of health literacy is subject to constant construction through social, cultural, and political processes. In fact, there is no independent, objective presence of health literacy. The history of defining health literacy is a social history and definitions are among the richest artifacts for examination and learning. Through the latter process we strive to continually improve our understanding of health literacy as the basis for interventions to improve health and well being in a cost-effective and sustainable manner. Hence, in lieu of debating which health literacy definition is 'correct,' we suggest the challenge is to find a definition that provides a basis for effective evidence-based approaches to improve health and well being as well as a foundation for future measurement.

A more evidence-based foundation and approach are especially needed in low-income and marginalized communities around the world. Ideally, health literacy should be perceived as one of the underpinnings to improve health and well being, which subsequently enhances global health equity. As a result, we suggest research evidence should determine the direction of evolving health literacy definitions as we continue to improve individual and public health.

While defining health literacy is a quest that will continue to challenge all stakeholders, once the socially-constructed complexity of the term is acknowledged and accepted as a common ground for action, current confusion should generate future clarity, a more cohesive field, and effective approaches to improving health, well being, and health equity.

References

[1] Mackert M, Champlin S, Su Z, Guadagno M. The many health literacies: advancing research or

fragmentation? Health Commun. 2015; 2;30(12):1161–5. DOI:10.1080/10410236.2015.1037422.

[2]   Oxford Dictionaries. Definition of definition in English | [Internet]. Oxford Dictionaries. 2017
      Available from: https://en.oxforddictionaries.com/definition/definition. Retrieved April 27, 2017.

[3]   Simonds S. Health education as sociol policy. Heal Educ Monogr. 1974;2:1–25.

[4]   PubMed. Health literacy search in PubMed [Internet]. 2017. Available from:
      https://www.ncbi.nlm.nih.gov/pubmed?term=%22health literacy%22. Retrieved April 27, 2017.

[5]   Bröder J, Okan O, Bauer U, Bruland D, Schlupp S, Bollweg TM, et al. Health literacy in childhood and
      youth: a systematic review of definitions and models. BMC Public Health. 2017; 17(1):361. DOI:
      10.1186/s12889-017-4267-y.

[6]   Cadman KP. Lay worker health literacy: a concept analysis and operational definition. Nurs Forum.
      2017; Apr 13. DOI:10.1111/nuf.12203.

[7]   Malloy-Weir LJ, Charles C, Gafni A, Entwistle V. A review of health literacy: definitions,
      interpretations, and implications for policy initiatives. J Public Health Policy. 2016; 37(3):334–52.
      DOI: 10.1057/jphp.2016.18.

[8]   Massey PM, Prelip M, Calimlim BM, Quiter ES, Glik DC. Contextualizing an expanded definition of
      health literacy among adolescents in the health care setting. Health Educ Res. 2012; 27(6):961–74.

[9]   Sørensen K, Van den Broucke S, Fullam J, Doyle G, Pelikan J, Slonska Z, et al. Health literacy and
      public health: a systematic review and integration of definitions and models. BMC Public Health. 2012;
      12:80. DOI: 10.1186/1471-2458-12-80.

[10] Zarcadoolas C, Pleasant A, Greer DS. Elaborating a definition of health literacy: a commentary. J
      Health Commun. 2003; 8 Suppl 1(781062704):119–20. DOI: 10.1080/713851982.

[11] Pleasant A, Kuruvilla S. A tale of two health literacies: public health and clinical approaches to health
      literacy. Health Promot Int. 2008;23(2):152–9. DOI: 10.1093/heapro/dan001.

[12] Nutbeam D. Health promotion glossary. Health Promot Int. 1998;1(1):113-27.

[13] Ad Hoc Committee on Health Literacy for the Council on Scientific Affairs, American Medical
      Association AMA, RD P, JA W, GR M, A F, B W, et al. Health literacy: report of the Council on
      Scientific Affairs. JAMA J Am Med Assoc. American Medical Association; 1999; 281(6):552–7.

[14] Nutbeam D. Health literacy as a public health goal: a challenge for contemporary health education and
      communication strategies into the 21st century. Health Promot Int. 2000;15(3):259–67.

[15] Fok MSM, Wong TKS. What does health literacy mean to children? Contemp Nurse. 2002; 13(2–
      3):249–58.

[16] Nielsen-Bohlman LT, Panzer AM, Kindig DA. Health literacy: a prescription to end confusion. San
      Fransisco: The National Academies Press; 2004.

[17] Kickbusch I, Wait S, Maag D. Navigating health. The role of health literacy. Alliance for Health and
      the Future, International Longevity Centre-UK; 2005.

[18] Zarcadoolas C. Understanding health literacy: an expanded model. Health Promot Int. 2005;20(2):195–
      203.

[19] Paasche-Orlow MK, Wolf MS. Literacy to health outcomes. Soc Sci. PNG Publications; 2007;31(Suppl
      1):19–26.

[20] Kwan B, Frankish J, Rootman I, Zumbo B, Kelly K, Begoray DL, et al. The development and
      validation of measures of "health literacy" in different populations. UBC Institute of Health Promotion
      Research and University of Victoria Community Health Promotion Research; 2006.
      http://blogs.ubc.ca/frankish/files/2010/12/HLit-final-report-2006-11-24.pdf. Retrived May 10 2017.

[21] European Commission. Together for health: a strategic approach for the EU 2008-2013. Brussels; 2007.

[22] Pavlekovic G. Health literacy. Programmes for training on research in public health for South Eastern
      Europe. Vol. 4: Health Promotion and Disease Prevention: A Handbook for Teachers, Researchers,
      Health Professionals and Decision Makers. 2008. p. 463–466.

[23] Rootman I, Gordon-El-Bihbety D. A vision for a health literate Canada report of the expert panel on
      health literacy. Ottawa; 2008.

[24] Ishikawa H, Yano E. Patient health literacy and participation in the health-care process. Health Expect.
      2008;11(2):113–22.

[25] Mancuso JM. Health literacy: A concept/dimensional analysis. Nurs Health Sci. 2008;10(3):248–55.
      DOI: 10.1111/j.1442-2018.2008.00394.x.

[26] Australian Bureau of Statistics. Adult literacy and life skills survey. Summary results. Australia.
      Canberra; 2008.

[27] Yost KJ, Webster K, Baker DW, Choi SW, Bode RK, Hahn EA. Bilingual health literacy assessment
      using the talking touchscreen/la Pantalla Parlanchina: development and pilot testing. Patient Educ
      Couns. 2009;75(3):295–301.

[28] Adams RJ, Stocks NP, Wilson DH, Hill CL, Gravier S, Kickbusch I, et al. Health literacy--a new
      concept for general practice? Aust Fam Physician. 2009;38(3):144–7.

[29] Ross Adkins N, Corus C. Health literacy for improved health outcomes: effective capital in the

marketplace. J Consum Aff. 2009;43(2):199–222.

[30] Freedman D a, Bess KD, Tucker HA, Boyd DL, Tuchman AM, Wallston K. Public health literacy defined. Am J Prev Med. 2009;36(5):446–51.

[31] Paakkari L, Paakkari O. Health literacy as a learning outcome in schools. Simovska V, editor. Health Educ. 2012;112(2):133–52.

[32] Wu AD, Begoray DL, Macdonald M, Wharf Higgins J, Frankish J, Kwan B, et al. Developing and evaluating a relevant and feasible instrument for measuring health literacy of Canadian high school students. Health Promot Int. 2010;25(4):444–52.

[33] Dodson S, Good S OR. Health literacy toolkit for low and of middle-income countries: a series of information sheets to empower communities and strenghten health systems. 2015.

[34] Mårtensson L, Hensing G. Health literacy - a heterogeneous phenomenon: a literature review. Scand J Caring Sci. 2012;26(1):151–60. DOI: 10.1111/j.1471-6712.2011.00900.x

[35] Kickbusch I. Health literacy : addressing the health and and education divide. Online J Issues Nurs. 2001;16(3).

[36] St Leger L. Schools, health literacy and public health: possibilities and challenges. Health Promot Int. 2001;16(2):197–205.

[37] Abel T. Cultural capital and social inequality in health. J Epidemiol Community Heal. 2008;62(7):e13–e13.

[38] Baker DW. The meaning and the measure of health literacy. J Gen Intern Med. 2006; 8:878–83.

[39] Sørensen K, Brand H. Health literacy lost in translations? Introducing the European Health Literacy Glossary. Health Promot Int. 2014; 4:634-44. DOI. 10.1093/heapro/dat013.

[40] Kalichman SC, Benotsch E, Suarez T, Catz S, Miller J, Rompa D. Health literacy and health-related knowledge among persons living with HIV/AIDS. Am J Prev Med. 2000;18(4):325–31.

[41] Perrenoud B, Velonaki V-S, Bodenmann P, Ramelet A-S. The effectiveness of health literacy interventions on the informed consent process of health care users: a systematic review protocol. JBI database Syst Rev Implement reports. 2015;13(10):82–94.

[42] Friedman DB, Hoffman-Goetz L. Literacy and health literacy as defined in cancer education research: A systematic review. Health Educ J. 2008;67(4):285–304.

[43] Jorm AF. Mental health literacy. Public knowledge and beliefs about mental disorders. Br J Psychiatry. 2000;177:396–401.

[44] Pignone M, DeWalt DA, Sheridan S, Berkman N, Lohr KN. Interventions to improve health outcomes for patients with low literacy. J Gen Intern Med. Springer; 2005;20(2):185–92.

[45] Hironaka LK, Paasche-Orlow MK. The implications of health literacy on patient-provider communication. Arch Dis Child. 2008;93(5):428–32.

[46] Porr C, Drummond J, Richter S. Health literacy as an empowerment tool for low-income mothers. Fam Community Heal. 2006;29(4):328–35.

[47] Yin HS, Johnson M, Mendelsohn AL, Abrams MA, Sanders LM, Dreyer BP. The health literacy of parents in the United States: a nationally representative study. Pediatrics. 2009;124 Suppl(Supplement_3):S289–98. DOI:10.1542/peds.2009-1162E.

[48] Borzekowski DLG. Considering children and health literacy: a theoretical approach. Pediatrics. 2009;124(Supplement):S282-8. DOI: 10.1542/peds.2009-1162D.

[49] Abel T, Hofmann K, Ackermann S, Bucher S, Sakarya S. Health literacy among young adults: a short survey tool for public health and health promotion research. Health Promot Int. 2015; 3:725-35. DOI: 10.1093/heapro/dat096.

[50] Kutner M, Greenberg E, Jin Y, Paulsen C. The health literacy of America's adults: results from the 2003 National Assessment of Adult Literacy (NCES 2006–483). Washington DC; 2006.

[51] Tiller D, Herzog B, Kluttig A, Haerting J, Nutbeam D, Berkman N, et al. Health literacy in an urban elderly East-German population – results from the population-based CARLA study. BMC Public Health. BioMed Central; 2015;15(1):883. DOI: 10.1186/s12889-015-2210-7.

[52] 52. Peerson A, Saunders M. Health literacy revisited: what do we mean and why does it matter? Health Promot Int. Cortina; 2009;24(3):285–96. DOI: 10.1093/heapro/dap014.

[53] 53. Shieh C, Broome ME, Stump TE. Factors associated with health information-seeking in low-income pregnant women. Women Heal. Taylor & Francis Group; 2010;50(5):426–42.

[54] 54. Levin-Zamir D, Lemish D, Gofin R. Media Health literacy (MHL): development and measurement of the concept among adolescents. Health Educ Res. 2011;26(2):323–35. DOI: 1093/her/cry007.

[55] Duong T V., Aringazina A, Baisunova G, Nurjanah, Pham T V., Pham KM, et al. Measuring health literacy in Asia: Validation of the HLS-EU-Q47 survey tool in six Asian countries. J Epidemiol. 2017; 27(2); 80–86. DOI:10.1016/j.je2016.09.005.

[56] Sørensen K, Van den Broucke S, Pelikan JM, Fullam J, Doyle G, Slonska Z, et al. Measuring health literacy in populations: illuminating the design and development process of the European Health

Literacy Survey Questionnaire (HLS-EU-Q). BMC Public Health. 2013;13(1):948. DOI: 10.1186/1471-2458-13-948.
[57]   Parker RM, Ratzan SC. Health literacy: a second decade of distinction for Americans. J Health Commun. 2010;15 Suppl 2(November 2012):20–33. DOI: 10.1080/10810730.2010.501094.

Developments and New Directions in Health Literacy Research

Health Literacy
R.A. Logan and E.R. Siegel (Eds.)
IOS Press, 2017
doi:10.3233/978-1-61499-790-0-17

The State of the Science of Health Literacy Measurement

Tam H. NGUYEN[a], Michael K. PAASCHE-ORLOW[b,1], Lauren A. McCORMACK[c]

[a] *William F. Connell School of Nursing, Boston College, Chestnut Hill, Massachusetts*
[b] *Boston University School of Medicine, Division of General Internal Medicine, Boston, Massachusetts*
[c] *RTI International, Division of Public Health Research, Research Triangle Park, North Carolina*

Abstract. Advancing health literacy (HL) research requires high-quality HL measures. This chapter provides an overview of the state of the science of HL measurement: where the field started, currently is, and should be going. It is divided into eight key sections looking at (1) the history of HL measurement, (2) the relationship between HL definitions and measurement, (3) the HL conceptual domains most and least frequently measured, (4) the methods used to validate HL measures, (5) the characteristics of the participants in the measurement validation studies, (6) the practical considerations related to administering HL measures, (7) the advantages and disadvantages of using objective versus subjective HL measures, and (8) future directions for HL measurement.

Based on the material presented in this chapter, the following conclusions can be drawn. First, there is an enormous proliferation of HL measures and this growth presents both opportunities and challenges for the field. Second, to move the field forward, there is an urgent need to better align HL measurement with definitions of HL. Third, some HL domains, such as numeracy, are measured more often than others, such as speaking and listening. Consequently, it is important to think about novel mechanisms to measure HL domains that are rarely measured. Fourth, HL measures are most often developed, validated, and refined using classical measurement approaches. However, strong empirical and practical rationales suggest making an assertive shift toward using modern measurement approaches. Fifth, most HL measures are not well validated for use in minority populations; consequently, future validation studies should be mindful of validation samples. Sixth, HL measures can be administered using multiple modes, most frequently via paper-and-pencil surveys. Identifying which mode of administration is most suitable requires reflecting on the underlying measurement purpose and the characteristics of the participants being measured. These considerations should also be made when deciding between a subjective versus objective HL measure.

Cumulatively, this chapter provides tools to help readers select and use the most appropriate measures of HL for their needs. It also provides rationale and strategies for moving the science of HL measurement forward.

Keywords: Health literacy, measurement, conceptual domains, validation, psychometrics

---

[1] Corresponding author: *Boston University School of Medicine, 801 Massachusetts Avenue, 2nd Floor, Boston, MA 02118, USA*

"We owe all the great advances in knowledge to those who
endeavor to find out how much there is of anything."

— James Maxwell, Physicist (1831-1879)

1. Overview and History of Health Literacy Measurement

The 2004 seminal Institute of Medicine report *Health Literacy: A Prescription to End Confusion* identified the development of new measures of health literacy (HL) as a key priority for the field [1]. Numerous scientific calls and proposals followed to develop and test HL measures in support of that recommendation [2]. Now, more than a decade later, over 150 HL measures exist, demonstrating a sweeping response to the scientific calls and reflecting tremendous productivity in this area [3-5]. This growth presents both opportunities and challenges for the field [6, 7]. In one respect, each of these measures provides a degree of utility and valuable lessons as the field moves forward. Despite these efforts, however, no "gold standard" measure for HL has emerged, and the variety of measures has made comparing results across studies and populations a serious challenge.

This chapter distills the state of the science of HL measurement by addressing several key areas. In section 2, we examine the relationship, or lack thereof, between definitions and measurement. In section 3, we summarize the conceptual domains most and least frequently measured, using the most current and well-accepted definitions and theoretical frameworks guiding the field. In section 4, we synthesize current methods used to validate HL measures and discuss their relative strengths and limitations. In section 5, we evaluate characteristics of the participants in the validation studies used to establish HL measures. In section 6, we discuss the practical considerations related to the various modes of administering HL measures. In section 7, we identify measures that assess HL subjectively versus objectively and discuss the relative advantages and disadvantages. Finally, in section 8, we provide a road map for the future of HL measurement.

The overarching aims for this chapter are to help readers identify factors that contribute to stronger HL measures, provide tools to help readers select and use appropriate HL measures, and put forth a rational strategy for advancing HL measurement. An inventory of all the existing HL measures available has been omitted intentionally as an easy-to-use, publicly available Health Literacy Toolshed (www.healthliteracy@bu.edu) serves this purpose.

2. Relationship between Definitions and Measurement

In general, the HL field has promulgated separate discussions regarding the *definition* of HL and the *measurement* of HL [7]. Despite promising recent work developing tools in tandem with definitions, the disconnect between definitions and what the tools measure has been a persistent conceptual stumbling block, which has led to several conundrums that will need to be solved for the field to progress in a coherent manner.

Multiple definitions of HL exist; however, some are vague or inadequately specified to allow measurement. There are even more tools to measure HL, but many are loosely related to a definition [3-5, 8]. This section examines the interplay between HL definitions and measurement from a legacy perspective verses more recent HL tools. It also looks at the paradox and barriers that exist to more fully integrating HL definitions with measurement.

2.1. Legacy Tools

The large majority of empirical HL research has used the Rapid Estimate of Adult Literacy in Medicine (REALM) [9] and the Test of Functional Health Literacy in Adults (TOFHLA) [10], or some variant of these tools. These instruments, however, only align superficially to a definition of HL.

The REALM is a word pronunciation test that uses medical words, an extremely narrow lens through which to view the concept of HL phenomena. In fact, in English, because of the high level of grapheme-phoneme discordance, the REALM provides valuable information; for example, it is quite difficult to pronounce a term like *vitiligo* without any prior familiarity with it. Consequently, as pronunciation in English incorporates a vague notion of understanding, the REALM is slightly more complex than initially apparent. Yet, words can certainly be pronounced without being understood.

Alternatively, the full TOFHLA includes reading, numeracy, and document literacy, and the modified cloze approach to ensure that the TOFHLA tests a person's understanding. TOFLHA takes a broader view of HL, but with distinct limitations. For example, the TOFLHA numeracy testing items require reading skills, making it quite difficult to disentangle numeracy dimensions from reading. Over the span of many projects conducted using the TOFHLA, presentation of differential results for the three subscales is incredibly rare. It is possible that users did not consider examining the separate scales in their projects or that the results were always consistent, making the presentation of separate analyses uninteresting. It is more likely, however, that the test scales are insufficiently distinct at the fundamental level of the cognitive processes involved.

2.2. A Way Forward

A portion of the newer instruments that measure HL have been developed in a manner that was explicitly linked to a specific definition and theory. Investigators for tools such as the Health Literacy Skills Instrument (HLSI) [11] and the Numeracy and Understanding in Medicine Instrument (NUMI) [12] approached their work by using an explicit operational HL definition that would motivate the purpose and scope of the tool. All items were designed to fulfill these specifications. Consequently, for these instruments, it is clear how to map results from test items to HL dimensions.

Interestingly, this has presented a paradox. Although the most commonly used legacy instruments are not based on a particular definition and relate only in general terms to the concept of HL, they nonetheless have demonstrated a high volume of predictive validity. However, newer tools developed in explicit relationship to a specific HL definition have not *yet* demonstrated predictive validity. The lack of extensive evidence exhibiting predictive validity has, in turn, caused some users in the field to be reticent about shifting to the use of newer HL tools. Until there is a shift to using newer tools, the field will not be able to advance and determine, for example, which HL dimensions are critical and in which contexts.

Overall, the development of tools aligned with specific HL definitions has begun. However, now these tools will need to be used to help refine observational research and guide efforts to design interventions that align more specifically with the challenges faced by people with limited HL.

3. Conceptual Domains Measured and Those Rarely Measured

Conceptual frameworks can help formulate research questions and examine relationships among predisposing variables, mediators, moderators, and other relevant outcomes [13, 14]. Frameworks can also inform an understanding of the domains that comprise a complicated construct. Similar to the fact that the term "health literacy" is widely used but not always well understood or applied consistently—as suggested by the sizeable number of different definitions that exist [8, 15]—multiple HL conceptual frameworks have been put forth [8, 16-18]. Yet, no single framework has gained significant traction or is viewed as the gold standard.

Examining the conceptual domains included in existing HL measures can offer insight into the construct as a whole. The National Assessment of Adult Literacy (NAAL) [19], for example, included three broad domains when examining HL using a more skills-based approach than had been used previously. Specifically, the NAAL used health-related stimulus materials that reflect the type of materials adults encounter in real life to examine three domains: (1) prose literacy, measured as the knowledge or skills needed to search, comprehend, and use information from text organized into sentences or paragraphs; (2) document literacy, defined as the knowledge and skills needed to search, comprehend, and use information from noncontinuous text in various formats (such as job applications, payroll forms, transportation schedules, and maps); and (3) quantitative literacy, measured as the knowledge and skills needed to identify and perform computations using numbers embedded in print materials (such as balancing a checkbook, calculating a tip, or figuring the amount on an order form).

The Health Literacy Toolshed website launched in 2015 and houses over 120 instruments to measure HL, with a goal of increasing the number of instruments available over time. The Toolshed developers organized the initial set of instruments into the following domains: prose (both pronunciation and comprehension); numeracy; communication (both speaking and listening); information seeking in documents, in addition to interactive media navigation; and skills related to the application and function of health information.

Most of the instruments include more than one domain when measuring HL, illustrating the overall complexity of the construct (Table 1). About half of the instruments included the numeracy domain, suggesting a general consensus that it is a core HL component, although instruments that measure only numeracy also exist. A lower number of instruments include a pronunciation domain, reflecting some of the more historical approaches to measuring literacy and perhaps indicating a movement away from this measurement approach. The communication components of HL—including both listening and speaking—are rarely included.

A small but growing number of instruments (n=19) include an application or functional component. About one quarter (n=26) examine information seeking in documents, and fewer (n=13) examine information seeking via interactive media navigation, including websites. Taken together, the relatively large number of domains used across the array of existing instruments to measure HL confirm that it is a multidimensional construct that must be measured carefully and completely using multiple items and stimuli in which a user can demonstrate their ability to interact effectively.

Table 1. Domains of health literacy assessed in the 128 instruments in the Health Literacy Tool Shed

Health Literacy Domain	HL Tool Shed measures assessing this domain
Prose: pronunciation	20
Communication: listening	6
Communication: speaking	3
Numeracy	63
Application/function	23
Information Seeking: document	31
Information Seeking: interactive media navigation	14

Source: Analysis of the 2015 Health Literacy Toolshed data http://healthliteracy.bu.edu/

4. Limitations of Validation Methods

The limited utility and predictive validity of some HL measures may reflect the methods used to develop and validate them. Consequently, exploring how existing measures were validated will provide insight into potential limitations and directions for future work.

At its core, measurement consists of rules for assigning numbers to objects, or concepts, in such a way as to represent quantities of an attribute [14]. The term "rules" indicates that the method of assigning numbers to attributes must be stated explicitly. The construction, scoring, refinement, and validation of latent scales are most commonly guided by psychometric methods associated with Classical Test Theory. However, Modern Measurement Theories offer practical solutions for measurement problems found in health-related research that have been difficult to solve using classical approaches [20-22]. This section first examines the advantages of Modern Measurement Theory, then reviews methodological approaches (i.e., Classical Test Theory vs. Modern Measurement Theory) used to develop and validate current HL measures, and finally suggests approaches for moving HL measurement forward. For brevity, it is assumed that most readers have a basic understanding of Classical Test Theory. A short description of Modern Measurement Theory is provided. Resources are available for those who wish to learn more about both approaches [14, 23].

4.1. Advantages of Modern Measurement Theory

Modern Measurement theories include Item Response Theory (IRT) and Rasch modeling. IRT, which focuses on the item-level rather than the scale-level, is a general statistical theory that uses mathematical models to describe the relationship between an individual's trait level and how they *respond* to an *item* [23]. This relationship can be described using two main parameter estimates: the discrimination parameter and the location/difficulty parameter. The discrimination parameter, often denoted *a*, reflects the ability of an item to discriminate between different levels of underlying traits; higher *a* values indicate better discrimination. The main difference between IRT and Rasch modeling is that the discrimination parameter across all items is set to the same value when using Rasch models, whereas this parameter is allowed to vary by item when using IRT models. While Rasch modeling provides stronger measurement properties, the fit of real-life data to Rasch models is not often suitable. The location/difficulty parameter, often denoted *b*, indicates the location of the item on the underlying construct; higher *b* estimates indicate that greater amounts of the underlying trait are needed to answer the question correctly (i.e., harder questions).

The advantages that IRT and Rasch modeling confer over Classical Test Theory are well documented [20, 24, 25]. In particular, there are four key advantages to using these methods to construct and refine HL measures [26]. First, by evaluating the location/difficulty parameter estimates across all items, IRT provides the opportunity to examine the level of HL skills measured (e.g., low, medium, high) and where efforts to develop new items should be focused. Second, the precision, or reliability, of measurement tools can be more accurately modeled using IRT. Specifically, instead of assuming that a tool has equal reliability across the trait continuum (i.e., a Cronbach's alpha=0.98), IRT can be used to identify the variability in measurement precision for individuals of differing trait levels of HL. This can be done by evaluating the test information function curve, which ideally should take on the shape of a horizontal line and be associated with a low standard error value. Third, an underlying assumption of IRT and Rasch models is that the estimated item parameters values (i.e., *a* and *b*) should be consistent for different groups, such as females or males (i.e., population invariance). This is in contrast to Classical Test Theory where scale properties are sample dependent. Although strong evidence supports this property, it does not hold in all cases [20, 24]. When estimated item parameters are different across groups after controlling for ability, an item is considered to have differential item functioning (DIF). IRT-based analyses can help identify items with DIF that may need to be rewritten or excluded. Additionally, even if significant DIF has been identified in certain items, those items can be retained if a model that incorporates the identified DIF is used to mathematically correct for item bias when estimating scores. Fourth, IRT can be used to build and validate item banks, which can subsequently facilitate computer adaptive testing (CAT). IRT does this by calibrating all items within a bank onto the same underlying trait scale. Once items are mapped onto a common scale, it does not matter that different people take different sets of test items.

Given that there are now over 150 HL tools, this can help address the lack of standardization in the measurement of HL and facilitate the comparison of scores and results across studies [5]. Because of these measurement properties, an assertive shift toward these methods would be highly advantageous.

4.2. Methods Used to Develop and Validate Health Literacy Measures

Consistent with the pattern observed in the larger scientific community [22], an analysis of HL measurement validation studies found that the methods used to develop and test HL measures were primarily guided by Classical Test Theory [26]. Specifically, among the 109 measures identified by Nguyen et al. [5], 88% (n=96) used Classical Test Theory and 12% (n=13) used IRT or Rasch modeling [11, 12, 27-37]. For a more up-to-date list of HL measurement tools that used modern methods for validation, see the HL Tool Shed and use the "Modern Approach for Tool Development" option to filter the list accordingly.

Among the measures that used IRT or Rasch modeling, most (n=9) [11, 28-32, 36, 37] used data from estimated parameter values to strategically eliminate items that had low discrimination and items that targeted the same (difficulty) level of the underlying trait. When reviewing the range in trait levels across the items on measures where the *b* parameter estimate was reported, items ranged from *b*=-6.34 to 2.06 [26]. However, when examining the density of items across this range, most items clustered toward the lower difficulty ranges [26]. This provides strong empirical evidence for developing more items in the higher difficulty ranges.

Seven HL measures reported assessing for DIF across various groups. Three HL item banks were identified in the literature, each with varying levels of complexity and domains of HL measured [12, 27, 37]. Among the three item banks, only one uses CAT; however, it is proprietary [27].

4.3. Strengthening the Validity of Health Literacy Measurement

The vast majority of existing HL measures uses Classical Test Theory to construct and validate scales. While this method has led to useful HL measures, there are limitations to relying heavily on this approach; notably, the lack of item-level data to meaningfully assess the difficulty of items in a scale across the latent trait, the need to revalidate measures when using them in different populations, and the challenge of comparing results across studies that used different measures. When evaluating HL measures that use Classical Test Theory, examining their reliability and validity estimates (i.e., psychometric properties) can be used to judge their strength. Commonly used reliability and validity estimates and their interpretation have been well summarized [14, 38]. Readers can then search the Health Literacy Toolshed to compare and contrast the psychometric properties of existing HL tools. It is worth mentioning that tools are valid to the extent that they are consistent (i.e., reliable) and useful in uncovering relationships (i.e., concurrent and predictive validity). In other words, for an HL tool to be "strong," it should be both reliable and valid. A systematic literature review by Nguyen et al. [5] found that the evidence supporting the validity of HL tools was weaker than the evidence supporting reliability, which reinforces that caution should be taken when using tools that are developed, refined, and validated using Classical approaches.

Because of these limitations, assertively shifting toward Modern Measurement approaches would be highly advantageous. Early efforts to use this approach have yielded valuable insight. However, to date, the application of Modern Measurement among HL measures has not fully leveraged the advantages of this methodological approach. Building item banks that include an equal density of questions across a wider range of HL trait levels that can be used in CAT applications will strengthen this body of literature. Items included in test banks should ideally demonstrate adequate discrimination parameter estimate values (i.e., *a*>1). Including DIF free items will also improve measurement validity across more populations.

It is important to note that Modern Measurement approaches will not solve all of the issues in HL measurement. Ongoing work is critically needed to refine and align the definition of HL within a conceptual framework and to accurately measure the concept. Furthermore, expanding the focus of HL measurement into the healthcare context (i.e., the communication skills of providers and the complexity of health systems and public health systems) is an important and necessary evolutionary step. While expanding the consideration of HL into these arenas will likely be complex, understanding these elements will not only help move the HL field forward but also will provide critical insight into how IRT or Rasch models can inform measurement development and refinement. Efforts toward these achieving these goals will necessarily require strategic collaboration. Additionally, designing high-quality mixed-methods research studies that meaningfully integrate qualitative and quantitative findings will be essential.

5. Limitations of Validation Samples

Given that the vast majority of HL measures were validated using Classic Test Theory, examining the samples from which they were validated is necessary to understand how these findings may or may not be reasonably generalized. It is easy to forget about such limitations and then make inaccurate conclusions. For example, it would not make sense to develop and validate a tool exclusively with female participants and then to assume that it will perform the same way with males.

A systematic review of HL measures examined the racial and ethnic composition of participants in validation studies for 109 tools to measure HL [5]. Of the 72 English-language measures examined in this review, 17 did not specify the racial/ethnic characteristic of their sample. Of the remaining 55 measures, 10 (18%) did not include blacks, 30 (55%) did not include Hispanics, and 35 (64%) did not include Asians in their validation sample. When Asian Americans and Hispanic Americans were included, they accounted for small percentages and numbers in the overall sample; interquartile range=10%–34% (n=13–154) and interquartile range=3.5%–16% (n=5–36), respectively.

Consequently, it is likely that inappropriate assumptions have been made when using these tools in other contexts. Additionally, the nature of the bias introduced by such assumptions cannot be estimated. For example, if a tool misclassifies Hispanics because it was developed with a sample that did not have enough Hispanic participants to ensure validity, subsequent analyses for Hispanic participants in studies using this tool could be misinterpreted. Therefore, it is important to interpret much of the HL literature with caution. If a classical approach is used to validate future HL measures, it is imperative that sampling strategies reflect the needs of high-risk groups. Correspondingly, the characteristics of the sample should be described in sufficient detail because this information has implications for the generalizability of a given measure.

Among the 37 non-English-language measures, only two specified the racial/ethnic characteristics of their sample beyond simply describing the general population in which the measure was being validated. For instance, Ko et al. [39] specified that the sample used to validate their "Health Literacy Test for Singapore" was 52% Chinese, 22% Malay, 24% Indian, and 10% Other. In comparison, most other non-English-language measures were similar to the "Hebrew Health Literacy Test," which reported simply that 119 Israeli participants were sampled to validate their scale; it is unclear which ethnolinguistic groups were represented from this highly multicultural society. The ethnolinguistic and cultural diversity of a specified population will influence the extent to which this may be problematic. For example, this issue is less relevant for Korean-language HL measures because the population is relatively linguistically homogenous, whereas it may be a greater concern for the use of Hebrew-language or Hindi-language HL measures, as these populations are more linguistically and culturally diverse. Future validation efforts should take into account the cultural diversity of the target population and include such details in reports.

Using Modern Measurement approaches to validate HL measures will reduce some of the challenges associated with the need to revalidate measures when used in different populations. While this property of population invariance found in modern approaches is robust, it does not always hold across all items and populations. Consequently, it will remain important to characterize validation samples to allow for DIF testing. When using Modern Measurement approaches, however, the sampling goal should be to obtain an equal distribution of participants with varying abilities across a latent trait; for example, the sample should include a sufficient number of participants with low, medium, and high levels of HL. This will lead to more stable parameter estimates for each test item. Once the parameters are estimated using an ideal "reference" group, differential item functioning can be tested against any number of different "focal" groups. Additionally, when DIF is identified (e.g., by race), a particular item may be excluded or a correction factor can be introduced. For tools developed with classical methods, if an item does not work the same across groups of participants, investigators do not have recourse. Such results cannot be corrected *post facto*. Consequently, it would be better to extend the validation cohorts for these tools or to abandon these tools for new data collection *ex ante*. Racial and ethnic data for the validation samples for each tool listed in the Health Literacy Tool Shed can be reviewed by choosing the "Read all details" option for any specific tool.

6. Practical Considerations When Using Health Literacy Measures

Researchers and practitioners use HL measures for various reasons, including patient-level assessment, intervention activities, and surveillance. Each situation may invoke the need for a different type of HL tool. For example, clinicians and healthcare professionals may want to assess the HL level of a sample of their patients to understand the general needs of the population they serve, or they may want to assess all new patients and need a tool that is easy to implement in a clinical setting (though clinical screening has not been shown to benefit patients) [40]. Also, researchers may be implementing a public health or community-based intervention and need to measure HL before and after implementation, or use HL as a control variable in an analysis examining a specific health outcome. In both clinical and research settings, HL measurement may be used to trigger specific interventions or to ascertain the possible differential impact of various interventions across the HL strata. In some instances, large-scale periodic HL assessments are conducted at the health system level or even at the national level.

Selecting the right HL tool is critical because different HL measures and different data collection strategies may be needed in a given situation. For example, what is the age and racial/ethnic diversity of the target population, what languages are spoken in the target population, what resources are available, and what are the measurement goals? These factors may influence the data collection method used and should be considered carefully at the outset of any program and in conjunction with the decision about which HL tool is used. Data collection methods range from mail, telephone, web-based or computer-based, mobile device-based, to in-person, or some combination thereof. In-person data collection could use paper-and-pencil or computer self-report, interviewer-facilitated approaches, or face-to-face verbal communication. Based on the 128 measures currently in the Health Literacy Tool Shed, more measures were developed and validated using paper-and-pencil and in-person strategies. A limited number of measures have been validated for web-based data collection, and very few have been validated for telephone administration (Table 2).

Table 2. Mode of administration used by 128 measures in the Health Literacy Tool Shed

Mode of Administration	HL Tool Shed measures using this mode
Computer-based	22
Face-to-face	82
Mail survey	5
Paper-and-pencil	60
Phone-based	3

Source: Analysis of the 2015 Health Literacy Toolshed data http://healthliteracy.bu.edu/

Each mode of administration offers strengths and limitations that are also related to the design of the project or study. For example, with web-based data collection, tools can include visual and/or interactive stimuli as part of the HL assessment process, such as food labels, health insurance forms, or health-related websites. With computer-based data collection and computer-assisted telephone interviewing (CATI), responses are recorded automatically into a dataset for analysis and interpretation, making data entry unnecessary. Development and programming expenses reflect certain fixed costs for computer-based and telephone strategies, and items can be modified relatively easily. Print-based HL tools typically require fewer data-collection fixed costs but involve costs associated with mailing surveys to study participants and follow-up and data entry. Mail-only surveys generally have lower response rates, but they can be improved with telephone or other types of follow-up [41]. Neither mail nor telephone surveys allow for the use of interactive stimuli to assess HL. With mail surveys, participants can be asked to read and interpret text and visuals, which is not the case with telephone administration. Web-based and in-person data-collection modes can use aural approaches. Costs, including staff training, can vary greatly depending on the data-collection mode and instrument used. There can also be an impact on response rates and data quality depending on the data-collection method used [41].

Researchers and practitioners carefully consider the needs of the study population when measuring HL. Reading ability, visual and hearing abilities, computer skills, and access to computers should all be factored into the choice of an HL tool and addressed in data-collection planning. Staff training is required not only to ensure data quality, but also to reduce potential harms. For example, individuals collecting data should be sensitive not to give the impression of testing subjects, as this could promote shame or stigma, especially in lower HL populations [42-45].

In sum, researchers and practitioners may be interested in measuring HL for different reasons. Additionally, researchers need to be mindful of the increasing diversity within populations when measuring HL. Also, having a clear understanding of the measurement goal and the target audience will help identify the best data-collection mode and type of HL tool to use.

7. Subjective Versus Objective Health Literacy Measures

A complex phenomenon that has developed in HL measurement is the elaboration of objective versus subjective measures. In objective measurement, people are challenged by standardized test stimuli to measure an underlying trait; in subjective measurement, people self-report their responses to questions about their experience, typically on Likert scales. There are distinct benefits and limitations to each of these approaches.

One benefit of subjective measures is the ease of testing because these measures do not require in-person testing and typically involve less cognitive effort than objective measures. This may mean that the risk for stigma is lower for subjective measures than for objective measures. Similarly, most HL measurement tools have been developed for research purposes, but some institutions have implemented subjective HL testing in clinical care. Subjective measures are typically easier to work into the flow of clinical care because they survey peoples' opinions. Also, subjective HL measures have the potential for rapid application. Indeed, some of the most commonly used subjective measures comprise three questions; some use just a single question [46, 47]. At the same time, more elaborate versions of subjective measurement have been developed. For example, the European Health Literacy Questionnaire was developed with 47 subjective items evaluating the three domains of healthcare, disease prevention and health promotion, and a four-component structure reflecting the four dimensions of accessing, understanding, appraising, and applying health information [48, 49]. It is possible that with repeated measurement over time, subjective measurements such as this could provide a different judgment by showing at a broad societal level to what extent the healthcare system is meeting the needs of the population.

The main challenge with subjective measurement is that there is no ground truth; meaning there is no way to know how a person's responses relate to their actual skill level. This is most relevant for certain groups of people who are likely to systematically rate their experiences at a higher level than other people in a manner that does not relate to their actual HL skills. For example, people who have not had much exposure to the health system may not appreciate the high degree of complexity they may encounter, so they may have inflated responses. Alternatively, for example, if male respondents have better scores on a subjective measure in a given project, it would not be clear if this is because men truly have an easier time with the activities being reported or if this difference reflects a subjective phenomenon in the cohort whereby the men in that cultural setting express a higher degree of self-confidence than the women [50]. In some cases, however, subjective measurement may provide the information that is needed. For example, subjective measurement is likely to be more successful in predicting outcomes for populations that have enough experience and enough insight in their HL ability. However, empirical testing is needed to support this perspective, and without additional data it is difficult to interpret results within a given cohort.

The main benefit of objective testing is that it results in a direct measure of the person's skill. There is an inherent value to having empirically grounded data. While this is often useful, there are multiple complexities with this approach. First, objective testing can feel like a test. People know that their skills are being evaluated; this can cause stigma, especially for people who struggle with the test items. Second, these tests typically require in-person testing. Third, the test items may not directly relate to the HL skills needed for a given scenario; a person's test score in one domain or content area may not reflect their skill in another aspect of HL. For example, it would be a mistake to assume that getting a perfect score on the TOFHLA means that a person knows how to use an inhaler. Lastly, given the limitations in methodological approaches used to develop and validate most HL measures (i.e., Classical Test Theory vs. IRT), there are concerns around meaningful interpretation of scale scores. For example, under Classical Test Theory it is assumed that score intervals across the scale are equal (i.e., on a measure with scores that can range from 0–10, an individual who scores a 5 has half the ability of an individual who scores a 10). However, when applying IRT to test data, what is often revealed is that items cluster around certain areas of the latent trait; most often the middle region (i.e., items with moderate difficulty). Without modeling the density of items across a latent trait, the value of objective measurement is reduced; for example, if an individual's HL score improves from 5 to 8, and the 3- point gain comes from items of the same difficulty level, it would be important to ask how much did that individual's HL ability really improve.

The empirical relationship between objective and subjective HL testing has received limited attention [51]. Kiechle et al. reviewed papers that concurrently used both types of measures and related them to various outcomes. They identified four studies they rated to be fair-quality studies with pertinent data. Among these studies, one reported no difference between objective and subjective HL measures for a rheumatoid arthritis disease severity score; one showed no difference between objective and subjective HL measures for a range of self-reported disease states; one exhibited a difference between objective and subjective HL measures for a patient's ability to interpret their prescription medication name and dose from a medication bottle; and one provided mixed evidence about the consistency between objective and subjective measurements of numeracy for predicting colorectal cancer screening utilization. While insightful, these studies do not provide adequate reassurance to support the assumption that conclusions from objective and subjective measures could be interchanged. At a conceptual level, these tools measure different constructs. Though it would add a layer of complexity, ideally the HL literature that derives from objective measures should be interpreted separately from reports from studies that used subjective measures.

Overall, the choice to use an objective or subjective HL measure depends on the goals and structural parameters of the work. Currently, most phone-based survey research will need to use subjective measurement, as it is difficult to facilitate current objective tests over the phone. When the goals of testing relate to phenomena that are better served with objective testing, this should be done if feasible. Finally, objective tests (e.g., the NAAL) may be better suited for estimating an individual's skills, whereas subjective measures (e.g., the European Health Literacy Questionnaire) may be better suited to assess if the healthcare system is serving the population well.

8. Future Directions

Much has been learned from the progress made in HL tool development since the 2004 seminal Institute of Medicine Report. This chapter has provided a critical review of the state of the science of those measures across several dimensions, including (1) the relationship between HL definition and measurement, (2) the conceptual domains of HL most and least frequently measured, (3) the methodological approaches used to develop and validate HL measures, (4) the characteristics of the participants in the validation studies, (5) the practical considerations when using HL measures, and (6) the use of subjective versus objective HL measures. Important patterns emerged from this critical review that can be used to help set future directions for HL measurement.

First and foremost, we need to better align HL measurement with definitions of HL. Given the number of different HL definitions that exists, it is imperative that tool developers are clear about what definition they are using and how that definition influenced the operationalization of HL in the tool. This will not only help guide the purpose and scope of the tool, but also help end-users interpret scores. Additionally, as more people use tools guided by a clear HL definition, it will help the field to further identify which definitions and theoretical frameworks are useful for understanding the mechanisms through which HL operates and how they impact outcomes.

An evaluation of existing HL tools demonstrates that some HL domains are measured more often than others. Specifically, prose/pronunciation and numeracy are the most commonly measured domains, whereas listening and speaking are the least measured domains. Consequently, it will be important to think about novel out-of-the-box mechanisms to measure these rarely measured HL domains. Novel approaches could also be used to address common issues of shame and the lack of time that is often associated with HL measurement. An example of an innovative approach is the use of gaze tracking technology while participants read a standard document [52]. It is hypothesized that the gaze patterns of individuals with high HL differ from individuals with moderate and low HL. Ongoing research is testing this hypothesis.

When reviewing the methodological approaches used to develop, validate, and refine HL measures, classical measurement approaches dominate the literature. This is consistent with patterns seen in measurement development and validation for most other patient reported outcomes [22]. However, there are strong empirical and practical rationales for making an assertive shift toward using modern measurement approaches to develop, validate, and refine HL tools. It is critical that the refinement and alignment between the definition of HL and measurement comes first before the full benefits of Modern Measurement approaches can be realized. Once refining and aligning the definition of HL is achieved, there is a valuable opportunity to build a robust HL item bank for CAT applications given the number of HL measures that exists. Creating a robust item bank has tremendous potential for addressing the lack of standardization in HL measurement, reducing participant burden, and addressing the challenge of making comparisons across studies. Achieving this will require skillful coordination, cooperation, and political will among the developers of HL tools and key stakeholders.

As HL tools continue to be developed, validated, and refined, it is critical to be mindful of validation samples. In situations where classical approaches are used, it is imperative that populations at highest risk for low HL are included in the validation sample because this has implications for the generalizability of the tool. A review of most existing HL measures demonstrates that Hispanic Americans and Asian Americans are rarely included in the validation samples of English-language HL measures, despite the fact that these groups have among the highest rates of low HL. In situations where modern approaches are used, the validation sample should aim to have an equal distribution of participants with varying abilities across a latent trait. This will ensure more stable item parameter estimates. Once a strong focal validation sample is obtained, testing for DIF across a number of different reference groups can be done.

Given the stock of currently available HL tools, a question commonly posed is, what tool should be used? Ultimately, the answer depends on the context of why HL is being measured. This chapter highlighted the differences between subjective and objective measures. Objective measures are generally better for situations when it is important to have a reliable estimate for an individual or set of individuals that are "grounded" in some verifiable way. Subjective measures are more strategically feasible for large-scale measurement of populations or systems over time. Various modes of measurement were also highlighted, including mail, telephone, web-based or computer-based, mobile device-based, in-person, or some combination thereof. Each mode of administration offers strengths and limitations. Identifying which administration mode is most suitable requires reflecting on the needs of the study population, including reading, visual and hearing abilities, and computer skills and access to computers. Considerations should also be made based on cost, desired response rate, and data quality. The Health Literacy Tool Shed is a valuable resource that can be used to filter existing tools based on their mode of measurement and whether they are subjective or objective in nature.

Finally, two parting reflections warrant brief mention. First, it is important to recognize that HL is a dynamic concept, and the rate at which this concept evolves is affected by language, culture, an increasingly global and mobile world, and sweeping health system changes taking place in many countries. Consequently, it will be necessary to have a more informed and sophisticated understanding of ethnolinguistic nuances and changes that occur naturally in most languages; particularly among languages spoken by people who are highly mobile and global. Ignoring these ethnolinguistic changes may decrease the content validity of HL measures over time. Likewise, to expand the focus of HL measurement into the healthcare context, a more informed and sophisticated understanding is needed of how health systems are evolving, as well as the complexities within and across different health systems that may influence HL and patient outcomes.

Second, many of the measurement-related issues identified in this chapter are not unique to HL. It is quite common for conceptual and operational definitions to evolve for emerging concepts of high scientific and social value. The increased recognition and inquiry often leads to a proliferation of new measures. However, even after several decades of study, this has not resulted in a gold standard.

For example, coping as a construct has a long history. Initial studies focused on psychopathology. Later, researchers moved toward positive behavior and the role of emotions. Significant concerns were identified in clarifying the concept and matching it with measurement [53]. After providing an updated review of the swiftly widening literature on stress and coping [54], the authors noted that measurement was still the most controversial issue in the field. One way researchers addressed this problem was to develop coping measures specialized by situations; for example, coping with sexual trauma. While measures multiplied in number, clarity of the concept of coping in health did not advance.

Lengthy theses can be written to discuss solutions for overcome these challenges. Two broad suggestions are offered. First, it is vital to overcome disunity by moving toward unified, integrative work; both in conceptualizing the definition of HL and operationalizing it into measurement tools. Second, it is imperative that we continue to build from where we are toward higher quality psychometric studies that include both classic and modern measurement approaches. Continuing to engage in the status quo will do more harm than good for the field.

In closing, much progress has been made in HL tool development, which has led to a number of useful HL tools and to measurement challenges for the field. It is important to contextualize the commonality of the measurement problems unearthed in this chapter rather than be discouraged by them. Learning from past lessons provides a hopeful path forward.

Acknowledgments: We would like to thank Rebecca Moultrie for her assistance with Table 1 and Jeffrey Novey for his careful review of this chapter.

References

[1]   Nielsen-Bohlman LN, Panzer AM, Kindig DA, editors. Health Literacy: A Prescription to End Confusion. Washington, DC: National Academies Press; 2004.

[2]   National Institutes of Health, Agency for Healthcare Research and Quality, Centers for Disease Control and Prevention. Understanding and Promoting Health Literacy (R01). Washington, DC: National Institutes of Health, Agency for Healthcare Research and Quality, and Centers for Disease Control and Prevention; 2004 [updated 2010 March 12; cited 2012 January 12]; Available from: http://grants.nih.gov/grants/guide/pa-files/PAR-07-020.html.

[3]   O'Neill B, Goncalves D, Ricci-Cabello I, Ziebland S, Valderas J. An overview of self-administered health literacy instruments. PLoS One. 2014;9(12). DOI:10.1371/journal.pone.0109110.

[4]   Haun JN, Valerio MA, McCormack LA, Sorensen K, Paasche-Orlow MK. Health literacy measurement: an inventory and descriptive summary of 51 instruments. J Health Commun. 2014;19(Suppl 2):302-33. DOI:10.1080/10810730.2014.936571.

[5]   Nguyen TH, Park H, Han HR, Chan KS, Paasche-Orlow MK, Haun J, et al. State of the science of health literacy measures: validity implications for minority populations. Patient Educ Couns. 2015. DOI:10.1016/j.pec.2015.07.013.

[6]   McCormack L, Haun J, Sorensen K, Valerio M. Recommendations for advancing health literacy measurement. J Health Commun. 2013;18(Suppl 1):9-14. DOI:10.1080/10810730.2013.829892.

[7]   Pleasant A. Advancing health literacy measurement: a pathway to better health and health system performance. J Health Commun. 2014;19(12):1481-96. DOI:10.1080/10810730.2014.954083.

[8]   Sorensen K, Van den Broucke S, Fullam J, Doyle G, Pelikan J, Slonska Z, et al. Health literacy and public health: a systematic review and integration of definitions and models. BMC Public Health. 2012;12:80. DOI:10.1186/1471-2458-12-80.

[9]   Davis TC, Long SW, Jackson RH, Mayeaux EJ, George RB, Murphy PW, et al. Rapid estimate of adult literacy in medicine: a shortened screening instrument. Fam Med. 1993;25(6):391-5.

[10] Parker RM, Baker DW, Williams MV, Nurss JR. The test of functional health literacy in adults: a new instrument for measuring patients' literacy skills. J Gen Intern Med. 1995;10(10):537-41.

[11] Bann CM, McCormack LA, Berkman ND, Squiers LB. The Health Literacy Skills Instrument: a 10-item short form. J Health Commun. 2012;17(Suppl 3):191-202. DOI:10.1080/10810730.2012.718042.

[12] Schapira MM, Walker CM, Cappaert KJ, Ganschow PS, Fletcher KE, McGinley EL, et al. The numeracy understanding in medicine instrument: a measure of health numeracy developed using item response theory. Med Decis Making. 2012;32(6):851-65. DOI:10.1177/0272989X12447239.

[13] Glanz K, Rimer BK, Viswanath K. Health Behavior and Health Education: Theory, Research, and Practice 4th ed. San Francisco: Jossey-Bass; 2008.

[14] Nunnelly J, Bernstein IH. Psychometric Theory. 3rd ed. New York: McGraw-Hill; 1994.

[15] Berkman ND, Davis TC, McCormack L. Health literacy: what is it? J Health Commun. [Historical Article]. 2010;15 Suppl 2:9-19. DOI:10.1080/10810730.2010.499985.

[16] Manganello JA. Health literacy and adolescents: a framework and agenda for future research. Health Educ Res. 2008;23(5):840-7. DOI:10.1093/her/cym069.

[17] Paasche-Orlow MK, Wolf MS. The causal pathways linking health literacy to health outcomes. Am J Health Behav. 2007;31(Suppl 1):S19-26. DOI:10.5555/ajhb.2007.31.supp.S19.

[18] Squiers L, Peinado S, Berkman N, Boudewyns V, McCormack L. The health literacy skills framework. J Health Commun. 2012;17(Suppl 3):30-54. DOI:10.1080/10810730.2012.713442.

[19] Kutner M, Greenberg E, Jin Y, Paulsen C. The Health Literacy of America's Adults: Results from the 2003 National Assessment of Adult Literacy (NCES 2006-483), U.S. Department of Education. Washington, DC: National Center for Education Statistics; 2006.

[20] Embretson SE. The new rules of measurement. Psychol Assess. 1996;8(4):341-9.

[21] Gulliksen H. Theory of Mental Tests. New York: Wiley; 1950.

[22] Hambleton RK. Emergence of item response modeling in instrument development and data analysis. Med Care. 2000;38(Suppl 9):II60-5.

[23] Hambleton RK, Swaminathan H, Rogers WH. Fundamentals of Item Response Theory. Newbury Park: Sage Publications; 1991.

[24] Hambleton RK, Jones RW. Comparison of Classical Test Theory and Item Response Theory and their applications to test development. Instructional Topics in Educational Measurement. 1993:38-47.

[25] Nguyen TH, Han HR, Kim MT, Chan KS. An introduction to Item Response Theory for patient-reported outcome measurement. Patient. 2014;7(1):23-35. DOI:10.1007/s40271-013-0041-0.

[26] Nguyen TH, Paasche-Orlow MK, Kim MT, Han HR, Chan KS. Modern measurement approaches to health literacy scale development and refinement: overview, current uses, and next steps. J Health Commun. 2015;20 Suppl 2:112-5. DOI:10.1080/10810730.2015.1073408.

[27] ETS. Health Activities Literacy Scale. 2012 [cited 2016 23 September]; Available from: http://www.ets.org/literacy/about/content/health_activities_content.

[28] Guttersrud O, Dalane JO, Pettersen S. Improving measurement in nutrition literacy research using Rasch modelling: examining construct validity of stage-specific 'critical nutrition literacy' scales. Public Health Nutr. 2014;17(4):877-83. DOI:10.1017/S1368980013000530.

[29] Lee SY, Bender DE, Ruiz RE, Cho YI. Development of an easy-to-use Spanish Health Literacy test. Health Serv Res. 2006;41(4 Pt 1):1392-412. DOI:10.1111/j.1475-6773.2006.00532.x.

[30] Lee SY, Stucky BD, Lee JY, Rozier RG, Bender DE. Short Assessment of Health Literacy-Spanish and English: a comparable test of health literacy for Spanish and English speakers. Health Serv Res. 2010;45(4):1105-20. DOI:10.1111/j.1475-6773.2010.01119.x.

[31] Leung AY, Cheung MK, Lou VW, Chan FH, Ho CK, Do TL, et al. Development and validation of the Chinese Health Literacy Scale for Chronic Care. J Health Commun. 2013;18(Suppl 1):205-22. DOI:10.1080/10810730.2013.829138.

[32] Nakagami K, Yamauchi T, Noguchi H, Maeda T, Nakagami T. Development and validation of a new instrument for testing functional health literacy in Japanese adults. Nurs Health Sci. 2014;16(2):201-8. DOI:10.1111/nhs.12087.

[33] Osborne RH, Batterham RW, Elsworth GR, Hawkins M, Buchbinder R. The grounded psychometric development and initial validation of the Health Literacy Questionnaire (HLQ). BMC Public Health. 2013;13:658. DOI:10.1186/1471-2458-13-658.

[34] Sauceda JA, Loya AM, Sias JJ, Taylor T, Wiebe JS, Rivera JO. Medication literacy in Spanish and English: psychometric evaluation of a new assessment tool. J Am Pharm Assoc (2003). 2012;52(6):e231-40. DOI:10.1331/JAPhA.2012.11264.

[35] Steckelberg A, Hulfenhaus C, Kasper J, Rost J, Muhlhauser I. How to measure critical health competences: development and validation of the Critical Health Competence Test (CHC Test). Adv Health Sci Educ. 2009;14(1):11-22. DOI:10.1007/s10459-007-9083-1.

[36] Stucky BD, Lee JY, Lee SY, Rozier RG. Development of the two-stage rapid estimate of adult literacy in dentistry. Community Dent Oral Epidemiol. 2011;39(5):474-80. DOI:10.1111/j.1600-0528.2011.00619.x.

[37] Yost KJ, Webster K, Baker DW, Choi SW, Bode RK, Hahn EA. Bilingual health literacy assessment using the Talking Touchscreen/la Pantalla Parlanchina: Development and pilot testing. Patient Educ Couns. 2009;75(3):295-301. DOI:10.1016/j.pec.2009.02.020.

[38] Netemeyer RG, Bearden WO, Sharma S. Scaling Procedures. Thousand Oaks, CA: Sage; 2003.

[39] Ko NY, Darnell JS, Calhoun E, Freund KM, Wells KJ, Shapiro CL, et al. Can patient navigation improve receipt of recommended breast cancer care? Evidence from the National Patient Navigation Research Program. J Clin Oncol. 2014;32(25):2758-64. DOI:10.1200/jco.2013.53.6037.

[40] Paasche-Orlow MK, Wolf MS. Evidence does not support clinical screening of literacy. J Gen Intern Med. 2008;23(1):100-2. DOI:10.1007/s11606-007-0447-2.

[41] Dillman DA, Smyth JD, Leah MC. Internet, Phone, Mail, and Mixed-Mode Surveys: The Tailored Design Method. 4th ed. New York: Wiley; 2014.

[42] Easton P, Entwistle VA, Williams B. How the stigma of low literacy can impair patient-professional spoken interactions and affect health: insights from a qualitative investigation. BMC Health Serv Res. 2013;13:319. DOI:10.1186/1472-6963-13-319.

[43] Farrell TW, Chandran R, Gramling R. Understanding the role of shame in the clinical assessment of health literacy. Fam Med. 2008;40(4):235-6.

[44] VanGeest JB, Welch VL, Weiner SJ. Patients' perceptions of screening for health literacy: reactions to the newest vital sign. J Health Commun. 2010;15(4):402-12. DOI:10.1080/10810731003753117.

[45] Wolf MS, Williams MV, Parker RM, Parikh NS, Nowlan AW, Baker DW. Patients' shame and attitudes toward discussing the results of literacy screening. J Health Commun. 2007;12(8):721-32. DOI:10.1080/10810730701672173.

[46] Chew LD, Bradley KA, Boyko EJ. Brief questions to identify patients with inadequate health literacy. Fam Med. 2004;36(8):588-94.

[47] Morris NS, MacLean CD, Littenberg B. Literacy and health outcomes: a cross-sectional study in 1002 adults with diabetes. BMC Fam Pract. 2006;7:49. DOI:10.1186/1471-2296-7-49.

[48] Sorensen K, Pelikan JM, Rothlin F, Ganahl K, Slonska Z, Doyle G, et al. Health literacy in Europe: comparative results of the European Health Literacy Survey (HLS-EU). Eur J Public Health. 2015;25(6):1053-8. DOI:10.1093/eurpub/ckv043.

[49] Sorensen K, Van den Broucke S, Pelikan JM, Fullam J, Doyle G, Slonska Z, et al. Measuring health literacy in populations: illuminating the design and development process of the European Health Literacy Survey Questionnaire (HLS-EU-Q). BMC Public Health. 2013;13:948. DOI:10.1186/1471-2458-13-948.

[50] Lee SY, Tsai TI, Tsai YW. Accuracy in self-reported health literacy screening: a difference between men and women in Taiwan. BMJ Open. 2013;3(11):e002928. DOI:10.1136/bmjopen-2013-002928.

[51] Kiechle ES, Bailey SC, Hedlund LA, Viera AJ, Sheridan SL. Different measures, different outcomes? A systematic review of performance-based versus self-reported measures of health literacy and numeracy. J Gen Intern Med. 2015;30(10):1538-46. DOI:10.1007/s11606-015-3288-4.

[52] Mele ML, Federici S. Gaze and eye-tracking solutions for psychological research. Cogn Process. 2012;13 Suppl 1:S261-5. DOI:10.1007/s10339-012-0499-z.

[53] Schwarzer R, Schwarzer C. A critical survey of coping instruments. In: Zeidner M, Endler NS, editors. Handbook of Coping: Theory, Research, Applications. New York: John Wiley & Sons, Inc.; 1996. p. 107–32.

[54] Aldwin CM. Stress, Coping, and Development: An Integrative Perspective. New York: The Guilford Press; 2007.

Health Literacy
R.A. Logan and E.R. Siegel (Eds.)
IOS Press, 2017
doi:10.3233/978-1-61499-790-0-34

Measuring Health Literacy in General Populations: Primary Findings from the HLS-EU Consortium's Health Literacy Assessment Effort

Juergen M. PELIKAN[ab], Kristin GANAHL[a]

[a] *Gesundheit Oesterreich GmbH (Austrian Public Health Institute), Vienna, Austria*
[b] *Department of Sociology, University of Vienna, Austria*

Abstract. This chapter is concerned with the difference of measuring health literacy of general population for purposes of public health as differentiated from measuring personal health literacy of individuals within health care services. The evolution of concept, measurement and empirical research of health literacy in the last decades is discussed, and the position of measuring comprehensive health literacy in general populations, especially by the European Health Literacy Survey (HLS-EU) study, is defined.

Main features of the HLS-EU conceptual and logic model, definition, instruments and study design are described. General results of the HLS-EU study are presented on the distribution of health literacy, its determinants and health related consequences, for the eight involved European countries as well as the total sample. These results principally confirm findings of earlier studies with somewhat different instruments and other kinds of samples, but also demonstrate considerable differences in distributions of health literacy and its relationships with relevant variables among and between the eight countries in a standardized comparative international study.

Follow-up studies based on the original HLS-EU study are mapped. In addition, the factors for the relative easy and widespread use of the instrument and research methodology by similar studies in other countries in Europe and Asia are discussed. This chapter closes with an outlook on the challenges of further developments and take-ups.

Keywords. Health Literacy, Measurement, Population Health Literacy, Health Literacy Survey Europe (HLS-EU)

1. Introduction

The measurement of health literacy (HL) in general adult populations undergirded by a comprehensive concept and literature-based, assessment instrument remains an underdeveloped area within HL research. However, the relevance of HL for health, the health gap, and outcomes of health service treatment frequently has been assessed, mainly for patient populations by instruments measuring functional HL. From these previous studies, HL has become of interest for public health policy, disease prevention, and health promotion. Hence, measuring HL also in general populations with a more comprehensive measure of HL has gained attention in HL research. The European Health Literacy Survey (HLS-EU) is an outcome of this development.

First, based on the HLS-EU study this chapter puts measuring comprehensive HL in general populations in context with a historical perspective by describing three traditions of the evolvement of HL research and the relations of the HLS-EU study to these traditions. Second, the developments of a comprehensive conceptual definition and generic model of HL - as well as an equivalent measurement instrument by the HLS-EU consortium - are described. Third, the main features of the study design of HLS-EU are characterized: the results from the HLS-EU study are presented for the distributions of HL, for social determinants of HL, and for health related associations of HL in the eight countries included in the HLS-EU study. In addition, construction and some characteristics of two short forms for the HLS-HL measurement instrument are presented. The take-up of HLS EU instruments and methodology in follow-up studies is described and the chapter concludes with a discussion of lessons learned and future challenges in measuring comprehensive HL within general populations.

2. Background and Research History of Measuring Comprehensive Health Literacy in General Populations

Health literacy still is an "evolving concept" [1], and there is only limited consensus on its definition [2], but certain trends can be identified characterizing its evolution [3] or its change of paradigm [4] to a more comprehensive concept of HL within the last two decades. There is an extension concerning the meaning of the term "health:" (disease *and* positive health; or health in relation to health care, *and* disease prevention, health protection, health promotion or public health in general) and of "literacy" (understanding as well as accessing, appraising and applying health relevant information) [5], or not just functional but also interactive and critical aspects of HL [6]. By that, the tasks, roles, settings and systems for which HL is conceptually relevant have been extended. HL is needed not just for the patient role in health care, but nearly for all roles in most of the settings or organizations where people are engaged in everyday life in contemporary societies [7].

Parallel to these extensions, the internal differentiation of a more comprehensive conceptualization of HL occurred. This resulted in a number of more specific concepts and measures for sub-dimensions or specific aspects of health literacy [8, p.82]. Examples for this internal differentiation are: disease-specific HLs, e.g. for asthma, diabetes, hypertension and heart failure or focusing on dentistry, cancer, or HIV; [9, 10], but also HL for different aspects of HL (oral, numeracy, media HL, e-HL); different stages in the life cycle (e.g. children and adolescents); or different life-style aspects (e.g. nutrition).

Perhaps more important, an understanding of HL conceptually as relational or interactive, dual [11] or contextual [1], individual vs. system related [2] or organizational [12] has developed and been widely accepted [5]. It is acknowledged that an individual's health literacy does not depend alone on his/her personal skills or competencies, but also on the demands and resources or the complexity of the situations in which health literate decisions or actions have to occur. By this understanding not only personal HL can be measured, but also situational/organizational or settings and systems specific HL. To put this another way,

HL cannot be improved only by learning of individuals or users alone, but also by developing more HL sensitive situations, settings, organizations and systems [12-15].

Historically the development of HL as a topic in research, but also in practice and policy, mainly followed three different traditions. First, there is a longer line of *literacy* research on youth (UNSCO 2016)[1] and in general populations of adult citizens, especially in countries who define themselves as immigration societies, like the US, Canada, or Australia. "Rigorously designed and carefully sampled surveys of the literacy skills of adults in industrialized nations were launched in the 1990s [16], expanded and repeated between 2003 and 2006 [17] and further expanded and repeated in 2011" [18, 4, p.19].

The National Assessment of Adult Literacy (NAAL) Survey[2] first was used in the U.S. in 1992; the International Adults Literacy Survey (IALS)[3] was used initially in 1994 in Canada, Ireland, Germany, the Netherlands, Poland, Sweden, Switzerland and the U.S. "Overall, all of the surveys examined how well people were able to use commonly available materials to accomplish everyday tasks with accuracy and consistency. ... These adult literacy surveys, supported by the Organization for Economic Cooperation and Development (OECD), provide needed information for economic and education policy makers. However, the first publication of findings in the 1990s [19] also drew attention of researchers from the health sector. Health literacy studies began with the dissemination of these findings and were spurred by the research question: "Are there health consequences?" [4, p.19-20].

Based on health related items – both materials and tasks - from the adult literacy surveys through the 2003 Adults Literacy and Lifeskills Survey (ALLS)[4] instrument, a research team led by Rima Rudd developed a scale labeled the Health and Literacy Scale (HALS), which "is a direct measure of literacy skills, focusing on adults' ability to use health related materials to accomplish an array of health related tasks. ... Subsequently, 230 health related items from international surveys were coded as belonging to one of five categories of health activities (health promotion, health protection, disease prevention, health care management, systems navigation and policy) and supported analyses of population health literacy for any country that participated in the surveys of the 1990s or the early 2000s [20]....The first such analyses were conducted in the U.S. and Canada [21]....Findings indicate that the distribution of health literacy is not independent of general literacy skills at a population or subpopulation level. ... These findings set the foundation for examinations of health literacy as a mediating factor in health disparities." [4, p.21]. However, the latter tradition to measure HL in adult populations via tests has not been followed up because of a lack of resources [22-23].

In line with this *literacy* tradition it is common for research to use performance based measures or tests because of its proximity to education and to educational institutions' preference to test student success via examinations. In relation to *health*, there also is a link to health education, where the term health literacy was used first [24]. Being supported by international agencies (UNESCO or OECD), literacy research has focused on inter-cultural or international comparisons, which from the beginning used appropriate instruments. The tradition of using performance tests for international comparisons was used in OECD programs such as the Programme for International Student Assessment (PISA) and the Programme for the International Assessment of Adult Competencies (PIACC) etc. However, performance tests cannot be developed to the same degree to measure respondents' access to or use of health information compared to respondents' understanding and appraisal. As a result, existing performance-based instruments for measuring health literacy exhibit limits in their scope to comprehensively assess the meaning of "health" and of "literacy" (including the full information cycle of finding, understanding, judging and applying information). However, the deficiency of "objective" performance-based instruments can be compensated by using perception based instruments, or "subjectively" self-reporting and self-assessing HL.

Second, measuring HL occurred - mainly in the US - within the healthcare sector by health professionals to identify patients who experienced difficulties to use or functionally adapt to the health care delivery system [25]. For this purpose, parallel to common physical testing of patients in health care (e.g. measuring blood pressure or fever), mental tests on understanding health relevant information and materials (e.g. REALM, TOFHLA, NVS) have been developed [e.g. 26, 27, 28]. Furthermore, short forms of these tests (e.g. S-TOFHLA, REALM-SF) [e.g. 29], and later short self-assessment instruments [30, 31], were developed in order to better integrate the measuring of patients′ HL within the tight time schedules of clinical practice. These tests enabled the identification of individual patients with low or limited HL in clinical practice. Similarly, when assessed on patient populations, the results suggested low HL is a widespread problem [32, 33], and evidenced the detrimental effects of low health literacy on health care utilization as well as patients′ clinical outcomes [34, 35]. Subsequent, short functional HL tests also were implemented for general populations [36, 37] with similar results.

Interestingly, "The 2004 Institute of Medicine report 'Health Literacy: A Prescription to End Confusion' offers insight into the weaknesses of these tools as ′true health literacy assessments` and into the simultaneous value of the tools for exploring and predicting health outcomes" [4, p.21, 38]. While critiques of HL instruments have continued [39-40], the association of low HL with worse health outcomes had practical consequences, and led to assessments of the difficulty and complexity of health materials [41-46]. "For the most part, studies across an array of health topics indicate that health materials are written at level that exceed the average reading skills of the public [47, 48]. … A recent study of the match or mismatch between health materials on critical topics and the documented skills of adults in the UK found such a mismatch [49]. However, studies related to the ′accessibility` of health materials were rarely part of or cited within inquiries focused on health outcomes." [4, p.23].

Furthermore, action and implementation HL studies often were stimulated. "A number of studies focused on enhanced information, the notion of universal precautions, and the application of the teach-back method in the clinical encounter [50, 51]. In addition, many initiatives (not yet studies) are underway to improve the communication skills of those in contact with patients and residents such as for students in medical school in Chicago Illinois-U.S. [52], practitioners in ten hospitals in the Reggio Emilia region of Italy [53], and for public health nurses in Fukushima Japan [54, 4, p.23]. Overall, in the last decade, these results (together with the relational understanding of HL) have led to the concept of health literate (health care) organizations, advanced by the US National Academy of Medicine, [12, 55] which has been advanced similarly in Europe [13, 56-58] and Australia [59].

Third, and more recently, the concept was adopted conceptually by theoreticians and researchers within the fields of health promotion [6, 60, 61] and public health in general, but without specific empirical research efforts. Within this tradition, a broad understanding of health and health relevant tasks is advisable and general populations or citizens are of interest rather than just single patients or specific patient populations.

These kinds of studies are important to diagnose and monitor the development of levels of HL within a larger population, and to identify vulnerable or disadvantaged sub-populations with specific capacities and needs and to evaluate the impact of health policy interventions and health promotion measures to improve population health. An initial empirical study in this tradition in Europe was conducted in Switzerland - HLS-CH in 2006 [62]. The multinational, HLS-EU study builds on the latter tradition.

However, performance measures in general adult populations have to be done in specific interactive surveys, and when they are more comprehensive like the Health Activities Literacy Scale (HALS) they take significant time[5] and therefore may be costly. In addition, the HALS instrument furthermore is not free of charge! As a result, the development of *comprehensive self-assessment* instruments to measure HL in general populations started in Europe first by the Swiss and later the HLS-EU survey team [62, 63] by building on both the tradition of HALS, i.e. measuring difficulty of relevant tasks, as well as the tradition of Chew et al.[30], i.e. measuring via self-assessment questions.

Again supported by an international institution (in this case the European Commission - EC), the HLS-EU started as a coordinated project in several countries, which enabled a multicultural perspective to design instruments and for international comparison and benchmarking of HL results. In a way, HLS-EU combined two traditions of HL research including the first tradition of literacy research dealing with general populations in addition to the third tradition to assess a public health or health promotion perspective. For serving the latter orientation, a comprehensive conceptual understanding of HL needed to be used and an instrument representing this broad understanding needed to be constructed. To guarantee a wide range of included health relevant tasks the instrument had to be perception instead of performance-based. Hence, a much shorter and more efficient (but comprehensive) instrument to measure HL resulted, which made it much easier for countries which were not included into the original partly EC sponsored project to later do studies on their own.

3. Measuring of Comprehensive Health Literacy in General Populations – the European Health Literacy (HLS-EU) Study

The HLS-EU study has been supported by the executive Agency for Health and Consumers (EAHC) of the European Union. It was implemented between 2009 and 2012 by a consortium of research institutions of eight European member states (Austria, Bulgaria, Germany, Greece, Ireland, Netherlands, Poland, Spain), coordinated by the University of Maastricht.

The HLS-EU study had five goals: (1) adapt a model instrument for measuring health literacy (HL) in Europe, (2) generate first-time data on HL in European countries, providing indicators for national and EU monitoring, (3) make comparative assessment of HL in European countries, (4) create National Advisory Bodies in countries participating in the survey and to document different valorization strategies following national structures and priorities, and (5) establish a European HL Network. While the study successfully also achieved goals four and five, this chapter focuses on how goals one to three have been advanced.

To fulfill goal one, i.e. to measure HL in an adequate way for public health oriented surveys of general population, the HLS-EU Consortium initially developed a multidimensional, integrative, conceptual and generic model and definition of comprehensive HL based on 12 published models and 17 definitions of HL [5]. "Health literacy is linked to literacy and entails people's knowledge, motivation and competences to access, understand, appraise, and apply health information in order to make judgments and take decisions in everyday life concerning healthcare, disease prevention and health promotion to maintain or improve quality of life during the life course" [5]. Conceptually this definition is based on a matrix (cf. table 1) that defines three domains for which HL is relevant (health care, disease prevention, health promotion) and four stages of managing information (accessing, understanding, appraising and applying) for taking health relevant decisions or actions.

Table 1: HLS-EU health literacy matrix

	access/find/obtain information relevant to health	Understand information relevant to health	Appraise/judge/ev aluate information relevant to health	Apply/use information relevant to health
Healthcare	Ability to access information on medical and clinical issues	Ability to understand medical information and derive meaning	Ability to interpret and evaluate medical information	Ability to make informed decisions on medical issues
Disease prevention	Ability to access information on risk factors for health	Ability to understand information on risk factors and derive meaning	Ability to interpret and evaluate information on risk factors for health	Ability to make informed decisions on risk factors for health
Health promotion	Ability to update oneself on determinants of health in the social and physical environment	Ability to understand information on determinants of health in the social and physical environment and derive meaning	Ability to interpret and evaluate information on health determinants in the social and physical environment	Ability to make informed decisions on health determinants in the social and physical environment

By the four stages of information management within this definition, the widely accepted typology of functional, interactive and critical [1] is partly extended and also made easier to analytically operationalize. The WHO definition of HL also underscores that knowledge is only one component of HL, in addition to motivation and competences, and skills. In addition, the HLS-EU integrated definition clarifies that HL is needed in many roles in everyday life in different settings (not just in the role of a patient in health care) [7] and that is necessary during the whole life course for the purpose of maintaining or improving ones quality of life. As a basic precondition for HL only fundamental literacy is mentioned explicitly, but literacy is expandable to include more specific literacies or competences such as language competency and science, civic, and cultural literacy as e.g. discussed in the Zarcadoolas et al. model [64], or to digital [65, 66], or media literacy [67, 68]. What is *not* explicit in the HLS-EU integrated definition is the relational character of HL that is provided within a definition from Kwan et al. [69]. However, the form of instrument by which HL is operationalized within the HLS-EU study takes HL's relational character into account. Overall, the HLS-EU integrated definition fulfills the specific expectations well and was seen as a requisite to comprehensively assess HL within general populations.

In order to operationalize a measurement instrument for HL (that represented the comprehensive definition), a number of concrete decisions had to be taken by the

HLS-EU consortium, in addition to selecting a perception-based way to assess comprehensively, feasible and efficient. What evolved in this consensus process [63] was an instrument with the following qualities:

- An unified *format* of items, but modularized for diverse content areas in lieu of having differing formats for different dimensions that cannot be integrated into one general measure of comprehensive HL, what holds true for some other HL instruments [30, 31, 62, 70]. In addition, a unified format allows for a number of specific directly comparable sub-measures.
- *Scope* and *content* of the instrument follows the health literacy *matrix*, to guarantee that the three dimensions and four stages of comprehensive HL and their combinations were each equally represented.
- The *content* of the items follows the example of the HALS [20], including partly complex and concrete *tasks* of health relevant *decisions* or *actions*, which are part of everyday life. To fulfill such tasks successfully a combination of motivation, knowledge and competences, as defined by the HLS-EU definition [5], was required.
- As an underlying dimension, *difficulty* of these different tasks as experienced by the respondents was defined for allowing comparability of single items and of aggregated sub-measures based on these.
- For format of items, *questions* (instead of rhetorical statements) were chosen, since questions can be more easily and directly answered than statements.
- A Likert scale of just four *symmetrical answer categories* was chosen. This kind of categorization avoids a nebulous middle category and meaningfully can be dichotomized in later statistical analysis of data, if preferred or necessary. ("Don't know" was not offered as an answer category, but no explicit answer was coded as "no answer" by the interviewer.)
- To avoid a response set overstating assessed difficulty of items, categories were *ordered* from very easy to very difficult.

Together these decisions resulted in 47 items within a common format such as: On a scale from very easy to very difficult, how easy would you say it is to *understand, what your doctor says to you?* "Very easy" - "fairly easy" - "fairly difficult" - "very difficult", (no answer).

Besides operationalizing the *conceptual* model of HL into 47 items, the questionnaire also had to encompass adequate indicators to represent selected determinants and consequences of HL as defined by the *generic/logical* model [5, figure], which in total contained 86 items. The original generic/logical model was further differentiated to analyze the survey data (cf. figure 1). It distinguishes between personal and situational factors influencing personal HL and between direct and indirect effects of HL on health relevant behaviors, health status, and some respondent illness behaviors. In the generic/logical model, a main direction for causality is hypothesized and also the possibility of reciprocal or cyclical causality. In this model HL also is conceptually understood either as a specific social determinant of health [71, 72] or as a mediator for the impact of other social determinants of health [73-74]. Effects of HL as a moderator [75] can be added as well [76, 77].

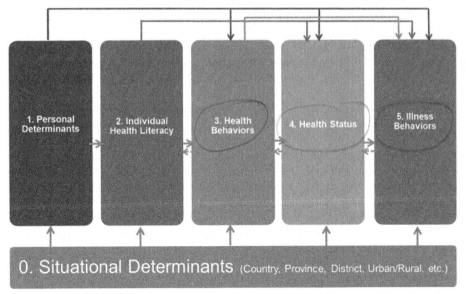

Figure 1: Generic Vienna Model of Health Literacy Defining Principal Determinants & Consequences of HL [3]

The questionnaire including the comprehensive HL measurement instrument has been translated by the HLS-EU-Consortium into seven languages and checked for plain language [63], and later was translated also into several European and Asian languages.

4. The European Health Literacy Survey (HLS-EU) - Data Collection in Eight Member-States of the EU

The European Health Literacy Survey was conducted in eight member-states of the EU - Austria, Bulgaria, Germany (North-Rhine-Westphalia), Greece, Ireland, the Netherlands, Poland and Spain - by a market research company according to Eurobarometer standards. Data was collected by Computer Assisted Personal Interviewing (CAPI) or Paper Assisted Personal Interviewing (PAPI) [78].

Data collection was based on multistage random samples of about 1000 EU-citizens aged 15 or older. National sampling points were selected randomly after stratification for population size and population density (metropolitan, urban and rural areas). Within each sampling point, a random sample of households (addresses) was visited by interviewers (applying random-walk procedures). In case of noncontact, interviewers re-visited the address for a second or a third time. The response rates by country varied from 36% in the Netherlands to more than 70% in Bulgaria[6]. A somewhat differing recruitment process can probably explain the considerable low response rate in the Netherlands: Dutch participants were pre-recruited by telephone or email in order to make appointments for the interview, rather than approached directly, as is often done in surveys within the Netherlands.

To increase representativeness, national samples were weighted by gender, age group, and size of locality based on national census data. Due to financial restrictions, only eight of the 27 EU countries participated in the study and a number of large EU countries and important regions are missing. As a result, no values for the 'average European citizen' were calculated. Instead, to have an average benchmark for the participating countries its total sample was used, but without a weighting for country size. Consequently, total sample values represent a 'country average' where all countries are represented with equal weights regardless of their population size.

5. Main Results of Measuring Health Literacy by the HLS-EU Instrument in Eight Member-States of the EU

Results of the original HLS-EU study have been published and presented at international conferences. The results compare the eight countries [78, 79] or are presented for single countries -- e.g. Ireland [80], the Netherlands [81], Poland [82] or for an extended sample in Austria [83]. The Solid Facts - Health Literacy of WHO-EURO [15] (available also in Russian 2014[7], Mandarin 2015[8] and in German 2016[9]) rely heavily on the HLS-EU study concerning HL definition, instrument and present results for general populations.

In this chapter, just some of the main results are highlighted, which often confirm and partly detail known HL trends in general and in patient populations.

5.1. Analysis of Single Items

Using the criterion of no answer rates, all 47 items worked well, except one plausible exemption with an elevated no answer rate ("find out about efforts to promote your health at work?" where the non-response rate was 17.1%). The difficulty of items varied considerably by content and for many items additionally by country, which suggests the instrument's sensitivity. All items were positively and partly significantly correlated with each other. The results for the single items present a good diagnostic opportunity to identify concrete topics where citizens have low HL, i.e. difficulties to deal with specific health related tasks, for purposes of planning of practical interventions to improve health policy measures. But for more detailed and complex analysis of distributions and associations of HL, the 47 items are too extensive, but can be reduced via aggregated indices or scales.

5.2. Building and Validation of Indices and Levels for Sub-dimensions and Comprehensive Health Literacy

The underlying matrix to operationalize the theoretical concept of comprehensive HL enables building a number of specific theoretically-based sub-indices. Besides one general comprehensive index, three sub-indices for domains of application of HL and four for specific stages in health relevant information management are available and 12 sub-sub-indices encompass combinations of these. Indices add the values for the answer categories of single items (very easy = 4, rather easy = 3, rather difficult = 2, very difficult = 1) for persons answering at least 80% of items included in the specific index. Following this procedure, elevated index values suggest higher HL. To ease comparability between indices, the general index and the sub-indices were standardized into a scale from 0 to 50 and the sub-sub-indices into a scale from 0 to 5.

$$Index = (mean - 1) * \left(\frac{50}{3}\right)$$

The reliability of indices, measured by Cronbach´s alphas for general index and sub-indices, was considerably above 0,7 and for most of the sub-sub-indices as well, only for few it was at least near to 0,7 [84, slide 23].

Distributions of index values for general index and sub-indices represent a normal distribution with some ceiling effects for higher HL, which for sub-sub-indices is more pronounced [84, slide 24-26]. The somewhat skewed normal distributions indicate that the HLS-EU-Q indices are more sensitive and provide more information for lower than higher HL scores, which makes sense for most research questions.

Differences between mean values and standard deviations of indices are considerable by country, e.g. between 30.5 for Bulgaria and 37.1 for the Netherlands, whereas with 9.2, Bulgaria has the highest and the Netherlands had the second lowest standard deviation at 6.4. In addition, there are HL differences by sub-dimensions. For example, tasks relating to health promotion or disease prevention are perceived as more difficult than those for health care, and tasks related to "appreciation" or "accessing" of information are perceived as more difficult than "understanding" or "applying" information [3, 84: slide 24-26].

Pearson correlations among and between indices are rather high, for the 7 sub-indices with the general index between $r = .89$ and $r = .93$, for the sub-indices among each other between $r = .70$ and $r = .81$, for the sub-sub-indices with the general index between $r = .72$ and $r = .82$, respectively with the sub-indices between $r = .54$ and $r = .84$ and within each other between $r = .42$ and $r = .69$ [3]. These correlations suggest that all indices measure HL, or something in common, but there also is variation in experienced difficulty of tasks by specific sub-dimensions of HL. Yet, the measures for comprehensive HL correlated moderately (but significantly) with a measure for functional HL, the New Vital Sign (NVS) test, which was included in the study. Pearson correlations with NVS were $r = .27$ for the general index, for the domain specific sub-indices $r = .24$ respectively $r = .25$. For the stages of information management correlation with NVS was somewhat higher with $r = .29$ for "accessing" or "understanding", than for "appraising" $r = .18$ or "applying" $r = .22$. A similar pattern additionally was found for the respective sub-sub- indices. Hence, functional HL measured by a performance test explained a certain amount of variation of the comprehensive self-assessed HL measure, but not significantly more than the level of education of the respondents.

Means and standard deviations enable comparative differences well within the same measure of HL, but not between different measures, and differences of numeric values of means are difficult to intuitively interpret. Thus, for the HLS-EU measures some levels have been defined as for to some other HL measures (e.g. the HALS or NVS, which enables comparing the percentages of the distributions of levels [20, 26].

5.3. The Distribution of Four Health Literacy Levels

Levels of HL have been defined for comprehensive general HL and for domain specific sub-indices and for stage specific sub-indices, but for sub-sub-indices (due to their small number of items and skewed distributions) it was *not* advisable to construct levels. Guiding the criterion for fixation of thresholds was a likelihood to experience tasks as difficult. In addition, for constructing the general comprehensive HL index, thresholds were set to minimize 'external' information loss to guarantee that categorized and metric HL indices produced similar correlation strengths and patterns (with NVS, age, financial deprivation, social status, self-assessed health and frequency of doctor use). Thresholds also were set to minimize 'internal' information loss by maximising their correlations with their corresponding metric indices. Similar to the four categories, of the original items four levels of HL were defined: inadequate level (0-25 pts. or 50%), problematic level (>25-33 pts. or 66%); sufficient level (>33-42 pts. or 80%), and excellent level (>42-50 pts. or top 20%). For some analyses, the levels of "inadequate" and "problematic" HL were combined to "limited" HL [cf. 78, pp. 28-30, respectively 79].

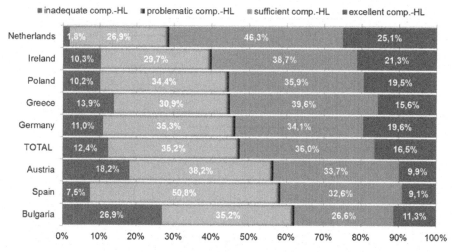

Figure 2: Percentages of Comprehensive Health Literacy Levels Thresholds for Countries and HLS-EU Total Sample

The percentage distributions of HL levels suggest two overall results (cf. figure 2). Limited HL is not just a problem for a minority of citizens, since nearly every second citizen in the total sample of all researched countries had limited HL. However, the percentage of limited HL differed considerably between the surveyed countries; it was lowest for the Netherlands (29%) and highest for Bulgaria (62%). Consequently, the HLS-EU study confirmed what other studies (with only partly similar instruments and for a variety of populations) previously suggested: limited HL is of considerable magnitude in populations of contemporary societies, and there is significant variation between countries, even when the same instrument and methodology are used.

Taking percentage of limited HL as a measure, by using the HLS-EU instrument, suggests limited HL is operant within up to 75 percent within vulnerable or disadvantaged groups, again with considerable variation among and between countries. Vulnerable and disadvantaged groups include senior citizens, persons with low education or financial difficulties, low self-assessed social status, as well as those with low self-assessed health status, or a high use of health care services.

5.4. Social Determinants of Health Literacy

In most studies, mainly in the U.S. and mostly using measures of functional HL, it has been suggested that HL is unequally distributed in relation to indicators of socio-demographic or socio-economic status [32, 33, 85]. The results of the HLS-EU study confirm this finding for general populations and for comprehensive HL.

Five measured and analyzed indicators (gender, age, education[10], financial deprivation[11], self-assessed social status[12]) in a multivariate regression model indicate a social gradient for HL [table 2/model 1; 78, p. 46]. With a value of 17% of explained variance the social gradient is significant, but somewhat less than for explained self-assessed health (25%) (cf. table 3/model 1) [78, p.53, 55]. The explained variance of HL varies considerably between the included countries, and was lowest in the Netherlands (8%) and highest in Bulgaria (25%), which can be interpreted as a difference in health related inequality between these countries. For the total HLS-EU sample, all five indicators are significant predictors of HL. The more robust effect was found for financial deprivation (β = -.24), followed by self-assessed social status (β = .14), level of education (β = .13), age (β = -.09) and gender (β = .06), which suggests that women have somewhat better HL than men. These effect parameters vary considerably between the eight countries (cf. table 2/model1) [78, p.53].

By introducing functional HL, measured by the NVS-test, into the model, the explained variance was increased to 19%. Financial deprivation (β = -.23) remained the strongest predictor, followed by functional HL (β = .13). The order of the other included predictors remained the same, but with somewhat lowered effect parameters, especially for education and age (cf. table 2/model 2) [3]. Hence, it is advisable to understand functional HL as an additional social determinant of comprehensive HL.

Table 2: Two multiple regression models for comprehensive HL as dependent variable and socio-demographic indicators as predictors, for HLS-EU Total Sample

Model 1	Coef.	STD. Coef.			95% CI for B		Pearson Corr.		
	B	Beta	t	Sig.	Lower	Upper	Raw	Partial	Semi-partial
(Constant)	28.78		62.43	.00	27.86	29.67			
Gender	1	.06	5.86	.00	.67	1.33	.05	.07	.06
Age	-.04	-.09	-8.52	.00	-.05	-.03	-.16	-.10	-.09
Education	.79	.13	11.33	.00	.65	.93	.25	.13	.12
Financial deprivation	-.192	-.24	- 19.91	.00	-2.11	-1.73	-.34	-.23	-.21
Social Status	.69	.14	11.39	.00	.57	.81	.31	.13	.12
Adj R²	**.174**								
Model 2									
(Constant)	27.47		58.32	.00	26.55	28.39			
Gender	.92	.06	5.43	.00	.59	1.25	.05	.06	.06
Age	-.03	-.06	-5.59	.00	-.04	-.02	-.16	-.07	-.06
Education	.60	.10	8.48	.00	.46	.74	.25	.10	.09
Financial deprivation	-1.85	-.23	- 19.33	.00	-2.04	-1.66	-.34	-.22	-.21
Social Status	.59	.12	9.77	.00	.47	.71	.31	.11	.10
NVS Score	.51	.13	11.23	.00	.42	.60	.27	.13	.12
Adj R²	**.188**								

HLS-EU TOTAL [N=7085]
Health Literacy: Comprehensive-HL-Index from 0=minimal HL to 50=maximal HL; Gender from 0=male to 1=female; Age in years; Education in ISCED levels == low education to 6 = high education; Financial deprivation from low deprivation to high deprivation; Social status from 1=lowest place in society to 10=highest place in society; NVS Score 0=low to 6= high functional HL

5.5. Health Relevant Consequences or Associations of Health Literacy

Following the literature and the generic causal model (cf. figure 1), the HLS-EU consortium expected to find effects or at least relationships or associations (due to the cross-sectional design of the study) of HL with health behaviors, as well as with indicators of health and sickness behavior. As a result, selected indicators for these variables were included in the HLS-EU questionnaire.

Concerning *health behavior* or *health risks* four variables or indicators were chosen: frequency of physical activity, [13] body-mass index (BMI [14]), alcohol consumption [15] and smoking behavior. [16] The strongest significant associations of HL were found for frequency of physical activity (for total sample $\rho = -.19$, varying between $\rho = -.04$ and $\rho = -.21$ for countries) [78, p. 63]. The frequency of physical activity increased continuously with grouped categories of the index of general HL.

In a multiple regression model, including the five social indicators and general HL, 8% of the variation of frequency of physical activity were explained and HL was the strongest predictor ($\beta = -,13$), followed by financial deprivation, social status, education, age, and gender [3]. Body mass index and amount of alcohol consumption were slightly significantly associated with HL as well, but smoking behavior was only associated with HL in some countries and sign of association was inconsistent [78, p.63].

For measuring *health status,* the three indicators of Minimum European Health Module (MEHM) were chosen, self-assessed health with an item of SF 36, (for which a strong correlation with objective assessments of health was suggested [e.g. 86], and number of chronic diseases and existence of disease related restrictions. For all three indicators there were significant associations with HL for the total sample and within the majority of countries [3, 78, p.71]. Association was strongest for self-assessed health ($\rho = -.27$ for total, varying for countries from $\rho = -.15$ to $\rho = -.33$), followed by number of chronic diseases ($\rho = .16$ for total, varying from $\rho = .05$ and $\rho = .26$ for countries), and for disease related restrictions ($\rho = .17$ for total, varying from $\rho = .08$ to $\rho = .32$ for countries). The relationship of HL with self-assessed health was continuous, for all eight countries with a differing degree of correlation and differing levels of self-assessed health within the assessed nations [78, p. 72-73].

The aggregated social gradient of the 5 social indicators in a multivariate regression model explained 25% of variance of self-assessed health in the total sample (variation for countries between 8% (Netherlands) and 42% (Poland)) (cf. table 3/model 1) [78, p. 55]. If additionally general comprehensive HL and functional HL (NVS) were in included into the model (cf. table 3/model 2) [3], 27% of the variance of self-assessed health was explained. Following age, comprehensive HL is the second strongest predictor ($\beta = -.17$, varying from $\beta = -.10$ to $\beta = -.21$ for countries), but NVS has no significant effect ($\beta = -.03$).

In a more complex model additionally including indicators for chronic illness and for health behaviors, considerably more variation of self-assessed health (44%) was explained. Chronic diseases were the strongest predictor ($\beta = .44$), followed by age ($\beta = .17$), while comprehensive HL was third ($\beta = -.13$) (cf. table 3/model 3).

Table 3: Three multiple regression models for self-assessed health as dependent variable and multiple indicators (social determinants, health literacy and health behavior) as predictors, for HLS-EU Total Sample

Model 1	Coef.	STD. Coef.			95% CI for B		Pearson Corr.		
	B	Beta	t	Sig.	Lower	Upper	Raw	Partial	Semi-partial
(Constant)	1.81		35.74		1.71	1.91			
Gender	.05	.03	2.82	.00	.02	.09	.06	.03	.03
Age	.02	.39	37.96	.01	.02	.02	.44	.40	.38
Education	-.05	-.07	-5.98	.00	-.06	-.03	-.23	-.07	-.06
Financial deprivation	.11	.11	10.00	.00	.09	.13	.22	.12	.10
Social Status	-.08	-.14	-11.88	.00	-.09	-.07	-.27	-.14	-.12
Adj R²	**.249**								
Model 2									
(Constant)	2.41		37.89	.00	2.29	2.54			
Gender	.07	.04	3.83	.00	.04	.11	.05	.05	.04
Age	.02	.37	34.14	.00	.02	.02	.43	.37	.34
Education	-.03	-.04	-3.23	.00	-.04	-.01	-.22	-.04	-.03
Financial deprivation	.07	.07	6.07	.00	.05	.09	.22	.07	.06
Social Status	-.06	-.11	-9.36	.00	-.08	-.05	-.27	-.11	-.09
HL	-.02	-.17	-15.00	.00	-.02	-.02	-.30	-.17	-.15
NVS Score	-.01	-.03	-2.28	.02	-.02	.00	-.24	-.03	-.02
Adj R²	**.268**								
Model 3									
(Constant)	1.81								
Gender	.06	.03	23.76	.00	1.66	1.95			
Age	.01	.17	3.35	.00	.02	.09	.05	.04	.03
Education	-.01	-.02	16.24	.00	.01	.01	.42	.19	.15
Financial deprivation	.02	.03	-1.79	.07	-.03	.00	-.22	-.02	-.02
Social Status	-.06	-.10	2.48	.01	.01	.04	.22	.03	.02
HL	-.02	-.13	-8.97	.00	-.07	-.04	-.26	-.11	-.08
NVS Score	-.01	-.03	12.37	.00	-.02	-.01	-.29	-.15	-.11
Long-term illness	.86	.44	-2.81	.01	-.02	.00	-.24	-.03	-.03
Physical activity	.06	.08	43.96	.00	.82	.90	.57	.47	.40
BMI	.01	.07	8.43	.00	.05	.07	.22	.10	.08
Adj R²	**.437**								

HLS-EU TOTAL [N=7224-7452]
Self-assessed health 1= very good to 5=very bad; Gender from 0=male to 1=female; Age in years; Education in ISCED levels == low education to 6 = high education; Financial deprivation from low deprivation to high deprivation; Social status from 1=lowest place in society to 10=highest place in society; HL: Comprehensive-HL-Index from 0=minimal HL to 50=maximal HL; NVS Score 0=low to 6= high functional HL; Physical activity time from almost every day to never; Long-term illness 0=no 1=yes; BMI low to high.

Overall, the findings suggest comprehensive HL can be understood as an independent, direct social determinant of self-assessed health, even when other relevant determinants are controlled for. However, an ongoing discussion remains in the literature about the specific ways HL may influence health, such as whether HL is a mediator between other social determinants of health, or whether HL is moderator of the impact of other health social determinants [72, 77]. A complex path model using data from the HLS-EU study suggests HL is a mediator of other social determinants and also is mediated by health behaviors in its impact on health. Hence, the path model results suggest HL has direct as well as indirect effects on health. In addition, the study's logistic regression models suggest HL moderates the association of age and education with self-assessed health [87]. Thus, an analysis of cross-sectional data provides insights about the different kinds of impacts of HL on health. However, more robust tests of the causal relationships of HL on health require longitudinal research and more comprehensive panel data sets, as well as the inclusion of diverse, relevant variables.

For measuring *disease behavior*, the frequency to use four different kinds of professional health care services (emergency units[17], hospitals[18], doctors[19] and other health care professionals[20] (such as dentists, physiotherapists, psychologists, dieticians or opticians) were selected as indicators. The associations of comprehensive HL with all four indicators were significant within the HLS-EU data, but only of moderate degree. Although the use of emergency units, hospitals and doctors decreased with higher HL, the use of other health care professionals increased slightly. This result seems plausible, since in most countries use of the aforementioned professionals demands co-payments, or has to be financed privately. The association with HL was strongest (and rather continuous) for visits of doctors ($\rho = -.11$, for total sample, varying from $\rho = -.01$ (Netherlands) to $\rho = -.19$ (Austria) [78, p.87]. In a multivariate regression model including the five social indicators and comprehensive HL, which explained 13% of variance of doctor's visits, HL also was a significant predictor ($\beta = -.07$) at the third position following age ($\beta = .29$) and gender ($\beta = .13$). The latter suggests women are visiting doctors more often [3, table 8]. But used in a model including additionally chronic diseases and self-assessed health, HL had no significant direct effect on doctor's visits [78, p. 88]. Correlations with use of emergency units ($\rho = -.06$) and hospitals ($\rho = -.06$) were significant as well for the total sample and most countries, but lower in value. Similarly there was an inverse association of HL with the use of other health professionals ($\rho = .06$) [78, p. 85].

In summary it can be said, that the associations of HL with usage of the professional health care system that have been found in the U.S. (with instruments measuring functional HL) [34, 77, 88], were confirmed in the HLS-EU survey for general populations and comprehensive HL. However, the findings were not as robust as U.S. studies suggest -- and did not occur for every indicator in all eight countries. But the HLS-EU study, (a general population oriented study of citizens' HL) did not assess associations of comprehensive HL with clinical outcomes, as many US studies have suggested [77]. The findings also suggest health literacy's impact on health care utilization may be inconsistent between Europe and the U.S. probably because European health care delivery systems differ so significantly with their US peers.

In summary, the results of a theory-based benchmarking study that included several European countries and a comprehensive conceptual understanding and an explicit generic model of HL provide a robust case for the relevance of HL in health research, practice and policy, although more longitudinal research is needed.

6. Development of Short Forms for the HLS-EU-Q47

Compared to a performance based comprehensive test of HL, like the HALS, the HLS-EU-Q47 is an efficient instrument. But even a battery of 47 Likert scaled items (needing about 10 minutes interviewing time), which also can be self-administered [89] or placed on the internet [90], is regarded as too time-consuming for some HL research intended for general or specific populations. As a result, two short forms, short-scale HLS-EU-Q16 (3 minutes) and short-short scale HLS-EU-Q6 (1 minute), were developed for the HLS-EU measure.

For the short instrument psychometric properties of a one-dimensional scale to measure comprehensive HL were demanded and representation of the scope and underlying theoretical content of the long-form as far as possible. To guarantee one-dimensionality, a one-parametric dichotomous Rasch model was used to select items. For that, items have been dichotomized into two categories, "easy" ("fairly" or "very" easy = 1) and "difficult" ("fairly" and "very" difficult = 0).

Accordingly, Rasch analyses were operationalized for every country and for the total sample. Three split criteria were used: median, gender and dichotomized level of education within each country. By that a sub-set of the same 16 items for all countries satisfied Rasch characteristics for each country, but the item order occasionally varied. Altogether, these 16 items represented the HLS-EU matrix well, with the exception that no item of the cell "applying information" for "health promotion" of the matrix fulfilled the Rasch criteria. Hence, this cell was not represented by an item in the short-form HLS-EU-Q16. Scale values were calculated as simple sum scores and varied between 0 and 16. It was recommended to only calculate scale values for respondents who answered at least 14 items. Correlations with the index of the long form were very high, r = .82 for total sample, varied for the countries between r = .73 and r = .88. Correlations with functional HL (NVS-test) were similar to these of the index of the long form (r = .25 for total, varying between r = .14 and r = .38 for the countries).

The distribution of HLS-EU Q-16 was J-shaped, with a clear ceiling effect for better HL. Therefore only three levels were defined, inadequate HL (scale values = 0-8), problematic HL (9-12) and adequate HL (13-16).

As expected, the short form was a less robust measure than the long form, having fewer items as well as dichotomized answer categories. Overall, the levels of long and short form were in accordance for 76% of all cases (varying for countries between 68% and 79%) [84]. It was possible to calculate score values for sub-scales of the short form, but levels could not be defined. Correlation patterns with important determinants and possible consequences of HL were very similar for the short and the long form of the instrument. In further studies, the Rasch homogeneity of the 16 items were confirmed e.g. for Austrian adolescents [91] and migrant populations in Austria [92], as well as in studies of general populations, e.g. for the Czech Republic and for Hungary.

The HLS-EU-Q16 short-form contained about a third of the original items and consequently took only a third of the interviewing time, about 3 minutes on average. Nevertheless, even this was regarded as too long for some types of studies. Therefore, another 'short-short-form,' containing 6 of the 16 items, was constructed and validated, which took about a minute of interviewing time [for details see 84].

With these two short forms, the HLS-EU instrument to measure comprehensive HL became available for efficient studies with some possibility to benchmark with studies that use the long form of the instrument.

7. Use of the HLS-EU Health Literacy Instruments in Further Research

During and after the HLS-EU research project, the HLS-EU survey questionnaire and the HL measure itself were translated into and validated for other languages (e.g. Albanian, Czech, Danish, French, Hebrew, Hungarian, Italian, Maltese, Portuguese, Russian, Serbo-Croatian, and Turkish). The translated questionnaires have been used in population surveys and smaller research projects in different countries and languages also outside Europe (including Indonesian, Japanese, Kazakh, Russian, Malay, Myanmar/Burmese, Traditional Mandarin, and Vietnamese). As a reminder, the eight original languages were: Bulgarian; Dutch; English; German; Greek; Polish; and Spanish).

A number of European countries started national population surveys by translating and using the HLS-EU-Q47 respectively HLS-EU-Q86[21] instrument. Albania [93], the Czech Republic [94], Denmark[22], Germany [96], Hungary [97], Italy [98], Portugal [99], and Switzerland [100] completed national HL Survey using the HLS-EU-instrument. In a number of other countries, e.g. France and Russia national surveys are in preparation.

In some of these countries, the instrument also has been applied to specific populations, e.g. in Austria to 15-Year-Old adolescents [91], in Germany to young and elderly populations [101], as well as to immigrant populations in Austria[23] [92], Germany [102], Sweden [103], and Switzerland [100].

In addition to replicating the HLS-EU-Q86 further relevant variables (e.g. information behavior, health perception) have been included and associated with HL, e.g. in Portugal [99], and in Germany [104].

The *short from* of the HL instrument, the HLS-EU-Q16, was used in Israel[24] [105], Belgium [106], Germany [107], Malta [108] or Sweden [103] and also in smaller research projects [e.g.109].

Furthermore, some specific clinical studies used the *short-short form* (HLS-EU-Q6) to measure HL as a relevant variable for their research question, e.g. a diabetes project [110] and a street youth project in Ghana [111].

The philosophy and the format of the items of HLS-EU-Q47 also have been used to develop specific batteries; e.g. of migrant-relevant tasks based on focus-groups [92].

HLS-EU data also has helped develop and validate a HL prediction model [112]. Some critical research has been conducted concerning the validity or interpretation of the instrument in Austria [113] and the instrument's validity among German adolescents [114].

Outside of Europe, an Asian coalition lead by Taiwan started to coordinate a number of Asian countries (Indonesia Kazakhstan, Malaysia, Myanmar, Taiwan and Vietnam) that used the translated HLS-EU-Q47 instrument in population surveys and started to benchmark data and results [115]. In Taiwan, the questionnaire was used via self-administered questionnaire and further questions were added to the HLS-EU-Q86 [115]. Independent of this coalition, the HLS-EU-Q47 was applied in Japan [90]. The survey was administered via an online questionnaire to internet users that closely matched the demographics of Japan's general population.

All of these studies suggested an operant need for a comprehensive, but efficient and perception-based instrument to measure HL. There was no coordinated strategy to propagate the HLS-EU design and instruments systematically. Researchers discovered HLS-EU from publications and presentations and independently decided to use its concept, model and instruments to do their own (follow-up) research. Interestingly, the translation into new languages, the fidelity of instrument application, and its amendments followed an evolutionary and un-coordinated pattern.

8. Lessons Learned and Future Challenges for Measuring Health Literacy in General Populations

Why has HLS-EU been accepted to followers in the scientific community of health research and health policy and similarly, why has some ensuing dissemination of the conceptual and logic model and the instruments been possible?

Of course, the evolving hyperbole of HL as a concept, and research showing its relevance for health care and for health and by that for public health and health promotion policy, helped set an agenda to measure population HL. But what were critical features of the HLS-EU study that made its methodology attractive to execute studies on comprehensive HL of general populations of citizens outside the original study?

First, it was important that the international HLS-EU consortium, which was supported by the Agency for Health and Consumers (EAHC) of the European Union, developed (in a consensus process) a comprehensive theory-based conceptual model and definition of HL that fit the broader meaning of the concept of health and HL used in public health and health promotion. Also, it was important that an explicit logic model of HL was used to undergird the research instrument. Peer acceptance also advanced because both models and the definition were based on existing already published materials and featured an integrative approach. In social and health sciences, concepts and definitions frequently are introduced from scratch and existing constructs unfortunately are not taken into account. Hence, social science sometimes does not build on what has already been published, which undermines the growth of an evidence-based discipline.

Second, it was important to operationalize a complex, multi-dimensional, but efficient, instrument of standardized meaningful items that assessed HL in terms of difficulty of concrete tasks and by that as the relation between personal competencies and situational demands. By using a standardized format of items and categories, the modularized instrument permits comparable standardized indices for a number of aspects of HL as well as a general measure of HL. It was important that these measures also were simultaneously validated within an international comparative study from eight countries. When the two short forms of the instrument were constructed and validated, it also supported their diffusion.

Third, it helped that model, definition and instrument were immediately used in a survey with a study design and questionnaire containing a number of indicators for HL relationships. These were predefined by a logic model and comparative data were collected in parallel for eight countries with the same methodology, which enabled a benchmarking of results. In turn, this suggested that the HLS-EU instrument enabled an array of interesting HL findings, which could be replicated and confirmed. It also suggested that a standardized international comparative study could assess interesting variation among and between countries concerning HL's distribution as well as HL's strength of association with other health determinants and consequences. These results also were a reason that the HLS-EU study was taken up as a relevant source for the Solid Facts – Health Literacy by WHO-EURO, which reinforced the findings' international diffusion.

These characteristics of the HLS-EU study led to a number of studies using the instrument, which quickly adopted the study design within different countries in Europe and Asia after the finalization of the original study. Since its introduction, the instrument has been used by HL researchers and by public health policy practitioners. In most of the countries where national surveys were done, their results stimulated public debate on limited health literacy (HL) and led to policy planning of intervention measures to improve a newly, diagnosed population deficit. In addition, research efforts based on HLS-EU instruments enabled additional international benchmarking of results, and lead to a number of interesting developments, such as suggesting the relationships of HL to other variables, and identifying critical questions regarding some aspects of the instrument.

On the other hand, many of the ensuing developments were not coordinated or well-documented. As a result, the principle future challenge is to create a sustainable institutionalized consortium, best supported by one or more international agencies, to regularly monitor and benchmark comprehensive HL over time, across countries and to jointly develop the instrument and research methodology. While the latter has been recommended by WHO-EUROs Solid Facts – Health Literacy, it still has to be practically accomplished.

Endnotes

---

[1] http://www.uis.unesco.org/literacy/Pages/international-literacy-day-2016.aspx

[2] https://nces.ed.gov/naal/

[3] https://nces.ed.gov/statprog/handbook/ials.asp

[4] https://nces.ed.gov/surveys/all/

[5] HALS full length test approximately 1 hour, respectively the "locator" version 30 – 40 minutes [2, p.4]

[6] Response rates: Netherlands 36%, Germany NRW 53%; Spain 62%; Greece/ Athens 65%, Austria and Poland 67%, Ireland 69%, Bulgaria 75%

[7] http://www.euro.who.int/__data/assets/pdf_file/0010/254377/Health_Literacy_RU_web.pdf?ua=1

[8] http://www.ahla-asia.org/main.php?fid=01&page_name=news_detail&news_id=310

[9] http://www.careum.ch/documents/20181/140554/WHO_2016_Gesundheitskompetenz_Fakten/1b5693 c2-cfa7-4c8c-82a1-e6edf4dab1db

[10] What is the highest level of education you have successfully completed (usually by obtaining a certificate or diploma? Use ISCED 97 – Showcard. ISCED levels rang von 0 = pre-primary education or now school education to 6= second stage of tertiary education.

[11] The financial deprivation index consists of three variables: (1) Are you able to pay for medication if needed to manage your own health? It is…Very easy/Fairly easy/Fairly difficult/Very difficult), (2) Are you able to afford to see the doctor? Is it … (Instructions: time, health insurance, cost, transport) Very easy/Fairly easy/Fairly difficult/Very difficult) and (3) During the last twelve months, would you say you had difficulties to pay your bills at the end of the month…? Most of the time/from time to time/Almost never-never. The financial deprivation score (z-scores) range from low to high financial deprivation

[12] On the following scale, step '1' corresponds to 'the lowest level in the society'; step '10' corresponds to 'the highest level in the society'. Could you tell me on which step you would place yourself?

[13] How often during the last month did you exercise for 30 minutes or longer e.g. running, walking, cycling? (1) Almost every day (2) A few times a week (3) A few times this month (4) Not at all (5) I haven't been able to exercise (SPONTANEOUS) (5) DK (SPONTANEOUS)

[14] Calculated index of weight-for-height: How tall are you? (Approximately) and How much do you weigh? (Approximately).

[15] Self-reported alcohol drinking behavior was measured by five questions and summarized to an index following a quantity-frequency approach. Ranging from very excessive alcohol consumers to no alcohol consumers (5 categories).

[16] Three variables were summarized to one smoking habits variable: classifying: nonsmokers, occasional smokers and smokers.

[17] How many times have you had to contact the emergency service in the last 2 years? (Instruction: Ambulance, out of hours clinic, emergency department) (1) 0 (2) 1 - 2 times (3) 3 - 5 times (4) 6 times or more (5) DK/ Refusal (SPONTANEOUS)

[18] How many times have you used a hospital service in the last 12 months? (1) 0 (2) 1 - 2 times (3) 3 - 5 times (4) 6 times or more (5) DK/ Refusal (SPONTANEOUS)

[19] How many times have you been to the doctor in the last 12 months? (1) 0 (2) 1 - 2 times (3) 3 - 5 times (4) 6 times or more (5) DK/ Refusal (SPONTANEOUS)

[20] How many times have you used services from other health professionals, such as dentist, physiotherapist, psychologist, dietician, or optician in the last 12 months? (1) 0 (2) 1 - 2 times (3) 3 - 5 times (4) 6 times or more (5) DK/ Refusal (SPONTANEOUS)

[21] The HLS-EU-Q86 is the full HLS-EU-survey questionnaire. It includes the HLS-EU-Q47 for comprehensive HL, the NVS for functional HL, and also indicators for social determinants, health behavior, health status, usage of the health care system.

[22] The HLS-EU-Q47 was used in parallel to the HLQ [95], but HLS-EU-Q results have not yet been published.

[23] Only by HLS-EU-Q16.

[24] Hebrew, Arabic and Russian

References

[1] Nutbeam D. The evolving concept of health literacy. Soc Sci Med 2008;67(12):2071-78. DOI: 10.1016/j.socscimed.2008.09.050.

[2] Baker DW. The meaning and the measure of health literacy. J Gen Intern Med. 2006;21(8): 878-883. DOI: 10.1111/J.1525-1497.2006.00540.X.

[3] Pelikan JM, Ganahl K. Die europäische Gesundheitskompetenz-Studie Konzept, Instrument und ausgewählte Ergebnisse.[The European Health Literacy sSudy : concept, instrument and selected results]. In: Schaeffer D, Pelikan JM, editors. Health Literacy Forschungsstand und Perspektiven. Bern: hogrefe; 2017. p.93-125.

[4] Rudd RE. Health literacy developments, corrections, and emerging themes. In: Schaeffer D, Pelikan JM, editors. Health Literacy Forschungsstand und Perspektiven. Bern: hogrefe; 2017. p.19-31.

[5] Sorensen K, Van den Broucke S, Fullam J, Doyle G, Pelikan J, Slonska Z, Brand H. for HLS-EU Consortium Health Literacy Project European. Health literacy and public health: a systematic review and integration of definitions and models. BMC Public Health. 2012;12(80). DOI:10:1186/1471-2458/12/80.

[6] Nutbeam D. Health literacy as a public health goal: a challenge for contemporary health education and communication strategies into the 21st Century. Health Promot Int. 2000;15(3):259–67. DOI: 10.1093/heapro/15.3.259.

[7] Kickbusch I, Maag D. Health Literacy. In: Heggenhougen K, Quah S, editors. International Encyclopedia of Public Health, Vol.3. San Diego; 2008. p. 204-211.

[8] Schulz PJ, Hartung U. The future of health literacy. In: Schaeffer D, Pelikan JM, editors. Health Literacy Forschungsstand und Perspektiven. Bern: hogrefe; 2017. p.79-91.

[9] Nguyen TH, Park H, Han H-R, Chan KS, Paasche-Orlow MK, Haun J, Kim MT. State of the science of health literacy measures: validity implications for minority populations. Patient Educ Couns. 2015;98: 1492-512. DOI: 10.1016/j.pec.2015.07.013.

[10] Haun JN, Valerio MA, McCormack LA, Sorensen K, Paasche-Orlow MK. Health literacy measurements: an inventory and descriptive summary of 51 instruments. J Health Commun. 2014 19(Suppl 2):302–33. DOI: 10.1080/10810730.2014.936571.

[11] Parker R. Measures of health literacy. Workshop summary: what? so what? now what?; Washington: The National Academies Press; 2009.

[12] Brach C, Keller D, Hernandez LM, Baur C, Parker R, Dreyer B, Schyve P, Lemerise AJ, Schillinger D. Attributes of health literate health care organizations. Washington DC: Institute of Medicine of the National Academies, 2012.

[13] Dietscher C, Pelikan JM. Health-literate hospitals and healthcare organizations - results from an Austrian feasibility study on the self-assessment of organizational health literacy in hospitals. In: Schaeffer D, Pelikan JM, editors. Health Literacy Forschungsstand und Perspektiven. Bern: hogrefe; 2017. p.303-313.

[14] Osborne R, Beauchamp A. Optimising health literacy, equity and access (Ophelia). Osborne R, Beauchamp A. Optimising Health Literacy, Equity and Access (Ophelia). In: Schaeffer D, Pelikan JM, editors. Health Literacy Forschungsstand und Perspektiven. Bern: hogrefe; 2017. p.71-78.

[15] Kickbusch I, Pelikan JM, Apfel F, Tsouros AD, editors. Health literacy: the solid facts. WHO Regional Office for Europe : Copenhagen, 2013.

[16] Tuijnman A, editor. The International Adult Literacy Survey (IALS). Results and highlights from an international perspective: IALS in relation to economies and labour markets. Workshop on literacy, economy and society; 1997; Calgary, Canada.

[17] Desjardins R, Murray TS, Tuijnmann AC. Learning a living: First results of the adult literacy and life skills survey. Ayer Publishing, 2005. Report No.: 9264010386.

[18] OECD. First results from the survey of adult skills. OECD Publishing, 2013.

[19] Kirsch IS, Jungeblut A, Jenkins L, Kolstad. Adult literacy in America: a first look at the findings of the national adult literacy survey. New Jersey: National Center for Education Statistics, 2002. Report No.: 065-000-00588-3.

[20] Rudd R, Kirsch I, Yamamoto K. Literacy and health in America. Policy Information Report. Educational Testing Service. Princeton; 2004.

[21] Murray T, Hagey J, Willms D, Shillington R, Desjardins R. Health literacy in Canada: a healthy understanding 2008. Ottawa, 2008.

[22] Jordan JE, Osborne RH, Buchbinder R. Critical appraisal of health literacy indices revealed variable underlying constructs, narrow content and psychometric weaknesses. J Clin Epidemiol. 2011;64(4): 366-379. DOI: 10.1016/j.jclinepi.2010.04.005.

[23] Guzys D, Kenny A, Dickson-Swift V, Threlkeld G. A critical review of population health literacy assessment. BMC Public Health. 2015; (15). DOI: 10.1186/s12889-015-1551-6.

[24] Simonds SK. Health education as social policy. Health Education Monographs. 1974;2(1_suppl): 1-10.

[25] Parker R. Health literacy: a challenge for American patients and their health care providers. Health Promot Int. 2000;15(4): 277-83.

[26] Weiss BD, Mays MZ, Martz W, Castro KM, DeWalt DA, Pignone MP, Mockbee J, Hale FA. Quick assessment of literacy in primary care: the newest vital sign. Ann Fam Med. 2005;3(6): 514-22. DOI: 10.1370/afm.405

[27] Davis TC, Crouch MA, Long SW, Jackson RH, Bates P, George RB, Bairnsfather LE. Rapid assessment of literacy levels of adult primary care patients. Fam Med. 1991;23(6): 433-5.

[28] Parker RM, Baker DW, Williams MV, Nurss JR. The test of functional health literacy in adults: a new instrument for measuring patients' literacy skills. J Gen Intern Med. 1995;10(10): 537-41.

[29] Davis TC, Long SW, Jackson RH, Mayeaux EJ, George RB, Murphy PW, Crouch MA. Rapid estimate of adult literacy in medicine: a shortened screening instrument. Fam Med. 1993;25(6): 391-5.

[30] Chew LD, Bradley KA, Boyko EJ. Brief questions to identify patients with inadequate health literacy. Fam Med. 2004;36(8): 588-594.

[31] Chew LD, Griffin JM, Partin MR, Noorbaloochi S, Grill JP, Snyder A, Bradley KA, Nugent SM, Baines AD, Vanryn M. Validation of screening questions for limited health literacy in a large VA outpatient population. J Gen Intern Med. 2008;23(5): 561-6. DOI: 10.1007/s11606-008-0520-5

[32] Paasche-Orlow M, Parker R, Gazmararian J, Nielsen-Bohlman L, Rudd R. The prevalence of limited health literacy. J Gen Intern Med. 2005;20(2): 175-184. DOI: 10.1111/j.1525-1497.2005.40245.x.

[33] Gazmararian JA, Baker DW, Williams MV, Parker RM, Scott TL, Green DC, Fehrenbach SN, Ren J, Koplan JP. Health literacy among Medicare enrollees in a managed care organization. JAMA. 1999;281(6): 545-51.

[34] Baker DW, Gazmararian JA, Williams MV, Scott T, Parker RM, Green D, Ren J, Peel.J. Functional health literacy and the risk of hospital admission among Medicare managed care enrollees. Am J Public Health. 2002;92(8): 1278-1283.

[35] DeWalt DA, Berkman ND, Sheridan SL, Lohr KN, Pignone M. Literacy and health outcomes: a systematic review of the literature. J Gen Intern Med. 2004;19(12): 1228-1239. DOI: 10.1111/j.1525-1497.2004.40153.x.

[36] Barber MN, Staples M, Osborne RH, Clerehan R, Elder C, Buchbinder R. Up to a quarter of the Australian population may have suboptimal health literacy depending upon the measurement tool: results from a population-based survey. Health Promot Int. 2009;24(3): 252-261. DOI: 10.1093/heapro/dap022

[37] Carthery-Goulart MT, Anghinah R, Areza-Fegyveres R, Bahia VS, Brucki SMD, Damin A, Formigoni AP, Frota N, Guariglia C, Jacinto AF, Kato EM, Lima EP, Mansur L, Moreira D, Nóbrega A, Porto CS, Senaha ML, Silva MN, Smid J, Souza-Talarico JN, Radanovic M, Nitrini R. Performance of a Brazilian population on the test of functional health literacy in adults. Revista de Saúde Pública. 2009;43(4): 631-8. DOI:10.1590/S0034-89102009005000031.

[38] Institute of Medicine of the National Academies. Health literacy: a prescription to end confusion. Washington, D.C.: The National Academies Press; 2004.

[39] Hernandez LM. Measures of Health Literacy. Workshop Summary; Washington: The National Academies Press; 2009.

[40] Dumenci L, Matsuyama RK, Kuhn L, Perera RA, Siminoff LA. On the validity of the shortened rapid estimate of adult literacy in medicine (REALM) scale as a measure of health literacy. Commun Methods Meas. 2013;7(2): 134-43. DOI: 10.1080/19312458.2013.789839

[41] Baur C, Deering M, Hsu L. eHealth: federal issues and approaches. In: Rice RE, Katz JE, editors. The Internet and Health Communication. Thousand Oaks, CA: Sage Publications; 2000. p. 355-384.

[42] Baur C, Prue C. The CDC Clear Communication Index is a new evidence-based tool to prepare and review health information. Health Promot Pract. 2014;15(5):629-37. DOI: 10.1177/1524839914538969.

[43] Doak CC, Doak LG, Root JH. Teaching patients with low literacy skills. Philadelphia: Lippincott Williams and Wilkins.

[44] Eysenbach G, Köhler C. How do consumers search for and appraise health information on the world wide web? Qualitative study using focus groups, usability tests, and in-depth interviews. BMJ. 2002;2002(324): 573-7. DOI:10.1136/bmj.324.7337.573.

[45] Gemoets D, Rosemblat G, Tse T, Logan R. Assessing readability of consumer health information: an exploratory study. Medinfo. 2004;11(2): 869-73. DOI: 10.3233/978-1-60750-949-3-869.

[46] Shoemaker SJ, Wolf MS, Brach C. Development of the Patient Education Materials Assessment Tool (PEMAT): a new measure of understandability and actionability for print and audiovisual patient information. Patient Educ Couns. 2014;96(3): 395-403. DOI: 10.1016/j.pec.2014.05.027.

[47] Rudd RE, Moeykens BA, Colton TC. Health and literacy: a review of medical and public health literature. Office of Educational Research and Improvement; 1999.

[48] Rudd R, Anderson J, Oppenheimer S, Nath C. Health literacy: an update of public health and medical literature. Review of Adult Learning and Literacy. 2007; Vol.7. p.175-204.

[49] Rowlands G, Protheroe J, Winkley J, Richardson M, Seed PT, Rudd R. A mismatch between population health literacy and the complexity of health information: an observational study. Br J Gen Pract. 2015;65(635): e379-e86. DOI: 10.3399/bjgp15X685285.

[50] Schillinger D, Piette J, Grumbach K, Wang F, Wilson C, Daher C, Leong-Grotz K, Castro C, Bindman AB. Closing the loop : physician communication with diabetic patients who have low health literacy. Arch Intern Med. 2003;2003(163): 83-90. DOI:10.1001/archinte.163.1.83.

[51] Brown DR, Ludwig R, Buck GA, Durham MD, Shumard T, Graham SS. Health literacy: universal precautions needed. J Allied Health. 2004;33(2): 150-5.

[52] Harper W, Cook S, Makoul G. Teaching medical students about health literacy: 2 Chicago initiatives. Am J Health Behav. 2007;31(1): 111-4. DOI: 10.5555/ajhb.2007.31.supp.S111.

[53] Gazzotti F. Health literacy in Italy's Emilia Romagna region. Health Literacy: Improving Health, Health Systems, and Health Policy Around the World: Workshop Summary. Washington DC: National Academies Press; 2013.

[54] Goto A, Rudd RE, Lai AY, Yoshida-Komiya H. Health literacy training for public health nurses in Fukushima: a case-study of program adaptation, implementation and evaluation. Japan Med Assoc J: 2014;57(3): 146-153.

[55] Rudd RE, Anderson JE. The health literacy environment of hospitals and health centers. Boston: Health and Adult Literacy and Learning Initiative, Harvard School of Public Health, 2006.

[56] Pelikan JM, Dietscher C. Gesundheitskompetenz im System der Krankenversorgung. [Health literacy in the health care system]. Journal Gesundheitsförderung. 2014;1(2): 28-33.

[57] Pelikan JM, Dietscher C. Warum sollten und wie können Krankenhäuser ihre organisationale Gesundheitskompetenz verbessern? [Why should and how can hospitals improve their organisational health literacy?]. BundesGesundheitsblatt-Gesundheitsforschung-Gesundheitsschutz. 2015;58: 989-95. DOI: 10.1007/s00103-015-2206-6.

[58] Groene RO, Rudd RE. Results of a feasibility study to assess the health literacy environment: navigation, written, and oral communication in 10 hospitals in Catalonia, Spain. J Commun Healthc. 2011;4(4): 227-37. DOI :10.1179/1753807611Y.0000000005.

[59] Dodson S, Good S, Osborne R. Health literacy toolkit for low- and middle-income countries: a series of information sheets to empower communities and strengthen health systems; New Delhi: World Health Organization, Regional Office for South-East Asia; 2014.

[60] Nutbeam D, Kickbusch I. Advancing health literacy: a global challenge for the 21st century. Health Promot Int. 2000;15(3): 183-184. DOI: 10.1093/heapro/15.3.183.

[61] Kickbusch I. Health literacy: addressing the health and education divide. Health Promot Int. 2001;16(3): 289-97. DOI: 10.1093/heapro/16.3.289.

[62] Wang J, Thombs BD, Schmid MR. The Swiss Health Literacy Survey: development and psychometric properties of a multidimensional instrument to assess competencies for health. Health Expect. 2012: 17(3). DOI: 10.1111/j.1369-7625.2012.00766.x.

[63] Sorensen K, Van den Broucke S, Pelikan JM, Fullam J, Doyle G, Slonska Z, Kondilis B, Stoffels V, Osborne R, Brand H. Measuring health literacy in populations: illuminating the design and development process of the European Health Literacy Survey Questionnaire (HLS-EU-Q). BMC public health. 2013;13: 948. DOI: 10.1186/1471-2458-13-948.

[64] Zarcadoolas C, Pleasant A, Greer DS. Understanding health literacy: an expanded model. Health Promot Int. 2005;20(2): 195-203. DOI: 10.1093/heapro/dah609.

[65] Norman C. eHealth literacy 2.0: problems and opportunities with an evolving concept. J Med Internet Res. 2011;13(4): e125. DOI: 10.2196/jmir.2035.

[66] van der Vaart R, Drossaert C. Development of the digital health literacy instrument: measuring a broad spectrum of health 1.0 and health 2.0 skills. J Med Internet Res. 2017;19(1): e27. DOI: 10.2196/jmir.6709.

[67] Levin-Zamir D, Lemish D, Gofin R. Media Health Literacy (MHL): development and measurement of the concept among adolescents. Health Educ Res. 2011;26(2): 323-35. DOI: 10.1093/her/cyr007.

[68] Hobbs R. The seven great debates in the media literacy movement. J commun. 1998;48(1): 16-32.

[69] Kwan B, Frankish J, Rootman I. The development and validation of measures of "Health literacy" in different populations. University of British Columbia, Institute of Health Promotion Research, 2006.

[70] Osborne RH, Batterham RW, Elsworth GR, Hawkins M, Buchbinder R. The grounded psychometric development and initial validation of the Health Literacy Questionnaire (HLQ). BMC Public Health. 2013;2013(13): 658. DOI: 10.1186/1471-2458-13-658.

[71] Marmot M. Social determinants of health inequalities. The Lancet. 2005;365(9464): 1099-104. DOI: 10.1016/S0140-6736(05)71146-6.

[72] Paasche-Orlow M, Wolf MS. The causal pathways linking health literacy to health outcomes. Am J Health Behav. 2007;31(50): 19-26. DOI: 10.5555/ajhb.2007.31.supp.S19.

[73] Friis K, Lasgaard M, Rowlands G, Osborne RH, Maindal HT. Health literacy mediates the relationship between educational attainment and health behavior: a Danish population-based study. J Health Commun. 2016;21(sup2): 54-60. DOI: 10.1080/10810730.2016.1201175.

[74] Schillinger D, Barton LR, Karter AJ, Wang F, Adler N. Does literacy mediate the relationship between education and health outcomes? A study of a low-income population with diabetes. Public Health Rep. 2006;121: 245-54. DOI: 10.1177/003335490612100305.

[75] Wang C, Kane RL, Xu D, Meng Q. Health literacy as a moderator of health-related quality of life responses to chronic disease among Chinese rural women. BMC Womens Health. 2015;15: 34. DOI: 10.1186/s12905-015-0190-5.

[76] McCormack L, Haun J, Sørensen K, Valerio M. Recommendations for advancing health literacy measurement. J Health Commun. 2013;18(sup1): 9-14. DOI: 10.1080/10810730.2013.829892.

[77] Berkman ND, Sheridan SL, Donahue KE, Halpern DJ, Crotty K. Low health literacy and health outcomes: an updated systematic review. Ann Intern Med. 2011;155(2): 97-107. DOI: 10.7326/0003-4819-155-2-201107190-00005

[78] HLS-EU Consortium. Comparative report of health literacy in eight EU member states. (Second extended and revised version, Date July 22th, 2014) The European Health Literacy Survey HLS-EU. The international Consortium of the HLS-EU Project, 2012.

[79] Sorensen K, Pelikan JM, Roethlin F, Ganahl K, Slonska Z, Doyle G, Fullam J, Kondilis B, Agrafiotis D, Uiters E, Falcon M, Mensing M, Tchamov K, van den Broucke S, Brand H; HLS-EU Consortium. Health literacy in Europe: comparative results of the European Health Literacy Survey (HLS-EU). Eur J Public Health 2015; 25(6):1053-8. DOI: 10.1093/eurpub/ckv043.

[80] Doyle G, Cafferkey K, Fullam J. The European Health Literacy Survey: results from Ireland. Dublin, Ireland: University College Dublin. 2012.

[81] van der Heide I, Rademakers J, Schipper M, Droomers M, Sorensen K, Uiters E. Health literacy of Dutch adults: a cross sectional survey. BMC Public Health. 2013;2013(13): 179. DOI: 10.1186/1471-2458-13-179

[82] Słońska ZA, Borowiec AA, Aranowska AE. Health literacy and health among the elderly: status and challenges in the context of the Polish population aging process. Anthropol Rev 2015;78(3): 297-307. DOI: 10.1515/anre-2015-0023.

[83] Pelikan J, Roethlin F, Ganahl K. Die Gesundheitskompetenz der österreichischen Bevölkerung–nach Bundesländern und im internationalen Vergleich. [Health literacy of the Austrian population]. Vienna: Ludwig Boltzman Institute Health Promotion Research, 2013.

[84] Pelikan JM, Roethlin F, Ganahl K, Peer S. Measuring comprehensive health literacy in general populations - the HLS-EU instruments. International Conference of Health Literacy and Health Promotion; Taipei/Taiwan2014.

[85] Howard DH, Sentell T, Gazmararian JA. Impact of health literacy on socioeconomic and racial differences in health in an elderly population. J Gen Intern Med. 2006;21(8): 857-61. DOI: 10.1111/j.1525-1497.2006.00530.x.

[86] Mackenbach JP, Simon JG, Looman CW, Joung IM. Self-assessed health and mortality: could psychosocial factors explain the association? Int J Epidemiol. 2002;31(6): 1162-8.

[87] Pelikan JM, Ganahl K. Determinant, mediator, moderator? How does health literacy influence self-assessed health? Results from the HLS-EU-study. 8th Annual Health Literacy Research Conference; Bethesda 2016.

[88] Mitchell SE, Sadikova E, Jack BW, Paasche-Orlow MK. Health literacy and 30-day postdischarge hospital utilization. J Health Commun. 2012;17(sup3): 325-38. DOI: 10.1080/10810730.2012.715233.

[89] Duong VT, Aringazina A, Baisunova G, Nurjanah, Pham TV, Pham KM, Truong TQ, Nguyen KT, Oo WM, Mohamad E, Su TT, Huang HL, Sorensen K, Pelikan JM, Van den Broucke S, Chang PW. Measuring health literacy in Asia: validation of the HLS-EU-Q47 survey tool in six Asian countries. J Epidemiol. 2017;27(2):80-86. DOI: 10.1016/j.je.2016.09.005.

[90] Nakayama K, Osaka W, Togari T, Ishikawa H, Yonekura Y, Sekido A, Matsumoto M. Comprehensive health literacy in Japan is lower than in Europe: a validated Japanese-language assessment of health literacy. BMC Public Health. 2015;15:505. DOI: 10.1186/s12889-015-1835-x.

[91] Roethlin F, Pelikan J, Ganahl K. Die Gesundheitskompetenz der 15-jährigen Jugendlichen in Österreich. Abschlussbericht der österreichischen Gesundheitskompetenz Jugendstudie im Auftrag des Hauptverbands der österreichischen Sozialversicherungsträger. [The health literacy of 15-year-old teenagers in Austria. Final report of the Austrian health competence teenager study on behalf of the Main Association of Austrian Social Security Organisations (HVSV)]. Wien: HVSVT, 2013.

[92] Ganahl K, Dahlvik J, Roethlin F, Alpagu F, Sikic-Fleischhacker A, Peer S, Pelikan, JM. Gesundheitskompetenz bei Personen mit Migrationshintergrund aus der Türkei und Ex-Jugoslawien in Österreich. Ergebnisse einer quantitativen und qualitativen Studie. [The Austrian health literacy immigrants study of people with migrationbackground in Turkey and Ex-Yugoslavia. Results from qualitative and quantitative study]. Vienna: Ludwig Boltzman Institute Health Promotion Research, 2016.

[93] Toçi E, Burazeri G, Sorensen K, Kamberi H, Brand H. Concurrent validation of two key health literacy instruments in a South Eastern European population. Eur J Public Health. 2014;2014(12): 482-6. DOI: 10.1093/eurpub/cku190.

[94] Kučera Z, Pelikan J, Šteflová A. Zdravotní gramotnost obyvatel cr⁻ Výsledky komparativního reprezentativního setrení. [Health literacy in Czech population results of the comparative representative research]. Casopis lekaru ceskych. 2016;155(5): 233-241.

[95] Bo A, Friis K, Osborne RH, Maindal HT. National indicators of health literacy: ability to understand health information and to engage actively with healthcare providers - a population-based survey among Danish adults. BMC Public Health. 2014;14: 1095. DOI: 10.1186/1471-2458-14-1095.

[96] Schaeffer D, Vogt Do, Berens E-M, Messer M, Quenzel G, Hurrelmann K. Health literacy in Deutschland. [Health literacy in Germany]. In: Schaeffer D, Pelikan JM, Eds. Health Literacy Forschungsstand und Perspektiven. Bern: hogrefe; 2017. p. 129-143.

[97] Koltai J, Kun E. Az egeszsegertes gyakorlati merese Magyarorszagon es nemzetkozi osszehasonlitasban. [The practical measurement of health literacy in Hungary and in international comparison]. Orv Hetil. 2016;157(50): 2002-6. DOI: 10.1556/650.2016.30563.

[98] Palumbo R, Annarumma C, Adinolfi P, Musella M, Piscopo G. The Italian Health Literacy Project: insights from the assessment of health literacy skills in Italy. Health Policy. 2016;120(9): 1087-94. DOI: 10.1016/j.healthpol.2016.08.007.

[99] Espanha R, Ávila P. Health Literacy Survey Portugal: A contribution for the knowledge on health and communications. Procedia Computer Science. 2016;100: 1033-41.

[100] Bieri U, Kocher JP, Gauch C, Tschoepe S, Venetz A, Hagemann M. Bevölkerungsbefragung "Erhebung Gesundheitskompetenz 2015". Studie im Auftrag des Bundesamts für Gesundheit BAG, [Populationsurvey „ Health literacy survey 2015" Survey on behalf of the Swiss federal office for public health]. Abteilung Gesundheitsstrategie. Bern: gfs.bern, 2016.

[101] Quenzel G, Schaeffer D. Health Literacy – Gesundheitskompetenz vulnerabler Bevölkerungsgruppen. Ergebnisbericht. [Health Literacy – health literacy of vulnerable groups. Report]. Bielefeld: Universität Bielefeld, 2016.

[102] Messer M, Vogt D, Quenzel G, Schaeffer D. Health Literacy und Prävention bei älteren Menschen mit Migrationshintergrund. [Health literacy and prevention among elderly people with migration background]. In: Schaeffer D, Pelikan JM, editors. Health Literacy Forschungsstand und Perspektiven. Bern: hogrefe; 2017. p.189-203.

[103] Wångdahl J, Lytsy P, Mårtensson L, Westerling R. Health literacy among refugees in Sweden – a cross-sectional study. BMC Public Health. 2014;2014(14): 1030-1041. DOI: 10.1186/s12889-015-2513-8.

[104] Schaeffer D, Vogt D, Berens E-M, Hurrelmann K. Gesundheitskompetenz der Bevölkerung in Deutschland.[Health literacy of the German population]. Bielefeld: Universität Bielefeld, 2016.

[105] Levin-Zamir D, Baron-Epel OB, Cohen V, Elhayany A. The association of health literacy with health nehavior, socioeconomic indicators, and self-assessed health from a national adult survey in Israel. J Health Commun. 2016;21(sup2): 61-8. DOI: 10.1080/10810730.2016.1207115.

[106] Vandenbosch J, Van den Broucke S, Vancorenland S, Avalosse H, Verniest R, Callens M. Health literacy and the use of healthcare services in Belgium. J Epidemiol Community Health. 2016;2016(0): 1-7. DOI: 10.1136/jech-2015-206910.

[107] Jordan S, Hoebel J. Gesundheitskompetenz von Erwachsenen in Deutschland. [Health literacy of adults in Germany]. BundesGesundheitsblatt-Gesundheitsforschung-Gesundheitsschutz. 2015;58(9): 942-50. DOI: 10.1007/s00103-015-2200-z.

[108] Office of the Commissioner for Mental Health. Health literacy survey. Malta 2014. 2014.

[109] Tiller D, Herzog B, Kluttig A, Haerting J. Health literacy in an urban elderly East-German population– results from the population-based CARLA study. BMC Public Health. 2015;2015(15): 883. DOI: 10.1186/s12889-015-2210-7.

[110]   Van den Broucke S, Van der Zanden G, Chang P, Doyle G, Levin D, Pelikan J, Schillinger D, Schwarz P, Sorensen K, Yardley L, Riemenschneider H. Enhancing the effectiveness of diabetes self-management education: the Diabetes Literacy Project. Horm Metab Res. 2014; 46(13):933-8. DOI: 10.1055/s-0034-1389952.

[111]   Amoah PA, Phillips DR, Gyasi RM, Koduah AO, Edusei J. Health literacy and self-perceived health status among street youth in Kumasi, Ghana. Cogent Medicine. 2017;4(1):1275091. DOI: 10.1080/2331205X.2016.1275091.

[112]   van der Heide I, Uiters E, Boshuizen H, Rademakers J. Health Literacy in Europe: the development and validation of health literacy prediction models. Eur J Public Health. 2015;25(suppl 3): 906-911. DOI: 10.1093/eurpub/ckw078.

[113]   Gerich J, Moosbrugger R Subjective estimation of health literacy - what is measured by the HLS-EU Scale and how is it linked to empowerment? Health Commun. 2016;29:1-10. DOI: 10.1080/10410236.2016.1255846.

[114]   Domanska O, Firnges C, Jordan S. Verstehen Jugendliche die Items des „Europäischen Health Literacy Survey Questionnaire "(HLS-EU-Q47)? Ergebnisse kognitiver Interviews im Rahmen des Projektes „Messung der Gesundheitskompetenz bei Jugendlichen "(MOHLAA).[Do adolescents understand the items of the European Health Literacy Questionaire" (HLS-EU-Q47)? Results from cognitive interviews with the framework of the project "Measurement of Health Literacy Among Adolescents" (MOHLAA)]. Das Gesundheitswesen. 2016;78(08/09): A200. DOI: 10.1055/s-0036-1586709.

[115]   Duong VT, Lin I-F, Sorensen K, Pelikan JM, Van Den Broucke S, Lin Y-C, Chang, PW. Health literacy in Taiwan: a population-based study. Asia-Pacific Journal of Public Health. 2015;27(8): 871-80. DOI: 10.1177/1010539515607962.

Health Literacy
R.A. Logan and E.R. Siegel (Eds.)
IOS Press, 2017
© *2017 The authors and IOS Press. All rights reserved.*
doi:10.3233/978-1-61499-790-0-60

Health Literacy: Insights and Issues

Rima E. RUDD[1]
Senior Lecturer on Health Literacy, Education, and Policy,
Harvard T.H. Chan School of Public Health, U.S.A.

Abstract. Definitions, by their very nature, establish a shared understanding of words and concepts but also set parameters for inquiry and measures. Health literacy, a term that emerged in the 1990s, has been defined in numerous ways over time and is still considered an evolving concept. This chapter provides a discussion of the difficulties inherent in restricted definitions that have led to research gaps. The discussion highlights the need for an expanded understanding of health literacy and it identifies missing elements. A call for new measures includes attention to a full range of literacy skills including calibrations of health professionals' communication skills. In addition, it argues for an in-depth understanding of health-related tasks and texts that will yield insights for a more thorough analysis of links between and among literacy skills, health system demands, and health outcomes. Finally, this chapter presents an argument for a careful consideration of institutional and system wide norms, policies, and regulations that facilitate or impede access to health information, services, and care. As the definition of health literacy expands so too can the scope and depth of health literacy research, practice implementation, and public policy.

Keywords. Health literacy contexts, health literacy definition, health literacy environments, literacy tasks

1. Introduction

Studies in health literacy have illuminated the well-documented pathway from educational achievement to health. More than two decades of studies indicate that literacy, a foundation stone of education, is linked to a variety of health outcomes and may be a more robust predictor of health than is a measure of educational attainment. The body of literature linking health and literacy is rigorous and the relationship between patients' literacy skills and a variety of health outcomes has been established [1,2,3]. Consequently, *health literacy* has emerged as a new variable for health researchers and as an important consideration for practitioners and policy makers. Analyses are yielding insight into health literacy as a determinant of health with implications for issues of equity as well as for health disparities. Indeed, literacy and its links to health outcomes have become the focus of a growing number of research studies as well as the inspiration for institutional and governmental policy initiatives in many industrialized countries.

The term *health literacy* was formally documented by Nutbeam in the World Health Organization's 1998 Health Promotion Glossary as *the cognitive and social skills which determine the motivation and ability of individuals to gain access to,*

---

[1] Corresponding author: Senior lecturer, Harvard T.H. Chan School of Public Health, 677 Huntington Avenue. Boston, MA. 02115 USA; E-mail: rrudd@hsph.harvard.edu

understand, and use information in ways which promote and maintain good health [4]. Over time, as is often true of many new concepts and areas of study, omissions or errors are corrected, research findings as well as insightful perspectives add to or reshape original ideas, and new paths of inquiry emerge.

The chapter is divided into five sections. The next section focuses on developments in health literacy studies and practice, beginning with links to adult literacy assessments and then, with insights from literacy research, to modifications to the concept of health literacy. The third section addresses research gaps due in part to unequal attention to the full panoply of literacy skills as well as to the initial omission of considerations for the communication skills of health professionals, the quality of health texts, and the context within which health literacy exchanges take place. The fourth section focuses on new directions in health literacy research as well as practice and policy. The concluding section calls for collaborative research, practice, and policy efforts among an array of professionals in health literacy, health communication, literacy, adult literacy, as well as in public health and health care development and reform.

2. The Development and Maturation of Health Literacy

Interest in health literacy had originally been inspired by the various waves of international surveys examining the literacy skills of adults in industrialized nations. Findings from 22 nations participating in the first assessments in the 1990s – the National Adult Literacy Survey (NALS) in the U.S. [5] as well as the International Adult Literacy Surveys (IALS) [6], indicated that general assumptions about literacy skills in industrialized nations were faulty. Indeed, the more recent Adult Literacy and Lifeskills Survey (ALLS) in the early part of this century [7] and from the PIAAC Survey of Adult Skills in 2011 [8] continue to offer problematic findings of limited literacy among large percentages of the population in many countries. Universal schooling, long assumed to secure a highly literate citizenry, did not yield expected skill levels. Instead, results indicated that a majority of adults in most industrialized nations have difficulty using everyday materials to accomplish mundane tasks with accuracy and consistency. Consequently, large numbers of people do not have sufficient literacy or numeracy skills to meet many of the demands and expectations of modern life.

2.1. A New Health Variable

Health literacy research in the U.S. began soon after the findings about adult literacy skills were published and disseminated. The initial National Adult Literacy Survey (NALS) conducted in the U.S. in 1992 involved a rigorous sampling schema with more than 26,000 participants [5]. Findings that a significant proportion of U.S. adults had limited literacy skills were greeted with dismay and generated headlines. They also drew the attention of a small group of health researchers who were curious about links to health outcomes. The initial question posed by these researchers was: *given the limited literacy skills of large numbers of adults in the U.S., are there health consequences*? The answer, now evident, is clearly *yes*. By the first decade of the 21st century, health literacy research studies indicated that those with limited literacy skills face more negative health outcomes than do those with better skills. Limited health literacy, as initially measured by reading skill components in health settings, was associated with limited participation in health promoting, disease prevention, and early detection activities; with diminished management of chronic diseases; with increased hospitalization and re-hospitalization; and with increased morbidity and mortality [1,2,3].

2.2. Population Based Measures and Findings

Population based measures of health literacy provided additional insight. The Health and Literacy Scale (HALS) was developed in 2002 to offer a direct measure of literacy skills focused on people's use of commonly available health materials to accomplish a variety of health-related tasks. The scale was comprised of items taken directly from the U.S. and international adult literacy assessments conducted between 1992 and 2005. All materials and tasks used in NALS, IALS, and ALLS were coded by Rudd and colleagues as health or non-health related and, if health related, assigned to one of five health activity categories: health promotion, health protection, disease prevention, health care management, system navigation and policy. As a result, the HALS was comprised of 191 health related items and tasks. Each item and every associated task was, of course, already calibrated for level of complexity. Thus, the HALS offered a measure of adults' ability to use a variety of health-related materials to accomplish an array of health-related tasks. The HALS supported analyses of population health literacy for any country that participated in the surveys of the 1990s or during the first decade of the 21st century [9].

HALS findings indicated that about half of U.S. adults, both those without a high school diploma and those who completed high school, have limited health literacy skills. Analyses indicate that the distribution of health literacy as well as general literacy are related to social factors such as employment, income, geography, access to resources, as well as majority or minority status. Adults who are members of a minority or marginalized group, who report living in poverty or without income from savings or retirement, and/or who are immigrants – have lower health literacy than do others with stronger access to resources [9,10]. Similar findings were reported in Canada [11], in the Netherlands [12], and Australia [13]. The HALS set the foundation for examinations of health literacy as a mediating factor in health disparities [10,12].

The U.S. Department of Education launched the National Assessment of Adult Literacy Skills [NAALS] in 2003 and, instead of applying the HALS analysis, inserted a small number of health- related items to be analyzed independently and so serve as a measure of health literacy and as a benchmark for further study [14]. Consequently, 28 new items related to 3 domains of health and health care information and services were added to the literacy assessment survey. The National Center for Education Statistics announced health literacy findings in September 2006. Twelve percent of adults scored in the proficient level and fully 53% of US adults scored in the *intermediate* range, a category indicating a need for literacy skill building. Fourteen percent of adults scored at below basic level and an additional 22% scored at the basic level. The report indicates that the average health literacy score for high school graduates was 232 on a 0 to 500 score range indicating low health literacy skills [14]. Findings, like those from the HALS analysis are troublesome.

Different in construct from the HALS and the NAALS but yielding similar findings, the European Health Literacy Survey (HLS-EU) questionnaire focused on self-perceived health literacy [15]. Participants were queried about their perceived difficulties related to accessing, understanding, appraising, and applying health information for health promotion, disease prevention, and health care related activities. Researchers found that close to half the population within participating countries of the EU had problematic or inadequate levels of health literacy [15,16]. Data analyses indicate that population groups with lower socioeconomic status and of lower social standing within any given country (due to minority or immigrant status, for example) have lower health literacy skills or perceived more difficulty with health literacy.

Each of the three population measures yielded similar and problematic findings that substantial numbers of adults in most industrialized nations have limited health literacy. Furthermore, each of the measures indicate that health literacy is linked to a variety of social factors.

Even with these strong findings of the prevalence of limited health literacy and with research findings of links between literacy and health outcomes – health researchers, practitioners, and policy makers were somewhat stymied. How, for example, could health professionals increase the literacy or health literacy skills of the public? Wasn't this more appropriately the responsibility of the education sector? Yet, inaction or even patience in face of the documented untoward health outcomes was clearly considered inappropriate. This awareness, coupled by insights from literacy experts, set the foundation for a paradigm shift in health literacy studies. As a result, the concept of health literacy has been changing and a more nuanced understanding of health literacy as a complex variable is emerging.

2.3. Evolving Definitions and Measures

Many researchers and practitioners in this relatively new area of study have revisited the definition of terms over the past decade. Some enthusiastically continue to do so – to the occasional dismay of others who feel that modifications to the concept of health literacy distracts from research efforts and from important work ahead. Yet, a wide variety of researchers and practitioners in medicine, health education, dentistry, nursing, pharmacy, and public health have been contributing to an on-going discussion of the concept of health literacy in reports, editorials, and on line discussion sites [17–20].

A variety of definitions of *health literacy* are currently on the table and need to be carefully examined to see which ones best serve a rigorous research as well as policy agenda. Nutbeam, who provided the first official definition in the WHO Health Promotion Glossary of 1998, noted in 2008 that *health literacy* is an evolving concept [21]. As the concept evolves, so too must the definitions and the measures linked to them. After all, a definition shapes research because it suggests a focus, determines the measures to be used, and specifies who or what is to be measured. To date, most of the measures in health literacy offer a fit with the initial definitions of health literacy focused on individual skills and abilities. Logically then, the focus of the 100 plus measures of health literacy is on the skills and deficits of the public [22]. While the definition and the measures together shaped the focus of work these early definitions also carried an underlying implication that responsibility for accessing, understanding, and applying available health information lies with the patient/lay public.

At the same time, early modifications to the concept, as articulated in the U.S. 2003 Health Communication Objectives for the Nation [23], the 2004 health literacy report from the National Academies of Science [1], and the 2010 National Action Plan [24] suggested that health literacy be understood as an interaction. These reports continue to inspire reflections about the many stakeholders involved in health literacy, the quality of health information, the skills of health professionals as well as the attributes of health institutions and systems. This broader understanding of health literacy as an interaction identifies other key variables or players, necessitates the development of new measures, and calls for more complex analyses. At the same time, it offers insight for change.

With this broader view comes an understanding that change can be effected through improved skills of the public and/or through a reduction on the demand side. Thus, the dilemma posed regarding action to be taken can be addressed by the education sector focusing on improving the literacy skills of the population and the health sector focusing on improving health information and removing literacy related barriers to services and care. As the field recalibrates focus, definitions, and measures, many research and practice gaps can be addressed.

3. Research Gaps

As noted above, a good deal of effort at the start of health literacy inquiry focused on establishing the links between literacy and health outcomes. In the initial excitement generated by this new variable for health analyses, researchers developed tools for measuring the health literacy skills and deficits of individuals (generally patients) without simultaneously measuring the difficulty of tasks as well as texts, the communication skills of those charged with presenting health information, or the context within which dialogues and interactions were taking place. The problem generated by initial conceptual limitations has let to serious gaps. This section explicates some of the missing components in health literacy. An identification of current limitations and gaps can provide insight and inspiration for further action and new discoveries.

3.1. Multiple Literacy Skills

The most commonly used early measures of individual's health literacy skills were comprised of short tests focused on reading (word pronunciation, reading comprehension skills) and, in a few cases, on use of numbers related to time and dosage [25,26]. These measures of individuals' literacy skills did indeed yield insightful finding and were powerful enough to help establish links between literacy skills and health outcomes [1]. However, because early discussions in health literacy primarily focused on and measured people's skills with the written word, discussion, interpretations, and suggestions for ameliorative action tended to focus on the written word as well. Consequently, little attention was paid to the oral exchange or to the burden of math in health discussions and decision-making. The conceptual error made in these early research efforts was, according to literacy experts such as Purcell-Gates, a limited understanding of literacy. While health literacy experts focused on print literacy, literacy scholars and educators generally think of five interrelated literacy skills: reading, writing, speaking, listening, and computation (math) as well as use of numeric concepts [27].

More recently, health researchers have been expanding the scope of inquiry to examine a broader range of literacy skills. In so doing, some researchers are using tools from other disciplines such as psychology for measuring presentation and listening skills [28,29] as well as developing new tools that help researchers look more closely at numeracy skills [30]. As a result, studies of listening skills [31], speaking and advocacy skills [32,33,34], and numeracy skills [35] may add further insight to analyses of the links between people's literacy skills and health outcomes. Findings are also providing insights for action and model building [36,37].

3.2. Analysis of Literacy Tasks

Missing from the health literacy inquiries is attention to what it is that people are expected to do – an examination of health-related tasks. In contrast, the adult literacy surveys referenced earlier analyzed the difficulty of tasks people were asked to undertake with the various materials provided them during the survey. Participants were asked to use a variety of commonly available materials as they might in everyday life such as: use a train schedule to determine which train would get them to a specific location at a specific time; complete a bank deposit slip to add funds to an account; use directions on an over-the-counter medicine to determine correct dosage for a child of a specific age; read a newspaper sports article to find the winning team from a recent game; make use of a grocery store sale sign to determine the cost of a food item after discount; read an editorial to determine the paper's perspective or bias; or consult a growth chart to see where a child ranked compared to others. These activities or tasks were analyzed for levels of complexity. The intent, in assessing the tasks, was to be able to focus on 'functional literacy' – to examine how well people are able to use commonly available materials in order to undertake mundane activities. In order to calibrate people's functional literacy skills, the first step was to calibrate the difficulty or complexity of texts and tasks. In so doing, the adult literacy assessments were not like school-based literacy tests with a focus on comprehension of information as presented in text books considered appropriate for a specific grade. Instead, the adult surveys measured the complexity of everyday texts and tasks and then focused on what people can do with texts [38].

Kirsch, one of the developers of the adult literacy surveys, explicates the reasoning and processes that went into the construction of the instruments. Materials were drawn from readily available texts related to six aspects of life: home and family, health and safety, consumer economics, community and citizenship, work, and leisure and recreation. A variety of tasks commonly associated with these materials were then developed. For example, a bus schedule handout would be used by someone seeking to travel to a specific location during a specific time. Thus, the task associated with this specific material focused on travel objectives. Overall, tasks were organized into three major categories with increasing levels of difficulty – locate information, integrate information, and generate information. Finding a specific piece of information (locate) in a simple or even complex text would be easier than finding and comparing several pieces of information (locate, integrate) in a simple or complex text. For example, finding the winning score in a sports article about one team is far less complex a task than finding and then comparing the scores of several teams in a league to determine who is ahead of whom. The ability to discern an underlying bias in a newspaper editorial requires a reader to 'read between the lines' and therefore presents an even more difficult task. First, it requires a more careful reading than does a sports article where the reader can scan for numbers (scores). Next, this task involves interpreting what has been provided and generating a conclusion. The development of the adult literacy survey items and the decisions underlying the scoring for difficulty and complexity of texts and tasks are delineated in a monogram by Kirsch that provides insight and assistance for health literacy researchers and practitioners wishing to more thoroughly understand barriers to information and action [38]. Evetts and Gauthier developed a workbook that directly applies this kind of analysis to a wide variety of materials [39] but such efforts have not yet been undertaken for an analysis of health materials and for health-related tasks related to the use of the health materials.

In addition, health researchers and practitioners may want to consider both proximal and distal tasks. We must certainly focus more than we have on identifying, analyzing, and simplifying the *proximal* tasks – those tasks involved in working with health texts. In addition, however, we need to consider the more *distal* tasks – those important health tasks people are expected to engage in – after they use the texts. This process would help us understand and perhaps reduce the challenges faced by people as they undertake health related actions. For example, proximal tasks for using a hospital discharge instruction sheet may include locating the section focused on cleaning a wound. The more distal tasks involve assembling needed materials and following the step-by-step procedure outlined in the directions. Needless to say, these activities rely on the clarity of the texts. However, they also involve the processes of moving literacy activities to action. Many health tasks or clusters of activities such as *taking medicine as prescribed* involve multiple *texts* (spoken and written), such as the dialogue with the doctor describing the need for and purpose of the medicine, the print prescription, the dialogue with the pharmacist, the label on the bottle, the marks on the measuring cup. Multiple tasks are involved with each of the texts such as understanding the need, recalling the purpose, filling the prescription, using the label to differentiation the new medicine from other similar bottles, noting the refill date, or calibrating the correct dose (counting or measuring). Filling the current gap in health literacy work with a deeper understanding of texts and associated tasks and of the literacy related burdens accompanying health actions sets the foundation for reducing demands on individuals. This kind of analysis can contribute to the design of more efficacious health materials, tools, and programs [40].

3.3. Conceptual Foundation

Health literacy had been primarily measured in terms of print literacy (word pronunciation, reading comprehension). Missing from the analyses were a simultaneous examination of the materials people were expected to use, as well as other important components of the literacy exchange including the skills of the health communicators – those responsible for crafting health information and delivering information through print materials or for postings on-line, as well as those engaged in interpersonal dialogue and/or in mass communication. Purcell-Gates, noted earlier for the call to expand an understanding of literacy skills, highlights the fact that literacy does not take place in a vacuum. Other players are involved and the context features large as well [1,27].

The early research studies did not contain discussions of conceptual models or theories that shaped the health literacy inquiry. Several such perspectives – from education, health communication, or the social sciences might have fostered an examination of a wider range of variables beyond patients' skills. For example, Kurt Lewin, long considered the 'grandfather' of the social sciences, envisioned and subsequently examined a force field containing both positively and negatively charged elements that influence the change process. These elements address individual as well as historic, social, and environmental constraints and facilitating factors. Lewin contends that it is imperative to consider these multilayered factors when one is trying to understand or foster change [41]. Applying Lewin's force field analysis, a researcher studying patient engagement, for example, would include measures of the health care institution's norms, policies, and regulations as central variables.

Bronfenbrenner's social ecological model, a theory shaping many educational as well as public health programs, expanded Lewin's notion of a force field and delineated categories for the multiple contexts to be considered. Bronfenbrenner's theory highlights the importance of various layers of personal, community, institutional, physical, social, and political contexts [42]. Here too, application of the social ecological model could contribute to broader health literacy research inquiries as well as to the design of health literacy programs to bring about efficacious change [43]. Such programs would incorporate efforts that address systemic issues and include institutional practices, professional competencies, as well as the individual's skills and deficits. Finally, from a public health perspective, insights can be gained from epidemiology, a foundation stone of public health grounded in the interplay among host, agent, and environment.

The value of such theoretical constructs is discussed in the report of the National Academies of Science's Committee on Science Literacy and Public Perception of Science. Convened in 2016, the committee grappled with the concept of science literacy and the social and political environment that fosters openness or hostility, support or suspicion, to science in general, to scientists, and to scientific findings. The committee focused on the need to understand science as a social process, shaped by scientific methods and practices and on the importance of the comprehension and dissemination of findings and content. The committee report builds on the premise that science is a way of knowing about the world. At the same time, social structures support or constrain the science literacy of individuals. An expanded concept of health literacy helped shape this discussion. The health literacy lens brought to bear on these issues included attention to system demands and content complexities as well as on individual skills and abilities – that of the lay public as well as that of scientists communicating with the public [44]. An understanding of these interplays must similarly shape future health literacy research, practice, and policy.

3.4. Accessible Information

The demand side of the literacy exchange includes health materials designed to help the public understand and use health information, directions, options, and calls to action. Early health literacy studies did include research efforts focused on the difficulty of health texts. However, these efforts were not integrated into the studies of links between health literacy and health outcomes. Instead, the focus was primarily on the 'readability' of health information. For almost five decades now, researchers have been reporting on the reading level or 'suitability' of health materials, tools, and messages designed for public use – primarily related to informed consent, health information, directions, preparations, and self-care.

More than two thousand studies primarily measured 'reading grade level' of a wide array of health materials from various disciplines and covering a variety of topics. Health materials were consistently found to be problematic -- assessed at reading levels or demands that far exceed the average reading skills of the public [45–47]. This represents a serious mismatch, making a good deal of health information relatively inaccessible. Unfortunately, reading grade tools only focus on word and sometime sentence length – indicative of difficulty in English language texts. This is now considered a relatively superficial indication of text difficulty. In contrast, the adult literacy surveys used commonly available materials, as noted above, that were all carefully analyzed and calibrated for level of complexity. Assessment criteria included attention to text type (such as narration, instruction, argument, description), to whether the presentation was in continuous (prose) or non-continuous (document) format, as well as to the presence or absence of distracting information [38].

For the health field, Doak, Doak, and Root introduced the Suitability Assessment Measurement (SAM) tool that was designed to enable health professionals to more fully analyze materials with attention to aspects of texts that facilitate or hinder reading, such as layout and design, vocabulary and sentence structure, passive or active voice, organization, cultural appropriateness, and use of visuals [48]. However, the vast majority of materials assessment studies reported in the health literature continued to focus on reading grade level, perhaps because the SAM was deemed too lengthy a process. New, shorter measures of text difficulty based on elements of the SAM are now widely available on line from the Centers for Disease Control [49] and the Agency for Healthcare Research and Quality [50].

Of course, health materials are not all prepared in prose format (full sentence and paragraph structure). Many health materials, such as labels, contain lists and many explanatory texts contain charts and graphs. Health information is also delivered via postings and videos. The PMOSE/IKIRSCH, developed by educators interested in the difficulty of lists, graphs, and charts [51], is a useful tool but, thus far, only occasionally used in health studies. In addition, several tools have been developed to help assess a wider variety of web sites and pages and have generated discussions about standards [52]. The report of Health Literacy Roundtable of the U.S. National Academies of Sciences, Engineering and Medicine's workshop on health literacy and technology offers examples of on-going developments that include evaluations of patient portals and eHealth postings [53].

Overall, the very substantial body of literature focused on the quality of health materials was not integrated into the studies of links between health literacy and health outcomes. Instead, in most health literacy studies, the health materials were often taken as a *given* and the focus was on patients' ability or inability to comprehend or use them. This might be appropriate for literacy development in schools, where an ability to read Shakespeare or Twain, for example, is considered a valuable cultural asset. However, health texts are developed for more mundane purposes. A critical research gap will be filled when all health materials are carefully examined and routinely assessed in research studies to make certain that they were developed with rigor and match the needs of the intended audience. Health materials comprise print as well as posted information, on-line information as well as mass and personal communication. Consideration need not be given only for assessing already produced or spoken health information. The readily available assessment tools are quite useful for formative research, in the development stages before health materials, messages, and postings are disseminated through appropriately designated channel of communication. Mass communication research has long indicated that the quality of a message as well as the appropriately chosen channel to be used predict audience comprehension, understanding, and perceived source credibility [54].

3.5. Health Discussions

Health information is often provided through presentations and discussion – delivered in face-to-face encounters, through in-person presentations, or over the airwaves. As indicated above, literacy experts often use the term 'texts' to refer to *talk* as well as to written and posted materials. The presentation of information delivered through dialogue in care settings, health related discussions, or public health announcements have not yet been thoroughly examined from a health literacy perspective.

A vast body of literature in health communication examines the relationship between the quality of the exchange in the patient/provider interaction and analyses consider links between the quality of these interactions and health outcomes. However, few studies offer a bridge between health literacy inquiry and provider-patient communication research. In order for health literacy research to expand and more thoroughly examine the oral exchange, existing measures must be adapted to address literacy related issues and thereby capture the ability of patients to articulate issues, listen to, and comfortably interrupt the provider. At the same time, the 'other side of the eoin' must be measured as well. Characteristics of talk related to literacy such as vocabulary, sequence, highlights, repetition, summary must be captured. Consequently, we need to work closely with communication experts to adopt and adapt existing tools for health literacy research. A richer understanding of the links between literacy and health outcomes might be gleaned from concordant analyses of the ability of patients to provide data, listen, and interact as well as the ability of providers to listen, respond, and present information in a coherent and easily accessible format.

Nouri and Rudd examined health literacy as well as provider-patient literature and found a paucity of studies that included attention to literacy related issues in the critical talk (oral) and listening (aural) that takes place in clinical encounters [55]. Among the few researchers to do so, Koch Weser focused on the use of rare and common words in the clinical encounter [56] and Roter, best known for in-depth analysis of the talk in clinical encounters, included literacy analyses, for example, in genetic testing discussions [57]. In addition, Roter offers a conceptual approach for capturing the oral literacy demand in health care dialogue, provides reviews of several studies that support the predictive validity of the framework and proposes ways to both diminish literacy demand and support more effective health care exchanges [58].

3.6. Professional Training

A recognition of the importance of texts and talks brings needed attention to the skills of those presenting health information in person, of those writing and delivering announcements, of those preparing print or on-line resources, and of those constructing graphic displays. With more balanced examinations of key players in the information exchange process, additional critical variables can be analyzed and influences on health outcomes more thoroughly understood. Unfortunately, the abilities or competencies of those who provide information in health care and public health have yet to be measured with a health literacy lens and the possible contributions to health outcomes are currently unknown. Several studies have begun to assess health literacy awareness and practice in dentistry and nursing, or pharmacy [59,60,61]. Leaders in this effort include Coleman and colleagues who have been examining needed health literacy competencies in medicine [62].

At the same time, the transformation of health data into vital information for the public has not been well documented. The skills and activities of health writers have not been examined. The components of rigorous formative research to be undertaken in the production of materials have been well articulated [48–52] but we lack evidence that such processes are regularly followed. Integration of health literacy insights with professional training for those responsible for the development and design of health texts can be beneficial. Regulations related to the design of both print and eHealth materials may be called for as well [52].

3.7. Health Contexts

Educators remind us that literacy has been found to vary by situation and will be influenced by contextual factors – such as time constraints, distracters, emotion laden circumstances, and the social as well as the physical environment. Literacy experts such as Purcell-Gates and LeVine insist that any measure of literacy must consider the context within which the literacy activities occur [27,63]. Many health activities take place in agencies and institutions such as hospitals, health centers, medical offices, dental clinics as well as in public health departments, workplaces, and social service agencies – all of which are professional workplaces and institutions of considerable complexity. From the educator's perspective, contextual factors will ease or hinder the application of literacy skills and, subsequently, the interactions. These factors must also be included in an examination of health literacy.

Institutions have expectations for those who come in from the 'outside'. They also determine the resources available and the actions of professionals within. Behaviors of visitors as well as of workers are encouraged or stymied by cultural norms and demands and, of course, time schedules and time constraints. Thus, the context within which patients, clients, and family members are filling out forms or making decisions, health professionals are providing information, materials are chosen and disseminated, and processes are designed to be carried out – is of prime importance. Contextual attributes and systemic policies affect agency and dignity and carry stress or support for patients, family members, and professionals. When the context is highlighted as a key component of health literacy, various institutional and system factors can be identified and measured and considered in analyses of health outcomes. This process can also yield insight and impetus for needed change.

Several pieces of work have set a strong foundation for this approach. Rudd and colleagues introduced the notion of a health care environment and developed a workbook for capturing key elements and developing a strategic plan for change [64]. Several researchers are using this tool to assess a variety of health care environments such as dental services within community health centers [65] and hospitals [66]. The Universal Tool Kit includes mechanisms for assessing clinical offices and tools for change [67]. Furthermore, the U.S. National Academies Roundtable on Health Literacy introduced the notion of institutional attributes and set out a list of ten attributes necessary for the development of health literacy [68]. This publication has garnered international interest and, as a result, a variety of practitioners, managers, and policy makers are engaged in discussions of needed cultural adaptations or modifications for use in their institutions.

These developments further expand the concept of health literacy. As we examine various definitions of terms and health literacy measures, we might ask: *to what extent does the definition of terms and the accompanying measures include the interactions among individuals, materials, and messages designed and delivered by health professionals, as well as the norms, policies, and practices within institutions?* A new definition could serve to shift away from a sole focus on the skills of the public to include the capacity of professionals and health institutions that support access to information and the active engagement of people [19,69].

3.8. Health Literacy Outside of Health Care Settings

A good deal of attention in health literacy studies was originally and is still focused on health care settings – the doctor's or dentist's office, the pharmacy, the community health center, the hospital. However, health related activities and decisions take place in a variety of contexts that include the home, the workplace, the community, and the voting booth. Health related deliberations and decisions accompany purchases, budgeting, insurance choices, work processes, political choices, as well as action in face of environmental hazards, natural or man-made disasters. However, health literacy studies have not ventured much outside of health care organizations and institutions. In 2000, Nutbeam suggested that health literacy include the development of skills that address social, economic, and environmental determinants of health [70].

Health literacy studies and applications can be expanded outside of the health care setting to play a vital role in each of the public health services of assessment, policy development, assurance, and research. For example, data collection and dissemination are core public health activities. If these efforts are better informed by health literacy insights, might more individuals participate in data collection efforts? If data findings are structured to be more accessible and understandable, might this enhance community action for change? Many health literacy insights and efforts could serve to inform public health programmatic work.

A greater integration of health literacy with health promotion and health protection activities can be fruitful as well [71]. In addition, insufficient attention has been paid to health literacy concerns with issues, policies, and actions related to occupational health, environmental health, or disaster management. A health literacy perspective can be brought to bear on a diverse set of topics, such as water quality, emergency response, food safety, air quality, preparedness, and policy decisions. Evaluation studies can examine efficacious change and outcomes in terms of civic engagement and community action. Research studies can inform the challenges to remove literacy-related barriers from the various local, state, regional, and national public health efforts to support and encourage the capacity of communities. One example of such an effort can be found in Japan where Goto and colleagues offered health literacy workshops for public health nurses charged with addressing community concerns in Fukushima City after the earthquake, tsunami, and power plant disaster [72].

4. New Directions in Health Literacy Research and Practice

As we explore new avenues of health literacy research and study possible ameliorative action, filling the gaps identified above can surely lead to stronger and more rigorous research and discovery as well as more efficacious practice and policies. Health literacy insights can enhance the design of patient portals, the posting of health information, the development of user-friendly consumer labels, the social and physical environment of health care institutions, the design and content of public health messages, disaster alerts as well as the public's understanding of air or water quality or climate change. In addition, the identification and removal of literacy related barriers to information, decision-making, care, and services will support agency and dignity. As a result, we may be more successful in our efforts to increase the active engagement of health professionals, patients, family members, workers, and community residents in collaborative decision-making, healthful action, and health promoting change. This may also improve individual and community health outcomes.

The current paradigm shift in health literacy studies began with a change from a focus on the skills of individuals to an understanding of the mismatch between the literacy skills of the public and the complexity of health information. Enriching this expanded purview is the current shift from a primary focus on patients' skills as a variable of interest to a research model that includes measures of health professionals' skills as well. Most recently, an additional force for change comes with the recognition that behaviors and practices of both patients and professionals are shaped by physical, social, and political contexts. This necessitates a shift in focus from skills and abilities of lay and professional people to examinations of organizational and system-wide norms, policies, and regulations that influence the actions and resources of those seeking assistance and of those providing needed information, help, and care [73].

4.1. Research to Practice

Many fields are grappling with the dilemma of how to disseminate research findings and how to translate these findings into practice. A long-standing issue related to the development and dissemination of information for the public continues to stymie health literacy efforts. While the use of assessment tools – ranging from reading level measures to the CDC Health Literacy Index, is reported with increasing frequency, insights derived from these same tools are not yet regularly shaping the development and design of health texts. Nor have practitioners consistently adopted plain language initiatives or rigorous formative research guidelines called for in the classic Doak, Doak, and Root work [48], in the planers guide for making health communication work, famously known as the 'pink book' issued by the U.S. National Cancer Institute [74], or in the mandate from the U.S. Congress in the Plain Language Act [75].

As a result, research findings have not yet fully influenced practice. Inquiries need to be launched to enable us to identify barriers and facilitating factors that could lead to change. Those responsible for contracting or developing health materials frequently cite time or budget constraints. Such explanations for omitting rigorous formative research and pilot tests for critical information designed for the public would not be tolerated from those developing medicine, medical devices, or tools. The U.S. Plain Language Act requires attention to language in government documents but there is not yet evidence in the literature that either public health or health care institutions have issued institutional policy mandates that require proof of plain language or other formative research undertakings for materials produced in-house or through contractors. On the other hand, many institutional review boards do now expect a calculation of reading grade level for informed consent documents and other research tools. Greater respect for the power of the word is needed and added rigor must be required through regulations.

In a review of health communication during the Anthrax episode in the U.S., Rudd and colleagues noted the unnecessarily complex words and concepts used in a short postcard mailed to all households. The authors acknowledged that times of chaos do put added stress on those agencies needing to develop rapid responses and alerts for the public. They suggested the development and training for 'first responders' who can be called upon to conduct rapid piloting and health literacy assessments to assure compliance with health literate communication strategies [76].

4.2. Professional Preparation

The early 2004 health literacy report from the National Academies of Science [1], called for raising awareness about health literacy and developing critical communication skills among health professionals in training and in practice. As was noted above, several researchers have examined the knowledge of health literacy amongst health care professionals and have consistently revealed limited knowledge of health literacy insights and findings. These efforts point to the need for awareness raising and skill building. Some professional schools are already engaged in the effort to raise awareness and provide mechanisms for addressing health literacy in practice and workshops are often available at local and national conferences [77,78].

4.3. Government Action and Policies

The U.S. and Canada were the first participants in the assessments of adult literacy in the early 1990s and findings inspired action on many fronts. In Canada, attention to program and policy issues were among the first steps [79]. Rootman and colleagues reviewed the early attention to health literacy in Canada and highlighted the early project on literacy and health undertaken by the Ontario Public Health Association and the establishment (in 1994) of the National Literacy and Health Program housed by the Canadian Public Health Association [80,81].

In the U.S., policy considerations followed the accumulation of research studies linking literacy to health outcomes. The first policy initiatives are evidenced in the inclusion of a health literacy objective in the health goals and objectives for the nation for 2010 [24], in the charge to examine and evaluate the findings in the field [2,3] and in the research funding earmarked for health literacy at the National Institutes for Health. Convened panels, workshops, and dissemination activities were undertaken to inspire policy development amongst professional organizations, regulatory agencies, and government institutions. For example, white papers related to the needed agenda in dentistry [82,83] and for hospitals [84] generated attention and spurred action. After the initial inclusion of improved health literacy among the goals and objectives for the nation, a U.S. Surgeon General's Workshop on Health Literacy was convened. The ensuing report concluded that limited health literacy is a systemic problem, not an individual deficit, and that health care and health information systems must be aligned with the needs of the public [85]. The report called on public health and health care professionals to provide clear, understandable, and science-based health information to the American people. The follow-up 2010 U.S. National Action Plan to Improve Health Literacy identified key stakeholders, suggested activities and contributions, and delineated seven goals to improve health literacy with a focus on information, communication, informed decision-making, access to services, research, and practice [24].

These and other policy initiatives were not confined to North America as international conferences increasingly included health literacy on the agenda. The U.S. National Academies Health Literacy Roundtable workshop on policy action highlighted numerous international activities undertaken [86]. Among them are the articulated health literacy goals in the Australian Safety and Quality goals for Health Care [87], the New Zealand Ministry of Health's guide: Building Health Literate Organizations in New Zealand [88]. These and other policy papers could set a foundation for future studies to examine a variety of systemic inhibiting and facilitating health literacy factors influencing health outcomes. Koh and colleagues argue that they also hold promise for moving nations beyond a focus on crisis care [89].

5. Conclusion

Finally, this delineation of gaps and new initiatives in research, practice, and policy highlight the need for collaboration with others well-schooled in fields with a rich and insightful literature, tested measures, and a history of efficacious change. The expanded agenda in health literacy calls for collaborative work with experts in literacy, researchers in health communication, and analysts focused on institutional change. In this way, contributors to health literacy can stand on the foundation set by others and together, forge new insights.

As noted at the outset, as a field of inquiry matures, new insights and perspectives bring about change and growth. Omissions or early errors are corrected, original ideas are reshaped, and new paths of inquiry emerge. As participants in health literacy studies and practice recalibrate definitions and measures and expand inquiry, research and practice gaps are being bridged.

References

[1]   Kindig DA, Panzer AM, & Nielsen-Bohlman L. editors. Health literacy: A prescription to end confusion. Washington D.C.: National Academies Press; 2004.
[2]   DeWalt DA, Berkman ND, Sheridan S, Lohr KN, Pignone MP. Literacy and health outcomes – A systematic review of the literature. J Gen Intern Med. 2004; 19:1228–39.
[3]   Berkman ND, Sheridan SL, Donahue KE, Halpern DJ, Crotty K. Low health literacy and health outcomes: an updated systematic review. Ann Intern Med. 2011; 155:97–107.
[4]   Nutbeam D. Health promotion glossary. Health Promot Intl. 1998; 13(4):349–64.
[5]   Kirsch IS. Adult literacy in America: A first look at the results of the national adult literacy survey. Washington D.C.: US Government Printing Office, Superintendent of Documents (Stock No. 065-000-00588-3); 1993.
[6]   Tuijnman A. The international adult literacy survey (IALS). Results and highlights from an international perspective: IALS in relation to economies and labour markets. A workshop on 'Literacy, Economy and Society.' Calgary, Canada; 1996.
[7]   Desjardins R, Murray TS, & Tuijnman AC. Learning a living: First results of the adult literacy and life skills survey. OECD. 2005.
[8]   OECD Skills Outlook 2013: First Results from the Survey of Adult Skills. Paris, France: OECD Publications; 2013.
[9]   Rudd RE, Kirsch I, & Yamamoto K. Literacy and health in America. Policy Information Report. Educational Testing Service. Princeton PA: ETS Publications; 2004.
[10] Rudd RE. Health literacy skills of US adults. Am J of Health Behav. 2007; 31(Supplement 1): S8–S18.
[11] Murray TS, Clermont Y, & Binkley M. Measuring adult literacy and lifeskills: new frameworks for assessments. Ottawa, Canada: Statistics Canada; 2005.
[12] van der Heide I, Wang J, Droomers M, Spreeuwenberg P, Rademakers J, Uiters E. The relationship between health, education, and health literacy: results from the Dutch adult literacy and life skills survey. J of Health Commun. 2013; 18(suppl):172–84. DOI: 10.1080/10810730.2013.825668.

[13] Barber MN, Staples M, Osborne RH, Clerehan R, Elder C, Buchbinder R. Up to a quarter of the Australian population may have suboptimal health literacy depending upon the measurement tool: results from a population-based survey. Health Promot Int. 2009; 24(3):252–61. DOI: 10.1093/heapro/dap022.

[14] Kutner M, Greenberg E, Jin Y, Paulsen C. In: The health literacy of America's adults: results from the 2003 national assessment of adult literacy. Education USDOE: National Center for Education Statistics, editor; 2006.

[15] Sørensen K, Van den Broucke S, Pelikan JM, Fullam J, Doyle G, Slonska, Z, Kondillis B, Stoffels V, Osborne RH & Brand H. Measuring health literacy in populations: illuminating the design and development process of the European Health Literacy Survey Questionnaire (HLS-EU-Q). BMC Public Health. 2013; 13(1), 948. DOI: 10.1186/1471-2458-13-948.

[16] Sorensen, K, Pelikan JM, Rothlin F, Ganahl K, Slonska Zl, Doyle G, Fullam J, Kondiis B, Agrafiotis D, Uiters E, Falcon M, Mensing M, Tchamov K, van den Broucke S, Brand H. Health literacy in Europe: comparative results of the European health literacy survey (HLS-EU). Eur J Public Health. 2015. DOI: http://dx/doi.org/10.1093/eurpub/ckO43.

[17] Peerson A, Saunders M. Health literacy revisited: what do we mean and why does it matter?. Health Promot Int. 2009 Sep 1;24(3):285–96. DOI: 10.1093/heapro/dap014.

[18] Berkman ND, Davis TC, McCormack L. Health literacy: what is it? J of Health Commun. 2010; 31(15 S2):9–19. DOI: 10.1080/10810730.2010.499985.

[19] Sørensen K, Van den Broucke S, Fullam J, Doyle G, Pelikan J, Slonska Z, Brand H. Health literacy and public health: a systematic review and integration of definitions and models. BMC Public Health. 2012;12(1):1. DOI: 10.1186/1471-2458-12-80.

[20] Pleasant A, Rudd RE, O'Leary C, Paasche-Orlow MK, Allen MP, Alvarado-Little W, Myers L, Parson K, Rosen S. Considerations for a new definition of health literacy. Perspective. Health Literacy Round Table. National Academy of Medicine. Washington DC: National Academies; 2016.

[21] Nutbeam D. The evolving concept of health literacy. Soc Sci Med. 2008; 67:2072–78. DOI: 10.1177/1359105313476978.

[22] Health Literacy Toolshed. http://www.healthliteracy.bu.edu. Retrieved March 1, 2017.

[23] Rudd RE. Health Literacy Objectives in U.S. department of Health and Human Services, Office of Disease Prevention and Health Promotion. National Action Plan to Improve Health Literacy. Washington, DC; 2003.

[24] U.S. Department of Health and Human Services. Baur C. (senior editor). National action plan to improve health literacy. Washington, DC: USDHHS. 2010.

[25] Davis TC, Long SW, Jackson RH, Mayeaux EJ, George RB, Murphy PW, & Crouch MA. Rapid estimate of adult literacy in medicine: a shortened screening instrument. J Fam Med. 1993; 25(6):391—95.

[26] Parker RM, Baker DW, Williams MV, Nurss JR. The test of functional health literacy in adults. J Gen Intern Med. 1995; 10(10):537–41.

[27] Purcell-Gates VE. Cultural practices of literacy: Case studies of language, literacy, social practice, and power. New York: Lawrence Erlbaum Associates Publishers; 2007.

[28] Woodcock R, McGrew KS, Mather N. Woodcock–Johnson III tests of achievement. Itasca, IL: Riverside Publishing; 2001.

[29] Fassaert T, van Dulmen S, Schellevis F, Bensing J. Active listening in medical consultations: development of the active listening observation scale (ALOS-global). Pat Edu Couns. 2007; 68(3):258–64. DOI: 10.1016/j.pec.2007.06.011.

[30] Osborn CY, Wallston KA, Shpigel A, Caanaugh K, Kripalani S, Rothman RL. Development and validation of the general health numeracy test (GHNT). Pat Edu Couns. 2013; 91(3):350–56. DOI: 10.1016/j.pec.2013.01.001.

[31] Rosenfeld L, Rudd R, Emmons KM, Acevedo-García D, Martin L, Buka S. Beyond reading alone: the relationship between aural literacy and asthma management. Pat Edu Couns. 2011; 82(1):110–16. DOI: 10.1016/j.pec.2010.02.023.

[32] Martin LT, Schonlau M, Haas A, Derose KP, Rosenfeld L, Buka SL, Rudd R. Patient activation and advocacy: which literacy skills matter most? J Health Comm. 2011;16:177–90. DOI: 10.1080/10810730.2011.604705.

[33] Katz MG, Jacobson TA, Veledar E, Kripalani S. Patient literacy and question- asking behavior during the medical encounter: a mixed-methods analysis. J Gen Intern Med. 2007; 22:782–86. DOI: 10.1007/s11606-007-0184-6.

[34] Rubin DL. Listenability as a tool for advancing health literacy. J Health Commun. 2012; 17(sup3):176–90. DOI: 10.1080/10810730.2012.712622.

[35] Rothman RL, Montori VM, Cherrington A, Pignone MP. Perspective: the role of numeracy in health care. J Health Commun. 2008; 13(6):583–95. DOI: 10.1080/10810730802281791.

[36] Apter AJ, Paasche-Orlow MK, Remillard JT, Bennett IM, Ben-Joseph EP, Batista RM, Hyde J, Rudd RE. Numeracy and communication with patients: they are counting on us. J Gen Int Med. 2008; 23(12):2117–24. DOI: 10.1007/s11606-008-0803-x.
[37] Ancker JS, Kaufman D. Rethinking health numeracy: a multidisciplinary literature review. JAMIA. 2007; 14(6):713–21. DOI: 10.1197/jamia.M2464.
[38] Kirsch IS. The international adult literacy survey (IALS): Understanding what was measured. ETS Research Report Series. 2001 Dec 1; 2001(2):i–61.
[39] Evetts J, Gauthier M. Assessing the complexity of literacy tasks. National Literacy Secretariat, Human Resources Development Canada. Ottawa CA; 2003.
[40] Rudd RE. Numbers get in the way. Health Literacy Roundtable Commentary. Washington DC: National Academy of Medicine. 2016. https://nam.edu/numbers-get-in-the-way. Retrieved March 1, 2017.
[41] Lewin K. Field theory in social science. New York: Dorwin Cartwright Publishers; 1951.
[42] Bronfenbrenner U. Ecological systems theory. London: Jessica Kingsley Publishers; 1992.
[43] McCormack L, Thomas V, Lewis MA, Rudd R. Improving low health literacy and patient engagement: A social ecological approach. Patient Edu and Couns. 2016. DOI: 10.1016/j.pec.2016.07.007
[44] National Academies of Sciences, Engineering, and Medicine. Science literacy: concepts, contexts, and consequences. Washington, DC: The National Academies Press; 2016.
[45] Rudd R, Anderson J, Nath C, Oppenheimer S. Health literacy: an update of medical and public health literature. In: Comings JBG, Smith C, editors. Review of adult learning and literacy: National Centre for the Study of Adult Learning and Literacy; 2007.
[46] Rudd RE. Needed action in health literacy. J of Health Psychol. 2013; 18(8):1004–10. DOI: 10.1177/1359105312470128.
[47] Rowlands G, Protheroe J, Winkley, J, Richardson M, Seed, PT, & Rudd RE. A mismatch between population health literacy and the complexity of health information: an observational study. *Br J Gen Pract*. 2015; *65*(635): e379–e386. DOI: 10.3399/bjgp15X685285.
[48] Doak CC, Doak LG, Root JH. Teaching patients with low literacy skills. 2nd ed. Philadelphia, Pa: Lippincott-Raven Publishers; 1996.
[49] Baur C, Prue C. The CDC Clear Communication Index is a new evidence-based tool to prepare and review health information. Health Promot Pract. 2014; 15:629–637. DOI: 10.1177/1524839914538969.
[50] Shoemaker SJ, Wolf MS, & Brach C. Development of the Patient Education Materials Assessment Tool (PEMAT): a new measure of understandability and actionability for print and audiovisual patient information. Patient Edu and Couns. 2014; *96*(3):395-403. DOI: 10.1016/j.pec.2014.05.027.
[51] Mosenthal PB, Kirsch IS. A new measure for assessing document complexity: The PMOSE/IKIRSCH document readability formula. J Adolescent & Adult Literacy. 1998; 41(8):638–57.
[52] Ford EW, Walls VU. Effective US health system websites: establishing benchmarks and standards for effective consumer engagement/practitioner application. J Healthcare Management. 2012; 57(1):47.
[53] National Academies of Sciences, Engineering, and Medicine. Health literacy and consumer-facing technology: Workshop summary. Washington, DC: The National Academies Press. 2015.
[54] McLuhan M, Understanding media: the extensions of man. New York: New American Library, 1964.
[55] Nouri SS, Rudd RE. Health literacy in the "oral exchange": an important element of patient–provider communication. Pat Edu and Couns. 2015; 98(5):565–71. DOI: 10/1016/j.pec.2014.12.002.
[56] Koch-Weser S, DeJong W, Rudd RE. Medical word use in clinical encounters. Health Expect. 2009; 12:371–82. DOI:10.1186/1472-6947-9-S1-S3.
[57] Roter DL, Erby LH, Larson S, Ellington L. Assessing oral literacy demand in genetic counseling dialogue: Preliminary test of a conceptual framework. Soc Sci Med. 2007; 65:1442–57. DOI: 10.1016/j.socscimed.2007.05.033.
[58] Roter DL. Oral literacy demand of health care communication: challenges and solutions. Nurs Outlook. 2011; 59(2):79–84.
[59] Maybury C, Horowitz AM, Yan AF, Green KM, Wang MQ. Maryland dentists' knowledge of oral cancer prevention and early detection. J Calif Dent Assoc. 2012; 40(4):341–50.
[60] Cafiero, M. Nurse practitioners' knowledge, experience, and intention to use health literacy strategies in clinical practice, J of Health Commun. 2013: 18 Suppl 1:70–81. DOI: 10.1080/10810730.2013.825665.
[61] Devraj, R. and Gupchup, G. V. Knowledge of and barriers to health literacy in Illinois, J American Pharmacists Assoc. 2012; 52 (6):183–93. DOI: 10.1331/JAPhA.2012.12011.
[62] Coleman CA, Hudson S, Maine LL. Health literacy practices and educational competencies for health professionals: a consensus study. J Health Commun. 2013;18(sup1):82–102. DOI: 10.1080/10810730.2013.829538.
[63] LeVine RA, LeVine S, Schnell-Anzola B, Rowe ML, Dexter E. Literacy and mothering: how women's schooling changes the lives of the world's children. Oxford University Press; 2011.

[64] Rudd RE, Anderson JE. The health literacy environment of hospitals and health centers. Partners for action: making your healthcare facility literacy-friendly. National Center for the Study of Adult Learning and Literacy (NCSALL). 2006. www.hsph.harvard.edu/healthliteracy. Retrieved March 1, 2017.

[65] Horowitz AM, Maybury C, Kleinman DV, Radice SD, Wang MQ, Child Q, Rudd RE. Health literacy environmental scans of community-based dental clinics in Maryland, Am J Public Health. 2014; 104(8): e85–e93. DOI: 10.2105/AJPH.2014.302036.

[66] Groene O, Rudd RE. Results of a feasibility study to assess the health literacy environment: navigation, written and oral communication in ten hospitals in Catalonia, Spain. J Commun Healthcare. 2011; 4(4):227–37.

[67] DeWalt DA, Callahan LF, Hawk VH, Broucksou KA, Hink A, Rudd R, Brach C. Health Literacy Universal Precautions Toolkit. AHRQ Publication No. 10-0046-EF. Rockville, MD. Agency for Healthcare Research and Quality; 2010.

[68] Brach C, Dreyer B, Schyve P, Hernandez LM, Baur C, Lemerise AJ, Parker R. Attributes of a health literate organization. Washington DC: National Academies of Science; 2012.

[69] Rudd RE, McCray AT, & Nutbeam D. Heath literacy and definitions of terms. Chapter 2. In: Health literacy in context: International perspectives. Hauppauge: Nova Science Publishers; 2012, p. 13–32.

[70] Nutbeam D. Health literacy as a public health goal: A challenge for contemporary health education and communication strategies into the 21st century. Health Promot Int. 2000; 15(3):259–67. DOI: 10.1016/S1054-139X(97)000009-8.

[71] Rudd RE. Public health literacy. In: Health Literacy Roundtable Workshop on Implications of Health Literacy for Public Health. Washington DC: National Academies of Science; 2013.

[72] Goto A, Rudd RE, Lai AY, & Yoshida-Komiya H. Health literacy training for public health nurses in Fukushima: A case-study of program adaptation, implementation and evaluation. JMAJ. 2014; 57(3):146–53.

[73] Koh HK, Rudd RE. The arc of health literacy. JAMA. 2015; 314(12):1225–26. DOI: 10.1001/jama.2015.9978.

[74] Arkin EB. Making health communication programs work: A planner's guide. DIANE Publishing; 1992.

[75] U.S. Congress. Plain language act. Public Law 111-274. October 13, 2010. Washington DC: U.S. Government Information Act; 2010.

[76] Rudd RE, Comings JP, and Hyde J. Leave no one behind: Improving health and risk communication through attention to literacy. J of Health Commun. 2003; 8(Suppl 1):104–15. DOI: 10.1080/713851983.

[77] Harper W, Cook S, Makoul G. Teaching medical students about health literacy: 2 Chicago initiatives. Am J Health Behav. 2007; 31:S111–14.

[78] Coleman C. Teaching health care professionals about health literacy: a review of the literature. Nurs Outlook. 2011; 59(2):70–78. DOI: 10.1016/j.outlook.2010.12.004.

[79] Vamos S. Health literacy programs and policy in Canada. In: Institute of Medicine, editor. Health literacy: improving health, health systems, and health policy around the world: Workshop summary. Washington DC: National Academies Press, 2013.

[80] Rootman I, Ronson B. Literacy and health research in Canada: Where have we been and where should we go? Can J Public Health. 2005; 96(suppl 2): S62–S77.

[81] Rootman I, Gordon-El-Bihbety D. A vision for a health literate Canada: report of the expert panel on health literacy. Ottawa CA: Canadian Public Health Association; 2008.

[82] [82] Whitepaper Workgroup Report, The invisible barrier: literacy and its relationship with oral health. J Public Health Dent. 2005; 65(3): 174-182.

[83] Rudd RE, Howowitz A. The role of health literacy in achieving oral health for elders. J Dent Educ. 2005; 69(9):1018–21.

[84] The Joint Commission. What did the doctor say? Improving patient literacy to improve patient safety. Oakbridge Terrace, Ill: The Joint Commission; 2007.

[85] Office of the Surgeon General (US); Office of Disease Prevention and Health Promotion (US). Proceedings of the Surgeon General's workshop on improving health literacy. Rockville MD: Office of the Surgeon General (US); 2006. https://www.ncbi.nlm.nih.gov/books/NBK44257/ Retrieved March 1, 2017.

[86] Health literacy: improving health, health systems, and health policy around the world: workshop summary Washingon DC: National Academies Press; 2013.

[87] Australia Clinical Excellence Commission (CEC) 2013. Clinical excellence commission programs and projects. 2nd edition. Sydney: CEC; 2013.

[88] New Zealand Ministry of Health. A framework for health literacy: a health literacy system response. http://www.health.govt.nz/publication/framework-health-literacy. Retrieved May 22, 2015.

[89] Koh HK, Berwick DM, Clancy CM, Baur C, Brach C, Harris LM, Zerhusen EG. New federal policy
      initiatives to boost health literacy can help the nation move beyond the cycle of costly 'crisis care'.
      Health Affairs. 2012;10–377. DOI: 10.1377/hlthaff.2011.1169.

Developments and New Directions in Health Literacy Theory

Health Literacy
R.A. Logan and E.R. Siegel (Eds.)
IOS Press, 2017
doi:10.3233/978-1-61499-790-0-81

Health Literary and the Arts: Exploring the Intersection

John D. IKE[a], Ruth M. PARKER[b,1], Robert A. LOGAN[c]

[a]Medical Student, Emory University School of Medicine, United States
[b]Professor of Medicine, Pediatrics, and Public Health, Emory University School of Medicine, United States
[c]Senior Staff, U.S. National Library of Medicine, United States

Abstract. Historically, study and implementation of health literacy mostly focused on text-based information with frequent attention to medical and health related content within an increasingly complex healthcare system. This chapter introduces visual literacy, particularly as it relates to the visual arts, as a potentially understudied and underutilized component of health literacy that might offer benefit to both patients and healthcare workers. Literacy is both content and context specific. We posit that interaction with the arts improves the ability to appreciate the context inherent within communication across cultures and belief systems.

Keywords: visual literacy, arts, visual arts, health literacy, moral imagination, empathy

1. Introduction

In the last decade, health literacy is viewed as aligning tasks and complexities with people's skills and abilities. Many health literacy efforts encourage providers and systems of care to make the information patients need understandable, navigable, and useful. A closer look at health literacy research reveals the challenges patients face when navigating and accessing healthcare; layers of unnecessary complexity are imparted onto patients by health systems. Research efforts increasingly underscore the need for health providers to improve their listening and communication skills. Rather than emphasizing the deficiencies of patients to understand health information, we as healthcare providers are to make ourselves and our delivery systems health literate by communicating essential information for acute and chronic health needs. This embodies the quality aim of being patient-centered.

Health literacy is also both content and context specific. Over the last two decades, health literacy research has predominantly focused on an exploration of textual literacy (the *written* and *spoken* word) as it relates to content – how health information is accessed, conveyed, and utilized. The study of context - how values, beliefs, and traditions affects content – is also fundamental to understanding and improving health literacy, but has been harder to define and explore than issues of content. Broadly speaking, we posit that the arts allow for exploration and understanding of context.

---

[1] Corresponding author: Professor of Medicine, Public Health, and Pediatrics, Emory University School of Medicine, Department of Medicine, 49 Jesse Hill Drive, Atlanta, GA, 30303; Email: rpark01@emory.edu

Furthermore, we argue that art is an underutilized tool of communication as it reflects our shared human experience and conveys critical information. Specifically, the arts communicate about healing, compassion, values, and health across time to patients and providers. The ability to *listen* and understand the elements the arts convey requires visual literacy. After searching the literature, we find the bridging of art, literacy, and health to be underexplored. In this chapter, we explore the underappreciated intersection of health literacy, visual literacy, and the arts in five subsections.

In Section 1, we provide an overview of visual literacy as a tool for exploring context. Section 2 addresses the question "why *listen* to the arts?" with emphasis given to the role the arts play in instructing us about a culture's values, traditions, and beliefs – the ideological lens of visual literacy. We use a case study on Santa Maria della Scala, a historic hospital in Siena, Italy, to illustrate this concept. Special attention is given to the role arts play in improving our moral and ethical imaginations, and the potential implications for patient care. Section 3 explores the role of the arts and visual literacy in addressing clinical practice and professional preparation. We reference literature on empathy with attention given to its decline in medical trainees and health care professionals, and the ways organizations are using art to counteract this trend. We also describe alternate means the arts have been used to improve clinical preparation and professional skills. Section 4 provides examples of where the arts are currently being utilized as an intervention to impact specific health outcomes. In the final section, we consider future directions for the use of the arts and visual literacy in advancing health literacy. We include a discussion of life skills progression (LSP) research and the role of "play." Perhaps our greatest conclusion rests on this central question: how is it that we can learn the *art* of medicine, without first listening to the *arts*.

2.   What is Visual Literacy?

In the introduction to his essay, "The History of Art as a Humanistic Discipline," Erwin Panofsky recounts Immanuel Kant's final interaction with his physician:

> Nine days before his death Immanuel Kant was visited by his physician. Old, ill, and nearly blind, he rose from his chair and stood trembling with weakness and muttering unintelligible words. Finally his faithful companion realized that he would not sit down again until the visitor had taken a seat. This he did, and Kant then permitted himself to be helped to his chair and, after having regained some of his strength, said, 'Das Gefühl für Humanität hat mich noch nicht verlassen' – 'The sense of humanity has not yet left me.' The two men were moved almost to tears. For, though the word *Humanität* had come, in the eighteenth century, to mean little more than politeness or civility, it had, for Kant, a much deeper significance, which the circumstances of the moment served to emphasize: man's proud and tragic consciousness of self-approved and self-imposed principles, contrasting with his utter subjection to illness, decay, and all that is implied in the word "mortality" [1].

The role of medicine and public health in history and our modern society extends beyond the 'hard' sciences of diagnosis and treatment. It demands and requires an appreciation of our collective humanity and the many *grey* and amorphous elements that define human relationships. The arts help us understand and appreciate our shared humanity and instill an appreciation for life's ambiguity. These lessons improve patient care through active listening and the engagement of the moral imagination. Effective communication, as Panofsky alludes to, requires a degree of shared ideas, a common vocabulary, a basic emotional literacy, and a mutual understanding of both content and context. Study of these elements and others in the healthcare setting as they relate to literacy gave rise to the field of health literacy.

Absent from the health literacy discussion and research is *visual literacy*. Visual literacy is generally defined as the ability to interpret, understand, and act upon visual information. It is distinct from text literacy (letters and numbers) as it is a 'sensory literacy' [2]. Research from the Kaiser Foundation states that in 2013, youth spent an average of seven hours and thirty-eight minutes engaged with visual content every day, a dramatic increase from the six hours and twenty-one minutes spent each day in 2009 [2, 3]. Such reports are not staggering when one considers the widespread use of image sharing platforms and social media websites which enable individuals to rapidly collect and share visual information. Since its inception in 2010, Instagram users alone have posted more than 20 billion images [2]. Despite the ubiquitous nature of images in our modern culture, structured teaching of how to interpret, and analyze these images is largely absent from formal education. Our education system, and as well as our healthcare system, champion textual literacy and computer literacy [2]. Similar trends are observed in health literacy research of the last two decades, as much of it is concentrated on the ability to interpret and act upon the written and spoken word.

In order to appreciate the importance of visual literacy in our modern society and in health-related fields, it is first important to review the tectonic shifts in the history of communication. Prior to the origin of the written word, prehistoric cultures used images to communicate ideas and beliefs. The Lascaux cave paintings of various animals and beasts in the Dordogne region of France are a prime example. Following this "dark age," the first revolution in communication was the introduction of Cunieform writing by the Sumerian Empire approximately 5,000 years ago [2]. After this time, cultures began to juxtapose symbols and images to signify meaning. The Egyptian hieroglyphics which juxtapose image and text are another well-known example. The second revolution in communication occurred in the 15th century with the introduction of the Gutenberg printing press and the ability to reproduce, rapidly and accurately, text and images [2]. Lastly, we are in the midst of the third revolution in communication – the digital age – which some would argue was born with the launch of the internet on Christmas Day, 1991 [2]. With each introduction of a new technology in communication, the cultural and social demands changed. Somewhere in the midst of these revolutions, the importance of visual literacy was overshadowed. Much effort has been put forth to restore visual literacy; to re-teach the population, particularly children, the 'alphabet' and 'grammar' of the visual world [2].

One arena where such techniques have been tested and employed is the visual art world. Brian Kennedy, the director of the Toledo Museum of Art in Ohio, and his team have spent considerable time and effort developing a visual literacy curriculum to reinforce the basic principles of interacting with visual content [4]. Broadly, Mr. Kennedy describes visual literacy as follows: "visual literacy is the ability to construct meaning from images. It's not a skill. It uses skills as a toolbox. It is a form of thinking that enhances your intellectual capacity" [5]. In order to cultivate one's visual literacy skills, one must first learn to *look*. The Art of Seeing Art™ curriculum is one formulaic and approachable method to engage visual content – to relearn the alphabet and grammar of the visual world. The system is predicated on six sequential elements: look, observe, see, describe, analyze, and interpret [4].

The first step is to 'look' which requires the viewer to slow down, get comfortable, and begin to visually dissect the image. Next, one must 'observe,' a step beyond looking that requires the viewer to begin to catalog the visual elements of the image. Once this is complete, the viewer is then 'seeing' the image by juxtaposing the cataloged visual elements against one's own cultural knowledge, awareness, and understanding of the image. In traditional textual literacy, looking is analogous to skimming while seeing is the equivalent of reading, and observation is the bridge between the two. Only after we 'see' the image, can we begin to 'describe' it – a method to organize one's thoughts, process, and then verbalize what we have seen. Next, one can begin to 'analyze' the image and determine how the catalogued descriptors and content of the image come together to tell a story. Last, we can 'interpret' the image by coalescing our previous knowledge and experiences with our analytical assessment of the image to determine its overall importance. It is also worth noting a metaphorical dotted line connects our final interpretation back to our initial act of looking: the process of engaging an image is cyclical and as we continue to grow and learn, looking a second time may offer a different interpretation [4].[2]

An additional well known method to interact with visual content is the Visual Thinking Strategies (VTS) method. This curriculum has been in existence since 1995 and was originally created to engage school-age children. The VTS methodology is predicated on three essential questions: What's going on in this picture? What do you see that makes you say that? What more can we find [6]? This methodology, while much more elementary than The Art of Seeing Art curriculum, is perhaps a more approachable method to engage art work quickly and effectively. As a result, many institutions including Harvard Medical School have adopted this strategy in their undergraduate and graduate medical education programs. One key example that will be reviewed later in this chapter is Harvard's Training the Eye: Improving the Art of Physical Diagnosis for undergraduate medical students & The Brigham and Women's Hospital Internal Medicine Humanistic Curriculum for internal medicine interns [7-8].

Outside of these formal approaches to interpreting and engaging with *individual* images, visual literacy is often approached through one of six distinct lenses: art history, form, iconology, ideology, semiotics, or hermeneutics. [2]. Art history traditionally focuses on the analysis of individual works of art as they relate to the history of a society or culture. Examples include exploring the cultural and social themes of the French Revolution through the lens of court painter, Jacques Louis-David. Study of form has primarily focused on the Elements of Art and Principles of Design outlined

---

[2] Of the above elements, the one most foreign to the visually illiterate person is the ability to describe an image using appropriate artistic concepts and vocabulary, not because it is difficult, but because we are seldom asked to do it. In order to tackle this issue, which is generally learned through formal art history instruction, The Art of Seeing Art™curriculum defines and illustrates the "Elements of Art" and the "Principles of Design" used to describe works of art. The Elements of Art are as follows: line, shape, color, space, and texture. When discussing how these elements relate to one another, one employs the Principles of Art: emphasis, balance, harmony, variety, movement, proportion, rhythm, and unity [4]

http://www.vislit.org/the-art-of-seeing-art/. Retrieved February 11, 2017.. These terms in isolation seem abstract, but their utility becomes more apparent when dissecting a visual image. We urge the reader to explore the Toledo Museum of Art's website for further discussion and application of these principles. With this logical method to dissect and discuss images, learners can begin to improve their visual literacy.

above with particular attention given to complexity and intricacies of the physical image [4]. Iconology focuses on the study of symbols and their meanings to different people at different times. Erwin Panofsky, the art historian whose quote opens this section, spent much of his career dissecting the complex iconography of the Italian Renaissance. Ideology focuses on an image's ability to communicate ideas, values, and beliefs of a culture, people, individual, or society. This lens will be the one we primarily employ in this chapter as we explore the role the arts play in informing us about health and, by association, health literacy. Semiotics is the study of signs and signifiers; the process by which images (and the objects/ideas they symbolize) are linked together to form complex systems of communication. For example, banks often employ floor to ceiling windows in their architectural design schemas to symbolize transparency, a value society demands from financial institutions. While relevant to the health literacy discussion, the complexity of semiotics and its relationship to the development of intricate hierarchal communication schemes will not be reviewed, though this is a potentially rich area for future research. Hermeneutics, the final lens through which visual literacy is often explored, deals with the literal and intended meanings of works [2].

For the purposes of this chapter, visual literacy can be viewed as an underexplored tool for health literacy. Through interaction with our visual world we expand our apperception; we begin to catalog the visual world into our own unique mental libraries whose volumes shape the way we engage and interact with our environment. This expansion of apperception, which results from improved visual literacy and awareness, is invaluable in healthcare. It improves a provider's ability to collect, interpret, and act upon diverse patient information to not only reach a diagnosis and treatment plan, but communicate, effectively, the relevant clinical information to a patient. Similar benefits from improved visual literacy are also likely found in peer-to-peer communication. In understanding our colleague's visual manifestation of self (the clothes they wear, the music they enjoy, the art they appreciate, the community they inhabit), we are better able to communicate because we are better in-in tune with their cultural values, beliefs, and traditions. Similarly, an appreciation of visual literacy might enhance how we approach and work to address a population with health literate communication.

3. Why *Listen* to the Arts?

The arts are a voice that reflect societal values, beliefs, and traditions with special attention given to both individual and collective experience. If we learn to *listen* effectively, the arts offer a means to meditate upon the past, present, and future simultaneously. The arts are a continuous and timeless source of reflection and perspective. Medicine and health, much like art, are inextricably linked to culture; a patient, a population, or a community cannot be effectively engaged if the content being discussed is not delivered using a common vocabulary which pays specific attention to context. The arts can help us learn to create shared vocabularies across cultures. Furthermore, the arts also instruct and challenge our emotional boundaries leading to an engagement of the moral imagination. Collectively, experience with the arts improves our ability to actively listen and understand our moral and ethical obligations. The arts also communicate key themes and ideas to our patients, effectively bridging the metaphysical boundary that exists between patient and provider.

The moral imagination is a thought methodology often employed when engaging the visual art world and other various liberal arts – poetry, literature, theater, and music. The origins of the "moral imagination" dates back to Enlightenment thinker Edmund Burke, an Irish statesman, political theorists, and orator, who in his book *Reflections on the Revolution in France* (1790) states the following:

> But now all is to be changed. All the pleasing illusions, which made power gentle, and obedience liberal, which harmonized the different shades of life, and which, by a bland assimilation, incorporated into politics the sentiments which beautify and soften private society, are to be dissolved by this new conquering empire of light and reason. All the decent drapery of life is to be rudely torn off. All the superadded ideas, furnished from the wardrobe of a moral imagination, which the heart owns, and the understanding ratifies, as necessary to cover the defects of our naked shivering nature, and to raise it to dignity in our own estimation, are to be exploded as a ridiculous, absurd, and antiquated fashion [9].

The quote defines, complexly, the moral imagination as a type of introspection into our own humanity that better enables us to recognize and understand the humanity of others. In the modern era, many writers, theologians and theorists have further clarified and explored Burke's original definition. However, an approachable and useful definition for our discussion was proposed by Jonathan Jones in his online publication – *First Things*: "[The moral imagination] can be defined as a uniquely human ability to conceive of fellow humanity as moral beings and as persons, not as objects whose value rests in utility or usefulness" [10].

To illustrate the use of the moral imagination as it relates to visual art and health, consider Santa Maria della Scala, a civic hospital that faces Siena's central cathedral [11]. Constructed in 1193, the "hospital" was originally designed to *host* pilgrims – those on physical and spiritual journeys with no permanent home – and provide them shelter, food, and friendship. Later this space was converted into a formal hospital which offered health services to the local poor, pilgrims, orphans, and the sick. In the central entrance hall is an impressive fresco cycle painted in the late 14th century shortly after the Black Death wiped out much of the European population. The cycle is composed of multiple large-scale frescoes that reference the founding of the hospital, its association with the church, its role in caring for orphaned children, and important to our conversation, images of healthcare providers intimately caring for and hosting the sick and dying. There are also depictions of caretakers sharing a meal and fellowship with their patients, which was customary at that time.

Walking into this space, we can engage our moral imaginations: If I were a starving and sick pilgrim in the 14th century, what would these frescoes communicate to me? As a healthy member of the Sienese society in the 14th century, what would this fresco cycle say about the values of my community? Would it instill providers and citizens with a personal responsibility to care for those in need? As a 21th century viewers involved in healthcare, what can we infer about the role of the physicians and caregivers in this society? Has this role changed? The fresco cycle is a tour de force that illustrates instances of true compassion and communicates a message of warming embrace to those in need. It communicates, visually, to a textually illiterate population that they will be cared for, clothed, fed, and loved. It reflects the origins of the word *hospital*, Os'pedale, which means "to host" and demonstrates in each image the meaning of hospitality. This fresco cycle is powerful and tells a story that still resonates.

It affords us an opportunity to draw contrast and reflect upon healthcare in our modern society.

Juxtapose this welcoming scene with the often sterile feel of many hospitals and doctor's offices in the United States with overcrowded waiting rooms, walls devoid of art, and a healthcare system that incentivizes institutions to quickly discharge patients into a world they might be grossly unprepared to reenter. Strolling through the halls of many "community" hospitals throughout the United States, we are often confronted with design and decoration that communicate sterile institutionalism to patients, visitors, and staff. Walking the halls of many of these institutions, unlike the grand entrance hall in Siena, makes us ponder different questions: Is this a place I would come to *heal*? Do I feel welcomed by this austere design? What are this institution's values? We must be cognizant of design and the visual aesthetics of our created spaces and the messages they communicate.

Interacting with Santa Maria Della Scala's 14th century fresco cycle continues to make us wonder when, in the history of medicine, we lost our ability to host; to welcome with open arms the sick and needy with kindness, shelter, and friendship. When did we lose our ability to truly care for those who feel the world has left them to suffer alone? The frescoes communicate to us that that before we can heal patients, we must host them. It reminds us that we must see ourselves in context of the societies who came and healed before us. We can use the arts as a moral guide to reflect, and our collective actions as a tool to exemplify altruism and *care* for patients [11]. Furthermore, we must remember that the arts can speak directly to and for our patients.

In essence, through the study and implantation of visual literacy into our repertoire of skills, we become keen observers of our natural and constructed world. The arts offer a means to mediate our values, the values of others, and the values of our community. Through such introspection, our ability to listen and communicate improves. It is important to note that one does not need to leave their home country and travel to have experiences like the one described above. Visits to local museums and other venues where the arts are displayed (including street art/graffiti) offer similar opportunities to reflect, learn, and integrate visual manifestations of diverse cultures with our preexisting knowledge and biases. We simply need to slow down and observe to reap the benefits of looking closely. The benefits as they relate to clinical preparation and practice will be reviewed in the next section.

4.   What Role Do the Arts and Visual Literacy Play in Clinical Practice and Professional Preparation?

Historically, the arts and medicine were inextricably linked. Some argue that it was only with the publication of the Abraham Flexner Report of 1910 in the United States that medical education shifted towards the "hard sciences," research, and basic biology, and away from the humanities and other tenets of professionalism. The implications of his report are still felt today throughout undergraduate and graduate medical education in the United States. In a recent New England Journal review article by Cooke *et al*, the authors highlight:

The academic environment has been transformed since Flexner's day. In academic hospitals, research quickly outstripped teaching in importance, and a "publish or perish" culture emerged in American universities and medical schools. Research productivity became the metric by which faculty accomplishment was judged; teaching, caring for patients, and addressing broader public health issues were viewed as less important activities. Thus, today's subordination of teaching to research, as well as the narrow gaze of American medical education on biologic matters, represents a long-standing tradition [12].

While it is important to recognize The Flexner Report as a pivot point for medicine and medical education, it is also helpful to review examples of the historic link between the arts and medicine.

The arts and medicine were not always so distant. The medical training at the University of Padova in the Veneto region of Italy is one such example. Established in the year 1399 AD, but with historical records dating to 1222 AD, the medical program at the University of Padova is one of the earliest medical centers in all of Europe [13]. At this historic university, those wishing to pursue a doctorate of medicine were first required to earn a doctorate in philosophy. To the Italians in the 14th and 15th centuries, medicine was inextricably linked to the study and appreciation of the human condition - to the moral and ethical dilemmas of the day, to the arts, and lastly, to the sciences. Furthermore, Andreas Vesalius, author of one of the most important anatomical texts in the history of medicine, *De humani corporis fabrica* (*On the Fabric of the Human Body*) published in 1543, was an esteemed professor at the University. The text is known for both its artistic genius as well as its medical content, something particularly notable considering Leonardo da Vinci was making similar strides in the realm of anatomical dissection and drawing at the time [14]. Similar to the Vesalius text, Leonardo's drawings similarly highlight the nonexistent boundary between art, medicine, and anatomy in 15th and 16th century Italy.

More recently, the arts were an important medium to explore the complexities of physical diagnosis. Jean-Martin Charcot, the "father of neurology," used the arts, specifically sketching and drawing, to process clinical information in the late 19th century. Julien Bogousslavsky notes in his article that, "one of the best achievements of Charcot in correlating the clinic with art includes his thorough study of artistic representations of 'possessed states', which allowed him to refine his work on hysteria. The artist and scientist are two facets of Charcot, whose permanent coexistence help [us] to understand his legacy" [15]. Other related review articles have further explored the role the arts played in the development of key neurological theories by Charcot [16, 17]. Charcot's prestige and reliance on art highlight that medicine and art, historically, have relied heavily on one another for guidance. Medicine is a 'human science' that demands an appreciation and recognition of the human experience. The arts inform us of this experience and better enable us to serve as medical professionals.

While the arts and humanities are not a requirement in our 21st century medical education system, many programs are turning to the arts for guidance. Two well-known examples are Harvard's "Training the Eye: Improving the Art of Physical Diagnosis" curriculum for undergraduate medical students and its humanistic curriculum for internal medicine residents at the Brigham and Women's Hospital in Boston, Massachusetts [8].

In Harvard's "Training the Eye Curriculum," students in their first and second year of medical school may choose to enroll in a course that uses visual art at the Museum of Fine Arts in Boston paired with clinical didactics to improve observational skills utilizing the Visual Thinking Strategies (VTS) curriculum highlighted above. Over the course of 9-weeks, students meet weekly to analyze and describe works of art and study images related to clinical diagnosis. A randomized controlled trial of this curriculum found a statistically significant difference in the number of descriptions, both artistic and clinical, amongst student participants compared to controls [7-8]. Amongst physicians in training, the arts also offer benefit. The BWH Internal Medicine Humanistic Curriculum began in 1992 and is now required for all first-year internal medicine residents. The curriculum's purpose is to foster resident well-being and humanistic qualities while preventing trainee burnout that can compromise personal and professional satisfaction [8]. Secondary goals of the program, composed of monthly sessions and "Night at the Museum of Fine Arts", include addressing empathy, compassion, humanism, and burnout.

A separate program at The Cleveland Museum of Art, *Vital Signs*, was launched in February 2012 as a partnership between the museum and the Cleveland Clinic, University Hospitals, VA Center for Excellence in Primary Care Education, Cleveland State University and NEO-Med [18]. The Vital Signs program, which underwent significant change in 2015 and is currently implemented under a different name, sought to engage medical students, nursing students, physical therapy students, medical residents, psychiatry residents, and pharmacy students [18]. The program seeks to build the following skills: observation and the ability to notice details in context; critical thinking through the ability to integrate multiple perspectives, aan appreciation for ambiguity; and, communication through active listening and analysis of a work of art with a diverse team [18]. Through these skills, the program aims to improve two core competencies: (1) cultural competence and awareness of personal, professional and society boundaries and, (2) self-knowledge through recognition of habits and beliefs that effect self-care, empathy, focus, and reflection [18].

Harvard's two programs – one for medical students, the other for training physicians – and the program at the Cleveland Museum of Art are only three examples of art related programs and interventions in professional medical training. Numerous other studies and programs related to the arts in undergraduate and graduate medical education have suggested a benefit in tolerance for ambiguity and increased positive views towards colleagues and the healthcare system. The importance of these training opportunities is especially important given the noted decline in empathy amongst undergraduate medical students and other health professionals [19-20]. Additional reported benefits of the arts include: emotional recognition, identification of story and narrative, and the awareness of multiple perspectives [21]. On the whole, these studies and educational curricula indicate that the arts offer value to physicians and healthcare providers in their ability to promote self-care, physical diagnosis, tolerance for ambiguity, and the ability to communicate effectively [22-28]. Encouraging visual literacy and engagement with the arts amongst those interested in health is an emerging field whose benefits deserve further quantification and exploration.

5. Where Are the Arts Being Utilized as an Intervention to Impact Health Outcomes?

In addition to benefitting health providers, it is equally important to consider the role arts play in patient wellbeing and healing. Numerous reports and studies have explored the role of the arts in improving patient outcomes.

In a 2010 meta-analysis, Heather Stuckey and Jeremy Nobel reviewed quantitative and qualitative research from 1995-2007 regarding four artistic engagement modalities and their associated health benefits [29]. In one music engagement randomized controlled trial, Guzzetta et al. found that playing relaxation music to coronary artery disease patients resulted in improvements in apical heart rates and peripheral temperatures [30]. In a separate pretest-posttest study on coronary artery disease patients after a myocardial infarction in Wisconsin, White et al. found that music engagement led to reductions in heart rate, respiratory rate, myocardial oxygen demand, and anxiety following just twenty minutes of listening [31]. In a phenomenological visual arts study in England, Reynolds et al. found that art engagement and discussion amongst female chronic illness patients resulted in a filling of occupational voids and distracted thoughts of illness [32]. They furthermore reported improvements in flow and spontaneity, expression of grief, and social networks [32]. A randomized controlled trial of breast cancer patients by Puig et al. found that engagement with the visual arts led to improved well-being through decreased negative emotions and a strengthening of positive emotions [33].

In movement based creative expression studies in the Atlanta, Georgia, Greenspan et al. found in a randomized controlled trial of elderly adults that tai chi and other wellness interventions resulted in improvements in physical symptoms and ambulation [34]. In a creative writing randomized controlled trial of HIV patients in New Zealand, Petrie et al. demonstrated a reduction in CD4+ lymphocyte counts amongst the intervention group [35]. While this meta-analysis and its associated studies is by no means an exhaustive list, numerous other studies have shown similar health benefits through artistic engagement, further emphasizing the plethora of future research opportunities in this realm [36-43].

Beyond patient-specific outcomes, the arts offer a public health benefit as well. One such case study took place in the Sunnyside neighborhood of Portland, Oregon in the late 1990s. In his article, "The Intersection of Urban Planning, Art, and Public Health: The Sunnyside Piazza," Jan Semenza dives into the history of urban planning and the effects that a deteriorating and dilapidated physical space has on public health and the role the arts play in community restoration and determinants of health [44]. Semanza argues that while many historical developments in urban planning (e.g. water distribution, sanitation) have resulted in improved public health, many of our current zoning laws and urban landscapes give rise to unhealthy communities that contribute to epidemics of obesity, diabetes, and depression [45-47].

To illustrate the role of the arts in public wellbeing, Semenza tells the story of the Sunnyside community which over the course of 9-months, designated the central town piazza as the location for a large-scale sunflower mural and urban redesign to symbolize and promote cohesion and shared identity. Two years following its completion, "the Sunnyside Piazza remains a catalyst of sidewalk conversations, as passersby read the signs about the community project, tourists take photographs, children throw pennies into the wishing pond, joggers run an extra lap around the sunflower, and strangers pause to admire the art" [44]. An observation of 507 pedestrians in April 2003 demonstrated that 164 persons (32%) interacted with the piazza compared to 7% (p<0.01) in an unimproved piazza. Other similar statistics demonstrated that citizens living in close proximity to the piazza experienced higher satisfaction and rated their neighborhood an "excellent place to live" [44]. While the generalizability of this data is limited, its premise is worth noting – the arts can inject a sense of wellbeing, pride, and improved emotional and physical health into a community.

In addition to local projects, individuals in the public health community have also introduced the concept that museum spaces and art galleries are underexplored avenues to promote health and wellness in communities. In their article, "Museums and art galleries as partners for public health interventions," Camic and Chatterjee from the UK highlight the many benefits art museums bestow upon their visitors and propose a strategy for public engagement projects and partnerships [48]. In a comprehensive review of current literature the authors highlight that engagement with museum spaces leads to a reduction in social isolation and furthermore promotes a sense of connection and belonging; optimism and hope; moral values and beliefs; emotional capital and resilience; opportunity for success; support; quiet, rest, sanctuary; and social capital [48].

In summary, the arts bestow benefits upon patients and also afford a broader, more generalizable benefit to communities.

6.   Future Directions – Implications of Exploring the Intersection of the Arts and Health Literacy

In this chapter, we described several studies that suggest exposure to the arts can be therapeutic for patients and contribute to the process of healing. Two other chapters within this book discuss life skills progression (LSP) research, which suggests health literacy boosts the quality of life and confidence, most notably for mothers in vulnerable populations [49]. The LSP research notes health literacy is an important social determinant of health because it can impact healthier personal and family behaviors, enhance health outcomes, as well as more prudent use of the health care delivery system [49-50].

Among the activities that are surrogate measures of health literacy, LSP research suggests one of the most significant is self-reflection [49-50]. In other words, LSP research suggests health care professionals should encourage the development and sustainment of maternal self-reflection because self-reflection is an activating mechanism which helps participants reassess personal and family health status and make commitments to a more therapeutic lifestyle, better child care, and healthier behaviors [49-50].

Yet, before health care professionals intervene with music therapy or encourage patient self-reflection, there needs to be a conceptual foundation that explains why both activities are therapeutic. While some findings suggest exposure to the arts and encouraging self-reflection are associated with the activation of healing mechanisms, the larger question is why does this occur? We suggest an answer may come from mid-20th century research on the therapeutic elements of play, which is often referred to with the mass communication literature (where it was advanced) as 'play theory' [51-52].

In the 1960s, Stephenson (drawing on Huizinga) suggested people are more inclined to be open to new ideas, notions, emotions, experiences, behaviors, and commitments when they are at play compared to all other life experiences [51, 53].

While Stephenson and Huizinga noted playing games, sports, or immersion activities are commonly (and falsely) thought of as play, they re-defined 'play' as a uniquely individual experience that generates intrinsic self-enhancement [51, 53]. For example, while ballet, baseball, and knitting are beloved by some, Stephenson noted their enjoyment is difficult to share and disagreements about voluntary/involuntary participation in these (and most other) activities are ubiquitous among families, friends, peers, colleagues, and loved ones [51].

Alternatively, Stephenson noted most of our daily routines and lives are filled with demands to meet the expectations derived from family, work, social and professional roles, as well as pressure to conform/comply with social, professional, and cultural norms [51]. To Stephenson, 'play' is when we momentarily exit external influences to briefly live in (or experience) the domain of our inner-most thoughts, which is an experience that gestalt psychologists suggest represents the centrality of the 'self' [51, 54]. Stephenson noted play (as defined within a gestalt perspective) represents a psychological event that is associated with self-generated sense of well-being.

Stephenson explained the circumstances when we 'play' are unique to each of us. Play (as he and Huizinga defined it) especially is operant when we intrinsically relish an experience, lose track of time, and look forward to a return. Play is characterized by a degree of solitude and a momentary separation from the world around us [51, 53]. Stephenson explained when people 'play,' our mind wanders and we often are more likely to consider new ideas, notions, behaviors, and attitudes. Stephenson added the experience is enjoyable because it is one of the few interludes when we live and think for ourselves as well as have the opportunity to become lost in our own thoughts (however ephemeral or even embarrassing).

In terms of psychological theory, Stephenson explained play impacts our apperception (e.g. our ability to monitor the external world as well as consider our own feelings, impressions, emotions, hunches, expectations, notion, and opinions). The experience becomes rewarding because it is intrinsically practical and self-enhancing, which explains why we may return to it unconsciously as a highly routinized activity [51, 54-55]. To put this another way, within a gestalt framework, 'play' is therapy and self-reflection is an applied manifestation of wellness.

In addition to Stephenson, the resulting internalized experience eventually becomes more gratifying than its activating mechanism. So, music from a harp is less healing on its own (regardless of the medium of exposure) than the resulting solitude, relaxation, pleasure, reflection, and new commitments that may occur as one listens. Or more positively, the greater impact of paintings, films, music, sculpture, and other arts is their capacity to foster momentary, highly personalized, internalized experiences.

Overall, the arts can activate aspects of wellness and healing because for some they are linked to an underlying psychologically therapeutic process that generates more self-reflection and self-awareness. One challenge is to find the genre or type of art that provides an activating mechanism for individuals and understand that the same formats of artistic expression, such as music therapy or amusing films, may (or may not) generate similar internalized experiences among individuals or demographically diverse populations. Another challenge is to understand that self-reflection is a desired outcome of play and its therapeutic value needs to be better understood and more widely encouraged instead of being criticized as frivolous or a waste of time.

Hence, in Stephenson's conceptual framework, the associations among exposure to the arts and encouraging reflection and the advancement of one's health literacy, the development of self-efficacy, and ultimately, enhanced health behaviors and outcomes are linked imaginatively.

Moreover, Stephenson's ideas are similar to contemporary social science research on the formation of human resilience, which suggests the creation of individual happiness, optimism, purpose in life, gratitude, and mindfulness provide significant buffers against external stress, anxieties, trauma, and depression. Similar to

Stephenson's 50 year-old suggestion that the importance of play is frequently overlooked in psychological research, Kent, Davis, and Reich suggest contemporary assessments of psychological health emphasize the absence/presence of stress, depression, anxiety, and trauma without evaluating the impact (and cultivation of) happiness, optimism, purpose in life, gratitude, and mindfulness [56]. As a result, Kent, Davis, and Reich suggest social scientists undervalue the understanding of how therapeutic dimensions in human behavior are generated, cultivated, and sustained [56]. We add the latter may provide a framework to understand the therapeutic value of the arts and its impact to enhance health literacy and health outcomes. Certainly, Stephenson's as well as Kent, Davis, and Reich's conceptual frameworks provide a foundation as well as open opportunities for future research in the area of the arts and health literacy.

More than two decades of research now inform the field of health literacy, and the growing evidence base for building a health literate nation reflects this. Much of the work focuses on the content related to medicine, health, and healthcare although literacy experts readily acknowledge that literacy skills are context and content specific. The arts more directly address context and future efforts that incorporate the arts might help us better learn how to understand values, beliefs, traditions so that these are incorporated into what we communicate about medicine and health. Viewing the arts as communicators, especially seeing their messages related to context, can enhance our health literacy approaches that seek to address both content and context. The underexplored intersection of health literacy and the arts holds promise for advancing how we enhance our skills and abilities to help individuals and populations navigate, understand, and use all that is available to improve health.

References:

[1] Panofsky E. Meaning in the visual arts. Phoenix ed. Chicago: University of Chicago Press; 1982.
[2] http://www.vislit.org/visual-literacy/. Retrieved February 11, 2017.
[3] http://kff.org/disparities-policy/press-release/daily-media-use-among-children-and-teens-up-dramatically-from-five-years-ago/. Retrieved February 11, 2017.
[4] http://www.vislit.org/the-art-of-seeing-art/. Retrieved February 11, 2017.
[5] Visual literacy: why we need it TedX https://youtu.be/E91fk6D0nwM. Retrieved August 2, 2016.
[6] http://www.vtshome.org/what-is-vts/method-curriculum--2. Retrieved February 11, 2017.
[7] Naghshineh S, Hafler JP, Miller AR, Blanco MA, Lipsitz SR, Dubroff RP, et al. Formal art observation training improves medical students' visual diagnostic skills. J Gen Intern Med. 2008;23(7):991-7. DOI: 10.1007/s11606-008-0667-0.
[8] Katz JT, Khoshbin S. Can visual arts training improve physician performance? Transactions of the Americal Clinical and Climatologic Association. 2014;125.
[9] Burke E. Reflections on the revolution in France. Mineola, NY: Dover Publications; 2006.
[10] http://www.firstthings.com/blogs/firstthoughts/2009/07/defining-moral-imagination. Retrieved February 11, 2017.
[11] http://blogs.hospitalmedicine.org/Blog/hospitality-and-art-in-medicine-a-response-to-sarah-candler-mds-medical-map-making/. Retrieved February 11, 2017.
[12] Cooke M, Irby DM, Sullivan W, Ludmerer KM. American medical education 100 years after the Flexner report. N Engl J Med. 2006;355(13):1339-44. DOI: 10.1056/NEJMra055445.
[13] Zampieri F, Zanatta A, Elmaghawry M, Bonati MR, Thiene G. Origin and development of modern medicine at the University of Padua and the role of the "Serenissima" Republic of Venice. Glob Cardiol Sci Pract. 2013;2013(2):149-62. DOI: 10.5339/gcsp.2013.21.
[14] Leonardo and the reinvention of anatomy. Hektoen Institute of Medicine http://hekint.org/index.php?option=com_content&view=article&id=1158:leonardo-and-the-reinvention-of-anatomy-2&catid=63&Itemid=716. Retrieved February 12, 2017.

[15] Bogousslavsky J. Charcot and art: from a hobby to science. Eur Neurol. 2004;51(2):78-83. DOI: 10.1159/000076533.
[16] Bogousslavsky J, Boller F. Jean-Martin Charcot and art: relationship of the "founder of neurology" with various aspects of art. Prog Brain Res. 2013;203:185-99. DOI: 10.1016/B978-0-444-62730-8.00007-4.
[17] Goetz CG. Visual art in the neurologic career of Jean-Martin Charcot. Arch Neurol. 1991;48(4):421-5.
[18] Larson C. A Discussion of Art & Health. Toledo Museum of Art. By teleconference. November 14, 2016.
[19] Hojat M, Mangione S, Nasca TJ, Rattner S, Erdmann JB, Gonnella JS, et al. An empirical study of decline in empathy in medical school. Med Educ. 2004;38(9):934-41. DOI: 10.1111/j.1365-2929.2004.01911.x.
[20] Klugman CM, Peel J, Beckmann-Mendez D. Art rounds: teaching interprofessional students visual thinking strategies at one school. Acad Med. 2011;86(10):1266-71. DOI: 10.1097/ACM.0b013e31822c1427.
[21] Shapiro J, Rucker L, Beck J. Training the clinical eye and mind: using the arts to develop medical students' observational and pattern recognition skills. Med Educ. 2006;40(3):263-8. DOI: 10.1111/j.1365-2929.2006.02389.x.
[22] Dolev JC, Friedlaender LK, Braverman IM. Use of fine art to enhance visual diagnostic skills. JAMA. 2001;286(9):1020-1.
[23] Gonzales E, Morrow-Howell N, Gilbert P. Changing medical students' attitudes toward older adults. Gerontol Geriatr Educ. 2010;31(3):220-34. DOI: 10.1080/02701960.2010.503128.
[24] Hojat M, Axelrod D, Spandorfer J, Mangione S. Enhancing and sustaining empathy in medical students. Med Teach. 2013;35(12):996-1001. DOI: 10.3109/0142159X.2013.802300.
[25] Mullangi S. The synergy of medicine and art in the curriculum. Acad Med. 2013;88(7):921-3. DOI: 10.1097/ACM.0b013e3182956017.
[26] Parker RM, Labrecque CA, Candler SG, Newell-Amato D, Messler J, Wolf M, et al. Communicating through the arts: lessons for medicine and public health. J Health Commun. 2013;18(2):139-45. DOI: 10.1080/10810730.2013.763706.
[27] Sasser CG, Puchalski CM. The humanistic clinician: traversing the science and art of health care. J Pain Symptom Manage. 2010;39(5):936-40. DOI: 10.1016/j.jpainsymman.2010.03.001.
[28] Shea S, Lionis C. Restoring humanity in health care through the art of compassion: an issue for the teaching and research agenda in rural health care. Rural Remote Health. 2010;10(4):1679.
[29] Stuckey HL, Nobel J. The connection between art, healing, and public health: a review of current literature. Am J Public Health. 2010;100(2):254-63. DOI: 10.2105/AJPH.2008.156497.
[30] Guzzetta CE. Effects of relaxation and music therapy on patients in a coronary care unit with presumptive acute myocardial infarction. Heart Lung. 1989;18(6):609-16.
[31] White JM. Effects of relaxing music on cardiac autonomic balance and anxiety after acute myocardial infarction. Am J Crit Care. 1999;8(4):220-30.
[32] Reynolds F, Prior S. 'A lifestyle coat-hanger': a phenomenological study of the meanings of artwork for women coping with chronic illness and disability. Disabil Rehabil. 2003;25(14):785-94. DOI: 10.1080/0963828031000093486.
[33] Puig A LS, Goodwin L, Sherrard PAD. The efficacy of creative arts therapies to enhance emotional expression, spirituality, and psychological well-being of newly diagnosed stage I and stage II breast cancer patients: a preliminary study. Arts Psychotherapy. 2006;33(3):218-28.
[34] Greenspan AI, Wolf SL, Kelley ME, O'Grady M. Tai chi and perceived health status in older adults who are transitionally frail: a randomized controlled trial. Phys Ther. 2007;87(5):525-35. DOI: 10.2522/ptj.20050378.
[35] Petrie KJ, Fontanilla I, Thomas MG, Booth RJ, Pennebaker JW. Effect of written emotional expression on immune function in patients with human immunodeficiency virus infection: a randomized trial. Psychosom Med. 2004;66(2):272-5.
[36] Carlson LE, Bultz BD. Mind-body interventions in oncology. Curr Treat Options Oncol. 2008;9(2-3):127-34. DOI: 10.1007/s11864-008-0064-2.
[37] Carruthers HR, Miller V, Morris J, Evans R, Tarrier N, Whorwell PJ. Using art to help understand the imagery of irritable bowel syndrome and its response to hypnotherapy. Int J Clin Exp Hypn. 2009;57(2):162-73. DOI: 10.1080/00207140802665401.
[38] Chancellor B, Duncan A, Chatterjee A. Art therapy for Alzheimer's disease and other dementias. J Alzheimers Dis. 2014;39(1):1-11. DOI: 10.3233/JAD-131295.
[39] Hughes EG, da Silva AM. A pilot study assessing art therapy as a mental health intervention for subfertile women. Hum Reprod. 2011;26(3):611-5. DOI: 10.1093/humrep/deq385.
[40] Nainis N, Paice JA, Ratner J, Wirth JH, Lai J, Shott S. Relieving symptoms in cancer: innovative use of art therapy. J Pain Symptom Manage. 2006;31(2):162-9. DOI: 10.1016/j.jpainsymman.2005.07.006.

[41] Nanda U, Eisen S, Zadeh RS, Owen D. Effect of visual art on patient anxiety and agitation in a mental health facility and implications for the business case. J Psychiatr Ment Health Nurs. 2011;18(5):386-93. DOI: 10.1111/j.1365-2850.2010.01682.x.
[42] Walsh SM, Martin SC, Schmidt LA. Testing the efficacy of a creative-arts intervention with family caregivers of patients with cancer. J Nurs Scholarsh. 2004;36(3):214-9.

[43] Wood MJ, Molassiotis A, Payne S. What research evidence is there for the use of art therapy in the management of symptoms in adults with cancer? A systematic review. Psychooncology. 2011;20(2):135-45. DOI: 10.1002/pon.1722.
[44] Semenza JC. The intersection of urban planning, art, and public health: the Sunnyside Piazza. Am J Public Health. 2003;93(9):1439-41.
[45] Hu FB, Manson JE, Stampfer MJ, Colditz G, Liu S, Solomon CG, et al. Diet, lifestyle, and the risk of type 2 diabetes mellitus in women. N Engl J Med. 2001;345(11):790-7. DOI: 10.1056/NEJMoa010492.
[46] Kumanyika SK. Minisymposium on obesity: overview and some strategic considerations. Annu Rev Public Health. 2001;22:293-308. DOI: 10.1146/annurev.publhealth.22.1.293.
[47] Narrow WE, Rae DS, Robins LN, Regier DA. Revised prevalence estimates of mental disorders in the United States: using a clinical significance criterion to reconcile 2 surveys' estimates. Arch Gen Psychiatry. 2002;59(2):115-23.
[48] Camic PM, Chatterjee HJ. Museums and art galleries as partners for public health interventions. Perspect Public Health. 2013;133(1):66-71. DOI: 10.1177/1757913912468523.
[49] Smith SA. Health literacy and social service delivery. In: Estrine SA AH, Hettenbach RT, Messina MG, editor. New directions in behavioral health: service delivery strategies for vulnerable populations. New York: Springer Publishing; 2011.
[50] Smith SA, Moore EJ. Health literacy and depression in the context of home visitation. Matern Child Health J. 2012;16(7):1500-8. DOI: 10.1007/s10995-011-0920-8.
[51] Stephenson W. The play theory of mass communication. Chicago: Transaction Press; 1988.
[52] Glasser T. Play, pleasure and the value of newsreading. Communication Quarterly.1982;30(2):101-7.
[53] Huizinga J. Homo ludens. Boston: Beacon Press; 1950.
[54] Stephenson W. Scientific creed: the centrality of self. The Psychological Record. 1961;11:18-25.
[55] Stephenson W. Play theory and value. In: Thayer L, editor. Communication: ethical and moral issues. New York: Gordon and Breach; 1973.
[56] Kent M, Davis MC, Reich JW, editors. The resilience handbook: approaches to stress and trauma. New York: Routledge; 2013.

Health Literacy
R.A. Logan and E.R. Siegel (Eds.)
IOS Press, 2017
doi:10.3233/978-1-61499-790-0-96

Seeking an Expanded, Multidimensional Conceptual Approach to Health Literacy and Health Disparities Research

Robert A. LOGAN[1]

Senior staff, National Library of Medicine, U.S.A.

Abstract. This chapter compares the conceptual foundations of health literacy and health disparities. It details some of the conceptual differences between health literacy and health disparities and explains some similarities that suggest the need for increased research collaboration. The chapter is among the first to address the structural and social determinants of health together and explain that future research needs to assess their interactions.

Overall, the chapter creates a conceptual foundation as well as challenges future scholars/practitioners to take more multidimensional approaches to assess health's determinants. The chapter also attempts to demonstrate there is nothing more practical than good theory, or clear conceptual foundations.

The chapter is divided into four sections that address the following topics: three conceptual frameworks about the determinants of health; opportunities in health disparities and health literacy research; seeking an expanded, multidimensional conceptual approach to health literacy and health disparities research; as well as a conclusion. The chapter suggests there are vacuums in current research knowledge that need future attention – especially regarding the integration of health literacy and health disparities research.

Keywords. Health literacy, health disparities, social determinants of health, structural determinants of health

1. Introduction

This chapter attempts to provide a broader conceptual framework within an ongoing discussion about the integration of health literacy and health disparities research in the U.S. [1]. The chapter attempts to demonstrate there is nothing more practical than a good theory, or clear conceptual foundations.

The chapter is written for future researchers and encourages them to set research agendas that will move the health literacy discipline forward. The chapter suggests there are gaps in current research knowledge that need future attention – especially regarding the integration of health literacy and health disparities research.

Although the chapter emphasizes health literacy research and developments in the U.S., some international health literacy work is included. The chapter's intent is not to review or summarize the health literacy and health disparities research literature, or

---
[1] Corresponding author: Senior staff, U.S. National Library of Medicine, 8600 Rockville Pike, Building 38, Room 2s22, Bethesda, MD. USA; E-mail: logan@nlm.nih.gov.

provide a systematic review of research findings – as these have been published recently [2–5].

The chapter is divided into four additional sections that address the following topics: three conceptual frameworks about the structural and social determinants of health; opportunities in health disparities and health literacy research; seeking an expanded, multidimensional conceptual approach to health literacy and health disparities research; as well as a conclusion.

Within the second section, 'three conceptual frameworks about the structural and social determinants of health,' three subtopics are addressed. They are: the structural determinants of health fostered within the health care delivery system (or health risks generated by patient care and the medical research process); some of the social determinants of health from a health disparities perspective; as well as some of the social and structural determinants of health from a health literacy perspective.

The second section also addresses the possible integration of health disparities and health literacy research as well as their conceptual differences.

The third section, 'opportunities in health disparities and health literacy research,' discusses some of the specific challenges that have been identified as gaps within the current health literacy and health disparities research.

The fourth section, 'seeking an expanded, multidimensional conceptual approach to health literacy and health disparities research,' addresses rationales to integrate the structural and social determinants of health in research and interventions. The conclusion summarizes the chapter's primary findings and makes suggestions about additional challenges for future researchers.

Before moving to these topics, the Calgary Charter's definition of health literacy provides the operational definition of health literacy used in this chapter. While Sorensen, Broucke, Fullam, Doyle, Pelikan, Slonska, and Brand note there is not a consensus definition of health literacy, they find diverse definitions of the term health literacy reflect perspectives from different disciplines, including clinical medicine and public health [6]. A recent perspective from the National Academies of Sciences, Engineering, and Medicine Roundtable on Health Literacy attests that it is difficult to define the term 'health literacy' because the field traverses an array of disciplines [7].

Until a new, consensus definition of health literacy is furnished by National Academies or others, the Calgary Charter, proposed at an international meeting in 2012, probably provides the most comprehensive, multidisciplinary perspective. The Calgary Charter's definition of health literacy suggests:

Health literacy allows the public and personnel working in all health-related contexts to find, understand, evaluate, communicate, and use information.

Health literacy is the use of a wide range of skills that improve the ability of people to act on information in order to live healthier lives.

These skills include reading, writing, listening, speaking, numeracy, and critical analysis, as well as communication and interaction skills [8].

A definition of health disparities is provided in the chapter's second section.

Also, the U.S. Institute of Medicine (IOM) changed its name to the National Academies of Sciences, Engineering, and Medicine in 2016 and will be referred to in the chapter as the National Academies. The clarification is needed because the

IOM/National Academies of Sciences, Engineering, and Medicine commendably generate significant publications about health literacy, health disparities, and many of the areas are discussed in this chapter. A chapter on the IOM's and National Academies' contribution to health literacy research appears elsewhere within this book.

2. Three Conceptual Frameworks: The Structural and Social Determinants of Health

This section discusses three conceptual frameworks that expand the clinical triangle that often are associated with the etiology of illness and its prevention (genotype, phenotype, and lifestyle behaviors). The section suggests one of the contributions of 21st century research is the increasing recognition that prevailing health disparities and poor health literacy across the U.S., as well as the health risks which occur within the U.S. health care delivery system, are significant determinants of individual and population health.

This section partially reflects a salutogenic framework about health, which suggests individual and population health and illness are not limited to disease diagnosis, treatment, and prevention [9]. While a salutogenic conceptual framework suggests illness and health represent a multidimensional continuum, the research about the determinants of health cites specific biopsychosocial or structural areas where health risks are generated, or where risks might be lowered by diverse prevention or intervention efforts.

The first of the three conceptual frameworks discussed here focuses on a few, selected structural determinants of health that are fostered within the U.S. health care delivery system, or some activities within health care delivery, which impact health risks, health care outcomes, and health care utilization. The research in this area suggests higher or lower health risks can be generated as a result of specific events generated by the health care delivery system that may or may not be related to the routine diagnosis and treatment of diseases or conditions.

The second conceptual framework focuses on the health risks fostered by health disparities that influence health outcomes and the utilization of the health care delivery system. Within the U.S.-based health disparities literature, the aggregate toll of health disparities on the nation's health is suggested as exemplifying some of the social determinants of health [10,11].

The third conceptual framework focuses on the risks fostered by low health literacy that impact health outcomes and the utilization of the health care delivery system. Within the health literacy literature, the toll of low health literacy also is suggested as an illustration of a social determinant of health in the U.S. as well as other nations [12].

A National Academies perspective recently noted while poor health literacy and ongoing health disparities each illustrate social determinants of health, the fields of health literacy and health disparities evolved independently [1,13]. The National Academies perspective also suggests health literacy and health disparities research have not been collaborative or integrated, which suggest they need to be discussed as two different domains of health's social determinants [1].

To backup, one of the important 21st century perspectives on health's underpinnings, as attested by the foci in the U.S. National Institutes of Health's Precision Medicine Initiative, suggests individual health and disease prevention are the byproducts of a triangular interaction among: phenotype (an individual's prior medical history and physical traits); genotype (an individual's genetic/genomic inheritance); and an individual's lifestyle (or behaviors known to impact health, such as smoking, exercise, substance abuse, and body mass index). One of the significant contributions of 21st century health care may be an increasing capacity to assess how the interactions among genotype, phenotype, and individual behaviors impact the health and disease prevention of individuals and perhaps diverse demographic populations [14,15].

However, another significant contribution of 21st century health research is an increasing understanding that illness and wellness also are impacted by: a) the social, cultural, economic, and geographical environments in which one lives, b) one's health literacy, and c) the challenges, errors, and oversights that occur as a result of exposure to the health delivery system [16,17,13,11].

Health literacy, health disparities, and 'quality chasm' research suggest the determinants of health should not be limited to the assessment of phenotype, genotype, and lifestyle patterns. Instead, health literacy, health disparities, and 'quality chasm' research suggest health and illness also are significantly influenced by diverse social and structural factors.

2.1. Structural Determinants of Health

Turning first to some structural determinants represented by the latent health risks generated by the health care delivery system, the U.S. National Academies 'quality chasm' reports suggest medical research processes, patient care, and other byproducts of exposure from routine care can significantly impact individual and population health [18,19,16].

In identifying one of specific health challenges derived from medical research processes, Unger, Cook, Tai, and Bleyer explain insufficient clinical trial participation impedes the development of the evidence-based foundation used to treat cancer as well as other diseases and conditions.[20] Unger, Cook, Tai, and Bleyer suggest insufficient clinical trial participation fosters long range health risks, which provides an example of an indirect, structurally-generated determinant of health [20].

Hartung, Zarin, Guise, McDonaugh, Paynter, and Helfand suggest the knowledge gaps between the published findings in refereed journals – and the more comprehensive datasets from which findings are derived – also may foster health risks (especially if medications and medical products are assessed on the basis of incomplete data) [21]. In turn, Hartung et. al infer the gaps between comprehensive data sets and published findings are a potentially detrimental byproduct of medical research processes, which represent an indirect, structurally-generated determinant of health [21].

More recently, Baker describes how the irreproducibility of some medical research poses foundational health risks because irreproducibility undercuts the reliability and validity of biomedical research, which means interventions may or may not evidence-based [22,23]. One recent estimate suggests 70 percent of lab experiments cannot be replicated by the original or other investigators [22]. The lack of reproducibility is perceived as a significant underlying challenge in biomedical and other research by 52 percent of respondents to a survey of biomedical research scientists [22]. Similar to the previous examples, the issues surrounding research reproducibility suggest routine medical research procedures can foster inadvertent but potentially detrimental health risks, which also may be characterized as a structural determinant of health.

Regarding some structural determinant issues generated within routine patient care, Demoly, Passalacqua, Pfaar, Sastre, and Wahn suggest poor patient adherence to provider directions is an enduring byproduct of provider-patient interaction [24]. Poor patient adherence is an acknowledged, underlying, significant barrier to better health outcomes throughout the health care delivery system as well as an enduring structural challenge, which is sometimes characterized an indirect, system-generated, structural determinant of health.

Similarly, the prior authorization of patient-provider care decisions (by insurers or others) provides an ongoing, significant source of patient and provider stress. Shah adds the prior authorization of patient-provider care decisions is ubiquitous within the U.S. health care system and carries with it significant health risks because it may undermine clinical efforts to strive for the highest standards of patient care [25]. The potential inability to pursue state-of-the art care is another indirect, system-generated structural determinant of health in the U.S.

In addition, recent findings suggest there may be 250,000 annual medical errors, or human and health care delivery system mistakes within U.S. clinical venues [26]. Makary and Daniel suggest the frequency of estimated medical errors may be the third highest cause of death in the U.S. In other words, self-generated clinical errors are linked to higher mortality rates than all existing diseases and conditions with the exceptions of heart disease and cancer [26]. Makary and Daniel's research updates a 1999 National Academies report that projected between 49,000–98,000 annual deaths from medical errors. Yet, the actual number of clinical errors and deaths remain uncertain because there is not a diagnostic related group (or a systematic way) to classify them [27]. Regardless of the extent of deaths from clinical errors, HealthNewsReview.org suggests self-generated mistakes within the health care delivery system are underappreciated and represent a direct structural determinant of health that is self-generated within the health care delivery system [28].

Some other structural determinants of health that have been identified as embedded within the U.S. health care delivery system include significant differences in the costs of similar treatments among different medical care institutions (within the same city) as well as significant dissimilarities in medical outcomes for the same diagnoses among and between peer health care delivery centers throughout the U.S. [29–33,18]. The inconsistencies regarding medical costs often are seen as barriers to improved utilization of the health care delivery system and curbing medical costs [34,29–31]. Significant inconsistencies in patient outcomes for the same diagnosis (among and between peer medical centers) also are an acknowledged impediment to better overall health care in the U.S. [35]. While cost and care disparities partially are addressed by periodically revising the standards of care set by the Joint Commission, and the recommendations of evidence-based groups, such as the National Center for Quality Assurance, Agency for Health Research Quality, the National Preventive Services Task Force, and the Centers for Medicare & Medicaid Services, the need for these efforts are a de facto acknowledgement of the role dissimilar costs and outcomes play in influencing the quality of health care in the U.S.

Overall, the degree that internally-generated issues associated with patient care, medical research, and clinical operations impact patient and population health suggest each are a contributor within a broad web of health's structural determinants. While the Kaiser Family Foundation notes each area represents a significant opportunity for research, the Foundation encourages researchers to differentiate between what they term 'health care disparities' (such as the structural determinants introduced above) and health disparities, which is suggested to be a different research field (reflecting a different perspective about health's determinants) [36].

The Kaiser Family Foundation operationally defines health care disparities as differences between groups in health insurance coverage, access to and use of care, quality of care, as well as some of the structural problems within the health care delivery system outlined above [36]. In contrast, the Kaiser Family Foundation suggests health disparities research focuses on a different conceptual dimension – the higher burden of illness, injury, disability, or mortality experienced by one population group relative to others [36].

Briefly, a health disparities research perspective focuses on the socio-economic, cultural, demographic, and geographical variables associated with health risks and health outcomes. Although health disparities research does not challenge that structural health determinants can emerge within the health care delivery system or the aforementioned phenotype, genotype, and behavioral biopsychosocial triangle, health disparities research seeks to identify and assess some of the socially-derived factors that are associated with health outcomes.

2.2. Health Disparities

More specifically, the field of health disparities suggests socially-derived demographic, socio-cultural, and environmental variables, such as gender, educational attainment, income, geography, public safety, housing and neighborhood quality, food security, and stressful living conditions, are statistically associated with comparative differences in health status across the U.S. [4,5,11]. The field of health disparities also can be extended to differences in health status among and between populations in other nations [37,38,11].

While the identification of socially derived variables that impact health status may be historically tied to social discrimination or exclusion issues in the U.S. (such as race, ethnicity, religion), the intent of health disparities research is to evaluate the associations between diverse variables and health status and note comparative differences in population health.

The U.S. National Institutes of Health operationally defines health disparities as the "difference in the incidence, prevalence, mortality, and burden of disease and other adverse health conditions that exist among specific population groups in the United States" [39]. The NIH definition seems to partially meet Braveman and Gruskin's criteria that a health disparities definition should focus on socially or structurally-derived patterns where a population group – already disadvantaged in terms of opportunity or resources – becomes increasingly more vulnerable to illness [40]. Adler adds the latter differences distinguish the field of health disparities from a focus on other population health inequalities, such as the superior health of young adults compared to senior citizens [41]. Adler infers the priority in health disparities research and practice should be more socially-generated, systematic, avoidable, and preventable population differences [41]. Interestingly, this important distinction may be partially buried in an operational definition of health equity as an ideal where people have the same and equal opportunities in order to reach their full health potential [42].

To backup, while the terms health equity, health disparities, and health care disparities are contemporary, the recognition that poverty, unemployment, deficient public safety, poor environmental conditions and diminished educational opportunities adversely impact a neighborhood's quality of life and health outcomes (compared to wealthier areas) is a leitmotif in some celebrated 19th and 20th century literature and films. While Sir Charles Chaplin's films and Charles Dickens' books sometimes end happily (based on a twist of fate that transforms the life of a vulnerable youth or person), their characters depict an anomie, angst, struggle, and stress (and a significant vulnerability) to remain healthy, safe, and sane compared to better opportunities in wealthier areas across town.

It is difficult to read Dickens or watch the Little Tramp without reaching an emotional appreciation of the sharp contrasts in health and safety and other aspects of life when comparing the lives of adults and children who live in vulnerable versus upscale neighborhoods. Dickens' novels and Chaplin's films also frequently convey an implicit understanding that while some social inequalities are inevitable, social indifferences about preventable disparities are reprehensible.

Fittingly, the specific focus of contemporary health disparities research is to empirically assess the extent of the sociological, demographic, geographic, and environmental associations in the U.S. with health status indicators and provide an unprecedented, evidence-based foundation for social interventions (presumably intended to improve the quality of life and health within nested vulnerable populations). While health disparities research is diverse and was recently summarized by Barr and Halvorson, four types of health disparities research findings are introduced here [4,5].

First, most health disparities research findings identify the demographic, socio-economic, and environmental variables that may impact health outcomes. Some of the frequently assessed independent (or predictor/control) variables that are associated with health outcomes include: race; ethnicity; gender; sexual orientation; age; disability; socio-economic status (SES); education; and geographic location. A second type of health disparities findings sacrifices some methodological range to provide more empirically robust (and generalizable) associations among fewer demographic predictor variables and health outcomes.

A third type of health disparities research findings assess if some socially-derived variables have a moderating effect on the associations among sociological, demographic, geographic, and environmental predictors with health outcomes. The latter is an important contribution because it identifies SES variables that potentially improve the health of vulnerable populations – and provides some evidence-based strategies that can be used in community-based interventions.

A fourth type of research findings are conceptually more multidimensional and identify how the health of vulnerable populations is impacted by interactions among socially-derived as well as structural variables. Within the latter type of findings, socially-derived health determinants (regardless if they are sociological, demographic, geographic, or environmental) are seen as working in conjunction with some of the structural health determinants described earlier in this section. In turn, these findings suggest health outcomes are associated with diverse social and structural health variables that may be more intermediate than primary influences. Overall, the fourth type of findings suggest future health disparities research should strive to be more multidimensional, and include variables with an emerging evidence-base of health efficacy, such as health literacy.

Each of these four types of research findings is introduced below. Some individual studies fit within more than one of the aforementioned categories, which suggests some of the categories are not mutually exclusive. The first type of health disparities research seems to have many more examples in the literature than the other three. The review is followed by a brief discussion of health disparities interventions and the lack of integration of health literacy within health disparities research.

First, most health disparities research findings identify a range of sociological, demographic, geographic and environmental variables (often as independent variables) that are associated with significant differences in comparative health status or outcomes (often the dependent variables) across segments of the U.S. population. These research findings may identify one or more independent, or predictor/control variables and assess their impact on one or more types of health outcomes (or dependent measures).

For example, Nakaya and Dorling found two demographic variables (income and geography) were associated with one health outcome (mortality rates) [43]. In an overview of extant health disparities research, the U.S. Centers for Disease Control and Prevention (CDC) reported race, ethnicity, sex, sexual orientation, age, disability, socio-economic status (SES), and geographic location – both as singular or combined independent variables – were associated with single as well as diverse health outcomes [11]. Some of the diverse acute health outcomes identified by the CDC include: colorectal cancer; heart disease; stroke; HIV infection; preterm births; tuberculosis; and health related quality of life [11]. Some of the diverse chronic health outcomes identified by the CDC include: obesity; diabetes; and hypertension [11]. Some of the diverse behavioral health outcomes identified by the CDC include: cigarette smoking; binge drinking; suicide; as well as fatal and non-fatal work related injuries [11].

Barr also found SES, a multifaceted demographic variable, was associated with diverse health outcomes, including lung cancer, other cancers, coronary heart disease, other cardiovascular disease, stroke, chronic bronchitis and other respiratory disease, as well as gastrointestinal disease [5].

The CDC adds other research suggests a community's environment (e.g. access to green space, or local air and/or water quality) similarly is associated with skewed health outcomes among vulnerable populations [11]. In an example of research using an independent variable derived from sociological measures, researchers assessed if the use of community coalitions (within health disparities reduction campaigns) impacted desired health outcomes [44]. In a somewhat rare systematic review of health disparities research findings, a Cochrane review found common data elements, operational definitions, and measures to assess community coalitions were missing, which made it challenging to assess overall efficacy [44].

Most important, the CDC has reported there is an evidence-base to confirm hypotheses that an array of sociological, demographic, geographic, and environmental variables are associated with diverse, skewed health outcomes (that adversely impact vulnerable populations). However, many of the latter findings are derived from studies where comprehensive independent (or predictor) variables are not assessed simultaneously and may not be compared [11].

In examples where clusters of independent variables are evaluated simultaneously, Currie and Schwandt note health disparities researchers have assessed if one health outcome (mortality rates) is impacted by SES (based on educational attainment, geographic area, and income levels) combined with demographic variables (based on race and ethnicity) singularly, or in aggregate [45]. Currie and Schwandt conclude: 'Some studies investigating mortality across educational groups and geographic areas argue not only that inequality in life expectancy is widening, but that overall life expectancy is actually falling among the most disadvantaged groups' [45, p. 708]. Barr adds some health disparities research assesses the associations among a range of demographic and sociological variables (e.g. ethnicity, low position within a social hierarchy, low social capital, and exposure to discrimination) – with several, dependent health status measures (such as the formation of high individual stress, the subsequent development of injuries to tissues and organs, and significantly increased risks of illness and death) [5, p. 140].

A second type of health disparities findings sacrifices some methodological range in order to assess more empirically robust (and generalizable) associations among fewer demographic predictor variables and health outcomes. For example, Chetty, Stepner, Abraham, Lin, Scuden, Turner, Bergeron, & Cutler recently found two demographic predictor variables (income and geography) are robustly associated with one health outcome (life expectancy rates in the U.S.) [46]. Chetty et. al. suggest the top one percent in income (who live in wealthier communities) live 15 years longer than the poorest one percent of Americans who live in impoverished areas [46]. Chetty et.al. add the wealthiest Americans (who live in wealthier communities with more social, environmental, and cultural amenities) gained more than three years of life expectancy during the first 14 years of the 21st century – while no other demographic group (based on income and neighborhood clusters) experienced similar results [46]. From 2001–2014, changes in life expectancy ranged from gains of more than four years to loses of more than two years comparing wealthier to lower income neighborhoods [46].

The Chetty et.al. study has been touted as a landmark because its findings are based on a quasi-universe rather than a sample of American adults, which means the results may be generalizable to the U.S. adult population. In an editorial accompanying the results, Woolf and Purnell suggest the results are a 'call to arms' for health care professionals to collaborate to improve population health [47]. Yet, in contrast to the first type of health disparities research, the Chetty study's findings are based on a comparatively narrow range of demographic and related independent variables as well as health outcomes. While the study's focus provides robust statistical power, its comparatively limited range suggests a distinctive type of health disparities research as well as a calculated tradeoff [46].

A third type of health disparities research assesses if some socially derived demographic variables have a moderating effect on the associations among sociological, demographic, geographical, environmental predictors and health outcomes. Returning to the Chetty et. al. study, the findings suggest the impact of income and geography as predictive variables in skewed life expectancy can be moderated by community-based efforts that impact specific health behaviors, such as curbing smoking, improving weight control, and fostering exercise [46]. In a review of meta-analyses, Pascoe and Richman found perceived discrimination and resulting stress may be moderated by emotion-focused strategies, changes in healthy eating habits, increased social support, and group identification [48]. In turn, the identification of moderating variables are helpful to future health disparities researchers because they identify evidence-based SES, or other factors, that might contribute to more successful community-based interventions for vulnerable communities. Simultaneously, the identification of moderating effects yield distinctive insights that are not necessarily raised in other health disparities research findings.

A fourth type of health disparities findings identifies how the health of vulnerable populations is impacted by interactions among socially-derived as well as structural variables. In other words, these studies evaluate how sociological, demographic, geographical, or environmental variables interact with structural health determinants.

For example, Currie and Schwandt recently found life expectancy disparities may be influenced by (and associated with) recent improvements in access to health insurance among young Americans [45]. (The access to health insurance among young Americans provides an example of the integration of a structural variable into health disparities research). Currie and Schwandt suggest if declining differences in insurance access are projected to a future adult population, comparative mortality rates (a key dependent variable measure of health disparities) may become less significant [45].

Similarly, the Chetty et.al. study suggests socially-derived SES variables work in conjunction with clinical variables (in this case smoking, exercise, weight control) to impact individual and community health [46].

Overall, these examples (among others) suggest population health outcomes sometimes are associated with multidimensional social and structural health variables – and all may work in conjunction with each other to impact health outcomes. This type of research provides an alternative to health disparities findings where specified independent (or primary, control, or predictor) variables (based on social, environmental, and other predictors) are seen to more directly impact health outcomes.

In addition to the interaction among variables, the fourth type of health disparities research findings suggest extant variables (sociological, demographic, geographical, environmental and structural) may be an intermediate compared to a direct or primary influence on health outcomes.

In short, the fourth type of health disparities findings provides an alternative, conceptual framework to understand the dynamics of health disparities. While some research may narrow the sociological, demographic, geographical, or environmental variables that predict health outcomes, the fourth research genre suggests the range of social and structural variables should be expanded – and researchers should expect most variables to have an intermediate (as opposed to a primary) impact on health outcomes.

To backup momentarily, a variable is classified as 'intermediate' when it results in empirical variation within both a study's dependent and independent research variables. In the Chetty study, the intermediate variables (smoking, exercise, weight control) interact and influence both the dependent variable (mortality) and the independent variables (income/geography SES variables) [46]. Hence, an intermediate association among and between variables in health disparities research suggests there is a degree of variation as well as a conceptual interdependence in modeling how health outcomes interact with social and structural determinants of health.

The finding that both social and structural variables may be interdependent as well as intermediate variables suggests two of the pressing challenges in health disparities research are to holistically conceptualize and assess the empirical associations among social and structural health determinants. Overall, the research provides a foundation to suggest conceptual advances in health disparities research might be enhanced by the addition of evidence-based social and structural determinants of health. In turn, this suggests future health disparities research might strive to be more multidimensional and include variables where there is an emerging evidence-base of health efficacy, such as health literacy.

Before we turn to an overview of health literacy, current initiatives such as the Robert Wood Johnson Foundation's (RWJ) community-based interventions, demonstrate how health disparities research is applied within community-based settings [49]. The RWJ intervention includes diverse initiatives designed to address community education, provide employment, augment food security, build or expand public parks, as well as enable access to better health care, and programs to modify specific health behaviors, such as smoking, obesity, and exercise [49]. While RWJ programs to address community education, provide employment, augment food security, build or expand public parks, and similar efforts are grounded in social (or sociological, demographic, geographical, environmental) determinants of population health, efforts to improve access to health care, and address smoking, weight control, and exercise are grounded in structural and clinical determinants of population health [49].

While a National Academies perspective recently identified the combined RWJ interventions as an example of applied, comprehensive health disparities research, the National Academies perspective added the RWJ initiative additionally illustrates the missing opportunities for collaboration between health disparities and health literacy researchers [1]. The National Academies perspective reports the RWJ interventions do not include health literacy initiatives despite evidence that health literacy interventions have an intermediate impact on health outcomes and the utilization of the health care delivery system (or represent an evidence-based social determinant of health) [1].

On the other hand, the National Academies perspective acknowledges the disciplinary gap is reciprocal – health literacy research often fails to include health disparities research in creating health literacy conceptual frameworks, methodological approaches, and initiatives [1].

While the National Academies perspective notes more research collaboration should be a priority, the perspective adds the lack of cooperation probably is derived from different research funding streams as well as some comparative differences in health literacy's genesis and development [1].

Health literacy's genesis and expansion will be reviewed in the next subsection. Since the author recently reviewed the development of health literacy research, the discussion within the following subsection is somewhat abbreviated [50].

2.3. Health Literacy

This subsection is divided into a discussion of health literacy's distinctive conceptual foundations and an overview of some major research findings is provided. We will explain how some early hypotheses about health literacy were confirmed by a national assessment of health literacy skills, which helped frame some of the current field's research approaches and its separation from health disparities research. The latter provides some additional reasons why health disparities and health literacy research have not been well integrated.

A recent systematic overview of health literacy's research findings suggests health literacy is a social determinant of health [2,3]. While the same systematic review notes health literacy research's future should feature an increased convergence of intermediate variables that include other social determinants of health (e.g. health disparities findings) and some structural determinants of population health, this section suggests the issue whether health literacy is a primary or intermediate variable is foundational to health literacy research's integration within related disciplines [2,3].

First, health literacy has become a self-contained area of study within the broader fields of adult literacy, health education, and health communication [51,52,12]. Health literacy's research interests also dovetail with other disciplines including: numeracy; consumer health informatics; cultural competence; eHealth, mHealth; patient activation; patient health self-management; health information seeking; shared health decision making; health prevention; adult literacy; risk assessment; mass media literacy; community-based health interventions; and the public understanding of science [53–56,51]. The relationships between health literacy and some of the latter areas are covered elsewhere in this book. PubMed's topic-specific query page on health literacy (that provides a gateway to research published in major medical/public health research journals) encompasses many of the aforementioned disciplines and expands as relevant research surfaces from related sub-disciplines [57].

Second, health literacy research and practice are designed to help address an array of enduring clinical and health care delivery system consumer communication challenges such as the understandability of: medical consent forms; medical insurance forms; hospital signage; medical terminology; as well as drug labeling and instructions. Other enduring challenges include the clarity of hospital discharge instructions, and fostering more meaningful patient/provider interpersonal communication interactions. Health literacy research and practice also are associated with broader issues such as: patient and consumer education; patient enablement and empowerment; patient-centered clinical practices; the education and development of health care professionals; plain language; patient adherence to clinical instruction; health care cost containment; palliative care; efficient use of the health care delivery system; and issues such as precision medicine and the public understanding of medical policy initiatives, such as the U.S. Affordable Care Act [58,59,50].

Third, while there is extant evidence that health literacy is a social determinant of health, a recent systematic review suggests health literacy is an intermediate (rather than a primary) as well as a probable moderating variable that impact health outcomes and the utilization of the health care delivery system [2,3]. The implications of these findings for future research are discussed at the end of this subsection.

Although health disparities research focuses on the demographic, sociological, geographic, environmental, and structural variables that skew differences in health outcomes (among vulnerable populations), health literacy's *raison d'etre* remains the challenges most adults have (regardless of demographic, socio-economic, or geographical underpinnings) to understand medical terms, seek information, as well as the enduring frustrations that are byproducts of utilizing the health care delivery system [50,52,53]. Health literacy's foundation also includes the residual socio-economic, clinical, and public health impact of consumer frustration, misunderstanding, disinterest, disengagement, anxiety, and anomie in dealing with personal illness and clinical care [50,52,53].

Other pressing reasons to improve the nation's health literacy (as well as address the impact of low health literacy on public health and medical care) are introduced within a recent executive order to create a health literacy partnership within a U.S. state [60]. The governor of Alabama's 2016 executive order explains almost nine out of ten Americans have difficulty understanding and actualizing the health information that is routinely available through the news media, advertising, commercial health products, and from health care facilities. The executive order notes adults with low health literacy are twice as likely as others to be hospitalized, are more likely to have chronic health issues, and are less likely to seek treatment. The executive order adds as health care costs rise, low health literacy is estimated to add as much as $238 billion to an overburdened U.S. health care system [60].

While a health literacy leitmotif may not be prominent within Dickens' novels or Chaplin's films, prior to the use of the term 'health literacy' Nelkin as well as Gregory and Miller explained the public's understanding of health and medicine was a latent barrier (as well as a potential facilitator) to improve U.S. public health and medical care [61,62]. While some generalizable findings in the late 20th century suggested a dearth of knowledge about science among most Americans, the first empirically rigorous assessment of the public understanding of health and medicine did not occur until the National Assessment of Adult Literacy (NAAL) in 2003 [63,64]. In short, the extent of the public's understanding of health and medicine was not empirically exposed until the early 21st century.

The NAAL, which remains the only generalizable evaluation of health literacy in the U.S., found 88 percent of Americans either had below basic, basic, or an intermediate understanding of basic medical terms and information. Only 12 percent of Americans were proficient in understanding medical terms or information [63,65]. Other international research findings suggest similar low levels of health literacy in diverse nations [65–67,53,6].

While most of the latter research provides demographic breakdowns, the findings are more generalizable to the full sample instead of demographic segments (or subpopulations) within many national and international health literacy assessments.

Prior to the NAAL and similar findings, Leonard and Ceci Doak (health literacy's U.S. pioneers) hypothesized that an adult's age, income, educational attainment, and adult literacy levels may not predict his or her understanding of medicine, medical terms, as well as consumer interest in seeking information about health and medicine [68,60,70,71]. The Doaks' informal hypothesis also suggested that demographics might be *less* associated with high literacy proficiency than the health disparities literature might suggest [68–71]. In other words, the Doaks' hypothesis inferred health literacy's diffusion within subpopulations was somewhat inconsistent with the patterns suggested in health disparities research. While the Doaks noted that low health literacy was omnipresent within vulnerable populations, they added low health literacy was ubiquitous among all social classes and backgrounds [68–71]. Since the mixed findings in the NAAL and similar international studies suggest a suboptimal health literacy proficiency is consistent among undifferentiated large populations with more mixed results for subpopulations, health literacy's dispersion seems to be characterized by *both* its population similarities and differences. In short as the Doaks suggested, health literacy's population distribution has some similarities as well as important differences compared to the skew towards vulnerable populations found in health disparities research.

Prior to the NAAL, the Doaks also suggested health literacy was conceptually distinctive from adult literacy and each should be measured as separate constructs (rather than co-mingled or used interchangeably as surrogate measures) to assess the capacity of the public to understand health and medicine [68–71].

In contemporary practice, *adult literacy* often is perceived as a combination of reading skills, document comprehension, writing skills, as well as functional abilities to understand pragmatic information, such as directions, instructions, numerical descriptions, and maps [72,52]. In contrast, *health literacy* focuses on a different set of abilities, skills, tasks, and conceptual underpinnings within clinical care, public health, health care management, patient/consumer, home, and other health information seeking contexts [72,52]. Nutbeam described health literacy skills within three categories: functional/technical skills (ability to read and understand numbers); interactive/social skills (listening, speaking); and critical thinking skills (the ability to integrate information within new life situations and challenges) [72]. The complexity of the latter additional skills suggests why adult literacy training sometimes is not perceived as surrogate for health literacy training among health educators and other practitioners.

In addition, the Doaks' suggestion that health literacy and adult literacy should be assessed as different research constructs (and not used interchangeably as surrogate measures) was operationalized within the NAAL's methodological approach – and partially bolstered by its findings. The NAAL findings suggested that health literacy, adult reading skills, as well as other literacy levels of U.S. adults were somewhat inconsistent [63,65,67]. The levels of health literacy proficiency (or the ability to understand medical terms and information) were somewhat differentiated from the other measures of adult reading skills [63,65,67]. So, besides a methodological separation of health and adult reading skills, the NAAL findings provided some initial evidence that the measurement of health literacy should be more grounded in measures tailored to assess health literacy than adult literacy. The latter distinction is noteworthy because adult literacy is significantly associated with educational attainment, which is a foundational demographic variable in health disparities research.

In recent years, the expansion of a literature that assesses health literacy instruments (quantitative, applied measures of health literacy) – and raises questions about which instrument to use – suggests a tacit consensus that health literacy is not a surrogate measure of adult literacy and suggests health literacy constructs should be utilized to measure the public understanding of health and medicine [73,50]. As a result, the separation of adult reading skills and health literacy into different constructs may have fostered a proliferation of 21st century, self-contained health literacy measures as well as a de-emphasis on the utilization of health disparities measures and approaches in health literacy interventions [73,53].

The separation of health literacy and adult literacy into self-contained research constructs also is conceptually important because it yields more insights about why some aspects of health disparities and health literacy research evolved separately in recent years.

Essentially, if health literacy and adult literacy are empirically independent constructs, this suggests adult literacy is not necessarily an integral component of an evidence-based health literacy conceptual framework. If adult literacy can be omitted, then, this justifies the possible exclusion of the demographic variables to which it is closely related, such as educational attainment, as well as some of the sociological, demographic, geographic, and environmental variables that are associated with both educational attainment as well as other disparate health outcomes. Hence, the exclusion of adult literacy and rejection of it as a surrogate measure of health literacy creates both conceptual as well as operationalized approaches that encourage researchers to adopt health literacy measures as self-contained independent variables. Conversely, if health literacy and adult literacy were analogous constructs, additional measures based on educational attainment (that are linked to variables used in health disparities research) might have been more valued and seen as part of an integrated, evidence-based, conceptual research framework.

Turning now to the reasons for the health care delivery system's 21st century burst of interest in health literacy, the appeal of health literacy initiatives and research was accelerated by a convergence of elements including: the aforementioned population research that suggested widespread, low health literacy levels; health information/communication technological developments (such as eHealth and mHealth); the initial research findings about health literacy's desirable impact on patient and health administrative outcomes; the comparative advantages of health literacy as a tactic of clinical, organizational, and social intervention; as well as a self-perpetuating momentum derived from increasing government and private health care organizational interest [74–76,50,12]. Regarding the latter example, the U.S. Joint Commission's (the National Committee for Quality Assurance) inclusion of health literacy within their accreditation standards in 2011 reinforced that health literacy initiatives and interventions represented pragmatic strategies to address clinical care and broader administrative health related issues [77]. In the U.S., recent innovations in the Affordable Care Act, such as Patient Centered Medical Homes and Accountable Care Organizations, also encouraged a new range of programs and institutional accountability that recommended some health literacy initiatives and evaluation research [78,79,12].

In addition, the comparative advantages of health literacy as a tactic of clinical, organizational, and social intervention was fostered by evidence that suggested therapeutic patient and public health outcomes might be generated by comparatively modest (e.g. less expensive) interventions designed to: boost patient and community understanding of health and specific conditions; foster more health self-management skills; improve quality of patient interaction at key points of health care interaction (such as prior to hospital discharge); and generate health information seeking (often using new, less costly digital technologies). In turn, health literacy interventions seemed to provide a portfolio of pragmatic and affordable strategies for health care organizations to consider – especially when planning health care delivery outreach initiatives and interventions [50].

The progress in health literacy research was described in a landmark systematic review from the U.S. Agency for Healthcare Research and Quality (AHRQ) published in 2011 [2,3]. Among other important findings, the AHRQ systematic review initially found low health literacy was associated with some important health challenges, such as improved health status and reduced mortality rates [2,3].

Koh et. al. and Bailey, Oramasionwu, and Wolf added some of the clinical benefits linked to health literacy interventions include: reduced mortality; improved patient adherence to medical instructions; and overall patient safety [79,80]. In a summary of research findings, the National Network of Libraries of Medicine noted health literacy interventions therapeutically assisted patients with cancer, diabetes, asthma, and hypertension [81].

In addition, the aforementioned AHRQ systematic review of health literacy research found an array of health care delivery challenges associated with low health literacy, such as: increased hospitalizations; more use of emergency care; and a reduced ability to understand both medication labels and health messages [2,3]. Koh et. al. added some health literacy interventions were linked to improved utilization of the health care delivery system [79]. Koh et .al. noted other specific health administrative benefits linked to health literacy interventions included: improved diabetes patient self-management skills; more use of preventive services; as well as a reduction in hospitalization and re-hospitalization rates (which in aggregate lower medical costs) [79].

In addition to noting some specific examples of health literacy's impact, the AHRQ systematic review suggested there is a sufficient evidence base to support the hypothesis that health literacy is a socially-derived determinant of population health [2,3].

Conversely, the evidence was more mixed whether health literacy (as an independent research construct) is a primary variable that influences outcomes, or whether health literacy is an intermediate variable that interacts with other social and structural determinants of health [2,3]. The issue is important to health literacy research's future because hypothetically, if health literacy is a primary, or robust, predictor of outcomes, then, this evidence justifies a continued separation of health literacy and health disparities research into self-contained research framing and methods. However, if health literacy is an intermediate variable that is interdependent with other socially-derived and structural determinants of health others (as discussed earlier), this suggests a need for more integration of health literacy and health disparities research framing and methods – and moving away from conceiving health literacy and health disparities as separate research challenges and questions.

Some evidence that health literacy might be a primary variable was suggested by Baker's findings in 2006 [82]. At a conference sponsored by the U.S. Office of the Surgeon General, Baker reported health literacy (measured as an independent construct) was a robust predictor of patient health, such as mortality and self-reported health status, as well as a few health care administrative outcomes, such as hospitalization rates, even when compared to traditional demographic predictors of health outcomes [82]. Moreover, Baker suggested health literacy was a robust predictor of desirable patient and health administrative outcomes even after controlling for social-demographic variables, such as income and educational attainment [82].

The evidence that health literacy may be an intermediate (as well as a moderating) variable was suggested by the more recent and comprehensive AHRQ systematic review [2,3]. The AHRQ systematic review suggested health literacy should be conceptually modeled as one among other possible social and structural variables that interact to predict health outcomes, or impact the use of the health care delivery system [2,3].

While acknowledging the current evidence is insufficient to provide a definitive position, the aforementioned National Academies perspective recently suggested that health literacy is: a) a social determinant of health and b) probably is an intermediate and moderating variable that interacts with other social determinants of health (often represented by the variables used in health disparities research) as well as the structural variables discussed earlier [1].

Assuming the National Academies perspective (and AHRQ systematic review) are reinforced by future research, it seems prudent to encourage researchers to seek an integration of social and structural determinants of population health in health literacy research rather than operationalize health literacy as a more singular, primary variable. Using the salutogenic conceptual foundation that was discussed at the start of this section, it also seems timely for research to take a multidimensional and multidisciplinary view when assessing social and structural determinants of population health in research planning, framing, methods, and implementation.

However, it also is important for future researchers to remain mindful that the larger topic of health literacy's integration or separation from health disparities research remains an important issue in advancing the research within both subdisciplines.

Finally, both health literacy and health disparities are challenged by an array of identified research gaps and methodological issues that undermine progress within both fields. Some of these research gaps and methodological issues research will be discussed in the next section. However, the intent is more to more to identify existing opportunities for researchers in both research areas rather than critique current shortcomings.

3. Opportunities in Health Disparities and Health Literacy Research

While overviews of health disparities and health literacy research describe some of the diversity and vitality of research in both fields, some significant evidence gaps and resulting needs in each area also have been identified [5,73,50]. This section introduces some of current evidence gaps that have been acknowledged in health disparities and health literacy research respectively. The intent is to encourage researchers to interpret the suggested evidence gaps or challenges as opportunities to elevate the authority and credibility of both disciplines.

Turning first to health disparities research, a U.S. National Academies health indicators report suggested revising an array of measures that provide foundational structural and demographic health information [83]. The National Academies report also suggests some current definitions and operationalization of variables within areas of structural and demographic health outcomes do not provide a foundation for high quality data that is needed in public and population health research, which includes health disparities [83]. For example, the National Academies report provided and defined revised measures of health outcomes, such as: life expectancy at birth; infant mortality; life expectancy at age 65; injury related mortality; self-reported health status; unhealthy days physical and mental; chronic disease prevalence; and serious psychological distress [83]. The report provided and defined revised measures of common health outcomes, such as: smoking; physical activity; excessive drinking; nutrition; obesity; and condom use [83]. The report provided and defined revised measures of health system activities, such as: health care expenditures; insurance coverage; unmet medical, dental, and prescription drug needs; use of preventive services; childhood immunization; and preventable hospitalizations [83].

While the National Academies health indicators report did not provide revised definitions of specific measures of the social determinants of health, the report emphasized future efforts were needed to create revised measures in both health disparities research and the larger field of population health [83]. Overall, the health indicators report strongly suggests the current measures of social and structural determinants of health are not optimal to provide needed insights about national trends especially for systematic reviews grounded in data aggregation and harmonization [83]. In turn, this suggests there are important challenges to improve basic research about population health and health disparities and the status quo of current research methods needs some reconsideration.

Similarly, the aforementioned AHRQ's health literacy systematic review suggested health literacy research needs more conceptual consistency, more research about its underlying measures, and a new emphasis on best research practices to generate data sets that provide a better foundation for future research as well as systematic analyses [2,3].

Regarding health literacy's current conceptual inconsistencies, most attention within this area focuses on the proliferation of health literacy definitions and the current lack of a consensus definition. For example, in a landmark paper, Sørensen et. al. outlined an array of health literacy definitions and noted how each reflected underlying differences in conceptual frameworks that included clinical practice versus public health and other perspectives [6].

While Sorensen et. al. and Pleasant agreed that the subtle differences among health literacy definitions and underlying conceptual models suggested the field's conceptual diversity, they countered the lack of a consensus about health literacy's definition –

coupled with diverse underlying conceptual models – inadvertently challenge the field's long range scholarly credibility and gravitas [6,73]. There is more discussion about this issue in Sorensen's and Pleasant's chapter within the current book.

Although the author adopted the Calgary Charter definition in this chapter's introduction, Pleasant adds the current inconsistencies among and between basic health literacy definitions can confuse researchers, and suggests the field lacks a sense of direction or scholarly leadership [84,8].

A recent National Academies perspective explains while it is difficult to reach a consensus definition of health literacy, the perspective outlines some of the underlying issues that need to be resolved in order to achieve a consensus definition [7].

To backup, one of health literacy's current research and conceptual gaps is to answer a foundational question: what is health literacy and how should it be defined?

In addition to a missing consensus definition, Pleasant notes there is a pressing need for more research regarding the quantitative rigor of health literacy's underlying measures [73,84]. Pleasant and others explained many of the health literacy field's diverse definitions and conceptual models fostered the use of diverse and sometimes incompatible research instruments [84–86,73]. Haun et. al. recently described the diversity of the 51 health literacy measures as 'instrument proliferation' [85, p. 301]. Similar to the Agency for Healthcare Research and Quality's systematic review, Pleasant explained current diverse and often incompatible research instruments make it difficult to aggregate research findings as well as compare results that might yield more systematic insights about conceptual models and instruments [2,3,84].

Pleasant and McCormack, Haun, Sorensen, & Valerio also found many health literacy quantitative research instruments have not been undergirded by basic research that demonstrates their psychometric rigor [87,73,84]. In a systematic review, Altin, Finke, Kautz-Freimuth, & Stock recently found only 17 articles focused on the development and validation of 17 health literacy instruments [88]. Pleasant suggests the latter issues inhibit investigators' abilities to make informed choices about which health literacy instrument (and underlying conceptual model) are optimal to use [73,84,85].

As a remedy, O'Neill, Goncalves, Ricci-Cabello, and Ziebland, Altin et. al., Haun et. al., McCormack et. al., and Pleasant noted a need for conceptual transparency as well as more basic research and validation studies about health literacy's diverse instruments [87–89,84,85,73].

Soon after these critiques were published, healthliteracy.bu.edu was launched to provide a clearinghouse of health literacy measures as well as links to the extant validation research undergirding each measure. While healthliteracy.bu.edu is a direct response to providing more transparency about the rigor of the common health literacy instruments, the site's future success depends on the expansion of basic research regarding health literacy's research instruments. Full disclosure: the author was involved in the creation of healthlitercy.bu.edu.

More broadly, Dewalt and Hink found while there is an abundance of health literacy initiatives, there is a comparative dearth of evidence-based assessments of health literacy interventions [90]. Abrams, Klass, and Dreyer found a similar dearth of evidence-based assessments of health literacy interventions especially within community-based interventions tailored to low literacy populations [91]. In aggregate, both findings suggest one of health literacy's most significant challenges is to increase the use of evidence-based research to assess the impact of clinical or community interventions.

The extant literature also identifies specific areas or topics within health care delivery and patient care where there is a dearth of health literacy evidence and scholarship. While the implication of much of this literature is health literacy cannot evolve as a field of study until these areas receive more scrutiny, each identified area opens an opportunity for future researchers.

For example, Koh et. al. identified a range of research needs in health care administrative settings such as: how intra-organizational communication affects the processes and outcomes for health care organizations that seek to be more health literate; what interpersonal and/or organizational strategies help reduce the burden on individuals to manage their own medical care, and how health information systems best engage patients and caregivers by providing easily understandable, personalized medical record data as well as other clinical information [78].

Koh et. al. added health administrators additionally need health literacy research about areas such as: how health literacy (in conjunction with health communication and health information technology) contribute to more shared decision making between patients and providers, and how health literacy strategies create personalized self-management tools and resources for patients [78]. Koh et. al. found more health literacy research is needed regarding the creation of accurate, accessible, and actionable health information that is targeted or tailored for specialized populations, such as medically underserved audiences [78].

For U.S.-based researchers, Koh et. al. added there are an array of health literacy needs and opportunities to evaluate how health literacy interventions and initiatives advance initiatives introduced within the U.S. Affordable Care Act, such as accountable care organizations and patient centered medical homes [78].

Turning to narrower clinical and health care organizational needs, Aldoory, Ryan and Rouhain recently reported a dearth of health literacy research (and evidence) to guide the creation of understandable informed consent forms provided to U.S. patients within clinical settings [92]. Aldoory et. al. implied the evidence gaps were surprising given the enduring importance of informed consent to patient safety and welfare [92].

Similarly, Rudd recently noted more health literacy research (and evidence) is needed in specific patient-clinical exposure areas such as: unnecessarily dense and complex forms (e.g. hospital entry, consent and discharge forms); clear signage; and enhancing the capacity of visitors to navigate building entrances, passageways, and destination points within hospitals, clinics, and other health care organizations [93].

Rudd noted there is little health literacy research about health care organizational/patient communication practices, such as the creation of a more cheerful, empathetic environment in which health care is delivered in medical offices, hospitals, clinics, and other health care organizations [93].

More broadly, still within health care organizations, Rudd added more health literacy research is needed in areas such as: the clarity of written and spoken clinical communication; assessments of the comparative degree of difficulty of written and posted health information routinely distributed by medical centers; the barriers that discourage people from health information seeking (such as problematic websites, phone interactions, poor maps and signage); and the mismatch between the literacy demands of health materials (written or on-line) and the literacy skills of adults with a secondary school education [93].

Rudd also explained more health literacy research is needed within specific areas of patient/provider communication such as: the reading tasks required of patients; understanding patient reading levels; enhancing the clarity of written and spoken communication; removing clinical jargon between health care organizations and culturally diverse audiences; as well as the impact of a health care professional's communication skills on health literacy and patient health outcomes [93]. Rudd added there are evidence gaps in diverse areas such as: the rigorous pilot testing of materials intended for consumers and patients; the measurement and ranking of the communication skills of clinical and health care professionals; and theory driven research based on assessments of consumer and patient interventions [93].

Regarding other scholarly frontiers, the author recently noted the need for research that bridges the conceptual overlaps and gaps among health literacy research and allied fields, such as health communication, and consumer health informatics [50,51]. As health information technology evolves and is used to monitor clinical biometrics, inform targeted audiences about health, as well as modify health-related behaviors, there is a pressing need for cross-disciplinary research that embraces consumer health informatics, health communication, and health literacy. There also may be a need to embrace research in related disciplines, such as the public understanding of science.

Overall, this section identifies specific topics and areas where health literacy and health disparities research is needed within diverse areas of clinical care, population health, and health care administration in addition to research that bridges multidisciplinary boundaries. The array of aforementioned topics suggests there are plentiful challenges for future health literacy and health disparities research, which provide opportunities to address existing questions, provide evidence, and furnish new frontiers.

4. Seeking an Expanded, Multidimensional Conceptual Framework of Health Disparities and Health Literacy Research

The fourth section, seeking an expanded, multidimensional conceptual approach to health literacy and health disparities research, begins with summaries drawn from the previous subsections and then, provides two examples where some integration has occurred. This is followed by a brief discussion of the similarities between the selected example of health literacy/health disparities expansion and a recent commentary that encourages more integrated research in population health and palliative care.

The previous sections of this chapter strongly suggest an expanded, multidimensional approach to health disparities and health literacy research is desirable partially because the diverse structural and social determinants of health are not mutually exclusive, and probably do not function in isolation. A tenet of the literature that describes structural and social determinants of health is that each of these areas are omnipresent, and each partially helps determine health, or may become part of the everyday experience that occurs when consumers access the health care delivery system.

This strongly suggests that conceptually and operationally, structural and social determinants of health overlap in matters of population and personal health. For example, a conceptual modeling of how demographic differences impact life expectancy probably is not limited to the identified, intervening variables of income and geography within health disparities research. Health disparities findings add there may be array of other sociological, demographic, geographic, and environmental factors that impact life expectancy and health outcomes. In addition, health literacy research suggests health and health care utilization outcomes (but not necessarily life expectancy) may be impacted by an array of underlying factors, such as: chronic misunderstandings of medical terms and instructions among users of the health care delivery system; poor tailoring of health materials to patient or caregiver needs; and the anxiety created by an illness and seeking treatment. Similarly, health outcomes (but not necessarily life expectancy) are indirectly impacted by quality of care issues, including: access to care; the quality of clinical research; as well other structural factors. While health disparities, health literacy, and structural challenges within the health care delivery system may or may not predict individual and population health, each may have a role in health's overall determination.

As structural and social determinants are omnipresent, this begs the broader question if they also are interdependent. The latter point is important since if structural and social determinants are interdependent then, research approaches and methods should encompass a range of interactions that traverse structural and social dimensions.

While the National Academies health indicators report did not suggest health literacy, health disparities, and structural dimensions are interdependent, the report recommends more inclusive research that integrates structural and social outcome variables [83]. The National Academies health indicators report suggests the horizon of future research is to conceive and operationalize population health in terms of more comprehensive approaches [83].

As aforementioned, some evidence that health literacy and health disparities (as social determinants of health and empirical variables) may be interdependent is suggested by the characterization of each dimension as representing intermediate and moderating variables. Since intermediate and moderating variables interact with independent and dependent research measures, this suggests that social and structural dimensions influence health's antecedents and outcomes both in quantitative findings and within research settings. Either way, an underlying research issue that needs to be addressed is the degree of interdependence as well as the interactions among health literacy and health disparities variables within specific settings, such as community based interventions, to improve the health and quality of life among vulnerable populations. The uncertainty about the interdependence among social and structural dimensions of health within community interventions or population health initiatives remains a core challenge in the future of health literacy and health disparities research both as individual and possibly collaborative areas of inquiry.

Currently, life skills progression (LSP) research and the NUKA health care approaches by the Southcentral Foundation provide at least two examples of interventions that combine social and structural dimensions as well as suggest future integrative research and practice pathways.

Using Wollensen and Peifer's life skills progression (LSP) conceptual framework, Smith focuses on a secondary analysis of social work, home visitation interventions for a vulnerable population (lower income homes often with single mothers) [94,95]. While LSP research is based on home visitation rather than community-based interventions and the research approach does not use conventional health literacy assessment tools, the LSP findings suggest how expanded conceptual approaches yield insights about the framing of interventions for vulnerable audiences as well as the contributions of structural and social dimensions to health outcomes [95].

For example, the dimensions within the research design in LSP interventions encompass some health disparities, health literacy, structural, as well as other variables. As a dimension, health disparities is assessed by variables such as: housing; food; transportation; insurance; language; education; employment; income; reading level;

and self-esteem [95–97]. Maternal health literacy is assessed by a composite of surrogate measures such as improvements in: health information seeking; reflective questioning about health; self care; enablement; and empowerment [95–97]. The structural dimensions of health are assessed by variables such as: use of health services and community resources; preventive practices suggested by a Healthcare Literacy Scale; prenatal care; maternal sick care; and child dental care [95–97].

Life skills progression research provides four tiers of findings that first, suggest improving maternal health literacy is associated with improvements in parental and child health [95–96]. Second, the findings suggest there are significant empirical associations (or interactions) among health disparities, health literacy, and structural variables [94]. Third, the findings suggest health disparities variables vary in their contribution to health outcomes [95–97]. Interestingly, immigration status, reading levels, and less than 12th grade education are less associated with outcomes than other demographic measures. Fourth, the findings suggest structural, health literacy, and health disparities dimensions may be interdependent, or statistically converge to improve family health outcomes [95–97].

Overall, the LSP findings demonstrate how a framework can be developed to assess some of the interactions across the social and structural dimensions that are discussed within this chapter. More details about the LSP findings and research approach are explained in a different chapter within this book.

While LSP focuses on interventions in non-clinical settings, the Southcentral Foundation's NUKA system of care integrates health's social, structural, and cultural dimensions within a medical center's routine health delivery to vulnerable populations (Alaska Natives) [98,99]. NUKA (a Native Alaskan word for 'giant structures and living things') tries to address health care's 'three aims' (improve patient experiences, health, and restrain costs) via screening for health's social, structural, and cultural dimensions and responding to operant individual and family needs [98].

The NUKA approach to integrated care is more than incorporating physical and mental health interdisciplinary teams within patient care. The NUKA approach includes routine health interventions that address structural health dimensions such as: significantly reducing patient waiting times; improving immediate access to clinicians and other specialists; creating innovative relationships among patients and providers; as well as rethinking how to listen to patients [98–99]. It includes routine interventions that address health disparities such as: strategies designed to revitalize treatments for mental and emotional health; and projects designed to build a sense of community heritage and pride [98,99]. NUKA includes routine interventions that address health literacy such as: learning circles that attempt to significantly boost patient engagement; education about specific issues such as spousal and child abuse, alcoholism, and obesity; and encouraging providers to help patients understand their diagnoses or condition [98,99]. NUKA also includes routine interventions that address individual and community health needs as well as conventional patient care [98,99].

Essentially, the NUKA approach to integrated care partially incorporates health disparities, health literacy, behavioral health, immediate clinical needs, prevention, wellness, and cost savings interventions simultaneously, depending on individual, family, or neighborhood requirements. As a result, the NUKA approach additionally provides a clinically based organizational template for some of the expanded research models and intervention assessments that are suggested within this chapter.

Moreover, the NUKA approach to care suggests a busy medical center and health care delivery system can frame care in terms of building relationships that seek to improve a patient's quality of life and personal development across their life course, foster community development, as well as treat a patient's disease or condition. Similarly, the LSP interventions are grounded in efforts to improve a client's quality of life as well as their personal development as a foundation to enhance the treatment of patient clinical needs.

In both the LSP and NUKA examples, the conceptual framing of individual and population health reflects 'a more comprehensive and holistic picture of life,' as recently discussed by Casarett and Teno [100]. Casarett and Teno add that a more comprehensive and holistic concept of life also fosters a foundation for the increased integration of population health and palliative care research and practice [100]. Hence, the links between the integration of health's social and structural dimensions that are identified in this chapter may parallel suggestions to integrate other population health fields. This additionally suggests an integrated conceptual framework is attracting interest as a strategy to enhance the future of research and practice within health care.

5. Conclusion

At present, there are foundational areas of clinical, public health, and health administration with evidence gaps and where health disparities and health literacy research has yet to occur, basic research needs to be conducted, and inconsistent results suggest a need for further research [92,73,87,2,3]. As research constructs, health disparities and health literacy also are currently best described as intermediate, moderating research variables that are associated with therapeutic individual, social, cultural, clinical, and health care organizational outcomes.

As aforementioned, the horizon for research is to integrate health's social and structural dimensions more holistically and assess the degree social and structural dimensions may or may not be interdependent in influencing health outcomes and care utilization. The NUKA and LSP examples additionally suggest social and structural dimensions can be part of a broader effort to nurture health and well being as well as integrate clinical care with services that often are currently seen as provided by social work, public health initiatives, educational development, public works, and other areas that impact human development.

Overall for health disparities and health literacy researchers, this is both a daunting and exciting time to enter fields where vital issues and questions are irresolute and the potential for imaginative research and practice is multidimensional and expansive. The future challenge of health disparities and health literacy research is to frame and assess interventions in diverse communities and provide more tailored, theory-based, and constructive interventions. At the same time, the chapter suggests the future challenge of health disparities and health literacy research is to advance as well as reinvent both fields via collaborative efforts and more integrated theoretical foundations, constructs, and operations.

Finally, a future opportunity for health disparities and health literacy researchers is the creation of international academic organizations that seek to foster collaborative research and practice. Currently, both health disparities and health disparities (as arenas of research and practice) need a member-based, international, academic infrastructure to host periodic meetings, publish refereed journals, provide news about research and practice to members, encourage practitioner-scholar, practitioner-practitioner, scholar-scholar dialogue, establish leadership, provide a clearinghouse for practitioner services, such as the Institute for Healthcare Advancement's health literacy listserv, and organize both fields into a more coherent whole [101].

While some of these needs may be served by existing international conferences and organizations, progress might be accelerated by the development of a focal point for interaction and diffusion among the world's health disparities and literacy researchers and practitioners. In addition, the lack of a central organization to define health literacy and health disparities research collaboration and professionalism lets the fields' future be defined externally – by clinical medicine, public health, and other disciplines its scholars and practitioners represent. Certainly, the development of an international health disparities and literacy disciplinary infrastructure to elevate research and practice standards (similar to professional societies in clinical, medical administration, public health, and social science disciplines) remains an area where future researchers can contribute to the evolution, growth, gravitas, and success of both fields.

References

[1] Logan RA, Wong WF, Villaire M, Daus G., Parnell TA, Willis E, Paasche-Orlow MK. Health literacy: a necessary element for achieving health equity. Discussion Paper. Washington, D.C.: National Academies of Sciences Engineering Medicine, 2015. http://www.nam.edu/perspectives/2015/Health-literacy-a-necessary-element-for-achieving-health-equity.

[2] Agency for Healthcare Research and Quality. Health literacy interventions and outcomes: an updated systematic review. Rockville, MD. Agency for Healthcare Research and Quality, Evidence report/technology assessment number 199; 2011. http://www.ahrq.gov/downloads/pub/evidence/pdf/literacy/literacyup.pdf

[3] Berkman ND, Sheridan SL, Donahue KE, Halpern DJ, Viera A, Crotty K, Holland A, Brasure M, Lohr KN, Harden E, Tant E, Wallace I, & Viswanathan M. Health literacy interventions and outcomes: an updated systematic review. Evidence Report/Technology Assessment No. 199. RTI International-University of North Carolina Evidence-based Practice Center under contract No. 290-2007-10056-I. AHRQ Publication Number 11-E006. Rockville, MD.: Agency for Healthcare Research and Quality; 2011.

[4] Halvorson G. Ending racial, ethnic, and cultural disparities in American Health Care. N. Charleston: CreateSpace Independent Publishing Platform; 2013.

[5] Barr DA. Health disparities in the United States: social class, race, ethnicity & health. 2nd ed. Baltimore: Johns Hopkins University Press; 2014.

[6] Sorensen K, Van den Broucke S, Fullam J, Doyle G, Pelikan J, Slonska Z, Brand H. HLS-EU Consortium Health Literacy Project European. Health literacy and public health: A systematic review and integration of definitions and models. BMC Public Health. 2012;12(80). DOI:10.1186/1471-2458/12/80.

[7] Pleasant A, Rudd RE, O'Leary C, Paasche-Orlow MK, Allen MP, Alvarado-Little W, Myers L, Parson K, Rosen S. Considerations for a new definition of health literacy. Washington: National Academy of Medicine; 2016. https://nam.edu/considerations-for-a-new-definition-of-health-literacy/

[8] http://www.centreforliteracy.qc.ca/health_literacy/calgary_charter. Retrieved August 4, 2016.

[9] Lindstrom B, Eriksson M. Salutogenesis. J Epidemiol Community Health. 2005; 59(6): 440–42.

[10] Penman-Aguilar A, Talih M, Huang D, Moonesinghe R, Bouye K, Beckles, G. Measurement of Health Disparities, Health Inequities, and Social Determinants of Health to Support the Advancement of Health Equity. J Public Health Manag Pract. 2016;22 Suppl 1:S33-42. DOI: 10.1097/PHH.0000000000000373.

[11] http://www.cdc.gov/minorityhealth/chdireport.html. Retrieved September 2, 2016.

[12] Parker RM, Ratzen SC. Health literacy: a second decade of distinctions for Americans. J Health Commun. 2010;15 Suppl 2:20–33. doi: 10.1080/10810730.2010.501094.

[13] Paasche-Orlow MK, Wolf MS. 2010. Promoting health literacy research to reduce disparities. J Health Commun. 2010; 15 Suppl 2:34–41. DOI: 10.1080/10810730.2010.499994.

[14] Collins FS, Varmus H. A new initiative on precision medicine. N Engl J Medicine. 2015;372 (9):793–795. DOI: 10.1056/NEJMp1500523.

[15] https://www.nih.gov/precision-medicine-initiative-cohort-program/scale-scope. Retrieved August 20, 2016.

[16] Weeks WB, Weinstein JN. Unraveled: prescriptions to repair a broken health system. N. Charlestown: CreateSpace Independent Publishing Platform; 2016.

[17] Nutbeam D The evolving concept of health literacy. Soc Sci Med. 2008; 67:2072–78. DOI: 10.1016/j.socscimed.2008.09.050.

[18] Institute of Medicine of the National Academies. Crossing the quality chasm: A new health system for the 21st century. Washington, D.C.: The National Academies Press, 2001.

[19] Berwick DM. A user's manual for the IOM 'quality chasm' report. Health Aff. 2002;21(3):80–90.

[20] Unger JM, Cook E, Tai E, Bleyer A. The role of clinical trial participation in cancer research: barriers, evidence, and strategies. Am Soc Clin Oncol Educ Book. 2015; 35:185–98. DOI: 10.14694/EDBK_156686.

[21] Hartung DM, Zarin DA, Guise JM, McDonaugh M, Paynter R, Helfand M. Reporting discrepancies between the ClinicalTrials.gov database and peer-reviewed publications. Ann Intern Med. 2014;160(7):477–83. DOI: 10.7326/M13-0480.

[22] Baker M. 1500 scientists lift the lid on reproducibility. Nature. 2016;533(7604): 452–54. DOI:10.1038/533452a

[23] Freedman LP, Inglese J. The increasing urgency for standards in basic biological research. 2014; Cancer Res.74(15):4024–9. DOI: 10.1158/0008-5472.CAN-14-0925.

[24] Demoly P, Passalacqua G, Pfaar O, Sastre J, Wahn U. Patient engagement and patient support programs in allergy immunotherapy: a call to action for improving long-term adherence. Allergy Asthma Clin Immunol. 2016; 29(12): 34. DOI: 10.1186/s13223-016-0140-2

[25] Shah MH. Prior authorization: undermining our health care system. J Med Assoc Ga. 2015;104(2):3.

[26] Makary MA, Daniel M. Medical error-the third leading cause of death in the US. BMJ. 2016; 353:i2139. DOI: 10.1136/bmj.i2139.

[27] Kohn LT, Corrigan JM, Donaldson MS, editors. To err is human: building a safer health system. Washington, D.C.: The National Academies Press, 2000.

[28] http://www.healthnewsreview.org/2016/05/superficial-coverage-of-medical-errors-could-leave-erroneous-impression-with-readers/. Retrieved September 1, 2016.

[29] Mitchell JJ Jr. The findings of the Dartmouth Atlas Project: a challenge to clinical and ethical excellence in end-of-life care. J Clin Ethics Fall. 2011; 22(3): 267–76.

[30] Gessert CE, Haller IV, Johnson BP. Regional variation in care at the end of life: discontinuation of dialysis. BMC Geriatr. 2013;13:39. DOI: 10.1186/1471-2318-13-39.

[31] O'Hare AM, Rodriguez RA, Halipern SM, Larson EB, Kurella TM. (2010). Regional variation in health care intensity and treatment practices for end-stage renal disease in older adults. JAMA. 2010;304 (2):180–6. doi: 10.1001/jama.2010.924.

[32] Tsai TC, Joynt KE, Orav EJ, Gawande AA, Jha AK. Variation in surgical readmission rates and quality of hospital care. N Engl J Med. 2013;369(12):1134–42. DOI: 10.1056/NEJMsa1303118.

[33] Nguyen OK, Halm EA, Makam AN. Relationship between hospital financial performance and public reported outcomes. J Hosp Med. 2016;11(7): 481–8. DOI: 10.1002/jhm.2570.

[34] Gawande A. Complications: a surgeon's notes on an imperfect science. New York: Metropolitan Books; 2002.

[35] Gawande A. The cost conundrum; what a Texas town can teach us about health care. http://www.newyorker.com/magazine/2009/06/01/the-cost-conundrum. 2009. Retrieved September 2, 2016.

[36] https://kaiserfamilyfoundation.files.wordpress.com/2013/01/8396.pdf. Retrieved September 2, 2016.

[37] Ratzan SC (2015). The future of health communication: innovating through partnerships. Metode Science Studies Journal. 2015; University of Valencia. DOI: 10.7203/metode.6.7096.

[38] Bambra C. Health divides: where you live can kill you. Bristol, UK: Policy Press; 2016.

[39] Carter-Pokras O, Baquet C. (2002). Viewpoint: what is a 'health disparity? Public Health Reports. 2002;117:426–34.

[40] Braveman P, Gruskin S. Defining equity in health. J Epidemiol Community Health. 2003; 57(4):254–8.

[41] Adler, NE. Overview of health disparities. In: Institute of Medicine Committee on the review and assessment of the NIH's strategic research plan and budget to reduce and ultimately eliminate health disparities; Thomson GE, Mitchell F, Williams MB, editors. Examining the health disparities research plan of the National Institutes of Health: Unfinished Business. Washington, D.C.: The National Academies Press; 2006.

[42] http://healthjournalism.org/core-topic.php?id=6&page=glossary#HealthEquity. Retrieved May 15, 2016.

[43] Nakaya T, Dorling D. Geographical inequalities of mortality by income in two developed island countries: a cross-national comparison. Soc Sci Med. 2005;60(12):2865–75. DOI:10.1016/j.socscimed.2004.11.007.

[44] Anderson LM, Adeney KL, Shinn C, Safranek S, Buckner-Brown J, Krause LK. Community coalition-driven interventions to reduce health disparities among racial and ethnic minority populations. Cochrane Database of Systematic Reviews. 2015; Issue 6. Art. No.: CD009905. DOI: 10.1002/14651858.CD009905.pub2.

[45] Currie J, Schwandt H. Inequality in mortality decreased among the young while increasing for older adults, 1990–2010. Science. 2016; 352(6286):708–12. DOI: 10.1126/science.aaf1437.

[46] Chetty R., Stepner M, Abraham S, Lin S, Scudent B, Tuner N, Bergeron A, Cutler D. The association between income and life expectancy in the United States, 2001–2014. JAMA. 2016;315(16):1750–66. DOI: 10.1001/jama.2016.4226.

[47] Woolf SH, Purnell JQ. The good life: working together to promote opportunity and improve population health and well-being. JAMA. 2016;315(16):1706–08. DOI: 10.1001/jama.2016.4263.

[48] Pascoe EA, Richman LS. Perceived discrimination and health: a meta-analytic Review. Psychol Bul. 2009;135(4):531–54. DOI: 10.1037/a0016059.

[49] http://www.rwjf.org/en/about-rwjf/newsroom/features-and-articles/Commission.html. Retrieved August 1, 2016.

[50] Logan RA, Health literacy research. In: Arnott-Smith C, Keselman A, editors. Meeting health information needs outside of healthcare: opportunities and challenges. Waltham, MA: Chandos; 2015. p.19–38.

[51] Keselman A, Logan RA, Smith CA, LeRoy G, Zeng-Treitler Q. Developing informatics tools and strategies for consumer-centered health communication. J Am Med Inform Assoc. 2008;15(4):475–83. DOI: 10.1197/jamia.M2744.

[52] Institute of Medicine of the National Academies. Health literacy: a prescription to end confusion. Washington, D.C.: The National Academies Press; 2004.

[53] Institute of Medicine of the National Academies. Health literacy: improving, health, health systems, and health policy around the world. Washington, D.C.: The National Academies Press; 2013.

[54] Hibbard JH, Mahoney ER, Stockard J, Tusler, M. Development and testing of a short form of the patient activation measure. Health Serv Res. 2005;40(6 Pt. 1): 1918–30.

[55] https://chirr.nlm.nih.gov. Retrieved September 8, 2016.

[56] Coulter A. Engaging patients in healthcare. Berkshire, England: Open University Press; 2011.

[57] https://www.nlm.nih.gov/services/queries/health_literacy.html. Retrieved July 11, 2016.

[58] National Academies of Sciences Engineering Medicine. Informed consent and health literacy: a workshop. Washington, D.C.: Washington, D.C.: National Academies of Sciences Engineering Medicine Health Literacy Roundtable, 2015.

[59] National Academies of Sciences Engineering Medicine. Precision medicine and health literacy: a workshop. Washington: National Academies of Sciences Engineering Medicine Health Literacy Roundtable, 2016.

[60] http://governor.alabama.gov/newsroom/2016/04/executive-order-number-18-2/. Retrieved June 20, 2016.

[61] Nelkin D. Selling science: How the press covers science and technology. New York: W. H. Freeman; 1995.

[62] Gregory J, Miller S. Science in public: communication, culture & credibility. New York: Perseus; 2000.

[63] http://nces.ed.gov/naal/health_results.asp. Retrieved May 16, 2016.

[64] Miller JD. Public understanding of, and attitudes towards, scientific research: what we know and what we need to know. Public Underst Sci. 2004;13(2):273–94. DOI: 10.1177/0963662504044908.

[65] Kutner M., Greenberg E, Jin Y, Paulsen C. The health literacy of America's adults: results from the 2003 National Assessment of Adult Literacy (NCES2006–483). U.S. Department of Education. Washington, D.C.: National Center for Education Statistics; 2006.

[66] Royal College of General Practitioners. Health literacy: report from an RCGP-led health literacy workshop. London, UK: Royal College of General Practitioners; 2014.

[67] White S. Assessing the nation's health literacy: key concepts and findings of the National Assessment of Adult Literacy (NAAL). Chicago: American Medical Association Foundation; 2008.

[68] Doak CC, Doak LG, Friedell GH, Meade CD. Improving communication for cancer patients with low literacy skills: strategies for clinicians. CA Cancer J Clin. 1998; 48(3):151–62.

[69] Doak CC, Doak LG, Root JH. Teaching patients with low-literacy skills. 2nd ed. Philadelphia: JB Lippincott; 1996.

[70] Doak LG, Doak CC, Meade CD. Strategies to improve cancer education materials. Oncol Nurs Forum. 1996;23(8):1305–12.

[71] Doak LG, Doak CC. (1987). Lowering the silent barriers for patients with low literacy skills. Promot Health. 1987;8(4):6–8.

[72] Nutbeam D. Health literacy as a public health goal: a challenge for contemporary health education and communication strategies into the 21st Century. Health Promotion Int. 2000;15:259–67.

[73] Pleasant, A. Advancing health literacy measurement: A pathway to better health and health system performance. J Health Commun. 2014;19(12):1481–96. DOI: 10.1080/10810730.2014.954083.

[74] Kreps GL, Neuhauser L. New directions in eHealth communications: opportunities and challenges. Patient Edu Couns. 2010;78:329–36. DOI: 10.1016/j.pec.2010.01.013.

[75] Neuhauser L, Kreps GL. Rethinking communication in the E-health era. J Health Psychol. 2003; 8(1): 7–22. DOI: 10.1177/1359105303008001426.

[76] Logan RA. Health campaigns research. In: Bucci M, Trench B, editors. Routledge Handbook of Public Communication of Science and Technology. 2nd ed. New York: Routledge; 2014. p.198–213.

[77] http://www.ncqa.org/Portals/0/Publications/Resource%20Library/NCQA_Primer_web.pdf. Retrieved May 11, 2016.

[78] Koh HK, Baur C, Brach C, Harris LM, Rowden JN. Towards a systems approach to health literacy research. J Health Commun. 2013;18(1):1–5. DOI: 10.1080/10810730.2013.759029.

[79] Koh HK, Berwick DM, Clancy CM Baur C., Brach C., Harris LM, Zerhusen EG. New federal policy initiatives to boost health literacy can help the nation move beyond the cycle of costly 'crisis care'. Health Aff. 2012;31(2): 434–43. DOI: 10.1377/hlthaff.2011.1169.

[80] Bailey, SC, Oramasion CU, Wolf MS. Rethinking adherence: A health literacy-informed model of medication self-management. J Health Commun. 2013;18 Suppl 1:20–30. DOI: 10.1080/10810730.2013.825672.

[81] http://nnlm.gov/outreach/consumer/hlthlit.html. Retrieved June 15, 2016.

[82] Baker DW. (2006). The associations between health literacy and health outcomes: self-reported health, hospitalization, and mortality. In: Office of the Surgeon General, Proceedings of the Surgeon General's workshop on improving health literacy. Rockville, M.D. Office of the Surgeon General (US); 2006. http://www.ncbi.nlm.nih.gov/books/NBK44260/#proc-healthlit.panel1.s14. Retrieved May 2, 2016.

[83] Institute of Medicine of the National Academies. Committee on the state of the USA health indicators. Board on population health and public health practice. Washington: The National Academies Press; 2009.

[84] Pleasant A. Health literacy measurement. Lecture 3 of 5 better health: evaluating health communication symposium. Bethesda (M.D.): National Library of Medicine. 2013; http://videocast.nih.gov. Retrieved June 16, 2016.

[85] Haun JN, Valerio MA, McCormack LA, Sorensen K, Paasche-Orlow MK. Health literacy measurements: An inventory and descriptive summary of 51 instruments. J Health Commun. 2014; 10 Suppl 2:302–33. DOI: 10.1080/10810730.2014.936571.

[86] Pleasant A. McKinney J, Rikard RV. (2011). Health literacy measurement: a proposed research agenda. J Health Commun. 2011;16 Suppl 3:11–21. DOI: 10.1080/10810730.2011.604392.

[87] McCormack L, Haun J, Sorensen K, Valerio M. Recommendations for advancing health literacy measurement. J Health Commun. 2013;18 Suppl 1: 9–14. DOI: 10.1080/10810730.2013.829892.

[88] Altin SV, Finke I, Kautz-Freimuth S, Stock S. The evolution of health literacy assessment tools: a systematic review. BMC Public Health. 2014; 14:1207. DOI:10.1186/1471-2458-14-1207.

[89] O'Neill B, Goncalves D, Ricci-Cabello I. Ziebland S. An overview of self-administered health literacy instruments. PLOS One. 2014; 9(12): e109110. DOI: 10:1371/journal.pone.0109110.

[90] Dewalt DA, Hink A. Health literacy and child health outcomes: A systematic review of the literature. Pediatrics. 2009; 124 Supp 3:S265–74. DOI: 10.1542/peds.2009-1162B.

[91] Abrams, MA, Klass, P, Dreyer, BP. Health literacy and children: Recommendations for action. Pediatrics. 2009; 124: S327–31. DOI: 10.1542/peds.2009-1162I.

[92] Aldoory L, Ryan KEB, Rouhain AM. Best practices and new models of health literacy for informed consent: Review of the impact of informed consent regulations on health literate communications. In: *Informed consent and health literacy: A workshop.* Washington, D.C.; National Academies of Sciences Engineering Medicine Health Literacy Roundtable, 2014.

[93] Rudd RE. Needed action in health literacy. Journal Health Psychol. 2013. DOI:10:1177/1359105312470128.

[94] Wollesen L, Peifer K. Life skills progression: an outcome and intervention planning instrument for use with families at risk. Baltimore, MD: Brookes; 2006.

[95] Smith SA, Moore EJ. Health literacy and depression in the context of home visitation. Matern Child Health J. 2012; 16(7): 1500–08. DOI: 10.1007/s10995-011-0920-8.

[96]   Smith SA. Health literacy and social service delivery. In: Estrine SA, Arthur HG, Hettenbach RT, Messina MG, editors. New directions in behavioral health: service delivery strategies for vulnerable populations. New York, Springer Publishing; 2011.

[97]   Carroll LN, Smith SA, Thomson NR. Parents as teachers health literacy demonstration project: Integrating an empowerment model of health literacy promotion into home-based parent education. Health Promot Pract. 2015; 16(2):282–90. DOI: 10.1177/1524839914538968.

[98]   Gottlieb K. The Nuka system of care: Improving health through ownership and relationships. Int J Circumpolar Health. 2013;5:72. DOI: 10.3402/ijch.v72i0.21118.

[99]   Gottlieb K, Sylvester I, Eby D. Transforming your practice: what matters most. Fam Pract Manag. 2008;15(1):32–8.

[100] Casarett D, Teno J. Why population health and palliative care need each other. JAMA. 2016;316(1):27–8. DOI: 10.1001/jama.2016.5961.

[101] http://listserv.ihahealthliteracy.org/scripts/wa.exe?INDEX. Retrieved April 23, 2016.

Health Literacy and Vulnerable Populations

Health Literacy
R.A. Logan and E.R. Siegel (Eds.)
IOS Press, 2017
doi:10.3233/978-1-61499-790-0-127

Assisting Vulnerable Communities: Canyon Ranch Institute's and Health Literacy Media's Health Literacy and Community-Based Interventions

Andrew PLEASANT[1]

Director of Canyon Ranch Institute and Global Health Literacy Research

Abstract. Canyon Ranch Institute and Health Literacy Media are a 501(c)3 non-profit public charity working to improve health based on the best evidence-based practices of health literacy and integrative health. As an organization, we offer a spectrum of health literacy work extending from plain language services to intensive community-based interventions. (See www.canyoranchinstitute.org & www.healthliteracy.media) In this chapter, we discuss the methodologies and outcomes of two of those community-based interventions – the Canyon Ranch Institute Life Enhancement Program and our Theater for Health program. Perhaps uniquely, an underpinning approach to both efforts is based on the increasing body of evidence of health literacy as a social determinant of health. Therefore, our research and evaluation of these programs captures not only changes in knowledge, attitudes, and beliefs but explicitly includes changes in informed behavior change and objective health outcomes as well. Our work makes it clear – that if you engage people in a health literate approach to informed behavior change (and respect their knowledge of their own lives and context) you can help people help themselves to better health. Further, from the perspective of health as a right and a resource for living, we find people who advance their health use this resource to continually better their own and their family's lives as well as the communities where they live. Hopefully, the examples provided in this chapter provide a sense of direction and motivation to others to fully explore the potential of health literacy to improve health and well-being, increase satisfaction with life, and produce health outcomes at a lower cost.

Keywords. Health literacy, health promotion, health education, Theater for Health, Theater of the Oppressed, health equity, health communication, informed behavior change, Calgary Charter on Health Literacy

1. Introduction

Canyon Ranch Institute (CRI) is 501(c)3 non-profit public charity founded with the mission to catalyze the possibility of optimal health for all people. In spring 2017, Canyon Ranch Institute joined with Health Literacy Media (HLM) to continue to improve our understanding of health literacy and put health literacy into action to improve health, well-being, and health equity around the world.

---

[1] Corresponding author: Canyon Ranch Institute. 8600 E. Rockcliff Road. Tucson, AZ. USA 85750; apleasant@healthliteracy.media

In particular, CRI and HLM focus on preventing, reducing, or reversing chronic disease in low-income communities across the United States and globally. The organization weaves together a robust approach to integrative health (mind, body, spirit, and emotion) and health literacy as the conceptual base for a suite of intervention designs.

According to the World Health Organization "Chronic diseases and conditions – such as heart disease, stroke, cancer, type 2 diabetes, obesity, and arthritis – are among the most common, costly, and preventable of all health problems [1]. In the United States, chronic diseases account for more than 75 percent of the over $2.3 trillion Americans spent on health care in 2008 [2]. That translates to $7,681 per person or 16.2 percent of the Gross Domestic Product of the United States [3].

Another goal of CRI/HLM is to build demonstration projects with valid and reliable evidence that address chronic disease in an effective and cost-effective manner. Theoretically, if an effective chronic disease prevention program (based on the best practices of health literacy and an integrative approach to health) can cost less than $7,681 per participant, the results suggest aligning health systems to focus on prevention is cost-effective. As a successful prevention program continues to reach more people over time, the benefits and savings compound and costs per participant continue to decline. Overall, CRI/HLM is working to bend the health care cost curve by slowing medical spending.

Historically, many efforts to improve individual and public health have primarily focused on delivering information to gain compliance with recommendations and guidelines. These efforts often were fundamentally premised on the incomplete and inaccurate assumption that simply providing information about health would be sufficient to change behavior [4,5,6,7,8]. Ongoing health care reform efforts in the U.S. are, in no small part, attempting to demonstrate that a focus on prevention, health literacy, and integrative approaches to health can help people live healthier lives and create a healthier and more efficient health care system [9,10,11].

2. Health Literacy

There are many diverse ways to conceptualize and operationalize health literacy. Initially, health literacy was a concept that focused on the public's misunderstanding and frequently confused navigation of complex health knowledge and health systems. Health literacy soon conceptually evolved to include the other challenges created by health systems and health care professionals. CRI/HLM employs health literacy as an evidenced-based path to behavior change for the public, health professionals, and health systems [4,12,13].

Health literacy is how people can – or how they can be helped and supported to – find, understand, evaluate, communicate, and use information to make an informed decision about their health and health behaviors [12,14]. Conceptually, the goals eclipse the historical approaches of health communication, health promotion, and health education that help people seek and understand health information. While helpful, the latter approach does not assist men and women to bridge the gap between what they know and what they do in practice.

The logic model – from finding/accessing information to actually using it – must always be built on a foundational awareness of literacy, culture, a scientific evidence base, and people's sense of empowerment (also known as 'civic literacy') [4,13].

If there is a golden rule to health literacy, it is to directly engage with people as early and often as possible. The best practices of health literacy should always align with the best practices of cultural competency and vice versa. This assures that interventions foster both an individual capacity to improve health and assist health systems and health care professionals.

CRI/HLM has designed, launched and evaluated a number of programs based on health literacy and an integrative approach to health over the years. In particular, these efforts include:

- **Canyon Ranch Institute Life Enhancement Program (CRI LEP)** – an evidence-based, multi-disciplinary program that transfers the best practices of Canyon Ranch to underserved communities to prevent, diagnose, and address chronic diseases. The CRI LEP uses an integrative approach to health that is grounded in the best practices of health literacy. See: http://canyonranchinstitute.org/program/cri-life-enhancement-program/

- **Canyon Ranch Institute Life Enhancement Program for Families** – The CRI LEP tailored for children in grades K-5 and their parents or guardians. See: http://canyonranchinstitute.org/program/cri-lep-for-families/

- **Canyon Ranch Institute Life Enhancement Program for Teens** – The CRI LEP tailored for teens and their parents or guardians. See: http://canyonranchinstitute.org/program/cri-lep-for-teens/

- **Healthy Community Program** – High stress, poor eating habits, and lack of regular physical activity have contributed to an epidemic of obesity and chronic disease, especially in low-income neighborhoods. CRI launched the CRI Healthy Community program to harness the strength of families and communities to make positive changes together. When families cook, learn, eat, and play together, they support each other in making lasting improvements to their health and wellness. When community resources are aligned in new ways, access to healthy ideas and habits increases for everyone. See: http://canyonranchinstitute.org/program/cri-healthy-community/

- **Healthy Garden Program** – Twenty percent of Americans report feeling extreme stress (ranking an 8 or 9 on a 10-point scale), which can lead to physical and emotional symptoms, including fatigue, irritability, and poor eating habits [15]. To combat these negative health effects, studies suggest open, outdoor spaces (such as gardens) can effectively manage stress [16]. Canyon Ranch Institute works locally with its partners to create open spaces to improve the health and well-being of individuals and communities. See: http://canyonranchinstitute.org/program/cri-healthy-garden/

- **Healthy Table Program** – Healthy eating is one of the most important components of a happy and vibrant life. Unhealthy eating habits can lead to a lifetime of chronic disease. CRI Healthy Table is based on the premise that healthy food can be the best medicine. See: http://canyonranchinstitute.org/program/cri-healthy-table

- **Healthy World Scholarship** – Canyon Ranch Institute has partnered with Canyon Ranch to create lasting change in the health and well-being of our nation's children through the Canyon Ranch Institute Healthy World Scholarship program. See: http://canyonranchinstitute.org/program/cri-healthy-world-scholarship

- **Theater for Health** – Storytelling through drama, music, and dance helps ideas memorably come to life. In CRI Theater for Health, a community collaborates with actors to develop a series of plays that explore solutions to health challenges they face. As people get involved in the story, see it acted out, and act it out themselves, they begin to incorporate new information into their decisions and adopt changes to live healthier lives. See: http://canyonranchinstitute.org/program/cri-theater-for-health/

This chapter focuses on two examples – the Canyon Ranch Institute's Life Enhancement Program (CRI LEP) and the Theater for Health program.

3. Canyon Ranch Institute Life Enhancement Program

The Canyon Ranch Institute Life Enhancement Program (CRI LEP) is an evidence-based, multi-disciplinary, integrative health program that increases health literacy while preventing, diagnosing, and addressing chronic diseases.

Although the CRI LEP has been conducted in partnership with a U.S. health care provider organization, we are confident the program would be successful in any cultural or geographic setting. Employees of our local partner – be it a hospital system, Federally qualified health care center, or other health care organization – are carefully selected to create a CRI LEP Core Team. The team is responsible for delivery of the program after thorough training in the model. The core team represents expertise in integrative health and medicine, nutrition, exercise, behavioral health, spirituality, pharmacology, and spirituality.

CRI LEP sessions include informational lectures, group fitness and stress-management activities, a grocery-shopping excursion, and planning sessions for setting health-related goals. These activities and experiences provide CRI LEP participants the opportunity to learn about and experience integrative health through seven core program elements including physical activity, nutrition, and stress management (Table 1).

Table 1. Core elements and related topics and activities in the CRI LEP

Core element	Selected examples of topics and activities
Nutrition	• The value of eating whole foods • How to identify and prepare whole foods • How to create balanced meals/a balanced approach to eating • Understand portion sizes • Experience mindful eating/the enjoyment of food • Experience a supermarket tour/learn to read food labels • Cooking demonstrations
Physical Activity	• Discuss core elements of fitness: heart rate, cardio, strength, flexibility, balance, and sense of play • Embrace movement as physical activity (e.g., dance, yoga, tai chi) • Incorporate culturally relevant movement into physical activity program (e.g.., salsa dancing, African dance, etc.) • Tailor exercise plans to the individual's needs (i.e., major muscle targets; exercises that can be easily done)
Behavior Change	• Set achievable goals reflecting the program's core elements and reality of each individual's life • Track progress and celebrate success • Help participants find, understand, evaluate, communicate, and use information related to their health goals
Sense of Purpose	• Find meaning in life • Find a sense of connection; not feeling isolated • Find a source of joy in life (having fun like a kid again) • Understand that not letting go of the past may be hurting the future • Incorporate meditation
Integrative Health	• Understand the four dimensions of health and well-being (physical, mental, spiritual, and emotional) and how they are interconnected • Train health professionals how to incorporate integrative health, wellness, and prevention into each clinical visit • Perform basic blood work, physical, and fitness assessments on all participants to help them better understand their own health
Stress Reduction	• Understand and apply stress management techniques • Understand and apply meditation and relaxation practices • Understand and apply yoga / Tai Chi practice
Social Support and Follow-up Services	• Establish trust among participants and facilitators • Incorporate a "buddy system" for participants to help support each other and maintain healthy living practices • Plan a graduation celebration for program participants • Follow up by facilitators with participants during and after the program to jointly set timelines for health goals and monitor progress

From a health literacy perspective, the components and approaches within the program are:

- Tailoring the program to each community and cultural setting.
- Training CRI LEP Core Team members in health literacy skills including:
  - o Use of (but not sole reliance upon) plain language,
  - o Building improved understanding, attitude change, and behavior change through scaffolding with language, and
  - o Proper use of the teach-back technique.
- Practicing with a simulated participant to assure delivery of the program is conducted in a health literate fashion.
- Hands-on practice sessions both with CRI LEP Core Team members and a live audience with feedback sessions.
- Seeking constant feedback and participation in program improvement from participants and CRI LEP Core Team members.

Each CRI LEP is tailored to a community and employs a multi-disciplinary team of health professionals. The team receives training from CRI staff about: health literacy; the content and approach of the CRI LEP; a simulated participant exercise focused on setting goals with participants; and how to collectively deliver the CRI LEP.

The CRI LEP does not recruit participants based upon any particular health status expect they must be at risk for or diagnosed with one or multiple chronic diseases. For example, some participants may not need to lower their HbA1c levels before entering the program while others may need to gain weight to reach their optimal health.

Although participation in the evaluation and research component of the CRI LEP is not required of participants, to date the effort has assessed Pre, Post, and Post + 3 months data from n=591 people. The research component of the program requires blood work before and three months after program participation. A three-month interval is hypothesized as the amount of time it takes for a healthy lifestyle change to impact the assessed indicators. Of n=591 who have consented to and participated in the research, 86 percent are female. At program entry, on average, participants have 12.4 years of formal education and an average of 2.9 self-reported chronic diseases. Forty-one percent of participants report an annual household income below \$15,000; 36% percent report full-time employment and 41% report they are unemployed.

In brief, the post-intervention, quantitative changes in knowledge, attitudes, beliefs, and behaviors include (but are not limited to) a:

- 49.7% decrease in depression based on the PHQ-9 scale
- 25.% decrease in self-reported stress levels
- 47.3% decrease in self-reported unhealthy days each month
- 30% increase in feeling better able to take care of their own health
- 20.8% increase in consuming water every day
- 60% decrease in daily consumption of full-sugar soda
- 40.1% decrease in the number of days their health prevents them from doing normal activities
- 15.2% decrease in frequency their body image prevents them from participating in physical activity
- 74.8% increase in weekly strenuous exercise

- 22% increase in the number of sit-ups they can perform
- 24.6% reduction in C-reactive protein levels

Underpinning these changes is a 10.2% increase in health literacy – as measured by the Calgary Charter on Health Literacy scale that was developed at Canyon Ranch Institute. In addition, using the Quality Adjusted Life Year (QALY) method for analysis of cost effectiveness, the CRI LEP is occurring at an average cost savings of $188,395.77 compared to the average cost of other interventions to produce the same health improvements. This is based on range of the average cost of a QALY in the United States using the Centers for Disease Control's Healthy Days Index to calculate EQ-5D scores [17].

Qualitatively, a post-intervention analysis of comments from participant focus groups identified themes that were consistent with the aforementioned quantitative changes. The themes included: improved health literacy; changes in a wide range of health-related attitudes and behaviors; weight loss; improvements in perceived health and well being; and increased awareness of the integrative aspects of health. One participant said, "I am a patient that has diabetes; I have had it just four years. I haven't had it normal but when I started this group, they helped me with the nutrition: eating vegetables, etc. I didn't eat breakfast; I didn't like breakfast. They taught me the importance of breakfast. They instilled the practice and that has helped me a lot. I now have my diabetes under control."

Participants also report improved health and well-being impacted some other aspects of their daily lives, which suggests the positive impact of an integrative health approach. For example, one participant said, "I think that I am going to be 200%. Well, I want to say that I am very thankful to be here in this group because like I said before…I feel good. When I began this program, everything bothered me; I felt bad. I am here, thanks to god and thanks to you all that I feel good now. Before, when I spoke with my daughter she would tell me, 'What's wrong? Why are you crying? What happened?' Now, I can feel the change that has happened; I talk with her and she says that something has changed in me; now I talk with her, whereas before I would say nothing. Before I didn't smile; now I smile. … I am happy because of the people in this group above all."

You can change your life forever. No U-turns! A CRI LEP participant's story.

"The Canyon Ranch Institute Life Enhancement Program (CRI LEP) saved my life.

The first few months of 2014 were my darkest days. I was recently divorced and learning how to be a part-time father. Then my mom, who I could always talk with about life's ups and downs, was diagnosed with dementia. I felt so alone, and so I turned to food to ease my emotional pain. When I saw that overeating wasn't helping me at all, I tried to eat healthy and lose weight. I didn't see results I wanted, so I felt like a further failure and turned to food all over again. Worst of all, I thought about suicide nearly every day. I told myself to think of how my death would affect my two beautiful kids. Those thoughts kept me alive.

Thankfully, I was serving on the board of directors of Curtis V. Cooper Primary Health Care when our health center started offering the CRI Life Enhancement Program, thanks to Charles H. and Rosalie Morris. I wanted to experience the CRI LEP myself to learn how it works and how best to spread the word about it. I also hoped it could help me turn around my own life.

Let me tell you, it was a wake-up call right from the start. The results from my CRI LEP baseline evaluation were a shock. My risks for heart attack, stroke, and type 2 diabetes were dangerously high. I sat in my car after getting my results from a CRI LEP Core Team member and thought, "I'm a dead man walking. I could be gone like that." Ten minutes later, I'd made up my mind to live. I knew I had to take full advantage of everything the CRI LEP offered.

The CRI LEP is health literacy in action. I learned how all parts of my life – food, exercise, my mental and spiritual well-being – affect all the other parts. I learned healthy new habits that will sustain me for the rest of my life. I learned how to share my life's challenges and successes with others. I made new friends and started to draw on old friends for social support. I found a glimmer of hope and followed it.

By the end of the CRI LEP, my blood results were really good, and I was on a path to a happier and healthier life. I lost 20 pounds during the program, but I've lost more than 50 pounds since then. When you're blessed with an experience like this, you want to share it with others. That's why the latest step in my journey has been to become a part of the Savannah CRI LEP Core Team. I'm here to show others what is possible and help us all move forward toward better health. My motto today is "No U-Turns" – for myself and every other participant in the CRI LEP."

Reginald Franklin
Savannah, GA

4. Theater for Health – Using the Arts to Advance Health Literacy and Improve Health

Theater for Health combines the arts – music, dance, theater, and visual arts – with the best practices of health literacy to reduce the risk of disease through improved personal and household hygiene. While exposure to arts previously has been associated with some health improvements, Theater for Health combines health literacy as a theory of behavior change with the arts (theater) to address public health challenges in which the audience interaction and proposed solutions additionally are grounded in scientific evidence [18,19,20].

To backup, innovative solutions to curb infectious diseases are needed to improve global population health and meet the United Nation's Millennium Development Goals. Initially, there are several easily adoptable and evidence-based behaviors that can reduce infectious episodes. These include: hand-washing; use of hand sanitizers; using bleach as a disinfectant; coughing and sneezing etiquette; and solar water disinfection. Often, the core public health challenge is not to develop a new science to address household hygiene issues but to foster innovative methods that expand how existing scientific knowledge is used to create and inform action – as well as bridge the gap between what people may know and what they actually do [21].

The Theater for Health initiative theorizes the most effective approach to support a community is to identify and select the exact practices that will be adopted as healthy behaviors [4,22,23]. To accomplish that end, Theater for Health was developed as a new form of community-based interactive theater.

In Theater for Health, the actors and the audience identify community health challenges and discuss viable solutions via a community dialogue that is fostered via a theatrical narrative. The audience members are encouraged to better find, understand, evaluate, communicate, and use health information to make informed decisions about their health as well as the health of their family and surrounding community. More foundationally, the goal is to improve health literacy [4,13,24,25].

Theater for Health integrates practices from the Theater of the Oppressed family of methods with best practices derived from health literacy. The Theater of the Oppressed was largely developed by Augusto Boal [26,27] who based his work upon Paulo Freire's [28] *Pedagogy of the Oppressed*. The well-known, yet seldom rigorously evaluated, Theater of the Oppressed family of methods seeks to empower communities to develop their own truths based on their lived experiences and interactions [26,27,28].

However, Theater for Health's conceptual underpinnings are a combination of health literacy's best practices coupled with an adaptation of Theatre of the Oppressed. Some of distinct differences between Theater for Health and Theatre of the Oppressed include:

- In Theatre of the Oppressed, the community is always treated as if their input, knowledge, beliefs, and behaviors are essentially correct.
- Theater for Health deliberately and explicitly incorporates evidence-based knowledge about health to help produce informed decisions.
- Similar to Theatre of the Oppressed, CRI Theater for Health encourages the audience to become 'spect-actors' and participate in development of the narrative. However, CRI Theater for Health focuses on supporting the community to identify and adopt evidence-based behavior changes. The stage becomes a safe place to propose and test new ideas and behaviors.

To reach the aforementioned goals (and unlike Theatre of the Oppressed), in Theater for Health evidence-based information is introduced into the dialogue between the performance and the community. At the same time, the power to reshape the narrative is determined by community participants, which reflects health literacy, Theatre of the Oppressed, and Freirean perspectives.

The transformation of Theatre of the Oppressed into Theater for Health requires an expansion of the role of the Facilitator, or 'Joker.' In Theater for Health, the person assuming the role of Facilitator (or 'Joker') must be able to help the audience find, understand, evaluate, communicate and use key evidence-based information about health [4,13,24,25). This individual also must be a skilled facilitator, who can engage and empower community members to play a vital and necessary role to identify health problems as well as offer solutions to improve personal, family, and community health.

Unlike traditional Theatre of the Oppressed approaches, such as Forum Theater, the 'Joker' in Theater for Health is a health professional who possesses the scientific knowledge to help improve the audience members' health literacy – so they are empowered to address the health challenges presented in the interactive performances. An extensive training workshop fosters health literacy and communication skills to facilitate the identification and adoption of behavior changes to improve health as well as the skills, attitudes, and willingness to encourage community participation and empowerment. Hence, the pilot program's 'Joker' was a physician with a master's degree in public health with extensive experience working in communities with health inequities.

The first pilot project of Theater for Health occurred in Lima, Perú and consisted of 12 collaboratively developed episodes structured as a tele-novela that were performed over 11 weeks (two performances were held the first week). While underwritten by The Clorox Company, the program was not branded. The participating community was not aware of the commercial sponsor, and specific products sold by the sponsor were not promoted. The primary goal of the partnership was consistent with The Clorox Company's corporate social responsibility efforts.

The primary goals were to improve health and well-being in the community and test the viability of Theater for Health.

The first pilot identified existing community conditions through formative research and introduced Theater for Health through live performances within the designated community. The intervention was intended to improve health literacy while interacting with people where they are based. Hypothetically, Theater for Health would individually and collectively help community members:

- **Find:** Community receives information through the performance narrative, workshops, and festivals of health that accompanied the performances.
- **Understand:** Performance narrative explains information – the science of health and household hygiene – and the process checks in on public understanding through interactions.
- **Evaluate:** Community members analyze the situations presented in the theatrical narrative to find issues relative to their own lives, and develop solutions.
- **Communicate:** Community discusses situations and solutions during and between performances.

- **Use:** Community members demonstrate behaviors during performances and adopt behaviors in their own lives.

To assess this series of hypotheses, (as is standard for Canyon Ranch Institute's approach to developing health literacy interventions), the process began with formative research in and with the community. This effort informed the initial drafting of the narrative tela-nova structure; the development of individual characters, and opportunities for interactions in each script. The process began with an intensive two-week workshop in Lima that involved local actors, directors, and stage personnel; scientific experts from Peru and the United States; and team members from the United States – with academic and professional backgrounds in arts, public health, health literacy, and communication. The tele-nova planning process educated artists about the science of household hygiene as well as scientists about the use of interactive, theatrical arts to address health issues. This process also identified and trained a local individual to transform the role of the 'Joker,' (in Boal's terms) into a source of valid scientific information for the community members before, during, and after each performance.

Artistic and scientific team members drafted four episodes during the preparatory workshop before program implementation began and the other eight episodes were drafted in process. The overall story line was adjusted weekly to incorporate participating community members' input and the reactions to previous episodes. After initial drafting, each script was reviewed for language appropriateness, content accuracy, and cultural relevance.

Every tele-nova episode was subject to continual refinement up to the moment of presentation in the community. Weekly rehearsals of the upcoming performance were videotaped and reviewed by a multidisciplinary and multicultural team drawn from the local actors and directors, and participants in the preparatory workshop including scientific and artistic experts from within and outside Peru. Adjustments were made prior to each performance. Live performances were videotaped and reviewed, with feedback going to the creative team in Lima on a timely basis to make weekly adjustments.

Input from participating community members also was incorporated each week. Feedback occurred during the opportunities for participating community members to interact during performances as well as post-performance qualitative interviews with 20 randomly selected audience members. The combined feedback efforts incorporated perspectives and information from community members and scientific experts that fostered continuous quality improvement. The overall approach also ensured consistent community engagement, which enhanced the diffusion and adoption of improved household hygiene behaviors.

The series of 12 performances was titled "*Siempre.*" *Siempre* translates to "Always" in English, and refers here to "always" being sick. The tele-novela structure – an approach very familiar to the audience and well-liked in Perúvian culture – was based on an overall story line about the life of two neighboring families who faced many health challenges and do not know how to proceed or what resources are available to them to address their health challenges. One family, the *Marañas*, (which translates roughly as tangled, messy, or unorganized) included a grandmother (age 60), grandfather (age 68), mother (age 42), twin girls (age 23), and a 5-month-old baby girl. The other family, the *Buendías*, (which translates roughly as "good days") included a mother (age 28), father (age 35), a daughter (age 8), two sons (ages 4 and 13), and a family dog called *Peluchín*.

The performances lasted between 30 and 45 minutes, and included at least 15 to 20 minutes of community interaction. The primary goals of the community interactions were: to review the main points of the script; identify correct and incorrect household hygiene practices presented in the narrative; ensure audience understanding of key scientific knowledge about household hygiene and outcomes of different behaviors; elicit suggestions of healthier household hygiene practices; and continually build the ongoing narrative structure.

Every episode introduced at least one, but often several, new household or personal hygiene practices or health-related messages, while reviewing and discussing the messages introduced in previous episodes. The overall focus was to encourage participating community members to discuss and demonstrate how to find, understand, evaluate, communicate, and use information to inform healthy home hygiene decision-making and behaviors.

The strategies used to encourage participation included: street parades; printed materials; mototaxi/megaphone announcements; community-based radio announcements; community meetings; bring-a-neighbor and get a reward incentives; direct incentives to attendees; empowerment workshops; arts workshops; knowledge contests; games; and a talent show. As a result of those efforts, the overall attendance at the performances of "*Siempre*" exceeded initial expectations, as average attendance across episodes was 172 adults and 59 children. At any single performance, the lowest attendance was 80 and the highest attendance was 500 people at the final performance and festival.

Baseline research included an in-depth individual interview administered in 250 households and a 90-minute observation protocol, which was conducted in n=50 randomly selected households within the two neighboring shantytowns. Process evaluation included individual interviews with n=20 randomly selected community members conducted immediately after each performance (for a total of n=240 individual interviews). Post intervention research included n=249 household interviews and n=50 household observations.

Overall, community members' participation in the performances increased as the effort progressed. While there was initial minimal participation, once trust and confidence were built, community members soon entered the performance space and suggested changes to the actors. Eventually, community members were able to summarize and accurately demonstrate on stage (via the teach-back technique) and in post-performance interviews the household and personal hygiene practices (e.g., use of bleach, importance of bleach dosage, proper hand washing) and the disease prevention messages (e.g., pneumonia, diarrhea, skin disease) discussed during previous episodes.

The following themes (gleaned through from the interview data) summarize what audience members reported they learned through the interactive artistic presentations:

- How and when to properly wash hands
- How to treat water (water for all purposes often arrived in the community already contaminated)
- How much bleach is needed for different purposes
- How to avoid infections and diseases
- How much teamwork is needed to solve community problems
- How to treat the in-ground hole (hueco) for disposal of dirty water
- What to do when symptoms of diseases appear

- How to clean vegetables, fruits, and kitchen utensils
- How to keep their houses clean
- How to prevent pneumonia, diarrhea, and skin diseases

The evaluation and research methodology also focused on understanding what participating community members would as a result of their involvement. Some of the responses to the question, "What would you change after attending the performance?" included:

- Practice at home what was learned from the actors
- Teach family members, especially children, how to wash their hands
- Keep community, house, and kitchen utensils clean
- Use soap for hand washing
- Supervise children when washing their hands
- Wash vegetables and fruits before eating
- Keep animals out of the cooking area
- Use bleach to treat water to make it safe for use
- Use the correct amount of bleach for specific purposes
- Boil water if no bleach is available
- Keep water containers clean
- Keep trash in a covered container
- Take sick relatives to a health center
- Stop smoking around children
- Clean the house more often
- Follow recommendations from health professionals
- Improve communication at home
- Improve communication in the community
- Organize people in the neighborhood to keep common areas clean

During post-performance interviews, researchers also asked participating community members about their perceptions of the Theater for Health performances. Some of the thematic responses included: how participants related to the dialogue within the performances, how participants perceived the collaboration and teamwork among the characters, and learning through theater and music. Participants also provided responses about the content that raised health issues such as: hand-washing; preventing disease; and the use of bleach as a good hygiene practice.

For example, community feedback included a 31-year-old female who said: "Everything I've seen (in the performances) is what I see in my community. What I have seen are examples that happen in this community in one or another kind of family ... We see our mistakes and it makes you look, think, and see what is going wrong. To me, it is very good." The quote is adapted from the participant's response in Spanish.

Similarly, a 19-year-old female who attended the performances said the main themes she recognized were, "Keeping our homes clean so that the bacteria do not concentrate in the environment and also to show solidarity between neighbors, is not it?"

Another participant, a 35-year-old female, said, "Well, I liked it because it is nice. The kids have fun and besides it teaches you many things to improve our home.

Sometimes we do not know what we do not know, but here we are taught how to use bleach, how children should wash their hands … Well, I liked everything."

Overall, a Pre/Post evaluation (that included microbiological sampling within the community) found audience members learned how and when to wash hands and how to avoid infections. Audience members also reported they learned the proper approach to oral rehydration therapy, the correct amount of bleach to treat water for different household purposes, and the importance of taking sick people to the health center. Some participants additionally reported they noticed some improved community organization that they suggested was initiated by a favorable public response to the theater performances.

Quantitatively, the participants in the post evaluation (derived from randomly selected members of the two adjoining communities) reported 97.6% were aware of the tele-novas. Among those surveyed, 69.6% attended tele-novas with mean attendance of 4.2 performances. Audience members attended a minimum of one and a maximum of 11/12. The distance people lived from the performance site negatively correlated with the number of performances attended -.194** (p=0.01).

Three months after the tele-novas, 57.4% reported changes in their family's household and personal hygiene behaviors as a result of the performances. An overall score of 3.15/4 on a scale also suggested the tele-novas resulted in therapeutic behavioral changes.

More specifically, participants reported the behavioral changes they made in their homes and lifestyles included: 83.8% of surveyed participants used household cleaners; 76% used bleach to treat water; 74.7% used bleach to clean water bins; 73.9% used bleach to clean utensils; 72.4 % began to protect food from flies; 76% cleaned utensils when cooking; 27.3% brought sick people to a doctor; 84.5% cleaned streets; 67% made home improvements; and 54.5% treated their water.

Regarding food preparation, samples taken in homes found a 34.4% overall decline in measured rates of *E. coli* and *listeria*. In other words, measurable *E. coli* and *listeria* disappeared from 34.4% of the sample of homes where it occurred prior to the tele-nova performances.

In addition, post-intervention health literacy levels were significantly correlated with several Pre/Post goals such as: an increase in health knowledge; the number of neighbors that participants spoke to about household hygiene; the frequency that household hygiene was discussed with community peers;

the frequency that participants washed their hands and brushed their teeth; an increased understanding of the connection between routine hygiene and one's health; as well as participant confidence to make changes in their household hygiene;

Similarly, more than n=100 people responded to all five statements (derived from the modified Calgary Charter on Health Literacy scale) that the tele-novas helped them better find, understand, evaluate, communicate, and use health information. The resulting Cronbach's alpha for the overall scale was an acceptable 0.87.

5. Conclusion

While health literacy is increasingly recognized as one of, if not *the*, most significant social determinant of health, health literacy remains a social construct. That is, health literacy is what the field collectively makes of the concept and how the field collectively arrives at a consensus on how to define and measure health literacy as a construct.

That said, the field of health literacy frequently strives to advance the understanding of a complex social determinant of health with diverse approaches. The approach that underpins all of Canyon Ranch Institute's and Health Literacy Media's initiatives is to help individuals, families, communities, and nations make informed behavior changes. The latter goal is based on conceptual and applied approaches initially outlined by the Calgary Charter on Health Literacy. Recent evaluation data suggests Calgary-based strategies provide an evidence-based foundation for program design as well as the measurement of health literacy.

Although some individuals and organizations hesitate to measure how informed behavior changes foster objective health status outcomes, this approach is a hallmark of the Canyon Ranch Institute's and Health Literacy Media's intervention strategies. Albeit expensive, by setting the bar at improved health status (as a result of sustained informed behavior change), we help define and advance an evidence-based consensus about health literacy's impact. If one believes, as we do, that health literacy is a social construct that can help improve health and well-being at lower costs (especially in low-income and neglected communities), then we need to evaluate our programs by measuring their specific impacts on community and individual health.

In addition, if there is a golden rule to design health literacy interventions it is to know your audience and engage them in the process. If people do not own their pathway to improved health and well-being, they are less likely to sustain any attempted change. One way to foster sustained and informed behavior change is to directly engage and empower individuals to identify the changes they wish to generate and support them to make and maintain a change. The latter requires innovative intervention approaches and a reevaluation about who is an expert. Essentially, Canyon Ranch Institute and Health Literacy Media's approach engages people as experts in their own lives. While we bring a host of skills and resources to an intervention, we should never value ourselves over the individuals and communities who participate in our programs.

Another overall goal of Canyon Ranch Institute and Health Literacy Media is to develop, evaluate, and share evidence via demonstration projects designed to envision a genuine 'health care' system. Conceptually, a health care system based on health literacy best practices as well as an integrative approach to health should embrace prevention as much, if not more, than treatment. Similarly, a health care system should create, improve, and build on evidence-based best practices. Only through a complete overhaul of the current 'sick care' system can an egregious reality be addressed: higher health care costs are occurring as health status declines in many nations. Through innovative work and dissemination of the outcomes, we hope diverse policy-makers are persuaded to support the type of transition we advance.

A transition also is more likely to occur if the health literacy community shifts its gaze and activities from inward to outward expansion. While work towards a stronger internal consensus about health literacy is needed in the community, what is equally if not more important is to demonstrate and communicate the evidence of health literacy's capacity to change behaviors through informed decision-making and improve health at a lower cost. Health literacy's outreach needs to include, but is not limited to all of clinical medicine and public health as well as other disciplinary and business communities including science, sociology, political science, religion, business, and civic organizations.

Hopefully, the examples provided in this chapter provide a sense of direction and motivation to fully explore the potential of health literacy to improve health and well-being, increase satisfaction with life, and produce health outcomes at a lower cost.

References

[1]   U.S. Centers for Disease Control and Prevention. Chronic Disease Prevention and Health Promotion 2015; updated Feb. 10, 2015. Available from: http://www.cdc.gov/chronicdisease/index.htm.
[2]   U.S. Centers for Disease Control and Prevention. Workplace health promotion: Reasons for investing Washington, D.C. 2010 Available from:
       http://www.cdc.gov/workplacehealthpromotion/businesscase/reasons/rising.html.
[3]   Center for Medicare and Medicaid Service Office of the Actuary U.S Department of Health and Human Services. National health expenditure data for 2008. Washington, D.C.; 2008 Available from: http://www.cms.gov/NationalHealthExpendData/02_NationalHealthAccountsHIst.
[4]   Zarcadoolas C, Pleasant A, Greer D. Advancing health literacy: a framework for understanding and action. San Francisco, CA: Jossey Bass; 2006.
[5]   Dierkes M, von Grote C, editors. Between understanding and trust: the public, science and technology. Amsterdam: Harwood Academic Publishers; 2000.
[6]   Pleasant A, Kuruvilla S, Zarcadoolas C, Shanahan J, Lewenstein B. A framework for assessing public engagement with health research. Technical Report. Geneva, Switzerland: World Health Organization; 2003.
[7]   Pleasant A. Health literacy around the world: Part 2 Health literacy within the United States and a global overview. Washington, D.C.: Institute of Medicine; 2013. Available from: http://nationalacademies.org/hmd/~/media/Files/Activity%20Files/PublicHealth/HealthLiteracy/Commi ssioned-Papers/Health%20Literacy%20Around%20the%20World%20Part%202.pdf.
[8]   Pleasant A. Health Literacy Around the World: Part 1 Health Literacy Efforts Outside Of the United States. Washington, D.C.: Institute of Medicine; 2013. Available from: https://www.ncbi.nlm.nih.gov/books/NBK202445/.
[9]   U.S. Department of Health and Human Services. HealthReform.gov Washington, D.C. Available from: http://healthreform.gov.
[10] U.S. Department of Health and Human Services. HealthCare.gov Washington, D.C. Available from: http://www.healthcare.gov.
[11] The patient protection and affordable care act, H.R. 3590 (2010).
[12] Coleman C, Kurtz-Rossi S, McKinney J, Pleasant A, Rootman I, Shohet L. Calgary Charter on health literacy 2009 Available from: http://www.centreforliteracy.qc.ca/Healthlitinst/Calgary_Charter.htm.
[13] Zarcadoolas C, Pleasant A, Greer D. Understanding health literacy: an expanded model. Health Promot Int. 2005;20:195–203.
[14] Pleasant A, Cabe J, Patel K, Cosenza J, Carmona R. Health literacy research and practice: a needed paradigm shift. Health Commun. 2015;30(12):1176–80.
[15] American Psychological Association. Stress in America™: Missing the health care connection. American Psychological Association; 2012 Feb. 7, 2013.
[16] Pleasant A, Scanlon M, Pereira-Leon M. Literature review: environmental design and research on the human health effects of open spaces in urban areas. Hum Eco Rev. 2013;20(1):36–49.
[17] Haomiao J, Zack M, Moriarty D, Fryback D. Predicting the EuroQol Group's EQ-5D Index from CDC's "Healthy Days" in a US sample. Med Decis Making. 2011;31:174–85.
[18] Van Erven E. Community theatre: global perspectives. New York, NY: Routledge; 2000.
[19] Stromberg PG. Caught in play: how entertainment works on you: Stanford University Press; 2009.
[20] Mwita M. Textualizing the HIV/AIDS motif in theater-against AIDS performances in Kenya. IN: Wachanga, D.N., ed. Cultural Identityand New Communication Technologies: Political, Ethnic and Ideological Implications. IGI Global; 2011.
[21] Pang T, Sadana R, Hanney S, Bhutta Z, Hyder A, Simon J. Knowledge for better health - a conceptual framework and foundation for health research systems. Bull World Health Organ. 2003;81:815–20.
[22] Pleasant A. Health literacy: An opportunity to improve individual, community, and global health. New Dir Adult Cont Educ. 2011;130:43–53.
[23] Pleasant A. A second look at the health literacy of American adults and the National Assessment of Adult Literacy. Focus on Basics. 2008;9B:46–52.
[24] Pleasant A. Health literacy: an opportunity to improve individual, community, and global health. Adult Education for Health and Wellness. 2011;130(Summer 2011):43–54.

[25] Pleasant A, Kuruvilla S. A tale of two health literacies: public health and clinical approaches to health literacy. Health Promot Int. 2008;23(2):152–9.
[26] Boal A. Games for actors and non-actors. London, New York: Routledge; 1992.
[27] Boal A. Theatre of the oppressed. New York: Theatre Communications Group; 1985.
[28] Freire P. Pedagogy of the oppressed. New York: Herder and Herder; 1970.

Health Literacy
R.A. Logan and E.R. Siegel (Eds.)
IOS Press, 2017
doi:10.3233/978-1-61499-790-0-144

Data-Driven Maternal Health Literacy Promotion and a Postscript on Its Implications

Sandra A. SMITH[a,1] and Lauren N. CARROLL[b]
a Center for Health Literacy Promotion, Seattle WA U.S.A.
b University of Washington, Seattle WA U.S.A.

Abstract. Scientific discovery and global health policy are moving health literacy promotion and maternal-child health from the fringes of research and public health to the forefront of healthcare reform [1]. In 2011 the United Nations General Assembly adopted the Shanghai Declaration [2]. The Declaration highlights new understanding of the origins of health and disease in early development. It calls on all nations to apply this knowledge to reduce the burdens of chronic disease and related disparities worldwide. The Declaration recommends a specific intervention strategy: *promote health literacy across the life course, particularly in parents and children, and empower women.*

This chapter explores findings and implications of the Life Skills Progression Maternal Health Literacy studies. These LSP-MHL studies evaluated implementations of an intervention designed to promote health literacy in parents and empower women in the U.S. First, the chapter reports findings of the most recent of five published LSP-MHL studies with discussion of its implications for future work in this line of inquiry. A postscript highlights two of many implications of the LSP-MHL intervention studies for health literacy research in the third era of modern healthcare.

Keywords. Health literacy, maternal health literacy, empowerment, Life Skills Progression, health promotion, home visitation, Shanghai Declaration

1. Introduction

Two research goals guided the present study. First, the authors aimed to assess progress toward maternal health literacy (MHL) *in the context of everyday life* among disadvantaged mothers of children aged 0 (pregnancy) to 3 years in the U.S. The authors hypothesized that MHL scores would show improvement and that the social determinants of health would influence progress. The second aim was to explore how data visualization methods might increase understanding of how MHL develops and what supports or impedes improvement. Of particular interest are visualizations that

---

[1] Sandra A. Smith, PhD, MPH Center for Health Literacy Promotion, 2821 2nd Avenue Ste. 1601, Seattle, WA 98121. USA; E-mail: sandras@u.washington.edu

could facilitate routine use of data by community-based, non-scientist health and social services providers as a guide to tailoring intervention for particular families and circumstances.

1.1. Overview of the Chapter

Section 2 of this chapter describes a sociocultural model of maternal health literacy (MHL) in contrast to the dominant clinical model and identifies gaps in the literature. Section 3 Methods details the research design, sample, intervention, measurement, and analytical methods of the present study. Section 4 Results presents findings along with data visualizations and notes on how to interpret them.

Section 5 Discussion considers results of this study confirming and challenging previous findings. New findings and data visualizations confirm that MHL improvement can be maintained and evolve over extended periods of changing HL needs and demands. Section 5.2 describes the utility of combined contextual and intermediate outcomes data to reveal pathways to progress and guide intervention tailoring. The negligible influence of reading skill in MHL improvement is discussed in Section 5.3. Section 5.4 outlines evidence that promoting MHL can reduce disparities due to literacy, young age and mental health. Discussion of MHL as an empowerment strategy, and an illustration of how data visualization documented health empowerment in the study population follow in Section 5.5. Section 5.6 examines the feasibility of data-driven practice in which practitioners routinely use data to personalize intervention. Next, in Section 5.7 an important new finding is discussed: the powerful influence of the social determinants of health on MHL as illustrated by the "Web of Interaction". Section 5.8 suggests MHL promotion can be scaled up through existing home-based interventions. Section 5.9 notes that new findings challenge earlier research which avoided the complexity of home contexts in favor of precision and parsimony. Embracing the complexity revealed pathways to progress and increased understanding of MHL improvement and empowerment. Section 6 suggests future directions for LSP-MHL research and practice.

The Postscript, presents a review of five published LSP-MHL studies and discusses two of their many implications. Section 7 outlines a brief history of the evolution of modern healthcare and describes the Developmental Origins of Health and Disease (DOHaD) and related theories that underpin the MHL concept, the LSP, and calls to promote health literacy as a pragmatic intervention to reduce disease and disparities. These theories have ushered in the third era modern healthcare and positioned maternal-child health and MHL at the very foundations of personal and public health worldwide. Section 8 outlines specific health promotion strategies shown to promote MHL and empowerment. Section 9 describes a comprehensive evaluation framework for health literacy interventions in child health. Section 10 closes the postscript with suggested topics for multidisciplinary dialogue on the challenges and promises of data-drive practice, evidence-based evaluation, and theory-based research in health literacy promotion, particularly in maternal and child health.

2. Maternal Health Literacy: personal asset, life skill, empowerment strategy

Maternal health literacy is a determinant of child [3] and adult health [4] and a source of health disparities [5] worldwide. In accordance with earlier research, the authors operationalized MHL using the World Health Organization definition [6] made specific to mothers [7]: the cognitive and social skills which determine the motivation and ability of mothers to gain access to, understand, and use information in ways that promote and maintain their health and that of their children.

In this sociocultural model, MHL is understood as a personal and community asset [8], a life skill required to navigate health systems and everyday choices that influence health [6]. Promoting MHL is an empowerment strategy to increase mothers' control over personal and child health [9] by increasing their capacity to function in three domains: 1) disease treatment and healthcare, 2) disease prevention and health protection, and 3) health promotion [10]. Each of these domains presents a different set of health literacy tasks in a different context requiring a different combination of skills.

Most health literacy research, especially in the U.S., has addressed the disease treatment and healthcare domain exclusively. Studies have taken a clinical approach focused on patients' lack of reading and numeracy skills needed to understand information related to clinical encounters. Scholars have described this construct as *health-related literacy* [11,12]. Associations are established between low health-related literacy and adverse clinical outcomes. However, results are mixed and the pathway linking reading skills to outcomes is unclear, especially the link between mothers' reading ability and child health outcomes [13]. Largely due to inadequate measures, intervention studies remain rare [3], especially community-based interventions customized to diverse low-literacy populations [14], interventions focused on improving skills [15], and interventions in child health [13]. Health literacy and empowerment rarely have been investigated together; and scant attention has been paid to the role of the social determinants of health in health literacy. The present study addresses these gaps in the evidence base.

3. Methods

3.1. Design

This study is a secondary analysis of a U.S. Agency for Healthcare Research and Quality/National Institutes for Health database combined for AHRQ/NICHD grant #R03HD055618-02.

3.2. Sample

Participating programs, parents and the intervention are described in detail elsewhere [16]. Briefly, of 2395 socio-economically disadvantaged primary caregivers in our database, 98.5% are mothers. Their average age is 24.2 years (sd 0.16); 37% are African American, 32% Caucasian, 18% Hispanic/Latino, and 13% other or unknown. A literacy screen validated with parents of children < age 6 in primary care

[17] indicated 27% of the mothers are below-average readers ($\leq$ 6th grade level) who would benefit from adult education. Children (N = 550) are aged 0 (pregnancy) to 3 years.

3.3. Intervention

The intervention was implemented by 69 home visitors in six programs representing five U.S. national models of home visitation. Home visiting is a preventive intervention to promote maternal-child health and support healthy child development and school readiness. The participating sites are located in California, Montana, Indiana, Georgia, and Virginia. The home visitors were paraprofessionals, public health nurses, nurse case managers, and social workers. These service providers addressed health and social issues together during visits to families in their homes for one to two hours weekly or monthly, for six to 36 months. The service providers were trained in health literacy and empowerment concepts. They integrated into their usual health education and skills development activities an empowerment approach to developing interactive and critical skills.

3.4. Measures - Life Skills Progression Instrument: LSP data guides practice

As part of their usual activities, the participating service providers collected data on mothers' preventive and healthcare-related practices and surrounding family conditions at baseline and six-month intervals for up to 36 months using the LSP [18]. To evaluate MHL and monitor improvement, the authors used the LSP measures of information seeking, use of health services and community resources, health behaviors, preventive practices, and maintenance of safe environments. In other words, they monitored changes in the degree to which mothers produced the theoretically identified consequences of increased health literacy: improvement in health services utilization, risk behaviors, and selfcare [19]. Two previously validated scales derived from the LSP assess different aspects of maternal health literacy [16,20].

The Healthcare Literacy scale (HcL) combines nine LSP item scores to evaluate mothers' use of information and healthcare for the dyad in the previous 6-month period. Sequential changes in the scale score indicate changes in skills that pertain to participation in healthcare. The Selfcare Literacy scale (ScL) combines seven LSP item scores to evaluate mothers' management of personal and child health at home. The ScL scale score indicates skills that pertain to everyday choices, preventive practices and health promoting behaviors that influence family health. See Table 1. In addition, to tie this study to research on health-related literacy, the authors used the LSP's optional health-related literacy screen [17].

Table 1. Summary of LSP Items, Categories, and MHL Scales
This table provides a listing of the items in the Life Skills Progression (LSP) instrument and their organization by categories and inclusion in Healthcare Literacy or Selfcare Literacy scale scores. Baseline scores for each item are listed, and the green box indicates that the average score at baseline was in the target range for a given LSP item.

Category	LSP Item	Avg. Baseline Scores (sd; n)	Health Literacy Scale
Relationships with Family and Friends	Relationships with Family and Extended Family	4.24 (0.02; 2367)	
	Relationships with Father of baby, Spouse, or Boyfriend	3.79 (0.02; 2328)	
	Relationships with Friends and Peers	3.59 (0.02; 2334)	
Relationships with Children	Attitudes towards Pregnancy	3.22 (0.03; 925)	Selfcare
	Nurturing	4.28 (0.02; 2014)	
	Discipline	4.15 (0.02; 1689)	
	Support of Child Development	3.63 (0.2; 2048)	Selfcare
	Safety	4.23 (0.01; 2023)	Selfcare
Relationships with Supportive Resources	Relationships with Home Visitor	4.00 (0.02; 2334)	
	Use of Information	3.93 (0.01; 2350)	Healthcare
	Use of Resources	3.85 (0.02; 2342)	Selfcare
Education	Language	2.82 (0.07; 511)	
	< 12th Grade Education	2.16 (0.05; 1120)	
	Education	2.04 (0.03; 2194)	
	Employment	1.87 (0.02; 2117)	
	Immigration	2.40 (0.07; 488)	

Category	LSP Item	Avg. Baseline Scores (sd; n)	Health Literacy Scale
Health and Healthcare	Prenatal Care	3.87 (0.03; 1129)	Healthcare
	Maternal Sick Care	3.74 (0.02; 1982)	Healthcare
	Family Planning	3.60 (0.03; 1942)	Healthcare
	Child Well Care	4.58 (0.02; 1969)	Healthcare
	Child Sick Care	4.33 (0.02; 1890)	Healthcare
	Child Dental Care	3.49 (0.04; 1032)	Healthcare
	Child Immunizations	4.75 (0.02; 1944)	Healthcare
Mental Health and Substance Use/Abuse	Substance Use/Abuse	4.73 (0.02; 2235)	Selfcare
	Tobacco Use	4.31 (0.02; 2281)	Selfcare
	Depression/Suicide	4.56 (0.02; 2295)	
	Mental Illness	4.77 (0.01; 2312)	
	Self-Esteem	4.12 (0.02; 2342)	Selfcare
	Cognitive Ability	4.75 (0.01; 2341)	
Basic Essentials	Housing	4.38 (0.02; 2369)	
	Food/Nutrition	3.57 (0.02; 2352)	
	Transportation	3.75 (0.02; 2355)	
	Health Insurance	2.83 (0.02; 2308)	Healthcare
	Income	2.54 (0.02; 2253)	
	Child Care	2.82 (0.04; 1954)	
Reading Level	Composite score showing < 6th grade reading level	0.27 (0.01; 2018)	

3.5. Analysis

Analysis and visualizations were completed with STATA [21] and R Studio [22]. In addition to descriptive statistics exploring changes in LSP item scores, paired t-tests were conducted to assess changes in MHL scores from baseline to 6 months of service, 6 to 12 months, 12 to 18 months, and from 18 to 24 months. Among mothers with three or more assessments, repeated-measures ANOVA was conducted to evaluate changes in LSP scores. Average MHL scale score, and LSP item score differences for each time period were calculated among mothers with scores for both time points, and are visualized as a heatmap. Hierarchical cluster analysis shows LSP item scores that display the same pattern of change over time. Bonferroni-adjusted pairwise correlations at baseline illustrate relationships between LSP items as a chord diagram.

4. Results

4.1. MHL Scores Improved Continuously

From initiation of service to 24 months, overall, Healthcare Literacy scores improved from below target into target range (mean score 3.9 to 4.03; n=2122 and 226, respectively). Overall, Selfcare Literacy scores started in target range and improved (mean score 4.09 to 4.23; n=2351 and 229, respectively) (repeated-measures ANOVA, p<0.01) See Figure 1. Healthcare Literacy scores showed greatest improvement from baseline to 6 months (paired t-test, p<0.01), with continued modest increases (repeated measures ANOVA, p<0.01). Selfcare Literacy scores showed greatest improvement later, in the 6-to-12-months period (paired t-test, p<0.01), with continued modest increases (repeated measures ANOVA, p<0.01).

4.2. Heatmap Shows What Changed When

Figure 2 illustrates the rate of average score change for each LSP item. The heatmap converts data to color to visualize patterns of change. Variations in color and intensity highlight the average differences in item scores from one observation to the next among mothers with both observations (e.g. "At 6 mo from baseline" shows the average score change among mothers with both a baseline and 6-mo observation). Observation points should not be confused with child age. Service typically began late in pregnancy or shortly after birth, so that at the end of 12 months of service the child may be aged 6 to 15 months. Orange indicates an increase in the overall average score from the previous observation; blue indicates a decrease. More intense color indicates greater score change since the previous observation. White indicates score maintenance; that is, no change between observations.

The upper heatmap showcases the two MHL scales, Healthcare Literacy and Selfcare Literacy. Healthcare Literacy shows early and steady improvement followed by maintenance. For Self-care Literacy, the heatmap shows delayed improvement followed by maintenance. The lower heatmap shows patterns of change for each LSP item. For example, in Prenatal Care (PNC), the last item listed, light orange in the

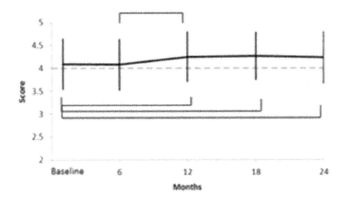

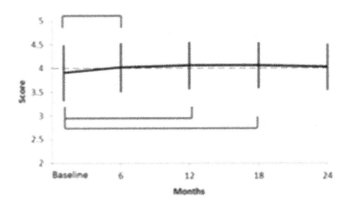

Figure 1. Average Maternal Healthcare Literacy and Selfcare Literacy Scores over Time

Figure 1 reports the average Healthcare Literacy and Selfcare Literacy scores over time. The bars indicate that the change in score is statistically significant (p<0.05).

leftmost column shows that in the first 6 months, prenatal care participation increased moderately from baseline as pregnant mothers enrolled in PNC. In the 6-12-months period, light blue indicates a moderate decline in PNC participation as some mothers gave birth and ended PNC. By 12-18 months of service, dark blue indicates a strong decline as the last of those who were pregnant at baseline delivered and obtained (or missed) a postpartum check-up. In the 18-24 month period, white indicates the near zero level of the previous observation was maintained, suggesting that mothers practiced birth spacing, an important intermediate outcome on the path to ultimate clinical outcomes.

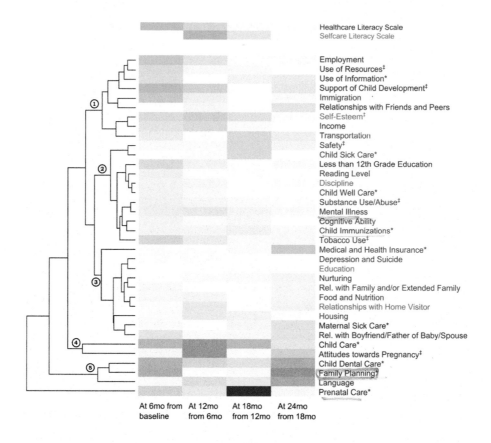

Figure 2. Differences in Average Scores over Time

Figure 2. This heatmap highlights changes in average LSP scores at each 6 month interval, calculated among mothers with both observations (e.g. 6mo to Baseline is based on mothers with both baseline and 6-mo observation scores). The Healthcare Literacy score shows early ample progress, followed by modest progress and near-maintenance. The Selfcare Literacy score shows delayed ample progress, followed by modest progress and near-maintenance. The dendrogram clusters the LSP items by pattern, providing insight into items that "behave" similarly over time. ① bracket shows LSP items that improved early and slowly continued to improve; ② bracket shows LSP items that demonstrated early slight decreases followed by modest improvements; ③ bracket shows LSP items with predominantly score maintenance or minor changes; ④ bracket shows LSP items with substantial and intermittent improvements; ⑤ bracket shows LSP items with substantial and ongoing improvements; last line shows an LSP item with a fluctuating progress.

4.3. Mothers Overcame Multiple Challenges

The heatmap also offers insight into challenges disadvantaged U.S. mothers faced to maintain health, and the timing and degree of improvements they achieved. Table 1 shows that overall 16 life skill indicators were rated below target range at baseline, and another four were borderline in target range (within 0.15 of target cut-off). Items rated below target range (challenges) include MHL indictors: Support of Child Development, Use of Information, Use of Resources, Prenatal Care, Maternal Sick Care, and Child Dental Care; along with contextual factors: Relationships with Father of Baby, Spouse, or Boyfriend; Relationships with Friends and Peers; Attitudes towards Pregnancy; Language; <12th Grade Education; Employment; Income; Child Care; and Reading Level. Of these 16 items, 12 demonstrated substantial improvement in the first year of service. Four remained below target: <12th Grade Education (rated for school-age mothers only), Maternal Sick Care (closely related to insurance status), Relationships with Father of Baby, Spouse, or Boyfriend; and Reading Level. Of the four borderline items (Self-Esteem; Discipline; Education; and Relationships with Home Visitor), average Self-Esteem scores showed continuous improvement throughout service.

4.4. Dendrogram Shows Factors that Changed Together

The dendrogram (numbered brackets on the left of Figure 2) clusters together items that display a similar pattern of change. Each of the numbered large brackets has sub-brackets that refine the groupings to smaller and more similar patterns. Here the authors discuss the major themes from the dendrogram, acknowledging nuanced differences within each bracket.

The top bracket ① shows LSP items that improved early and continued to improve at a slower rate. This bracket includes MHL indicators: Use of Information, Use of Resources, Self-esteem, and Support of Child Development; along with contextual factors that influence or are influenced by them: Immigration, Relationship with Friends and Peers, Employment, Income, and Transportation.

The next bracket ② shows items that demonstrated early slight decline in scores followed by modest score improvements including MHL indicators: Safety, Child Sick Care, Tobacco Use, Substance Use/Abuse, and Child Well Care; along with Discipline and contextual factors: Mental Illness, Cognitive Ability, Less than 12th Grade Education.

The third bracket ③ highlights items that showed predominantly score maintenance or minor shifts in average scores for each period, including MHL indicators: Child Immunizations, Parent Sick Care, and Medical/Health Insurance; along with contextual factors: Housing, Depression/Suicide, Education, Nurturing, Relationships with Family and/or Extended Family, Food/Nutrition, Relationships with Home Visitor, and Relationships with Boyfriend/Father of the Baby/Spouse.

The last brackets ④ and ⑤ show items that improved strongly early and sporadically, with slight decreases or score maintenance including MHL indicators: Child Dental Care, Prenatal Care, Child Care, Attitudes towards Pregnancy, and Family Planning; along with Language.

4.5. Correlations Weave a Web of Interaction

Figure 3 highlights the relationships among LSP items mapped in a chord diagram. The items with the most and strongest correlations include MHL indicators: Self-esteem, Use of Resources, Use of Information, Maternal Sick Care, and Child Sick Care; along with contextual items in Basic Essentials; Relationships with Family, Friends and Peers; and Relationships with Supportive Resources. The factors with the fewest and smallest correlations are Language, Immigration, Less than 12th Grade Education, and reading level.

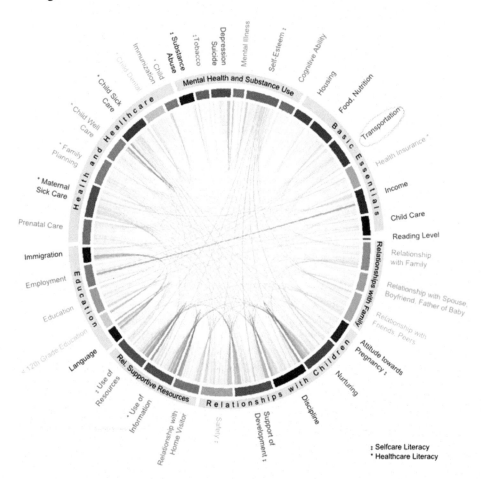

Figure 3. Web of Interaction

Figure 3. The Bonferroni-pairwise correlations mapped in a chord diagram highlight the complexity of health literacy concepts through their relationships with each other. The chord diagram draws a link for each significant pairwise correlation. The relative width of the colored bar representing each LSP item is proportional to the number of correlations with that item; a wider bar indicates the item has more correlations and/or stronger correlations than an item with a narrower bar.

5. Discussion

Analysis of LSP contextual and intermediate outcomes data from six home-based intervention programs in the U.S.enabled the research team to examine both the extent of MHL improvement and what influenced disadvantaged mothers' capacity to manage episodic and everyday challenges to family health. Contextual data provided a rare view of the home context in which mothers raising children in poverty use information for health and enabled the authors to probe the complexity of mothers' everyday lives as a guide to intervention. Results add evidence to findings from previous LSP-MHL studies, highlight the utility of contextual and intermediate outcomes data in health literacy practice and research, and suggest new directions for LSP-MHL research.

5.1. Results Confirm that MHL Develops and Improves

Overall, mothers achieved significant improvements in risk behaviors, preventive practices, and use of health services and community resources, indicating increased knowledge and skills. Figure 1 shows that progress continued throughout the study period with different patterns of change consistent with earlier findings [16].

Further, findings add evidence that improvements can be maintained and built on over an extended period marked by evolving health challenges. The heatmap, Figure 2, makes evident the developmental nature of health literacy. As mothers' and children's needs changed, mothers demonstrated new skills while maintaining progress in other areas. Improvement occurred across the domains of health literacy. These findings support Nutbeam's theory that the skills to use information and services for health can be developed through usual health promotion efforts [23].

5.2. Web of Interaction Maps Pathways to Progress

The Web of Interaction (Figure 3) underscores the inherent complexity of MHL in everyday life by visualizing the extent and magnitude of correlations among 36 factors that interact to influence mothers' progress toward optimal health functioning. All the correlations are statistically significant and positive, indicating that gains in one LSP item score correlate with gains in multiple related items. This new finding has significant implications for practice; it means that each item represents a point to start a positive chain reaction.

Data-informed service providers can tailor intervention to address almost any issue that motivates the mother, and reasonably expect to simultaneously or subsequently improve MHL, advance program priorities, and positively influence the health trajectory of the dyad. For example, one mother's goal to obtain a driver's license (transportation, a social determinant of health) initially seemed a distraction, but her efforts catalyzed MHL score improvement along with other positive changes. The license enabled her to participate in well-child preventive care, and to get a job, which increased her income and enabled her to provide better nutrition and a safer, more stable and stimulating environment, which in turn increased her self-esteem and capacity to improve risk behaviors and support child development.

5.3. Reading Skill Is Not an Important Factor in MHL

The Web of Interaction (Figure 3) shows estimated reading skill is the least influential of 36 factors in MHL. This result confirms a previous LSP-MHL study that found reading skill predicted MHL scores at baseline, but did not predict improvement [27]. Advanced HL skills developed even where functional skills were weak. Focus on developing interactive and critical skills, especially reflection, through a collaborative, mother-directed, problem-focused process consistently improved MHL scores [20,24,25,27].

5.4. Promoting MHL Reduces Disparities

Unskilled readers made greater progress in MHL than their more skilled counterparts [19], indicating that reading skill is neither necessary nor sufficient to manage health and healthcare. The intervention benefitted skilled and unskilled readers, and also reduced the gap between them. This has not been achieved by information improvement initiatives in child health [13]. Further, previous LSP studies showed reductions in disparities related to age [20] and mental health [16,24].

5.5. MHL Promotion Empowers Women

Previous LSP-MHL studies demonstrated that MHL improvement empowers mothers for health. Two studies [16,24] found that depressed mothers improved their MHL scores in part by obtaining treatment for depression, demonstrating increased understanding of information and services, and increased control over actions and decisions affecting the dyad's health. Another study found MHL also empowered service providers in three Parents as Teachers programs [25].

The heat map, Figure 2, further demonstrates empowerment. In the example of prenatal care described under Results, the figure shows a near zero level of prenatal care participation was maintained through the second year of service. The heatmap also shows a strong increase in Family Planning scores in the same period. These two MHL indicators together strongly suggest that, across the six programs, mothers achieved health empowerment as defined by the World Bank [26]: they made a health decision (to plan their next pregnancy); they transformed that choice into desired actions (choose, obtain, use a birth control method) and outcomes (control of their lives and health). These findings further demonstrate health literacy promotion as a pragmatic intervention to empower women and thereby improve infant health and future adult health.

5.6. Data-driven Health Literacy Promotion Is Feasible and Effective

This study demonstrates that data-driven, evidence-based health literacy promotion is feasible and effective. Non-scientist service providers working in uncontrolled home and community environments demonstrated ability to collect quality data, interpret and use it to personalize intervention for specific individuals and circumstances. Paraprofessionals [20,25] social workers [27], and nurse case managers [24] were shown to be effective catalysts to MHL improvement.

5.7. Strong Relationships Among Social Determinants of Health and MHL

Mobley and colleagues [16] found that rural mothers with low MHL scores had problems with housing and transportation. This finding suggested that the social determinants of health (SDoH) might be significant factors in MHL. In the present study, data visualization made clear the powerful influence of transportation and other SDoH, evidenced in the Web of Interaction by the large footprints of items in the Basic Essentials category. The role of SDoH in health literacy improvement is new vista for future research.

5.8. Integrate MHL Promotion into Existing Interventions

Results confirmed that MHL promotion can be integrated into the goals and usual activities of larger existing preventive interventions. The LSP-MHL studies evaluated implementations of the intervention in nine programs in disparate regions of the U.S. with overlapping goals and various service populations, models and providers. Consistently positive results support MHL promotion as a pragmatic intervention that could be scaled up through existing home-based programs.

5.9. Complexity Facilitates Intervention

This study challenges earlier LSP-MHL studies which concentrated on health literacy indicators with limited, selective attention to the contextual data. Results demonstrate that the complexity of dynamic, sometimes chaotic home environments does not preclude strategic intervention; nor does it reduce understanding of what impedes or promotes MHL. Rather, the complexity guides and facilitates intervention.

6. New Directions in LSP-MHL Research and Practice

6.1. Analyze Outcomes and Contextual Data Together

Future LSP-MHL studies should analyze full contextual data along with MHL indicators to further inform interpretation of findings and increase understanding of what impedes or promotes MHL. More studies are needed to fully understand the relationship of MHL and the SDoH and to evaluate interventions that directly address the SDoH as a strategy to increase capacity for MHL.

6.2. Facilitate Routine Use of Data by Service Providers

Technology and data visualization should be applied to facilitate routine use of data by non-scientist service providers. Additional studies are needed to determine how data visualization methods can be applied to elucidate progress in particular families, caseloads, and programs, and the degree to which they support evidence-based practice and policymaking by non-scientists.

6.3. Apply Implementation Science to Guide Scale-up

The U.S. Affordable Care Act [28] expanded home visitation nationwide, set standards of effectiveness, and required outcomes evaluation to identify promising practices and increase quality of service. This expansion and move to evidence-based practice suggest further evaluation of home visitation networks as existing infrastructure on which to mount a national initiative to improve health literacy in disadvantaged parents and empower women in the U.S.

6.4. Update, Expand the LSP Database

To facilitate such research, the LSP database should be updated and expanded. This can be rapidly accomplished by collecting existing LSP data now held separately by more than 400 programs using the instrument as of early 2017. Early adopters have up to 13 years of data.

An expanded database would overcome a limitation of this and other LSP-MHL studies, and increase their strengths. Additional data on male partners would enable evaluation of paternal health literacy progress. The variety of participating programs and service providers, and the size and diversity of the combined study population, along with repeated measures of intermediate outcomes and contextual factors would provide robust data to better understand and promote MHL and empowerment.

Further, the expanded and updated database would serve as the foundation for a national database to collect data as it is generated and establish norms, comparison groups, and performance reports for contributors. A national LSP database would support ongoing research to rapidly identify and disseminate best practices in MHL promotion, and in home visiting, while training the next generation of researchers for both fields.

7. Post Script: Health Literacy Research and Practice for the Third Era of Modern Healthcare

This postscript considers two of many implications of the LSP-MHL studies for future health literacy research and practice. First, in the broad view, the author traces the theoretical foundations of the LSP-MHL framework to global health policy, and further to its roots in the convergence of theory and evidence from multiple fields that is bringing heath literacy promotion to the forefront of global health. The potential of future health literacy research grounded in that theoretical foundation is discussed. Secondly, the LSP-MHL intervention studies address a specific identified need for research in health literacy and child health including, in addition to theoretical grounding and evidence, specific strategies and an evaluation framework.

7.1. Theoretical Foundations to Advance Research and Practice

Health literacy emerged as a field of research and health policy around 2000. In the same period, theory and empirical evidence from multiple fields converged into a new understanding of health and disease that ushered in the third era of modern healthcare [29]. However, health literacy research has yet to make the shift to the new paradigm. Consequently, two decades of research has produced scant data and little insight to inform intervention. The LSP-MHL studies can serve as a model to help align research with the theoretical foundations of the new era.

7.2. A Brief History of Healthcare

The first era of modern healthcare (1900s) began with germ theory and understanding of health as the absence of disease. Practice aimed to achieve survival from infectious diseases. The second era (1950–) started with discovery of gene theory and understanding of health as a combination of genetic makeup and adult lifestyle choices. First-era practice was overlaid with chronic disease treatment and emphasis on quality of life, patient activation, informed consent, self-care, and health promotion. The current third era of modern healthcare (2000–) began with discovery of the Developmental Origins of Health and Disease (DOHaD) [29].

Evidence of DOHaD led global health scholars and policy makers to view promoting health literacy as a pragmatic intervention to improve public health, empower women, and reduce disparities worldwide. U.S. policy documents call for health literacy intervention to improve maternal-child health and achieve the full benefits of health care reform [1]. Still, healthcare systems have been slow to respond. Research in U.S. academic medical centers continues to develop the science around second era concepts of health and literacy; an approach that has stymied intervention.

Two theories that grew out of DOHaD underpin the LSP, MHL and global health literacy policy. These theories offer new foundations for research to increase understanding of the broader concept of health literacy and inform intervention to promote it across the life course. Theory-based evaluation combining outcome measures with contextual data can shed light on both the extent of improvement and how the change occurred [30].

7.3. Life Course Health Development - Promote health literacy over the life course

Discovery of DOHaD led to new understanding of health as constantly developing and socially determined. Life course health development theory [1] describes how health develops over a person's lifetime. The primary challenges and tasks of health protection, promotion, and management evolve along a trajectory from early development in utero and childhood, to increasing function in adolescence, to maintenance of function in adulthood, to decline in old age. Health literacy challenges and skills change along the same trajectory, such that an individual's health literacy progression is lifelong and evolving; hence, the UN General Assembly's recommendation to promote health literacy across the life course.

7.4. The Social Determinants of Health - Focus on Parents

The Social Determinants of Health (SDoH) are factors that determine whether and how developmental predisposition to adult disease is expressed. Health influences and is influenced first by our parents' and then our own income, education, nutrition, transportation, and physical and social environments including healthcare access and health literacy [31]. Child development research shows that parents pass skills to their children in the course of everyday interactions [32]. Therefore, the benefits of parents' improved health literacy can be expected to extend to entire families across their life course; hence the United Nations' call to focus health literacy promotion efforts on parents. Findings of the latest LSP-MHL study confirm the logic that the SDoH also are determinants of health literacy.

7.5. Health Disparities Begin Before Birth - Prioritize Mothers in Poverty

Since the social determinants of health shape parents' health and health literacy, which in turn shape their children's early development and adult health, disparities are present even before birth and perpetuate. Therefore, health and health literacy follow the social gradient; disease and limited health literacy concentrate among the disadvantaged and disempowered; hence the research priority on parents raising children in poverty. The LSP-MHL studies found that lower functioning mothers made greater gains in MHL than their higher functioning counterparts and so reduced disparities related to literacy, young age, and mental health.

The LSP-MHL studies and other research with parents confirm that mothers remain the primary caregivers of children, and the primary managers of health and healthcare at home [33]. It is likely that fathers have MHL and perhaps other distinctly paternal health literacy skills; but available data on fathers is insufficient to assess those skills or their impacts. Improving MHL, and in the process empowering disadvantaged women, reduces disparities by enabling mothers to reduce health risks, maximize protective factors, and better obtain the benefits of accessible health and social services for themselves and their families.

7.6. Health Empowerment - Develop Interactive and Reflective Skills

Health literacy is empowering to the degree that it enables individuals to gain control of decisions and actions that affect their health. The second-era approach to health literacy research and practice views adequate health-related literacy as a prerequisite for health empowerment. Since low health-related literacy is considered to be pervasive and unmodifiable short of reforming education systems, research has generally ignored empowerment. Rather, patients' low literacy has been posited as an explanation for inequities and disparities, low quality, [34] poor outcomes [15], and high costs [35]. This deficit approach is disempowering to all concerned. It ignores the health literacy of those without current need or access to services. It positions those seeking care as cognitively inadequate or insufficiently motivated to obtain the benefits of that care. Without empowerment, improved understanding of healthcare information fosters dependence on health professionals to decide what to believe or do.

In contrast, in the LSP-MHL approach, service providers engaged mothers in reflection, a process through which mothers honed interactive and critical skills to decide themselves what to believe or do. By definition, they were empowered; they gained control over decisions and actions that affect their health [6].

The LSP-MHL studies show that theory-based evaluation combining intermediate outcomes measures with contextual data can elucidate both the extent of improvement and what facilitated or impeded it. By starting from the understanding that health and disease originate in early development and evolve over the life course in ways determined by social conditions, health literacy research can guide intervention across the life course and so reduce the burdens of disease and disparities worldwide in the third era of modern healthcare.

8. Evidence-based Evaluation of Health Literacy for Child Health

The LSP-MHL studies address an important specific research need identified by Dewalt and Hink [13]. In a systematic review of health literacy and child health, they found an abundance of information improvement initiatives, but a comparative dearth of evidence-based assessments of interventions to improve parents' health literacy, especially interventions that reduced disparities between skilled and unskilled readers. In addition to theoretical grounding, the LSP provides evidence, specific strategies, and a comprehensive evaluation framework for community, family, and child health interventions.

8.1. Health Promotion Strategies Improve MHL

Health literacy can be promoted through usual health promotion activities: health education, skills development, and direct information assistance. Health promotion planning typically is concerned with content, timing and teaching strategy. In the LSP-MHL intervention, content and timing are determined by the mother according to her interest and motivation and surrounding family and community conditions. The teaching strategy is reflective questioning.

8.2. Reflective Questioning: Teach by Asking

Rather than delivering standard content and answering questions, service providers were trained to use LSP data to prioritize needs, build on strengths, and tailor reflective questions to engage mothers in addressing a particular challenge. Reflective questions create opportunities to practice interactive and critical skills in the process of deciding what to believe or do. Reflective conversations led mothers to prioritize challenges, obtain information, plan actions, marshall resources, and progress toward their goals with increasing autonomy and confidence.

8.3. "I talk less; parents think more."

The use of reflective questioning, instead of traditional information-giving or educating, precipitates an essential change in practice. By leading reflective conversations, service providers shifted the focus of their visits from expert-defined content to the reflective process, so that learning became mother-directed, problem-based, collaborative, and therefore empowering. Reflective questioning shifts the intent of health education from information-giving for knowledge gain, to empowerment for making decisions and taking actions that affect health.

    Direct information assistance includes reflective conversation to evaluate and personalize information and apply it in context for personal benefit. Mothers were encouraged to discuss information from healthcare providers and other sources. To aid recall, trigger discussion, and encourage further learning, mothers were provided printed health education materials, including materials designed for low-skilled learners [36]. Print materials and other information were offered when requested, rather than according to a schedule, and were discussed as part of reflective conversations. More research is needed to determine the degree of improvement attributable to materials.

9. Evaluation Framework for Health Literacy Interventions in Child Health

What researchers measure and how they measure it matters because it determines what they find out about what works, what is worth doing, and who should do it [30]. The LSP approach to measuring health literacy and evaluating interventions in child health can advance research and practice by changing what researchers measure, how they measure it, and how *practitioners* use the data.

The dominant clinical approach asks *How poorly does this patient read?* It measures patients' and parents' health-related literacy by a single administration of a brief reading test. From these measures researchers have found out that nearly everyone, including an estimated one third of parents [37], has low health-related literacy. This "silent epidemic" [38] presents a risk to child safety, systems efficiency, and costs. Researchers have concluded that nothing short of reforming education systems can improve parents' health-related literacy; so improving information is the only available response. As the primary source of knowledge in healthcare organizations, clinicians are expected to manage the risks of parents' and other patients' low health-related literacy. Some argue for using the data to identify patients with low health-related literacy; but reading test scores suggest no viable response to those patients. Bennett validated a 3-question screen to identify parents of children to age 6 in pediatric care who would benefit by referral to adult literacy programs [17]. With this exception, health-related literacy testing is conducted only for research purposes since it leaves patients feeling embarrassed and alienated [39], disempowered.

In contrast, the LSP asks *What is this mother doing for health? What is helping; and what is in her way?* Rather than estimating skill level and inferring what a person at a given level of skill can or will do, the LSP monitors progress to optimal functioning through a continuum of characteristic actions, practices and behaviors indicative of increasing skill and autonomy. From measures of progress, researchers and practitioners see changes in what a mother (or a service population), actually does for health with the information, skills and support she has. With repeated measures, they can see the effects of both improved information and of efforts to increase capacity to use that information.

Since the LSP monitors changes in the home context, researchers and practitioners also gain insight into how the social determinants of health operate to influence a family's health and health literacy. The contextual data supports recommendations that pediatricians collaborate with home visitation programs [3,40] to monitor and improve child health. It might be more effective to address health and social problems together, rather than through separate systems [26].

By embracing the complexity, researchers find multiple pathways to progress, and multiple points from which practitioners can start a positive chain reaction. The challenge then is not to discover the one thing that works, but rather to discover the combination of factors that work for a particular mother and child in a particular situation. Whatever step a mother is willing and able to take now for her child's health is worth taking; it shifts her into action, sets the dyad on a positive trajectory, and builds confidence to take the next step.

Further, from measures of progress, researchers find that professional and paraprofessional health and social services providers of diverse backgrounds can be effective catalysts to improve maternal health literacy, and thereby improve child health and future adult health. Action research in health literacy and child health, like the LSP studies, in which practitioners undertake research activities to increase their own effectiveness, hones intervention and might reveal a universal process for identifying the effective combination of factors in a specific circumstance.

While the LSP is a data collection instrument, it also is integral to intervention and its evaluation. The LSP documents progress, regression, and maintenance that otherwise may not be evident, and guides practice in the field. Further, LSP data documents effectiveness for funders and policy makers, guides reflective supervision, and informs staff training and evaluation.

The LSP-MHL studies demonstrate the feasibility and effectiveness of health literacy intervention in child health. Intervention that is grounded in current theory and empirical evidence, community-based, and data-driven can improve maternal health literacy, empower women, and positively influence the health trajectory of families and communities.

10. Third-era Health Literacy Research: Multidisciplinary and Multinational

Additional implications of the LSP-MHL intervention studies provide a platform for future multidisciplinary dialogue on the challenges and promises of data-drive practice, evidence-based evaluation, and theory-based research in health literacy promotion, particularly in maternal and child health. Topics for ongoing discussion include incorporating MHL improvement into federal benchmarks of effectiveness in home visitation; how the LSP approach can be adapted for disease-specific home-based interventions and clinical settings; and how implementation science and big data methods can be applied to disseminate MHL promotion in community-based intervention programs. Collaborative multinational research may identify a universal method to adapt the LSP-MHL approach to cultures and conditions in poverty populations across the globe.[2]

References

[1]   Halfon N, Larson K, Lu M, Tullis E, Russ S. Lifecourse health development: past, present and future. Matern Child Health J. 2014; 18:344–365.
[2]   Hanson M, Gluckman P, Nutbeam D, Hearn J. Priority actions for the non communicable disease crisis. Lancet 378: 566–67; 2011. Shanghai Declaration available at http://www.thelancet.com/cms/attachment/2009245863/2032056526/mmc1.pdf. Retrieved October 4 2016.
[3]   Abrams MA, Klass P, Dreyer BP. Health literacy and children: Recommendations for action. Pediatrics. 2009; 124(Supplement): S327–S331. DOI:10.1542/peds.2009-1162i.
[4]   Halfon N, Hochstein M. Life course health development: An integrated framework for developing health, policy, and research. Milbank Q. 2002;80(3):433-79.
[5]   Kickbush I, Pelikan JM, Apfel F, Tsouros AD (Editors.). Health literacy: the solid facts. World Health Organization, Copenhagen; 2013. http://www.euro.who.int/__data/assets/pdf_file/0008/190655/e96854.pdf?ua=1. Retrieved October 4 2016.
[6]   Nutbeam D. Health promotion glossary. Health Prom Int. 1998;13(4):349–364. DOI: 10.1093/heapro/13.4.349.
[7]   Renkert S, Nutbeam D. Opportunities to improve maternal health literacy through ante-natal education: an exploratory study. Health Prom Int. 2001;16:381–388.
[8]   Nutbeam D. The evolving concept of health literacy. Soc Sci Med. 2008;67:2072–2078.

[2] This research was funded by the U.S. National Library of Medicine. The authors declare there is no conflict of interest.

[9]   Kickbush I, Maag D. Health Literacy. In: Heggenhougen K, Quah S, Editors. International encyclopedia of public health, 3rd ed. San Diego: Academic Press; 2008:204–211.
[10] Sørensen K, Van den Broucke S, Fullam J, et al. BMC Public Health. 2012;12(1):1. DOI: 10.1186/1471-2458-12-80. http://www.biomedcentral.com/1471-2458/12/80. Retrieved February 2 2016.
[11] Baker DW. The meaning and the measure of health literacy. J Gen Intern Med. 2006;21(8):878–883. DOI: 10.1111/j.1525-1497.2006.00540.x.
[12] Nutbeam D. Defining and measuring health literacy: What can we learn from literacy studies? Int J Public Health. 2009;54(5):303–305. DOI: 10.1007/s00038-009-0050-x.
[13] Dewalt DA, Hink A. Health literacy and child health outcomes: a systematic review of the literature. Pediatrics. 2009;124 (Supplement): S265–S274. DOI: 10.1542/peds.2009-1162b.
[14] Rudd RE. Mismatch between skills of patients and tools in use: Might literacy affect diagnoses and research? J Rheumatol. 2010;37(5):885–886. DOI: 10.3899/jrheum.100135.
[15] Berkman ND, Sheridan SL, Donahue KE, Halpern DJ, Viera A, Crotty K, Holland A, Brasure M, Lohr KN, Harden E, Tant E, Wallace I, & Viswanathan M. Health literacy interventions and outcomes: an updated systematic review. Evidence Report/Technology Assessment No. 199. RTI International-University of North Carolina Evidence-based Practice Center under contract No. 290-2007-10056-I.
[16] Smith SA, Moore EJ. Health literacy and depression in the context of home visitation. Matern Child Health J. 2012;16(7):1500–1508. DOI: 10.1007/s10995-011-0920-8.
[17] Bennett IM, Robbins S, Haecker T. Screening for low literacy among adult caregivers of pediatric patients. Fam Med. 2003; 35: 585–590.
[18] Wollesen L, Peifer K. Life Skills Progression: an outcome and intervention planning instrument for use with families at risk. Baltimore: Brookes; 2006.
[19] Sykes S, Wills J, Rowlands G, Popple K. Understanding critical health literacy: a concept analysis. BMC Public Health. 2013;13(1):150. DOI: 10.1186/1471-2458-13-150.
[20] Smith S. Promoting health literacy; concept, measurement, intervention [PhD]. Cincinnati, OH: Union Institute and University; 2009. Publication No. AAT 3375168.
[21] StataCorp. Stata statistical software: release 11. College Station, TX: StataCorp LP; 2009.
[22] RStudio Team. RStudio: integrated development for R., Boston: R Studio Inc; 2013.
[23] Nutbeam D. Health outcomes and health promotion: defining success in health promotion. Health Promo J of Austr. 1996: 658–60.
[24] Mobley S, Thomas S, Sutherland D, et al. Maternal health literacy progression among rural perinatal women. Matern Child Health J. 2014;18(8):1881–1892. DOI: 10.1007/s10995-014-1432-0.
[25] Carroll LN, Smith SA, Thomson NR. Parents as teachers health literacy demonstration project: integrating an empowerment model of health literacy promotion into home-based parent education. Health Promot Pract. 2014;16(2):282–290. DOI: 10.1177/1524839914538968.
[26] World Bank. Empowerment. PovertyNet. http://go.worldbank.org/S9B3DNEZ00. Retrieved June 15 2016.
[27] Haynes GW, Neuman D, Hook C, et al. Comparing child and family outcomes between two home visitation programs. Fam Consum Sci Res J. 2015;43(3):209–228. DOI: 10.1111/fcsr.12098.
[28] Patient Protection and Affordable Care Act, 42 U.S.C. § 18001 et seq. (2010)
[29] Wadhwa P, Buss C, et al. Developmental origins of health and disease: Brief history of the approach and current focus on epigenetic mechanisms. Sem Repro Med. 2009;27(05):358–68.
[30] Schorr L. Common purpose: strengthening families and neighborhoods to rebuild America. New York, NY: Anchor Books; 1997.
[31] Social Determinants of Health. https://www.healthypeople.gov/2020/topics-objectives/topic/social-determinants-of-health. Retrieved October 4 2016.
[32] National Research Council and Institute of Medicine. From neurons to neighborhoods: the science of early childhood development. Committee on Integrating the Science of Early Childhood Development. Shonkoff JP, and Phillips DA, editors. Board on Children, Youth, and Families, Commission on Behavioral and Social Sciences and Education. Washington, D.C.: National Academy Press; 2000.
[33] Matoff-Stepp S, Applebaum B, Pooler J, Kavanagh E. Women as health care decision-makers: implications for health care coverage in the United States. J Health Care Poor Underserved. 2014 Nov;25(4):1507–13. DOI: 10.1353/hpu.2014.0154.
[34] Agency for Healthcare Research and Quality. National Healthcare Disparities Report. Rockville, MD: U.S. Department of Health and Human Services, Agency for Healthcare Research and Quality; 2008. AHRQ Pub. No. 08-0041.
[35] Rasu RS, Bawa WA, Suminski R, Snella K, Warady B. Health literacy impact on national healthcare utilization and expenditure. Int J Health Policy Manag. 2015; 17;4(11):747–55. DOI: 10.15171/ijhpm.2015.151.
[36] Smith SA. Beginnings pregnancy guide and beginnings parents guide. Seattle: Practice Development Inc; 1989–2014.

[37] Yin HS, Johnson M, Mendelsohn AL, Abrams MA, Sanders LM, Dreyer BP. The health literacy of parents in the United States: a nationally representative study. Pediatrics 2009;124 (Suppl):S289–S298. DOI: 10.1542/peds.2009-1162e.

[38] Parker RM, Schwartzberg JG. Guest editorial. What patients do— and don't—understand: widespread ignorance has triggered a silent epidemic. Postgrad Med. 2001;109(5):13–16.

[39] Parikh N, Parker R, Nurss J, Baker, DW, Williams, MD. Shame and health literacy: the unspoken connection. Patient Educ and Couns.1996;27:33–39.

[40] American Academy of Pediatrics, Council on Community Pediatrics. The role of preschool home-visiting programs in improving children's developmental and health outcomes. http://www.pediatrics.org/cgi/DOI/10.1542/ peds.2008-3607. Retrieved October 4 2016.

Health Literacy Leadership

Health Literacy
R.A. Logan and E.R. Siegel (Eds.)
IOS Press, 2017
doi:10.3233/978-1-61499-790-0-169

Roundtable on Health Literacy: Issues and Impact

Lyla HERNANDEZ[a,1], Melissa FRENCH[b], and Ruth PARKER[c]

[a,b] *National Academies of Sciences, Engineering, and Medicine*
[c] *Emory University School of Medicine*

Abstract. In 2004 the Institute of Medicine (IOM) report, Health Literacy: A Prescription to End Confusion, highlighted that "efforts to improve quality, to reduce costs, and to reduce disparities cannot succeed without efforts to improve health literacy" [1]. The IOM report emphasized that poor health literacy is a major challenge for individuals who need to find, understand, and use information to make informed decisions for health. Following the publication of the 2004 report and in response to rising interest in health literacy in the U.S., the IOM established the Roundtable on Health Literacy. Roundtables convene a broad array of stakeholders from foundations, health plans, associations, government, private companies, and patient and consumer groups to discuss challenges and provide a forum for exchange of knowledge and expertise. The Roundtable does not make recommendations, rather its mission is to inform, inspire, and activate diverse U.S. (and potentially international) stakeholders. The Roundtable's activities support the development, implementation, and sharing of evidence-based health literacy practices and policies. The Roundtable's goal is to improve the health and well-being of Americans as well as persons in other nations.

Since its inception, the Roundtable has explored ways in which health literacy relates to a diverse array of topics from medications to oral health to public health to health equity and more. In particular the Roundtable has served to highlight the issues central to the alignment of system demands and complexities with individual skills and abilities. Roundtable workshops and discussions, no matter the specific topic, maintain a focus on identifying and illuminating evidence-based health literacy approaches that foster high-quality, patient centered care. The work of the Roundtable has been used throughout the United States and globally to foster health literate organizations and approaches to improving patient-centered care and the health of populations. Going forward the Roundtable's efforts will continue to build upon past work, strive to maintain relevance to the field, and encourage and engage others in advancing our nation's health.

Keywords. Health literacy, numeracy, oral health, health equity, informed consent, palliative care, precision medicine, health information technology, health literate organization

1. Introduction

In 2004 the Institute of Medicine[2] (IOM) report, Health Literacy: A Prescription to End Confusion, highlighted that "efforts to improve quality, to reduce costs, and to reduce

---

[1] Corresponding author: Board on Population Health and Public Health Practice, Health and Medicine Division, National Academies of Sciences, Engineering, and Medicine, 500 5th Street NW, Keck 813, Washington, DC 20001; Email: lhernandez@nas.edu.

[2] Please note that as of March 2016 the IOM was renamed the Health and Medicine Division of the National Academies of Sciences, Engineering, and Medicine. As such, it continues the consensus studies and

disparities cannot succeed without efforts to improve health literacy [1]." The IOM report emphasized that poor health literacy is a major challenge for individuals who need to find, understand, and use information to make informed decisions for health. The IOM report also provided a comprehensive strategy to improve health literacy in the U.S.

The publication of the IOM report and announcements of research funding opportunities from the Agency for Healthcare Research and Quality and the National Institutes of Health fostered interest in health literacy in the U.S. Within two years, the interest within the U.S. health care community resulted in the IOM's 2006 decision to establish the Roundtable on Health Literacy.[3] Unlike consensus studies by committees of the U.S. National Academies, Roundtables do not make recommendations. A major strength of the Roundtable is it gathers a broad array of stakeholders from foundations, health plans, associations, government, private companies, and patient and consumer groups to discuss challenges and provide a forum for exchange of knowledge and expertise. Accordingly, the mission of the Roundtable on Health Literacy is to inform, inspire, and activate diverse U.S. (and potentially international) stakeholders. The Roundtable's activities support the development, implementation, and sharing of evidence-based health literacy practices and policies. The Roundtable's goal is to improve the health and well-being of Americans as well as persons in other nations.

2. Issues and Activities

To achieve its mission, the Roundtable sponsors meetings and workshops where Roundtable members, invited participants, and the public discuss the challenges facing health literacy research and practice. The Roundtable identifies approaches to promote health literacy through mechanisms and partnerships in both the public and private sector in the U.S. (and potentially other nations). The Roundtable's products include peer-reviewed workshop summaries, commissioned papers, and individually authored discussion papers and commentaries. The Roundtable's commissioned papers may support a particular workshop or be stand-alone projects which explore specific topics in depth. Discussion papers and commentaries are prepared by individual members as well as non-members of the Roundtable. These submissions provide substantive, in-depth analysis of specific topics or illuminate issues through thought-provoking, concise essays.

The following discussion describes some areas of interest and activity undertaken by the Roundtable since its inception, which are outlined in Table 1.

2.1. Health Literate Organizations

The Roundtable examined issues related to aligning the demands and complexities of health care systems with individual skills and abilities (Figure 1) through a commissioned paper, two workshops, and two discussion papers (Table 1. Topic: Health Literate Organizations). The commissioned paper explored how health care

---

convening activities previously undertaken by the IOM. As a result, the Roundtable on Health Literacy may be referred to in the chapter as the IOM Roundtable, the National Academies Roundtable, or simply the Roundtable.

[3] http://nationalacademies.org/healthliteracyRT

organizations could reduce their health literacy-related complexities and developed a list of attributes of a health literate organization that was presented at a workshop during which reactions were given by individuals from a variety of organizations [2, 3].

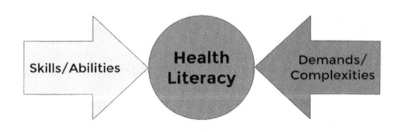

Figure 1. A Framework for Health Literacy [4]

Individual Roundtable participants revised the list of the proposed 18 attributes from the commissioned paper to ten, based on comments and reactions at the workshop and prepared two discussion papers. The first paper briefly describes ten attributes of a health literate organization (Figure 2), that is, an organization that makes it easier for people to navigate, understand, and use information and services to take care of their health [5]. The second paper provides an elaboration of the meaning of and basis for each of the ten attributes, followed by a set of implementation strategies that can be used to achieve the attribute [6].

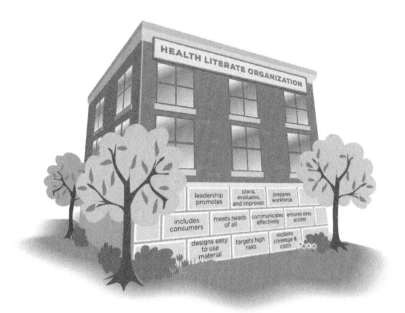

Figure 2. Attributes of a Health Literate Organization

2.2. Health Reform

"Although low health literacy is certainly not a featured concern of the health care reform legislation passed in early 2010, there are those who would argue that the law cannot be successful without a redoubling of national efforts to address the issue [9]." The Roundtable commissioned three papers, held three workshops, and individual authors prepared three discussion papers on U.S. health insurance reform. A list of all health reform-related publications is provided in Table 1 (Topic: Health Reform).

The Roundtable convened a workshop that examined how health literacy could facilitate the implementation of provisions of the ACA. The Roundtable commissioned two papers to be presented at the workshop to stimulate discussion. The first paper by Somers and Mahadevan explored how health literacy could apply to the provisions of the Act [10]. The second paper by Sanders explored various ways in which the Act affected children [11].

Many of those who became newly eligible for health insurance in the U.S. have poor health literacy, are more comfortable in languages other than English, or are unfamiliar with the U.S. health system and health insurance. Health insurance terms and, indeed, the concept of health insurance itself present communication challenges for health insurance exchanges. The Roundtable convened a second workshop on health insurance reform that focused on four topics: "lessons learned from existing state insurance exchanges; the impact of state insurance exchanges on consumers; the relevance of health literacy to health insurance exchanges; and current best practices in developing materials and communicating with consumers [12]."

Several members prepared discussion papers to further illuminate important issues in health insurance reform. One paper by Patel and colleagues provides basic information on health insurance including important terms, types of public and private health insurance options, an explanation of health insurance marketplaces, and the personnel available to provide help [13]. A second paper by Patel and colleagues describes how simplifying approaches to obtain and use health insurance can empower underserved communities to become involved in and take charge of their health [14]. Wu and colleagues prepared a paper that addressed the questions: What are my choices for health insurance? How do I get it? How do I use it? How much will it cost me [15]?

In 2014 the Roundtable commissioned an effort aimed at identifying major issues, other than information technology, encountered by health insurance exchanges when working to enroll individuals within their areas. The resulting paper describes 11 successful strategies for reaching hard-to-reach individuals in African American, Hispanic, and Asian populations, proposes a model for engaging hard-to reach populations, and makes recommendations for key stakeholders [16].

The Roundtable convened a third workshop in July 2016. That workshop focused on health insurance literacy including coverage and cost, the role of health literacy in accessing health care and remaining in treatment (including shared decision-making), delivery and financing system reforms that affect organizational health literacy, and quality and equity considerations. When the report of the workshop is completed it will be available on the Roundtable website.

2.3. Medications

Health literacy challenges regarding understanding and use of medications has been a long standing topic for the Roundtable. Activities include two workshops with planned future activities in this area (see Table 1, Topic: Medications). A 2007 Roundtable workshop examined what is known about how medication container labeling affects patient safety and approaches that could be used to address identified problems [17]. The Impact section of this chapter describes some far reaching action stimulated by this workshop.

The U.S. Food and Drug Administration launched the Safe Use Initiative in 2009 to address unnecessary adverse events associated with misuse of medications. A Roundtable workshop focused on challenges in educating consumers about over-the-counter medications and current drug safety efforts undertaken by numerous stakeholders. Participants also suggested ways to improve the Safe Use Initiative [18].

A 2016 workshop addressed the topic of providing clear written communications to patients and caregivers while focusing on the patient experience. The day began with a patient experience panel and moderated discussion that featured the experiences and insights of patients and caregivers. Later panels focused on human-centered design and its role in regulations, translating research into practice, and the future of health literate design. The proceedings of the workshop will be published on the roundtable website when completed.

2.4. Oral Health

The relevance of health literacy to oral health has been explored through a 2011 workshop, discussion papers, and development of an oral health collaborative (Table 1, Topic: Oral Health).

The workshop explored research in oral health literacy and how findings from the research inform oral health practice [19]. The Roundtable collaborative on oral health and health literacy is in the process of development. A collaborative is an ad hoc convening activity which enables Roundtables to involve additional stakeholders beyond the membership of the Roundtable. Collaboratives are groups of roundtable members and others in the field who work together to make progress toward the goals of the Roundtable. Their work can also focus on advancing recommendations from consensus studies of the National Academies of Sciences, Engineering, and Medicine.

The Action Collaborative on Health Literacy: A Potential Pathway to Connecting Dental Health with General Health focuses on exploring ways in which health literacy principles and practices can promote effective integration of dental health and general health into an actionable primary care model. The collaborative's ultimate goal is to catalyze action in the use of health literacy practices to promote integrated, coordinated, patient-centered care in the U.S. (and potentially internationally). An initial information gathering activity of the collaborative was commissioning an environmental scan of existing programs and practices that integrate dental and general health with descriptions of health literacy approaches employed. When the commissioned report is completed it will be available on the Roundtable website.

A discussion paper by Horowitz and colleagues explores why after-visit summaries could be an important tool for dentistry in providing patient-centered care [20]. The authors state "providing information to patients about their disease, including their individual risk for disease, along with health support tools, has the potential to benefit individual patients and patient populations overall." A commentary by Geiermann and colleagues discusses the role of community health representatives in improving oral health in communities on the Navajo reservation [21]. Slayton and colleagues produced a discussion paper that explores prevention and management of tooth decay through "person-centered approaches, such as individual risk assessment, active surveillance, oral health literacy and preventive interventions/therapies, supplemented, when necessary, by surgical care (drilling, filling, extraction) [22]."

2.5. State of the Science

Evidence-based approaches are central to the efforts of the Roundtable as it convenes discussions on various topics. Pursuing what is known, what evidence exists, is important to the field of health literacy and the efforts of the Roundtable. Several specific promising areas of the science of health literacy have been examined, including how to measure health literacy and challenges related to numeracy skills (Table 1, Topic: Research).

2.5.1. Research

Two workshops have been convened that focused on health literacy research issues. A 2009 workshop examined measures of health literacy. "Although research on health literacy has grown tremendously in the past decade, both in terms of assessing the level of health literacy of individuals and examining the relationship of health literacy to various health outcomes, a concern is that there is no widely agreed-on framework for health literacy as a determinant of health outcomes [23]."

In 2010 a Roundtable workshop explored promising areas for research including a report on presentations at the first Health Literacy Annual Research Conference, the role of health literacy in health disparities research, the relationship of health literacy to information technology applications, and professional development in health literacy research [24]. And in 2013, DeWalt and McNeil prepared a paper that describes how health literacy can be linked to quality performance measurement in the U.S. [25].

2.5.2. Numeracy

"[T]he ability to understand, evaluate, and use numbers is important to making informed health care choices [26]." The Roundtable explored numeracy issues as a major area of difficulty for consumers (Table 1, Topic: Numeracy). The Roundtable commissioned a paper on numeracy skills that addressed three major questions:

1. What does research show about people's numeracy skill levels in the U.S.?
2. What numeracy skills are needed by U.S. consumers to select a health plan, choose treatments, and understand medication instructions?
3. What do we know about how U.S. providers should communicate with those with low numeracy skills?

The commissioned paper by Peters and colleagues was presented at a Roundtable workshop that explored several topics related to numeracy including the effects of ill health on cognitive capacity, issues with communication of health information to the public, and communicating numeric information for decision making [26, 27].

Some Roundtable members prepared two discussion papers related to health literate communication about numerical information as a follow up to interest and questions generated by the workshop. A paper by Pleasant and colleagues provides guiding principles for communicating numbers in a clear, simple way [28]. The paper by Rudd explores what the science tells us about people's levels of numeracy, about numeracy in health interactions, and about health-related numeracy tools [29].

2.6. Other Issues

In addition to the activities described above, the Roundtable has engaged in numerous work in other areas (see Table 1, Other Issues.)

Table 1. Roundtable on Health Literacy-related Workshop Summaries, Commissioned Papers, and Discussion Papers and Commentaries

Topic	Workshop Summaries	Commissioned Papers	Discussion Papers and Commentaries
Health Literate Organizations	*How Can Health Care Organizations Become More Health Literate: Workshop Summary* [3] *Organizational Change to Improve Health Literacy: Workshop Summary* [7]	The Other Side of the Coin: Attributes of a Health Literate Health Care Organization [2] Measures to Assess a Health Literate Organization [8]	Attributes of a Health Literate Organization [5] Ten Attributes of a Health Literate Health Care Organization [6]
Health Reform	*Health Literacy Implications for Health Care Reform: Workshop Summary* [9] *Facilitating State Health Exchange Communication Through the Use of Health Literate Practices: Workshop Summary* [12]	Successfully Engaging Hard-to-Reach Populations in Health Insurance: A Focus on Outreach, Sign up and Retention, and Use [16]	Helping Consumers Understand and Use Health Insurance in 2014 [13] Amplifying the Voice of the Uninsured in the Implementation of the Affordable Care Act [14] Let's Ask 4: Questions for Consumers and

	Health Insurance and Insights from Health Literacy: Helping Consumers Understand: Proceedings of a Workshop—in Brief [30]	Providers About Health Insurance [15]
Medications	*Standardizing Medication Labels: Confusing Patients Less: Workshop Summary* [17] *The Safe Use Initiative and Health Literacy: Workshop Summary* [18]	
Oral Health	*Oral Health Literacy: Workshop Summary* [19]	After-Visit Summaries: A Tool Whose Time Has Come for Use in Dentistry [20] Health Literacy in Dentistry and Navajo Nation Community Health Representatives [21] Dental Caries Management in Children and Adults [22]
Research	*Measures of Health Literacy: Workshop Summary* [23]	Integrating Health Literacy with Quality Performance Measurement [25]

	Innovations in Health Literacy Research: Workshop Summary [24]		
Numeracy	*Health Literacy and Numeracy: Workshop Summary* [26]	Numeracy and the Affordable Care Act: Opportunities and Challenges [27]	Strategies to Enhance Numeracy Skills [28] Numbers Get In the Way [29]

Other Issues			
Defining Health Literacy			Considerations for a New Definition of Health Literacy [31]
Discharge Instructions	*Facilitating Patient Understanding of Discharge Instructions: Workshop Summary* [32]	Primary Care Implementation of After-Visit Summaries for Patients with Limited Health Literacy [33]	
Equity	*Toward Health Equity and Patient-Centeredness: Integrating Health Literacy, Disparities Reduction, and Quality Improvement: Workshop Summary* [34] *Integrating Health Literacy, Cultural*		Health Literacy: A Necessary Element for Achieving Health Equity [36] Health Literacy as an Essential Component to Achieving Excellent Patient Outcomes [37]

	Competence, and Language Access Services: Workshop Summary [35]		
Informed Consent	*Informed Consent and Health Literacy: Workshop Summary* [38]	Best Practices and New Models of Health Literacy for Informed Consent: Review of the Impact of Informed Consent Regulations on Health Literate Communications [39]	
International	*Health Literacy: Improving Health, Health Systems, and Health Policy Around the World: Workshop Summary* [40]	Health Literacy Around the World: Part 1: Health Literacy Efforts Outside of the United States [41] Health Literacy Around the World: Part 2, Health Literacy Efforts Within the United States and a Global Overview [42]	
Palliative Care	*Health Literacy and Palliative Care: Workshop Summary* [43]		Health Literacy and Palliative Care: What Really Happens to Patients [44]
Precision Medicine	*Relevance of Health Literacy to Precision*		Getting it Right with the Precision Medicine Initiative:

	Medicine: Proceedings of a Workshop [45]		The Role of Health Literacy [46]
Prevention	*Promoting Health Literacy to Encourage Prevention and Wellness: Workshop Summary* [47]		Integrating Health Literacy into Primary and Secondary Prevention Strategies [48]
Progress in Health Literacy	*Health Literacy: Past, Present, and Future: Workshop Summary* [49]		
Public Health	*Implications of Health Literacy for Public Health: Workshop Summary* [50]	A Prescription is Not Enough: Improving Public Health with Health Literacy [51]	
Statewide Efforts	*Improving Health Literacy Within a State: Workshop Summary* [52]		
Technology	*Health Literacy and Consumer Facing Technology: Workshop Summary* [53] *Health Literacy, eHealth, and Communication: Putting the Patient First: Workshop Summary* [54]		Designing Health Literate Mobile Apps [55]

3. Future Plans

3.1. Health Literacy, Cultural Competence, and Language Access

One of the six aims for improving health care in the U.S. is to provide care that is equitable, that is, "care that does not vary in quality because of personal characteristics such as gender, ethnicity, geographic location, and socioeconomic status [56]." "Increasing health equity and reducing health disparities requires aligning health care system demands and complexities with individual skills and abilities, and such alignment requires attention to the issues of health literacy, cultural competency, and language access in order to ensure high quality patient care [35]." The Roundtable held a workshop and commissioned a paper focused on integrating the domains of health literacy, cultural competence, and language access services.

A 2015 Roundtable workshop explored opportunities and incentives for integration of the three domains in U.S. health care (and potentially internationally); identified critical issues and challenges to their integration; discussed real-world approaches to integration; and examined needed actions on research, policy, and services and care related to integration of the domains [35]. Several speakers suggested it is difficult for health organizations to integrate health literacy, cultural competence, and language access services because germane quality performance measures are unavailable.

The Roundtable decided to undertake a project aimed at identifying measures for the integration of the three domains and describing how the measures can be used to improve quality and the patient-consumer experience. For the project two commissioned papers and a workshop are planned. The first paper will identify and analyze quality performance measures for health literacy, for cultural competence, and for language access. It will then propose an integrated approach to measurement across the three domains. A workshop will then be held in May 2017 at which the commissioned paper will be presented and reactions to the paper will be obtained from individuals representing a variety of perspectives. A second commissioned paper will use information obtained from the workshop as well as other sources to identify opportunities and rationales for inclusion of the integrated approach into value-based strategies to improve patient-consumer experiences. Both papers and the proceedings of the workshop will be available on the Roundtable website when completed.

4. Impact

It is now recognized that health literacy encompasses more than the skills and abilities of individuals. It also reflects the demands and complexities of the health and health care systems. Contributions of the Roundtable and its members to this understanding and to other issues of health literacy have helped advance the field both within the United States and internationally. Below are a few examples of the broad impact and reach of this collective work.

4.1. Health Literate Organizations

A great deal of work has centered on identifying and understanding the attributes of a health literate organization. The original work focused more on health care organizations than public health agencies. The list of ten attributes discussed earlier was slightly modified by the U.S. Centers for Disease Control and Prevention (CDC) to apply more closely to public health organizations. According to the CDC website, "The white paper, Ten Attributes of Health Literate Health Care Organizations, describes what healthcare organizations can do to lower barriers for people to get and use health information and services. Participants of the Institute of Medicine Roundtable on Health Literacy wrote the paper to inspire healthcare organizations to address health literacy issues. The Office of the Associate Director for Communication (OADC) has interpreted the attributes and offers a modified version to apply to organizations doing public health work [57]."

International attention also has been paid to the workshop summaries and discussion papers in this area. A German translation of the discussion paper by Brach and colleagues was posted on the website of the Austrian Network of Health Promoting Hospitals [6]. The paper was widely distributed and was used in defining measures for fulfilling the Austrian Health Goal No. 3 (out of 10) to improve the health literacy of the population.

Kowalski and colleagues used the discussion paper by Brach and colleagues to develop a set of ten questions measuring the extent to which organizations are health literate [58, 6]. The measures were implemented as part of a larger study in 51 German hospitals. They found that the instrument "provides a useful tool to assess the degree to which health care organizations help patients to navigate, understand, and use information and services [58]."

The Asian Health Literacy Association (AHLA) under the direction of Secretary General Dr. Peter Chang, is conducting an international survey to measure the health literacy of health care organizations. For the survey, they plan to base questions on the publication, Attributes of a Health Literate Organization and also will use the Health Literate Healthcare Organization 10-item questionnaire (HLHO-10), developed by Kowalski and colleagues [6, 58].

A report of the World Health Organization includes a chapter on the attributes of health literacy-friendly organizations and is based on the discussion paper by Brach and colleagues [59, 6]. The WHO report also includes an adapted infographic originally developed for the discussion paper.

Enliven, a registered charitable trust based in Auckland, New Zealand, obtained a contract from the Ministry of Health to review the health literacy environments and clinics in three District Health Boards. They incorporated the ten attributes described in the paper by Brach and colleagues into the review tool they developed [6]. Their report states that each of the ten attributes "has been operationalised within the Resource as a set of evidence-grounded processes, outputs or outcomes that together constitute an appropriate response to health literacy at the organisational level [60]."

4.2. Medications

The U.S. Pharmacopeia Convention (USP) is a nonprofit, scientific organization that sets drug standards that are enforceable in the U.S. by the Food and Drug Administration. The standards are also used internationally by more than 140 countries.

In 2007, Roger Williams (then Chief Executive Officer of USP) attended the Roundtable workshop described above on standardizing medication labels. After hearing presentations describing how patients routinely misunderstand medication instructions and warnings, he decided to convene a group to develop standards for prescription container labeling. In 2008 a USP advisory panel was formed and initial standards were published in 2011.

In 2013, the USP universal standards for simplifying the content and appearance of prescription labels became official. The USP credited the Roundtable's work in inspiring these new, patient-friendly standards.

4.3. Science Literacy

The Roundtable's work also has been used by other components of the National Academies of Sciences, Engineering, and Medicine. As described earlier in this chapter, the Roundtable has engaged in many activities aimed at illuminating the understanding that health literacy is an alignment of system demands and complexities with individual skills and abilities.

The Board on Science Education, Division of Behavioral and Social Sciences and Education of the National Academies of Sciences, Engineering, and Medicine recently completed a consensus study on the need to improve the understanding of science and scientific research in the United States. The report of that committee, Science Literacy and Public Perception of Science was released August 9, 2016 [61]. Conclusion 4 of that report states "Concerns about the relationship of health literacy to health outcomes have led to a reconceptualization of health literacy as a property not just of the individual but also of the system, with attention to how the literacy demands placed on individuals by that system might be mitigated." The report goes on to state, "This reconceptualization of health literacy informed the committee's understanding of science literacy. As a result, the committee supports expanding contemporary perspectives on science literacy to encompass the ways that broader social structures can shape an individual's science literacy. In addition, the committee questions the common understanding that science literacy is, or should be seen only as a property of individuals—something that only individual people develop, possess, and use."

5. Conclusion

The Roundtable benefits from the multiple lenses of its membership. It has an established record in exploring health literacy-related issues in a number of areas as discussed in this chapter. Roundtable workshops and discussions, no matter the specific topic, maintain a focus on identifying and illuminating evidence-based health literacy approaches that foster high-quality, patient centered care.

Issues central to the alignment of system demands and complexities with individual skills and abilities will continue to serve as a main focus of Roundtable efforts and work. These efforts will build upon past work, will strive to maintain relevance to the field, and will continue to encourage others to engage in advancing our nation's health literacy.

All Roundtable publications, webcasts of workshops, commissioned papers, discussion paper, and commentaries are available on the Roundtable webpage at http://nationalacademies.org/healthliteracyRT.

References

[1]   Institute of Medicine. Health Literacy: A Prescription to End Confusion. Washington, DC: The National Academies Press, 2004. DOI: 10.17226/10883.

[2]   Schillinger D., Keller D. The Other Side of the Coin: Attributes of a Health Literate Health Care Organization. Washington, DC: The National Academies Press, 2011. https://www.ncbi.nlm.nih.gov/books/NBK201219/. Retrieved October 3, 2016.

[3]   Institute of Medicine. How Can Health Care Organizations Become More Health Literate: Workshop Summary. Washington, DC: The National Academies Press, 2012. DOI: 10.17226/13402.

[4]   Parker R., Ratzan S., Health Literacy: A Second Decade of Distinction for Americans, J Health Commun. 15 (2010), 20-23. DOI: 10.1080/10810730.2010.501094.

[5]   Brach C., Dreyer B., Shyve P., Hernandez L., Baur C., Lemerise A., et al., Attributes of a Health Literate Organization. Washington, DC: The Institute of Medicine, 2012.

[6]   Brach C., Keller D., Hernandez L., Baur C., Parker R., Dreyer B., et al. Ten Attributes of Health Literate Health Care Organizations. Washington, DC: The Institute of Medicine, 2012.

[7]   Institute of Medicine, Organizational Change to Improve Health Literacy: Workshop Summary. Washington, DC: The National Academies Press, 2013. DOI: 10.17226/18378.

[8]   Kriplani S., Wallston K., Cavanaugh K., Osborn C., Mulvaney S., Scott A., et al. Measures to Assess a Health Literate Organization. 2014. http://www.nationalacademies.org/hmd/Activities/PublicHealth/HealthLiteracy/~/media/Files/Activity%20Files/PublicHealth/HealthLiteracy/Commissioned-Papers/Measures_to_Assess_HLO.pdf. Retrieved October 3, 2016.

[9]   Institute of Medicine. Health Literacy Implications for Health Care Reform: Workshop Summary. Washington, DC: The National Academies Press, 2011. DOI: 10.17226/13056.

[10] Somers S., Mahadevan R. Health Literacy Implications of the Affordable Care Act. 2010. http://www.chcs.org/media/Health_Literacy_Implications_of_the_Affordable_Care_Act.pdf. Retrieved October 3, 2016.

[11] Sanders L. Health Literacy and Health Reform: Where Do Children Fit In? 2011. http://nationalacademies.org/hmd/~/media/Files/Activity%20Files/PublicHealth/HealthLiteracy/Commissioned-Papers/Health%20Literacy%20and%20the%20Health%20Reform%20-%20Where%20Do%20Children%20Fit%20In.pdf. Retrieved October 3, 2016.

[12] Institute of Medicine. Facilitating State Health Exchange Communication Through the Use of Health Literate Practices: Workshop Summary. Washington, DC: The National Academies Press, 2012. DOI: 10.17226/13255.

[13] Patel K., West M., Hernandez L., Wu V., Wong W., Parker R. Helping Consumers Understand and Use Health Insurance in 2014. Washington, DC: The Institute of Medicine, 2013.

[14] Patel K., Parker R., Villarruel A., Wong W. Amplifying the Voice of the Underserved. Washington, DC: The Institute of Medicine, 2013.

[15] Wu V., Jacobson K., Wong W., Patel K., Hernandez L., Isham G., et al. Let's Ask 4: Questions for Consumers and Providers about Health Insurance. Washington, DC: The Institute of Medicine, 2013.

[16] Parker R., Wu V., Patel K. Successfully Engaging Hard-to-Reach Populations in Health Insurance: a Focus on Outreach, Signup and Retention, and Use. 2015. http://www.nationalacademies.org/hmd/~/media/Files/Activity%20Files/PublicHealth/HealthLiteracy/Commissioned-Papers/EngagingHardtoReachPopsinInsurance.pdf. Retrieved October 3, 2016.

[17] Institute of Medicine. Standardizing Medication Labels: Confusing Patients Less: Workshop Summary. Washington, DC: The National Academies Press, 2008. DOI: 10.17226/12077.

[18] Institute of Medicine. The Safe Use Initiative and Health Literacy: Workshop Summary. Washington, DC: The National Academies Press, 2010. DOI: 10.17226/12975.

[19] Institute of Medicine. Oral Health Literacy: Workshop Summary. Washington, DC: The National Academies Press, 2013. DOI: 10.17226/13484.

[20] Horowitz A., Robinson L., Ng M., Acharya A. After Visit Summaries: A Tool Whose Time Has Come for Use in Dentistry. Washington, DC: The Institute of Medicine, 2014.

[21] Geiermann S., Begay M.-G., Robinson L., Clough S. Health Literacy in Dentistry and Navajo Nation Community Health Representatives. Washington, DC: The Institute of Medicine, 2016.

[22] Slayton R., Fontana M., Young D., Tinaoff N., Novy B., Lipman R., et al. Dental Caries Management in Children and Adults. Washington, DC: The National Academies Press, 2016.

[23] Institute of Medicine. Measures of Health Literacy: Workshop Summary. Washington, DC: The National Academies Press, 2009.

[24] Institute of Medicine. Innovations in Health Literacy Research: Workshop Summary. Washington, DC: The National Academies Press, 2011.

[25] DeWalt D., McNeil J., Integrating Health Literacy with Health Care Performance. Washington, DC: The National Academies Press, 2013. https://nam.edu/wp-content/uploads/2015/06/BPH-IntegratingHealthLiteracy.pdf. Retrieved October 3, 2016.

[26] Institute of Medicine. Health Literacy and Numeracy: Workshop Summary. Washington, DC: The National Academies Press, 2014.

[27] Peters E., Meilleur L., Tompkins M. Appendix A: Numeracy and the Affordable Care Act: Opportunities and Challenges, in: Health Literacy and Numeracy: Workshop Summary. Washington, DC: Institute of Medicine, 2013.

[28] Pleasant A., Rooney M., O'Leary C., Myers L., Rudd R. Strategies to Enhance Numeracy Skills. Opportunities and Challenges, in Health Literacy and Numeracy: Workshop Summary, 2016. http://www.nationalacademies.org/hmd/~/media/Files/Activity%20Files/PublicHealth/HealthLiteracy/Commissioned-Papers/AVS%20for%20Patients%20with%20Limited%20Health%20Lit.pdf. Retrieved October 3, 2016.

[29] Rudd R. Numbers Get in the Way. Opportunities and Challenges, in Health Literacy and Numeracy: Workshop Summary, 2016.

[30] National Academies of Sciences, Engineering, and Medicine. Health Insurance and Insights from Health Literacy: Helping Consumers Understand: Proceedings of a Workshop in Brief. Opportunities and Challenges, in Health Literacy and Numeracy: Workshop Summary, 2016.

[31] Pleasant A., Rudd R., O'Leary C., Paasche-Orlow M., Allen M.P., Alvarado-Little W., Myers L., Parson K., and Rosen S. Considerations for a New Definition of Health Literacy. Opportunities and Challenges, in Health Literacy and Numeracy: Workshop Summary, 2016.

[32] Institute of Medicine. Facilitating Patient Understanding of Discharge Instructions: Workshop Summary. Opportunities and Challenges, in Health Literacy and Numeracy: Workshop Summary, 2014.

[33] Lyles C., Gupta R., Tieu L., Fernandez A. Primary Care Implementation of After-Visit Summaries for Patients with Limited Health Literacy. http://www.nationalacademies.org/hmd/~/media/Files/Activity%20Files/PublicHealth/HealthLiteracy/Commissioned-Papers/AVS%20for%20Patients%20with%20Limited%20Health%20Lit.pdf?la=en. Retrieved December 2, 2016.

[34] Institute of Medicine. Toward Health Equity and Patient Centeredness: Integrating Health Literacy, Disparities Reduction, and Quality Improvement: Workshop Summary. Washington, DC: The National Academies Press, 2009.

[35] National Academies of Sciences, Engineering, and Medicine. Integrating Health Literacy, Cultural Competency, and Language Access Services: Workshop Summary. Washington, DC: The National Academies Press, 2016.

[36] Logan R., Wong W., Villaire M., Daus G., Parnell T., Willis E., et al. Health Literacy: A Necessary Element for Achieving Health Equity. Washington, DC: The Institute of Medicine, 2015.

[37] Parnell T. Health Literacy as an Essential Component to Achieving Excellent Patient Outcomes. Washington, DC: The Institute of Medicine, 2014.

[38] Institute of Medicine. Informed Consent and Health Literacy: Workshop Summary. Washington, DC: The National Academies Press, 2015.

[39] Aldoory L., Ryan K., Rouhani A. Best Practices and New Models of Health Literacy for Informed Consent: Review of the Impact of Informed Consent Regulations on Health Literate Communications. 2014. http://www.nationalacademies.org/hmd/~/media/Files/Activity%20Files/PublicHealth/HealthLiteracy/Commissioned-Papers/Informed_Consent_HealthLit.pdf. Retrieved October 3, 2016.

[40] Institute of Medicine. Health Literacy: Improving Health, Health Systems, and Health Policy Around the World: Workshop Summary. Washington, DC: The National Academies Press, 2013.

[41] Pleasant A. Health Literacy Around the World Part 1: Health Literacy Efforts Outside the U.S. 2012. http://nationalacademies.org/hmd/~/media/Files/Activity%20Files/PublicHealth/HealthLiteracy/2012-SEP-24/WorldHealthLit.pdf. Retrieved October 3, 2016.

[42] Pleasant A. Health Literacy Around the World Part 2: Health Literacy Efforts Within the United States and A Global Overview. 2012. http://nationalacademies.org/hmd/~/media/Files/Activity%20Files/PublicHealth/HealthLiteracy/Commissioned-Papers/Health%20Literacy%20Around%20the%20World%20Part%202.pdf. Retrieved October 3, 2016.

[43] Institute of Medicine. Health Literacy and Palliative Care: Workshop Summary. Washington, DC: The National Academies Press, 2016. DOI: 10.17226/21839.

[44] Alves B., Meier D. Palliative Care: What Really Happens to Patients. Washington, DC: The Institute of Medicine, 2015.

[45] National Academies of Sciences, Engineering, and Medicine. Relevance of Health Literacy to Precision Medicine: Proceedings of a Workshop Washington, DC: The National Academies Press, 2016. DOI: 10.17226/23538.

[46] Parker R., Bakken S., Wolf M. Getting It Right with the Precision Medicine Initiative: The Role of Health Literacy. Washington, DC: National Academy of Medicine, 2016.

[47] Institute of Medicine. Promoting Health Literacy to Encourage Prevention and Wellness. Washington, DC: The National Academies Press, 2011. DOI: 10.17226/13186.

[48] Ratzan S. Integrating Health Literacy into Primary and Secondary Prevention Strategies. 2009. https://www.nationalacademies.org/hmd/~/media/Files/Activity%20Files/PublicHealth/HealthLiteracy/2009-SEP-15/02-Ratzan.pdf. Retrieved December 2, 2016.

[49] Institute of Medicine. Health Literacy: Past, Present, and Future: Workshop Summary. Washington, DC: The National Academies Press, 2015. DOI: 10.17226/21714.

[50] Institute of Medicine. Implications of Health Literacy for Public Health: Workshop Summary. Washington, DC: The National Academies Press, 2014. DOI: 10.17226/18756.

[51] Pleasant A., Cabe J., Martin L., Rikard R. A Prescription is Not Enough: Improving Public Health with Health Literacy. 2013. https://www.nap.edu/download/18756#. Retrieved December 2, 2016.

[52] Institute of Medicine. Improving Health Literacy Within a State: Workshop Summary. Washington, DC: The National Academies Press, 2011. DOI: 10.17266/13185.

[53] Institute of Medicine. Health Literacy and Consumer-Facing Technology: Workshop Summary. Washington, DC: The National Academies Press, 2015. DOI: 10.17226/21781.

[54] Institute of Medicine. Health Literacy, eHealth, and Communication: Putting the Patient First: Workshop Summary. Washington, DC: The National Academies Press, 2009.

[55] Broderick J., Devine T., Langhans E., Lemerise A., Lier S., Harris L. Designing Health Literate Mobile Apps. Washington, DC: The Institute of Medicine, 2014.

[56] Institute of Medicine. Crossing the Quality Chasm: A New Health System for the 21st Century. Washington, DC: The National Academies Press, 2001. DOI: 10.17226/10027.

[57] Centers for Disease Control and Prevention. Health Literacy Organizational Attributes 2016. 2016. http://www.cdc.gov/healthliteracy/planact/steps/index.html. Retrieved October 5, 2016.

[58] Kowalski C., Lee S.Y., Schmidt A., Wesselmann S., Wirtz M.A., Pfaff H., et al. The health literate health care organization 10 item questionnaire (HLHO-10): development and validation, BMC Health Serv Res **15** (2015), 47. DOI: 10.1186/s12913-015-0707-5.

[59] WHO Regional Office for Europe. The Solid Facts About Health Literacy: WHO (World Health Organization). 2013. http://www.euro.who.int/__data/assets/pdf_file/0008/190655/e96854.pdf. Retrieved October 5, 2016.

[60] Thomacos N., Zazryn T. Enliven Organisational Health Literacy Self-assessment Resource. Melbourne: Monash University Enliven & School of Primary Health Care, 2013.

[61] National Academies of Sciences, Engineering, and Medicine. Science Literacy and the Public Perception of Science. Washington, DC: The National Academies Press, 2016. DOI: 10.17226/23595.

Health Literacy
R.A. Logan and E.R. Siegel (Eds.)
IOS Press, 2017
© 2017 The authors and IOS Press. All rights reserved.
doi:10.3233/978-1-61499-790-0-186

The U.S. *National Action Plan to Improve Health Literacy*: A Model for Positive Organizational Change

Cynthia BAUR[a],[1] Linda HARRIS[b], Elizabeth SQUIRE[b]

[a] *U.S. Department of Health and Human Services, Centers for Disease Control and Prevention*

[b] *U.S. Department of Health and Human Services, Office of the Assistant Secretary for Health, Office of Disease Prevention and Health Promotion*

Abstract. This chapter presents the U.S. *National Action Plan to Improve Health Literacy* and its unique contribution to public health and health care in the U.S. The chapter details what the *National Action Plan* is, how it evolved, and how it has influenced priorities for health literacy improvement work. Examples of how the *National Action Plan* fills policy and research gaps in health care and public health are included. The first part of the chapter lays the foundation for the development of the *National Action Plan,* and the second part discusses how it can stimulate positive organizational change to help create health literate organizations and move the nation towards a health literate society.

Keywords. Health Literacy, National Action Plan to Improve Health Literacy, health literate organizations, health information

1. Introduction

In the last 30 years, many U.S. public and private sector organizations provided the research, evaluation, and strategic initiatives that raised awareness of the negative effects of limited health literacy on the public's health. At the federal government level, the U.S. Department of Health and Human Services (HHS), the agency in charge of enhancing and protecting the health and well-being of all Americans, supports a national objective to improve health literacy and a *National Action Plan to Improve Health Literacy* [1], as well as health literacy programs, activities, and research. Federal agencies collaborate with the country's National Academies of Sciences, Engineering and Medicine, Medicine and Health Division (National Academies), formerly the Institute of Medicine or IOM, the country's independent advisory body on health and medicine. The U.S. National Academies of Sciences, Engineering, and Medicine convenes a Roundtable on Health Literacy with participants from government, research, health, and medical organizations and businesses [2]. Many other organizations in health, medicine, education, information services, and social services, sponsor in-person meetings, electronic discussions, projects, and health information that raise awareness and provide resources to address health literacy issues in communities.

---

[1] Corresponding author: Endowed Chair and Director, Horowitz Center for Health Literacy, School of Public Health, University of Maryland, 4200 Valley Drive, College Park, MD. USA; email: cbaur@umd.edu

Compared to other industrially advanced countries, however, the U.S. has average school-aged and adult literacy and numeracy scores in domestic and international assessments [3,4,5,6,]. Modest skills are only part of the U.S. problem; they intersect with complex public and private sector systems for wellness, prevention, and healthcare and emergency services, as well as large amounts of readily available but often difficult-to-use health information materials. Collectively, this situation has led to U.S. Surgeons General declaring limited health literacy to be a major public health problem [7,8]. On the other hand, the country's robust research infrastructure; stable and relatively well-funded public health agencies; advanced healthcare services; large number of researchers and practitioners attracted to the health literacy topic; and an engaged civil society provide attention to and resources for health literacy work. Both Healthy People 2010 and 2020, a public-private partnership to establish U.S. public health priorities, have had objectives to improve the health literacy of the population [9].

This chapter reviews what the U.S. *National Action Plan to Improve Health Literacy (National Action Plan)* is and how and why it emerged in 2010 as a framework to bring together disparate public and private sector activities. The chapter also explains the significance and influence of the *National Action Plan* and puts it in the context of related developments in health literacy research and practice. The *National Action Plan*'s contents reflect the U.S.' unique public and private sector roles and responsibilities for health activities. However, the methods used to develop the *National Action Plan* reflect best practices in strategic planning, systems thinking, community engagement, and partnership building. Therefore, the *National Action Plan* can be a model for many organizations and countries interested in comprehensive, strategic approaches to health literacy improvement and positive organizational change.

The chapter begins with a comprehensive overview of the *National Action Plan.* This section of the chapter outlines the foundational initiatives, research and literature that contributed to the development of the *National Action Plan's* goals. Next, the chapter highlights the research gaps that the *National Action Plan* aimed to fill as well as how organizations within and outside the federal government are using the *National Action Plan* to create positive change.

The chapter later explores how the *National Action Plan* Stimulates and Reinforces Positive Organizational Change at HHS through initiatives including The Agency for Health Research and Quality's *Health Literacy Universal Precautions Toolkit* and the Health Literate Care Model. This section of the chapter ends with an overview of the existing challenges to implementing and tracking a health literacy organizational change model. Finally the chapter finishes with the emerging opportunities to implement an organizational change approach to health literacy such as the strategies highlighted in the *National Action Plan.* The chapter summary reflects on the progress of the National Action Plan.

2. What is the *National Action Plan to Improve Health Literacy*?

The *National Action Plan* is a comprehensive strategic plan for health literacy improvement work at federal, state, local (community), and individual organization levels [1]. The Healthy People definition of health literacy as people's capacity for obtaining, processing, understanding, and deciding on health information and services is one of the perspectives included in the document. The *National Action Plan*, however, was one of the first reports to position health literacy improvement as the result of effective organizational and professional practices to meet people's needs for useful health information and services. Because of this orientation toward health literacy as a systems-level concern, the *National Action Plan* presents a vision of a health literate society – not only health literate people – along with goals, strategies, and recommended actions that organizations and individuals can implement to help realize the vision [1]. Two core principles anchor the *National Action Plan*:

All people have the right to health information that helps them make informed decisions.

Health services should be delivered in ways that are easy to understand and improve health, longevity, and quality of life.

These principles are translated into seven goal statements (listed below) about what organizations and individuals can do to make health information and services effective for people with all levels of health literacy skills.

1. Develop and disseminate health and safety information that is accurate, accessible, and actionable

2. Promote changes in the health care system that improve health information, communication, informed decision-making, and access to health services

3. Incorporate accurate, standards-based, and developmentally appropriate health and science information and curricula in child care and education through the university level

4. Support and expand local efforts to provide adult education, English language instruction, and culturally and linguistically appropriate health information services in the community

5. Build partnerships, develop guidance, and change policies

6. Increase basic research and the development, implementation, and evaluation of practices and interventions to improve health literacy

7. Increase the dissemination and use of evidence-based health literacy practices and interventions

The goals and strategies are intended for professionals in multiple disciplines, such as medicine, public health, and communication; managers – senior and program level – in public and private sector organizations; researchers; community leaders; and policymakers because they are the ones who can organize, take action, and evaluate progress toward a health literate society. Professionals in various roles, such as clinicians, educators, administrators, and program managers, can generate public policies, organizational or individual priorities, and identify necessary actions; some actions may cut across boundaries and require collaboration [1,10].

2.1. Foundation for the National Action Plan to Improve Health Literacy

The multi-disciplinary nature of the *National Action Plan* reflects, in part, contributions from researchers, practitioners, and program staff in different fields who helped provide the evidence base as well as a rationale for a national plan. The diversity in perspectives enriched the plan development process but also revealed differences in understanding of the health literacy concept as well as gaps in coordination and collaboration in health literacy work that the plan aimed to address. Key activities that led to the plan's development ranged from research to understand limited health literacy's effects to translation of findings into consumer health information. The list below highlights main developments in the field prior to the *National Action Plan*.

> Published research studies, reports, and professional conferences highlighting the scope of adult literacy, numeracy, and health literacy problems in the U.S. and other countries [4,5,11,12,13]

> Published guidelines on how to create easy-to-read health communication materials [14,15,16]

> A privately funded communication campaign ("Ask Me 3") to promote clear communication between healthcare professionals and patients [17]

> Public comments in favor of a health literacy objective in Healthy People 2010

> An HHS cross-cutting Health Literacy Workgroup to support the Healthy People health literacy objective

> A Healthy People 2010 health literacy action plan [18]

> HHS and U.S. Department of Education collaboration to develop the first national health literacy measures in the National Assessment of Adult Literacy (NAAL) [19]

> The 2004 IOM expert committee and report on health literacy [20]

> U.S. Surgeons General workshops and reports on health literacy [7,8]

This constellation of activities in a relatively short time span – about 10 years from the mid-to-late 1990s to mid-2000s – generated attention to limited health literacy as a research, practice, outcomes, and policy issue. Simultaneously, this period also showed that although some key organizations and individuals participated and overlapped in multiple activities, individuals and groups had their own priorities, interests, and health literacy definitions.

In this same 10 year period, several U.S. federal health agencies drew attention to health literacy as a public health problem negatively affecting a range of health-related outcomes. Several agencies published their own plain language manuals, which they made publicly available. For example. the National Institutes of Health (NIH) National Cancer Institute published *Clear & Simple: Developing Effective Print Materials for Low Literacy Audiences* to help communicators apply health literacy insights [16], and the Centers for Disease Control and Prevention (CDC) issued *Simply Put*, a plain language guide for health communicators and health educators [15]. U.S. Agencies also recognized that consumers needed plain language health information and created websites with accessible materials. NIH's National Library of Medicine (NLM) created MedlinePlus, a web-based collection of easy-to-understand medical information from NIH institutes and centers, HHS agencies, and evidence-based external resources [21]. NLM also published an influential bibliography that provided a health literacy definition adopted by Healthy People 2010 and later by many other organizations [22]. The U.S. HHS Office of Disease Prevention and Health Promotion (ODPHP) contributed multiple resources, including the National Health Information Center and www.healthfinder.gov, first a clearinghouse for consumer health information and later a web-based collection of consumer health information designed according to health literacy principles. ODPHP also sponsored the report *Wired for Health and Well-being* that examined health literacy issues in the emerging digital environment [23]. ODPHP managed the Health Communication focus area in Healthy People 2010, including the health literacy objective, and established the HHS Health Literacy Workgroup to coordinate HHS agencies' health literacy activities [24]. ODPHP worked with the U.S. Department of Education on the NAAL health literacy measures, and ODPHP and the HHS Workgroup proposed that the national health literacy objective could be a focal point and unifying element within and across organizations, groups, and individuals, as well as the basis for a national plan.

In addition to government agencies' contributions, several key publications provided the scientific and policy basis for a national plan. The 1993 National Adult Literacy Survey (NALS) report on adult literacy skills showed that about one-half of the U.S. adult population had literacy skills at the two lowest levels [4]. Medical organizations, such as the American Medical Association, became interested in health literacy, and the 1999 American Medical Association's Ad Hoc Committee for the Council of Scientific Affairs' report summarized 30 years of research on literacy's effects on health, explained the relevance for clinical practice, and called for awareness, research, and policies to address limited health literacy [13]. The NLM health literacy bibliography contributed the initial health literacy definition as well as identified 479 relevant publications that documented the evidence base for health literacy programs and interventions. The bibliography defined health literacy as "the degree to which individuals have the capacity to obtain, process, and understand basic health information and services needed to make appropriate health decisions" [22].

The Healthy People 2010 health literacy objective preceded and provided a base for a national plan. The health literacy objective was part of the 2010 Health Communication focus area [24]. The inclusion of health communication objectives confirmed the importance of communication as an intellectual framework, a scientific endeavor, and a set of processes and interventions for health improvement in public health policy making. Given that the objective called for health literacy improvement for the entire U.S. population, the logical question was how to begin meeting the objective. A comprehensive national action plan seemed necessary to engage the large number of organizations that work in the health and education sectors and address the many factors that influence health literacy issues for different populations.

2.2. Process to Develop the National Action Plan

The *National Action Plan* emerged from a series of purposeful activities to make the case for health literacy improvement and suggest strategies and actions that organizations and individuals could take to help meet the objective of improving population health literacy. The U.S. HHS Health Literacy Workgroup, comprised of staff interested in and leading health literacy projects in their agencies, sponsored the *National Action Plan* preparation. The *National Action Plan* contents were based primarily on the 2006 U.S. Surgeon General's Workshop on Improving Health Literacy [7], a series of four public town hall meetings in 2007 and 2008, and feedback from stakeholder organizations on draft plans circulated in 2009. The Surgeon General's Workshop provided the scientific basis for the plan; the town hall meetings and stakeholder feedback provided the community perspective and examples of local activities. HHS released the plan in 2010 [1].

While the plan was under development, new research and publications added evidence that limited health literacy was a national problem; the research questions, findings, and publications informed the *National Action Plan's* contents. The U.S. National Academies Roundtable on Health Literacy published its report with multiple findings in 2004 and called for a "health-literate America" [20]. The U.S. Department of Education released the National Assessment of Adult Literacy data at the 2006 Surgeon General's Workshop [7]. The data provided the first population data on adults' health literacy skills [19]. The Agency for Healthcare Research and Quality commissioned and published the first of two systematic reviews of literacy and health literacy and their effects on different outcomes [25,26]. Individual research studies funded by the NIH health literacy program announcement continued to build the evidence base in key areas such as chronic disease management and provider-patient communication [27,28]. Collectively, the additional research and publications bolstered the argument for a national approach to a complex, society-wide problem and offered insights into the types of goals and strategies a national plan should include.

3. How a *National Action Plan* Fills Policy and Research Gaps

This chapter (as well as others in the edited volume) reflects that the U.S. has been and continues to be a fertile environment for health literacy improvement work. Yet, in the mid-2000s, the multiple activities lacked a common focus and purpose. The activities were often *about* an aspect of health literacy, but didn't necessarily generate sufficient scale to *improve* the health literacy of the population, as stated in the Healthy People objective [9]. Although the HHS Office of Disease Prevention and Health Promotion (ODPHP), the lead agency for the HHS Health Literacy Workgroup, worked collaboratively with public and private sector organizations, ODPHP and the Workgroup didn't have the resources to lead a broad-based national health literacy initiative. But, ODPHP and the Workgroup did have other resources, such as a partnership with the Surgeon General's office and its convening powers for a scientific workshop. In 2006, the U.S. Surgeon General's office declared that scientific evidence supported health literacy improvement as a public health priority [7]. The *National Action Plan* emerged because the Workgroup used the tools it had – a national health objective, scientific reviews, convening powers, and report writing – to channel disparate activities in a common direction and advance a national perspective on health literacy improvement.

Although the NLM bibliography [22], the IOM report *Prescription to End Confusion* [20], and the Surgeon General's Workshop [7] showed the extensive research supporting the negative effects of limited literacy and health literacy, the volume of research reflected the large number of disciplines working on health literacy-related topics. Researchers used their own theories, questions, and methods rather than a common research agenda and progression of knowledge-building. Much of the early research evaluated the readability of materials and associations between people's health literacy "levels" and a range of health and service outcomes [20,25]. NIH's 2004 release of a health literacy program announcement provided researchers the first set of common topics and questions to inform lines of inquiry [27]. The *National Action Plan* built on the program announcement questions and topics and highlighted priority areas for research and evaluation.

In addition to helping fill research gaps, the *National Action Plan* helped fill strategic planning and policy gaps in the emerging health literacy field. The U.S. was the first country to publish a national health literacy plan, and after its publication, the U.S. plan served as an example for other countries interested in writing their own strategic plans. Representatives from many countries and regions, including Australia, Canada, China, England, the European Union, the Netherlands, New Zealand, and Singapore, communicated with the HHS Workgroup leaders to learn about the U.S. process. Of course, each country's planning process reflects its culture, history, politics, and institutions [29,30,31]. The fact that professionals in other countries found value in the U.S. plan indicates, though, that the basic strategic plan structure of purpose, goals, strategies, and actions can transfer to other contexts.

The *National Action Plan* also was grounded in health policymaking activities that encompassed health communication components. For example, Healthy People 2010 was the first U.S. federal health policy document to substantively address health communication issues. The *National Action Plan* elaborated strategies and actions not provided in Healthy People 2010. The plan also served as a reference document for strategies and actions that could be transposed into other reports and policy documents, such as the National Healthcare Quality and Disparities Report [32] and National Prevention Strategy [33], as well as guidelines, such as the National Standards for Culturally and Linguistically Appropriate Services in Health and Health Care [34].

4. Examples of Organizations using the *National Action Plan* to Create Positive Change

To make sure the *National Action Plan* was used to improve organizational practices, the HHS Health Literacy Workgroup leadership committed to implementing the plan and creating positive organizational change. Because the *National Action Plan* contains a comprehensive set of goals, strategies, and actions intended to improve health literacy, organizations and professional groups can choose to implement those that best fit their organization or profession. Health, communication, and education professionals; managers; public and private sector organizations; communities; and policymakers are the intended users of the plan because they are the ones who can organize and take actions and evaluate progress toward a health literate society [1]. This section highlights how some organizations have used the plan as an inspiration and framework for their own actions.

The Wisconsin Health Literacy organization was an early supporter of the *National Action Plan* and used it to guide several activities. In 2009, Wisconsin Health Literacy Conference attendees reviewed and commented on a draft plan. Soon after the conference, Wisconsin Health Literacy held a planning session to set strategic priorities for the upcoming years. Two priorities that came out of that planning session were simplifying medication labels and health literacy training for healthcare professionals. Steve Sparks, Health Literacy Director of Health Literacy Wisconsin, credits the *National Action Plan* in helping to bring these two priorities to life. In a conversation with Steve Sparks (August 2016) he said, "The *National Action Plan* gave the Wisconsin Health Literacy organization ideas for outreach and fee for service activities we wouldn't have thought of otherwise." In 2011, Wisconsin Health Literacy held their biannual summit on health literacy, and the *National Action Plan* was the summit theme [35]. The plan's seven goals were highlighted throughout the presentations and topics at the summit. In the summit evaluation, over 80% of attendees agreed that the summit had provided tools and strategies to improve patient outcomes as outlined in the action plan.

The Institute for Healthcare Advancement (IHA) also used the *National Action Plan* to organize its 2012 annual conference. The conference provided workshops and tools that encouraged attendees to develop an action plan for their organization. Prior to the conference, IHA staff led an online discussion to learn how organizations were using the plan. Responses included the University of Washington Medical Center's effort to make patient education materials more accessible in line with Goal 1 of the *National Action Plan*, "Develop and Disseminate Health and Safety Information That Is Accurate, Accessible, and Actionable." The Center built a patient education library with materials such as 3D anatomical models, posters, laminated picture cards, videos, games, and interactive kits for patients to practice health literacy skills [36]. Medical Center staff at the University of Washington are encouraged to provide teaching aids from this library for those patients who prefer non-reading methods of learning, thereby fulfilling the intention of Goal 1 to provide health and safety information in ways that the public can understand.

The *National Action Plan* recommends several strategies and actions about including the target audience in the planning, development, and testing of health information. Several examples illustrate how organizations have implemented user testing approaches from the action plan.

- The California Medical Assistance Program (Medi-Cal) and the University of California–Berkeley School of Public Health used user testing approaches from the *National Action Plan* to help seniors and others with disabilities understand their Medi-Cal health care options [37]. The School of Public Health worked with Medi-Cal beneficiaries to design a guidebook in English, Spanish, and Chinese. In an evaluation of the program, the participants who used the guidebook experienced significant increases in knowledge, positive attitudes, and intentions to enroll in the Medi-Cal program [38].

- Other user testing initiatives include the Internal Message Testing Network established by the U.S. Food and Drug Administration (FDA) (on the advice of FDA's Risk Communication Advisory Committee) in 2010. The Internal Message Testing Network pragmatically addressed some of the limitations on U.S. federal agencies to survey the public. To advance user testing within a challenging environment, the Internal Message Testing Network asked FDA employees to provide feedback on some of the agency's drafts of intended messages. Currently, the network includes more than 700 FDA employee volunteers who can be screened to best match target audience demographics. Although the FDA's Message Testing Network is not a substitute for public input, the network provides timely feedback and uncovers flaws when time or resources are limited.

- One tool to help website developers and digital tool developers create health literate content is *Health Literacy Online (2nd Edition)* developed by the HHS Office of Disease Prevention and Health Promotion (ODPHP). *Health Literacy Online* is a research-based guide to developing intuitive health websites and digital health tools that can be easily accessed and understood by all users, including the millions of Americans who struggle to find, process, and use online health information [39]. *Health Literacy Online* synthesized lessons learned from ODPHP's original research with more than 700 web users. The guide helps developers operationalize the strategies highlighted within the *National Action Plan.*

Evidence-based strategies to address health literacy like the examples above are continually emerging from the fields of communication, health care, public health, and adult education. It is important for organizations to share interventions and strategies that work, so that organizations can learn from each other and as a nation we can meet everyone's information and communication needs.

5. The *National Action Plan* Stimulates and Reinforces Positive Organizational Change at HHS

In addition to promoting the *National Action Plan* for use outside HHS, the HHS Health Literacy Workgroup has used the *National Action Plan* to help HHS agencies change organizational policies and practices to support health literacy improvement. This section provides several examples of how the agencies are using the *National Action Plan* or have been influenced by it.

5.1. An Organizational Change Approach

The prevalence of limited health literacy and its relevance for a large number of HHS-supported programs and activities motivated the Workgroup to take a practical approach focused on organizational changes to improving health literacy. The goals and strategies in the *National Action Plan* align with an organizational change approach and identify health literacy as an integral component for effective functioning of the health care delivery and public health systems. The value of looking for problems and solutions in organizational practices is that this approach addresses the fact that the vast majority of Americans, almost 90% of the population according to the National Assessment of Adult Literacy (NAAL) survey, need clearer and more actionable health information [19].

An organizational approach to health literacy improvement means that organizations take responsibility for assessing and improving how they communicate with the public and the people they serve. For example, if an individual or a group doesn't understand a public health message about a preventive health action, the organization that created and distributed the message looks first at its own practices and how it created and distributed the message rather than blaming the individual or group for poor health literacy skills. The idea that organizations are responsible for changing their practices to communicate clearly with everyone, from the lowest to the highest health literacy skill level, has become known as the "universal precautions" approach, explained in more detail below [40]. An organizational approach to health literacy, led by HHS and other public health and health care organizations, has generated roadmaps for change aligned with the *National Action Plan* and can lead to improvements in the health literacy of individuals and groups served by public and private health sectors.

5.2. Health Literacy as an Organizational Quality Issue

The *National Action Plan* helped frame public discussion of health literacy and its related discipline of health communication, moving them from the sidelines of public health to a more valued role as an essential element of quality improvement in health and health care. In a 2012 *Health Affairs* article, Dr. Howard Koh (the former HHS Assistant Secretary for Health) and co-authors from the federal Centers for Medicare and Medicaid and the Agency for Healthcare Research and Quality noted how the failure of health care organizations to simultaneously address health literacy and quality of care issues harms consumers and patients and perpetuates poor health outcomes and higher medical costs [41]. The authors described a typical healthcare scenario when health literacy issues are minimized or ignored:

Mrs. Jones is without insurance and on a fixed income, and she suffers from diabetes and heart failure. She arrives a half-hour late for her appointment because the hospital signage confused her. Her confusion increases when she cannot understand the pile of forms the receptionist hands her. It rises even further in the examination room when she cannot understand the medical jargon that her provider uses. At that point, she is too overwhelmed to ask any questions and the doctor leaves her with a handful of prescriptions that she does not understand and referrals for laboratory work that she cannot quite comprehend. Not surprisingly, she fails to obtain the laboratory tests and some of her prescriptions go unfilled. Eventually, she ends up being hospitalized, treated, and discharged, again with little understanding of what she is supposed to do to best care for herself [41].

The authors highlighted evidence-based strategies to demonstrate that system-level changes focused on health literacy can remedy the mistakes and missed opportunities in the Mrs. Jones' scenario and support preventive and patient-centered care instead. As an example of the types of quality improvements organizations can expect, the authors reported findings from a study on simplifying and making written materials easier to understand through a plain language and pictogram based intervention. The intervention resulted in fewer medication dosage errors (5.4 percent versus 47.8 percent) and greater adherence compared to standard medication counseling (38 percent versus 9.3 percent) [42].

5.3. Health Literacy Universal Precautions

The U.S. Agency for Healthcare Research and Quality helped healthcare organizations work toward the healthcare improvement goal (Goal 2) in the *National Action Plan* with the *Health Literacy Universal Precautions Toolkit* [40]. The toolkit is intended to reduce the complexity of health care, increase patient understanding of health information, and enhance support for patients of all health literacy levels. The toolkit contains 20 specific steps for implementing "health literacy universal precautions" across a health care system. Health literacy universal precautions are the steps that healthcare practices take when they assume that all patients may have need help comprehending health information and accessing health services. The 20 steps include concrete suggestions, such as focusing on teach-back. Teach-back is a method for provider-patient dialogue to check for understanding on both sides of the oral exchange. Another technique is a brown-bag medication review with patients so they can gain understanding of what the medicines are for and how to take them.

5.4. The Health Literate Care Model

Former U.S. HHS Assistant Secretary for Health Dr. Howard Koh and former HHS colleagues followed up the 2012 Health Affairs quality article with a model for improving health literacy using the Universal Precautions approach. They developed the "Health Literate Care Model" based on the evidence-based Chronic Care Model [43]. The original chronic care model shows how to change health delivery systems to provide improved care for patients. One of the elements in the updated model with health literacy components is a set of patient-reported measures for evaluating health care organizations' level of success in engaging in clear and actionable communication (productive interactions) with their patients [43]. Health care organizations using this model make health literacy an organizational value that informs all components of the system including self-management support, delivery system design, shared decision-making support, clinical information systems, and connections to community resources [43]. The development of the Health Literacy Universal Precautions Toolkit [40] and the Health Literate Care Model [43] are examples of organizational level approaches aligned with National Action Plan goals.

5.5. Health Literate Organizations

To further help healthcare organizations recognize and implement health literacy strategies, members of the HHS Health Literacy Workgroup and the Health Literacy Roundtable of the National Academies collaborated on a list of ten characteristics or attributes that describe organizations where health literacy is a sufficiently high priority [44]. This collaboration introduced the concept of a "health literate health care organization." A foundational principle of health-literate health care organizations is that they make clear and effective patient communication a priority at all levels of the organization and for all communication channels [45]. This principle is in line with the National Action Plan's healthcare goal, which called for healthcare services organizations to address the health literacy needs of patients, family members, and caregivers.

Government agencies can also aim to be health-literate health care organizations. The HHS Health Literacy Workgroup encourages HHS agencies to model the ten attributes. The Workgroup began the process of tracking their own efforts to meet the goals of the National Action Plan and the Ten Attributes of Health Literate Health Care Organizations [44] when they developed the HHS Biennial Health Literacy Action Plan (2015–2017). The Workgroup sponsored the plan to raise leaders' and staff awareness about health literacy issues and track progress on health literacy improvement in HHS-funded activities. The Workgroup used the national plan as a framework and selected multiple strategies so that HHS' actions will advance the achievement of national goals and track progress toward becoming a health-literate organization. Through this work, the Workgroup has identified priority health literacy improving practices within their agencies and is in the process of implementing or changing the practices.

5.6. Challenges to implementing and tracking a health literacy organizational change model

Measuring changes in organizations focused on health literacy improvements can be difficult. Many public and private health organizations are large and complex with many competing demands and priorities. Leaders may see health literacy as just one more problem on a long list. Some patient populations may have multiple and challenging needs of which healthcare is only a part. Organizational improvement strategies are still developing, and despite the *National Action Plan* and the *Ten Attributes of Health Literate Health Care Organizations* [44] document, the field lacks a standardized way of defining and tracking progress toward health literate organizations and a health literate society.

For example, although the HHS Health Literacy Workgroup uses the *National Action Plan* in its own work and has collected many examples from other organizations, the full extent of the plan's effects is challenging to measure for several reasons. First, individual organizations may track their own health literacy improvement work, but they don't necessarily share that information with HHS or other organizations. Nor is organizational level data collected in a single place and reported in a comprehensive way. Second, systematically collecting and reporting data on the *National Action Plan's* effects takes financial and human resources that so far have not been available. Third, the health literacy field is only beginning to develop and test measures of organizational performance related to health literacy issues.

Some promising developments related to assessing organizational performance are emerging. For example, Rudd and Anderson developed a guide and accompanying tools for healthcare organizations to analyze health literacy-related barriers to healthcare access and navigation [46]. The guide can help chief executive officers, presidents, program directors, administrators, and healthcare workers at hospitals or health centers assess the health literacy environment of their healthcare facilities and analyze ways to better serve their patients and staff and ultimately to increase revenue [46]. This tool, as well as the *Ten Attributes of Health Literate Health ·Care Organizations* [44] and the *Health Literacy Universal Precautions Toolkit* [40], can help organizations focus on the system level challenges they face, but it is difficult to track which organizations use which tools and how often. Also, there is no mandate or even recommendation about which tools and measures to choose for different contexts nor organization to report to.

Hospital Compare, a consumer-oriented website that provides information on how well U.S. hospitals provide recommended care to their patients, provides another promising organizational measurement tool [47]. Hospital Compare was developed by the Centers for Medicare and Medicaid Services and the Hospital Quality Alliance. The tool empowers consumers to select multiple hospitals and directly compare U.S. hospital performance information. For example within Hospital Compare, users can assess how hospitals address several health literacy items, such as overall patient-reported experiences about communication with medical teams, communication about medicines, as well as communication about discharge information and care transitions. The tool's data are derived from the U.S. Hospital Consumer Assessment of Healthcare Providers and Systems Survey (HCAHPS). Although the site was developed for consumers to use performance measures to decide easily where to receive care, the tool can help healthcare organizations identify where they can improve their health literacy performance. To date, the tool applies only to Medicare-certified hospitals.

6. Emerging opportunities to implement an organizational change approach to health literacy

As healthcare organizations respond to federal and state health reform initiatives, they have the opportunity to integrate health literacy insights and *National Action Plan* strategies into their organizational improvements. For example, shared decision making and quality research that is easily understood and usable by people with different levels of health literacy are both provisions of prior health reform initiatives and may continue to be included in future health reform efforts [45,48]. The Agency for Healthcare Research and Quality (AHRQ) has implemented various health reform provisions in multiple ways, including developing easy-to-use guides on comparative effectiveness research findings and interactive tools, such as an online "question builder" that allow patients to assemble a set of questions for a healthcare visit [49]. The Office of Disease Prevention and Health Promotion (ODPHP), with support from AHRQ, developed a patient decision tool, myhealthfinder, to help people identify recommended clinical preventive services [50].

HHS has developed decision aids that facilitate shared decision making between patients and providers. ODPHP, AHRQ, the Centers for Medicare and Medicaid Services and other agencies have implemented shared decision making mandates by designing personalized decision support for clinical preventive services and a roadmap to help people understand the "coverage to care" continuum. Additionally, HHS has created primary care training grants with preference for applicants that provide training in enhanced communication with patients and cultural competency and health literacy [48]. Several HHS agencies have developed internal professional training in health literacy as well as grant programs to improve written and spoken communication among health professionals throughout the nation to fulfill this mandate.

As the laws and regulations for healthcare reform continue to evolve, new opportunities to connect health literacy improvement to other drivers of healthcare organizational changes may emerge. Health literacy researchers and practitioners can draw on the *National Action Plan* [1], *Ten Attributes of Health Literate Health Care Organizations* [44] and the Health Literate Care Model [43] for strategy ideas and models for positive changes.

Health literacy researchers and practitioners might use the following questions to explore how action plans have contributed to health literacy improvements in organizations.

> Do organizations with written health literacy plans implement moreeffective changes than those that insert health literacy changes in other initiatives?

Do organizations with health literacy training programs for healthprofessionals rate more favorably with their patients than organizations that don't have such programs?

Do countries with national health literacy plans show higher levels of patient satisfaction and engagement with healthcare professionals?

How do national health literacy objectives affect organizational commitments to health literacy improvements?

Do health care organizations that implement the health literate care model achieve improved quality outcomes?

7. Summary

The U.S. *National Action Plan to Improve Health Literacy* was one of the first documents outlining a path toward a health literate society envisioned in the 2004 IOM health literacy report [20]. The HHS Health Literacy Workgroup led the plan development process and sought input from many public and private sector organizations and individuals to make sure that the plan was relevant and practical. The plan helped inform and support the concept that health professionals and organizations bear the majority of responsibility for ensuring clear communication with the public. This approach focuses on improvements organizations can make to help people find and use health information and services effectively.

Although more documents and tools supporting an organizational change approach have emerged since the IOM's report, the *National Action Plan* is still a singular contribution because of its scope "beyond the clinic." The seven goals speak to a wide range of health activities, including public information and public health, as well as everyday life where people spend the majority of time managing their own health questions and concerns. The plan also envisions productive partnerships with many sectors, including education and community-based services. Even if the *National Action Plan* hasn't been implemented and tracked as fully as the HHS Workgroup envisioned, the plan has catalyzed attention to organizational responsibility for health literacy. It has spawned examinations of communication processes and products and the complexity of health information and services. The plan has inspired numerous organizations to implement its strategies, and it has inspired multiple models for how organizations, including HHS, can aspire to and track progress on becoming health literate organizations. National health literacy plans can establish benchmarks to foster assessments and gauge practice improvements. The plan can continue to inspire and expand a vision of what health literacy improvement means.

In the foreword to the *National Action Plan*, Dr. Howard Koh, former HHS Assistant Secretary for Health, wrote "when people receive accurate, easy-to-use information about a health issue, they are better able to take action to protect and promote their health and wellness. That is why health literacy is so critical to our efforts in the U.S. Department of Health and Human Services. It is the currency for everything we do" [1]. The *National Action Plan* provides a focus for these actions as well as a long view toward the many necessary changes that can move the country toward a truly person-centered health system and a health literate society.

References

[1] Office of Disease Prevention and Health Promotion, U.S. Department of Health and Human Services. National action plan to improve health literacy. Washington, DC: U.S. Department of Health and Human Services, Office of Disease Prevention and Health Promotion; 2010.

[2] Roundtable on health literacy [homepage on the Internet]. Washington, DC: The National Academy of Medicine [updated 2016 Aug 17; cited 2016 Oct 31]. Available from: http://www.nationalacademies.org/hmd/Activities/PublicHealth/HealthLiteracy.aspx

[3] National Center for Education Statistics. The nation's report card: 2013 mathematics and reading grade 12 assessments. U.S. Department of Education; 2014 May 7. Report No.: NCES 2014087.

[4] Kirsch I, Jungeblut A, Jenkins L, Kolstad A. Adult literacy in America: a first look at the results of the National Adult Literacy Survey. Washington, DC: U.S. Department of Education, National Center for Education Statistics; 1993.

[5] Kutner M, Greenberg E, Baer J. A first look at the literacy of America's adults in the 21st century. Washington, DC: U.S. Department of Education, National Center for Education Statistics; 2005.

[6] Goodman M, Finnegan R, Mohadjer L, Krenzke T, Hogan J. Literacy, numeracy, and problem solving in technology-rich environments among U.S. adults: results from the Program for the International Assessment of Adult Competencies 2012. Washington, DC: U.S. Department of Education, National Center for Education Statistics; 2013.

[7] U.S. Office of the Surgeon General, Office of Disease Prevention and Health Promotion. Proceedings of the Surgeon General's workshop on improving health literacy. Rockville, MD: Office of the Surgeon General; 2006.

[8] U.S. Office of the U.S. Surgeon General. National call to action to promote oral health. Rockville, MD: Office of the Surgeon General; 2003.

[9] Healthy People 2020 [homepage on the Internet]. Washington, DC: U.S. Department of Health and Human Services; 2010. Available from: www.healthypeople.gov. Retrieved October 28, 2016.

[10] Baur C. National Action Plan to improve health literacy. In: Thompson TL, editor. Encyclopedia of health communication. Thousand Oaks, CA: SAGE Publications.

[11] Baker DW, Gazmararian JA, Williams MV, Scott T, Parker RM, Green D, Ren J, Peel J. Health literacy and use of outpatient physician services by Medicare managed care enrollees. J Gen Intern Med. 2004;19(3):215–20.

[12] Howard DH, Gazmararian J, Parker RM. The impact of low health literacy on the medical costs of Medicare managed care enrollees. Am J Med. 2005;118(4):371–7.

[13] Health literacy: report of the Council of Scientific Affairs. Ad hoc committee on health literacy for the Council on Scientific Affairs, American Medical Association. JAMA. 1999;281(6):552–7.

[14] Doak CC, Doak LG, Root JH. Teaching patients with low literacy skills. 2nd ed. Philadelphia: J.B. Lippincott; 2007.

[15] Centers for Disease Control and Prevention. Simply put. 3rd ed. Atlanta: Centers for Disease Control and Prevention; 2010.

[16] National Cancer Institute, National Institutes of Health. Clear & simple: developing effective print materials for low-literate readers. Bethesda, MD: U.S. Department of Health and Human Services; 1998.

[17] National Patient Safety Foundation (US). Ask me 3: Good questions for Your Good Health [internet]. Boston (MA): National Patient Safety Foundation. Available from http://www.npsf.org/default.asp?page=askme3. Retrieved November 18, 2016.

[18] Rudd R. Improvement in health literacy. In: Baur C, editor. Communicating health: priorities and strategies for progress. Washington, DC: U.S. Department of Health and Human Services; 2003. p. 35–60.

[19] Kutner M, Greenberg E, Jin Y, Paulsen C, White S. The health literacy of America's adults. Washington, DC: U.S. Department of Education; 2006.

[20] Nielsen-Bohlman L, Panzer AM, Kindig DA, editors. Health literacy: a prescription to end confusion. Washington, DC: The National Academies Press; 2004.

[21] National Library of Medicine, National Institutes of Health. MedlinePlus [homepage on the Internet]. Bethesda, MD: U.S. Department of Health and Human Services. Available from: https://medlineplus.gov/. Retrieved October 31, 2016.

[22] Selden CR, Zorn M, Ratzan SC, Parker RM, compilers. Health literacy [bibliography online]. Bethesda, MD: National Library of Medicine; 2000.

[23] Office of Disease Prevention and Health Promotion, U.S. Department of Health and Human Services. Eng TR, Gustafson DH, editors. Wired for health and well-being: the emergence of interactive health communication. Washington, DC: U.S. Department of Health and Human Services; 1999.

[24] Healthy People 2010 [homepage on the Internet]. Washington, DC: U.S. Department of Health and Human Services; 2000. Available from: http://www.healthypeople.gov/2010/. Retrieved October 31, 2016.

[25] Berkman ND, DeWalt DA, Pignone MP, Sheridan SL, Lohr KN, Lux L, Sutton SF, Swinson T, Bonito AJ. Literacy and health outcomes. Evidence Report/Technology Assessment No. 87. RTI International – University of North Carolina Evidence-based Practice Center under contract no. 290-02-0016. AHRQ Publication Number 04-E007-2. Rockville, MD: Agency for Healthcare Research and Quality; 2004.

[26] Berkman ND, Sheridan SL, Donahue KE, Halpern DJ, Viera A, Crotty K, Holland A, Brasure M, Lohr KN, Harden E, Tant E, Wallace I, Viswanathan M. Health literacy interventions and outcomes: an updated systematic review. Evidence Report/Technology Assessment No. 199. RTI International – University of North Carolina Evidence-based Practice Center under contract no. 290-2007-10056-I. AHRQ Publication Number 11-E006. Rockville, MD. Agency for Healthcare Research and Quality; 2011.

[27] Understanding and promoting health literacy PAR-04-116 [page on the Internet]. Bethesda, MD: National Institutes of Health, U.S. Department of Health and Human Services; 2004. Available from: http://grants.nih.gov/grants/guide/pa-files/PAR-04-116.html. Retrieved October 31, 2106.

[28] Elwood W. The literature of health literacy: over 20 years of science to improve knowledge, skills and health. Bethesda, MD: Office of Behavioral and Social Sciences Research, National Institutes of Health; 2015. Available from: https://obssr.od.nih.gov/literature-health-literacy-20-years-science-improve-knowledge-skills-health/. Retrieved October 31, 2016.

[29] Developing a health literacy action plan. Wellington, New Zealand: New Zealand Ministry of Health; 2012. Available from: http://www.health.govt.nz/our-work/making-services-better-users/health-literacy/health-literacy-reviews/developing-health-literacy-action-plan. Retrieved November 8, 2016.

[30] An inter-sectoral approach for improving health literacy for Canadians [homepage on the Internet]. Victoria, British Columbia; 2012. Available from: http://www.cpha.ca/en/programs/portals/h-l/resources.aspx. Retrieved November 8, 2016.

[31] Amin H, Choo RM, Khoo G, Khan R, Koh JY, Loh HS, Thilagaratnam S, Vasquez K, Wadia S. The Singapore Action Plan to improve health literacy. Irvine, CA: 2015 Institute for Healthcare Advancement Annual Conference Poster; 2015. Available from: https://www.iha4health.org/wp-content/uploads/2015/03/The-Singapore-Action-Plan-to-Improve-Health-Literacy.pdf. Retrieved November 8, 2016.

[32] Agency for Healthcare Research and Quality. 2015 national healthcare quality and disparities report and 5th anniversary update on the National Quality Strategy. Rockville, MD: Agency for Healthcare Research and Quality; 2015.

[33] National Prevention Strategy [homepage on the Internet]. Rockville, MD: Office of the U.S. Surgeon General, U.S. Department of Health and Human Services; 2011. Available from: http://www.surgeongeneral.gov/priorities/prevention/strategy/index.html. Retrieved October 31, 2106.

[34] The National CLAS Standards. Rockville, MD: Office of Minority Health, U.S. Department of Health and Human Services; 2016. Available from: http://minorityhealth.hhs.gov/omh/browse.aspx?lvl=2&lvlid=53. Retrieved October 31, 2016.

[35] Wisconsin Health Literacy. Previous summits/videos. Wisconsin Literacy Inc. Available from: http://wisconsinliteracy.org/health-literacy/training-conferences/previous-summitsvideo.html. Retrieved September 30, 2016.

[36] Golley, Linda. National Action Plan stories from LINCS listserv: listserv [internet]. Message to: LINCS listserv. 2012. Retrieved November 21, 2016.

[37] Neuhauser L, Rothschild B, Graham C, Ivey SL, Konishi S. Participatory design of mass health communication in three languages for seniors and people with disabilities on Medicaid. Am. J. Public Health. 2009;99(12):2188-2195. DOI:10.2105/AJPH.2008.155648.

[38] Kurtovich E, Ivey SL, Neuhauser L, Graham C, Constantine W, Barkan H. A multilingual mass communication intervention for seniors and people with disabilities on Medicaid: a randomized controlled trial. Health Serv. Res.. 2010;45(2): 397–417. DOI: 10.1111/j.1475-6773.2009.01073.x.

[39] Office of Disease Prevention and Health Promotion, U.S. Department of Health and Human Services. Health literacy online 2nd Edition. Available from https://health.gov/healthliteracyonline/. Retrieved October 13, 2016.

[40] The Agency for Healthcare Research and Quality. AHRQ Health literacy universal precautions toolkit. Available from http://www.ahrq.gov/sites/default/files/wysiwyg/professionals/quality-patient-safety/quality-resources/tools/literacy-toolkit/healthlittoolkit2.pdf. Retrieved October 25, 2016.

[41] Koh HK, Berwick DM, Clancy CM, Baur C, Brach C, Harris LM, et al. New federal policy initiatives to boost health literacy can help the nation move beyond the cycle of costly 'crisis care'. Health Aff. 2012;31(2):434–43. DOI: 10.1377/hlthaff.2011.

[42] Yin HS, Dreyer BP, van Schaick L, Foltin GL, Dinglas C, Mendelsohn AL. Randomized controlled trial of a pictogram-based intervention to reduce liquid medication dosing errors and improve adherence among caregivers of young children. Arch Pediatr Adolesc Med. 2008;162(9):814–22. DOI: 10.1001/archpedi.162.9.814.

[43] Koh HK, Brach C, Harris LM, Parchman ML. A proposed 'health literate care model' would constitute a systems approach to improving patients' engagement in care. Health Aff. 2013Jan;32(2):357–67. DOI: 10.1377/hlthaff.2012.1205

[44] Brach C, Keller D, Hernandez L, Baur C, Parker R, Dreyer B, et al. Ten attributes of health literate health care organizations. National Academies Press; 2012.

[45] Schillinger D, Keller D. How can health care organizations become more health literate: workshop summary. National Academies Press. Available from: https://www.ncbi.nlm.nih.gov/books/NBK201212/

[46] Rudd, R., Anderson, J. The health literacy environment of hospitals and health centers. Boston, MA; 2006.

[47] Centers for Medicare & Medicaid Services. Hospital compare. Centers for Medicare & Medicaid Services. Available from: https://www.medicare.gov/hospitalcompare/search.html. Retrieved October 18, 2016.

[48] Patient Protection and Affordable Care Act, Public Law 148, 111th Cong., 2nd sess. (March 23, 2010).

[49] Agency for Healthcare Research and Quality. Question builder. United States: Agency for Healthcare Research and Quality. Available from: http://www.ahrq.gov/patients-consumers/question-builder.html. Retrieved October 26, 2016.

[50] healthfinder.gov. Office of Disease Prevention and Health Promotion. myhealthfinder. Available from: https://healthfinder.gov/. Retrieved November 10, 2016.

Health Literacy
R.A. Logan and E.R. Siegel (Eds.)
IOS Press, 2017
doi:10.3233/978-1-61499-790-0-203

The Journey to Become a Health Literate Organization: A Snapshot of Health System Improvement

Cindy BRACH[1]

Agency for Healthcare Research and Quality

Abstract. A health literate health care organization is one that makes it easy for people to navigate, understand, and use information and services to take care of their health. This chapter explores the journey that a growing number of organizations are taking to become health literate. Health literacy improvement has increasingly been viewed as a systems issue, one that moves beyond siloed efforts by recognizing that action is required on multiple levels. To help operationalize the shift to a systems perspective, members of the U.S. National Academies of Sciences, Engineering, Medicine Roundtable on Health Literacy defined ten attributes of health literate health care organizations.

External factors, such as payment reform in the U.S., have buoyed health literacy as an organizational priority. Health care organizations often begin their journey to become health literate by conducting health literacy organizational assessments, focusing on written and spoken communication, and addressing difficulties in navigating facilities and complex systems. As organizations' efforts mature, health literacy quality improvement efforts give way to transformational activities. These include: the highest levels of the organization embracing health literacy, making strategic plans for initiating and spreading health literate practices, establishing a health literacy workforce and supporting structures, raising health literacy awareness and training staff system-wide, expanding patient and family input, establishing policies, leveraging information technology, monitoring policy compliance, addressing population health, and shifting the culture of the organization.

The penultimate section of this chapter highlights the experiences of three organizations that have explicitly set a goal to become health literate: Carolinas Healthcare System (CHS), Intermountain Healthcare, and Northwell Health. These organizations are pioneers that approached health literacy in a systematic fashion, each exemplifying different routes an organization can take to become health literate. CHS provides an example of how, even when the most senior leadership drives the organization to become health literate, continued progress requires constant reinvigoration. At Intermountain Healthcare, the push to become a health literate organization was the natural consequence of organizational adoption of a model of shared accountability that necessitated patient engagement for its success. Northwell Health, on the other hand, provides a model of how a persistent champion can elevate health literacy to become a system priority and how system-wide policies and procedures can advance effective communication across language differences, health literacy, and cultures.

---

[1] Corresponding author: Center for Delivery, Organization, and Markets, Agency for Healthcare Research and Quality, 5600 Fishers Lane, Rockville, MD 20857; E-mail: cindy.brach@ahrq.hhs.gov

The profiles of the three systems make clear that the opportunities for health literacy improvement are vast. Success depends on the presence of a perfect storm of conditions conducive to transformational change. This chapter ends with lessons learned from the experiences of health literacy pioneers that may be useful to organizations embarking on the journey. The journey is long, and there are bumps along the road. Nonetheless, discernable progress has been made. While committed to transformation, organizations seeking to be health literate recognize that it is not a destination you can ever reach. A health literate organization is constantly striving, always knowing that further improvement can be made.

Keywords. Health literacy, health literate organization, organizational assessment, quality improvement, system perspective, organizational change, spread, transformation

1. Introduction

The Roundtable on Health Literacy, sponsored by the U.S. Academies of Sciences, Engineering, and Medicine, introduced the concept of a health literate health care organization – that is, an organization that makes it easy for people to navigate, understand, and use information and services to take care of their health [1, 2]. This chapter explores the journey that a growing number of health care organizations are taking to become health literate. Readers looking for a "how-to" guide may want to consult the publication, *Building Health Literate Organizations: A Guidebook To Achieving Organizational Change* [3].

Many organizations would state that making it easier for people to navigate, understand, and use information and services is an organizational priority, but would not describe themselves as health literate. They might, for example, describe that priority as being person-centered or striving for superior patient experiences [4, 5]. The aim of this chapter is not to distinguish health literate organizations from their similarly oriented counterparts. Rather, this chapter's objective is to trace the movement of the health literacy field towards a systems perspective – one that moves beyond siloed efforts by recognizing that action is required on multiple levels – and to document and learn from implementation experiences of those who have commenced the journey.

This chapter is informed by the framework posited by a participants in the National Academies Roundtable on Health Literacy, which identifies ten attributes of a health literate organization [2]. The organization of this chapter roughly follows the journey that organizations make when they aim to become health literate. After describing health literacy's emergence as a systems issue, the ten attributes of a health literate organization, and the external drivers of organizational health literacy, the chapter follows a naturalistic path, telling the story of organizational progress as it frequently unfolds. First, it discusses the steps that organizations take when they begin the journey: using health literacy assessment tools and focusing on written and spoken communication. Next, we look at what happens when an organization sets a goal of becoming health literate, covering the following topics: organizational leadership, strategic planning, health literacy workforce and structures, universal awareness and training; patient and family advisory councils, policies, information technology and monitoring, population health, and culture.

In addition to literature cited, the following data sources informed this chapter.
- Documents and interviews with multiple individuals who work at three systems that have declared becoming health literate as an organizational goal:

Carolinas HealthCare Systems, Intermountain Healthcare, and Northwell Health.
- Interviews with twenty organizations that were part of a study on organizational health literacy measurement.
- Conference presentations, including those at workshops of the National Academies Roundtable on Health Literacy and the Health Literacy Annual Research Conference.
- Site visits to health care organizations while making grand round presentations.

2. Emergence of Health Literacy as a Systems Issue

The field of health literacy was spawned by research that found that people with limited literacy skills were at risk of poor health and health care [6]. Many articles in the 1990's documented that individuals with low literacy are less likely to use preventive services or adhere to treatment, while they are more likely to be hospitalized and be in poor health [7]. It quickly became clear, however, that the problem was not constrained to the population of the poorest readers. Studies revealed that written health materials, such as patient education materials, exceeded the *average* person's ability to read and understand them [8-12]. The finding from the 2003 National Assessment of Adult Literacy that only 12 percent of the population could complete an array of tasks requiring comprehension of real world written health materials consolidated the growing sense that the literacy demands of health information had to be reduced [13].

The first decade of the 21st century saw health literacy expand beyond its roots in written communication to include spoken communication [14]. In addition, there was an ever-growing recognition of challenges associated with accessing services and navigating among facilities [15], providers, and settings. As a result, health literacy frameworks and calls to action came to incorporate the need to address the numerous complexities people face in accessing health care and managing their health [16-18]. Within this broader view of health literacy as a "systems" issue, it was understood that even the most skilled, well-intentioned clinician cannot single-handedly overcome the health literacy barriers people face [19]. Rather, as had already occurred in the patient safety arena [20], health systems rather than individual clinicians have come to be held responsible for addressing the underlying problem.

The importance of systems in addressing health literacy deficits was articulated in the 2004 landmark health literacy report from the National Academies of Science, Engineering, and Medicine (then known as the Institute of Medicine) [21]. It referenced the 2001 Crossing the Quality Chasm report that specified, among other things, that *systems of care* should be redesigned such that information available to patients and families allows informed decision making [22].

Paasche-Orlow and colleagues were among the first to offer a vision of how health care systems should transform themselves to respond to health literacy challenges [23]. In 2006 they advocated for reorganizing health care to make systems patient-centered and pointed to the Care Model as a foundation[24]. This concept was later expanded upon with the development of the Health Literate Care Model, which identifies specific health literacy strategies that should be integrated into the Care Model to improve patient engagement in prevention, decision-making, and self-management [25].

Paasche-Orlow and Wolf also pointed to the complexity of the health care system and its acute care orientation as factors driving poor health outcomes [26].

Since 2010, the emphasis on the need for organizational, rather than clinician-level, remediation has grown. The Joint Commission called for organizations to make effective communication a priority [27]. The National Action Plan to Improve Health Literacy, published in 2010, called upon health care executives to: train all staff; establish formal mechanisms to review all written information for patients; include members of patient communities in organizational assessments and health literacy improvement efforts; integrate health literacy and cultural and linguistic competence audit tools, standards, and scorecards into all quality process and performance improvement activities and metrics; and create welcoming, easy-to-navigate, shame-free environments [28]. A striking example of the shift toward a systems approach is the U.S. National Academies of Sciences, Engineering, and Medicine Roundtable on Health Literacy's adoption of a new mission statement in 2015 to include a vision of "a society in which the demands of the *health and health care systems* are respectful of and aligned with people's skills, abilities, and values" [29].

3. Attributes of Health Literate Health Care Organizations

To help operationalize the shift to a systems perspective, members of the National Academies Roundtable on Health Literacy set out to define the attributes of a health literate organization. The aim of the Roundtable was to create the health literacy equivalent of the National Standards for Culturally and Linguistically Appropriate Services (the CLAS Standards) [30]. The CLAS Standards had been issued by the DHHS' Office of Minority Health in 2000 and had gone on to become the template for organizations seeking to be culturally and linguistically competent. Toward this end, the Roundtable commissioned a white paper, held a workshop, and ultimately published an IOM Perspective that resulted in the forging of a set 10 attributes that exemplify health literate health care organizations [1, 2, 31]. (See Table 1.) In the years following its publication, the *Ten Attributes of Health Literate Health Care Organizations* has been used as a framework for both an assessment tool and a guidebook on building health literate organizations [3, 32]. It has served as a guidepost for organizations wishing to transform themselves to meet health literacy goals and has influenced health literacy efforts internationally [33, 34]. We will see later in this chapter how two large health care systems in the United States adopted the ten attributes framework as their organizing principle for health literacy improvement.

Table 1. Ten attributes of health literate health care organizations

A health literate health care organization:

1. Has leadership that makes health literacy integral to its mission, structure, and operations.
2. Integrates health literacy into planning, evaluation measures, patient safety, and quality improvement.
3. Prepares the workforce to be health literate and monitors progress.
4. Includes populations served in the design, implementation, and evaluation of health information and services.
5. Meets the needs of populations with a range of health literacy skills while avoiding stigmatization.
6. Uses health literacy strategies in interpersonal communications and confirms understanding at all points of contact.
7. Provides easy access to health information and services and navigation assistance.

8. Designs and distributes print, audiovisual, and social media content that is easy to understand and act on.
9. Addresses health literacy in high-risk situations, including care transitions and communications about medicines.
10. Communicates clearly what health plans cover and what individuals will have to pay for services.

In operational terms, being a health literate organization means moving beyond the project-based improvement mindset. For example, an organization that only addresses health literacy for one population (e.g., people with heart disease) is not a health literate organization. An organization can even have several health literacy improvement projects without being health literate. For an organization to be truly health literate, health literacy has to pervade the organization and be integral to all operations. As long as health literacy is seen as an add-on, struggling for a seat at the table, organizations will not be health literate.

4. External Drivers of Organizational Health Literacy in the United States

The shift from fee-for-service to value-based payments in the United States has buoyed health literacy as an organizational priority. Financial rewards for positive clinical and patient satisfaction outcomes have encouraged the adoption of population management methods and focused attention on the patient experience. Addressing health literacy – by increasing patients' understanding of health information, ability to get needed services, and self-management capabilities – can help health care organizations meet both clinical and patient satisfaction outcomes. Laws passed by the U.S. Congress in the second decade of this century have accelerated the movement towards value-based payments. Payment reform under the U.S. Patient Protection and Affordable Care Act and the U.S. Medicare Access and CHIP Reauthorization Act has been particularly important in re-shaping organizational priorities in the United States.

4.1. Patient Protection and Affordable Care Act (ACA)

In 2010, U.S. Congress passed the ACA, which includes provisions to promote a redesign of the health care delivery system [35]. Following passage of the ACA, the Centers for Medicare and Medicaid Services (CMS – part of the U.S. Department of Health and Human Services) made payment changes that shifted health care organizations from to focusing purely on the volume of services delivered to rewarding efficiency (through shared savings) and quality. More specifically, through Alternative Payment Models, such as Accountable Care Organizations, U.S. providers have incentives to actively manage the health care of an entire population of Medicare[2] beneficiaries rather than reactively delivering acute care for episodes of illness.

Similarly, through the Medicare Hospital Value-Based Purchasing (HVBP) Program, Medicare payments now depend in part on quality metrics, including patient experience surveys, readmission rates to hospitals, and clinical measures. For example, starting in federal fiscal year 2015, CMS reimbursement changes provided hospitals

[2] Medicare is a health insurance program operated by the U.S. government for people who are 65 or older and certain younger people with disabilities.

with incentive to reduce 30-day readmissions for patients with targeted conditions. This focused a great deal of attention on improving patient education and discharge process to ensure that patients with targeted conditions stayed away from the hospital for at least a month. Furthermore, for the first time hospitals are being paid, in part, based on their post-hospital outcomes and how patients rate the care they receive. Notably, patients' ease of understanding of their doctors and nurses is one of the metrics on which patients are asked to rate their experience.

Formerly health care organizations had patient relations departments focused on attracting and retaining patients. The new approach is to focus more on improving patients' experiences of their care. This in turn has given rise to a new profession – the Patient Experience Officer [36]. Patient Experience Officers, with their mission to sensitize the delivery system to patients' experiences, are a natural ally for health literacy.

The ACA also gave a boost to the patient-centered medical home model (PCMH) that already had been gaining currency in primary care circles. Accreditors that issued standards for organizations seeking certification as PCMHs required clear communication, enhanced access and coordination, patient education and self-management support, and culturally and linguistically appropriate care [37]. With the ACA's promotion of patient-centered care, internal health literacy advocates had another lever for health literacy improvement.

4.2. Medicare Access and CHIP Reauthorization Act of 2015 (MACRA)

The passage of the Medicare Access and CHIP Reauthorization Act of 2015 (MACRA) by the U.S. Congress spread value-based purchasing further. Starting in 2017, U.S. health care providers that are not participating in Advanced Alternative Payment Models are scheduled to participate in the Merit-based Incentive Payment System (MIPS) [38]. Like the above-described HVBP Program, MIPS will reward or penalize physicians based on their outcomes, including patient experience. If implemented, MIPS is likely to do for outpatient care what HVBP Program did for hospitals: focus attention on patients' experiences of care. In a 2016 environmental scan of organizations undertaking organizational health literacy improvement, the most common form of monitoring was found to be tracking patient experience data, either through CAHPS® or other surveys [39].

MIPs will also give incentives to address health literacy from a population health perspective. Previously, U.S. health care organizations had little financial incentive to make sure patients understood how to care for themselves and maintain their health. The system was geared toward delivering as many billable services as possible. Following the dictates of professionalism, which obliges clinicians to help patients manage their conditions, came at a cost. As the population became healthier, revenues would decline due to a reduction in the number of procedures or office visits. With MIPS and the expected increase value-based payments by private health plans in the U.S., investments to make health information more understandable and ensure that patients can navigate the health care system might actually pay off.

In sum, U.S. health care organizations are realizing that being held accountable for outcomes and satisfaction means they need to do a better job of engaging patients. Health care systems will have to depend on individuals becoming involved in their health and health care if they are to achieve such goals as controlling high blood pressure and blood sugar. Addressing health literacy is fundamental to engaging patients; people cannot actively participate in their health care and take responsibility for their health if they are stymied by the complexity of health information and health care systems [25].

5. Early Days: Commencing the Journey to Become a Health Literate Organization

Payment reform provides an incentive to organizations to address health literacy, but does not tell organizations **how** to become health literate. Organizations usually start out with limited health literacy projects before they make a decision to address organizational shortcomings in a systematic fashion. They may take advantage of opportunistic innovation, making inroads where they can, when they can. Typically, it is only after they make some progress that organizations can make the leap from project-based quality improvement to system transformation. This section reviews how systems have taken these first steps, including undertaking organizational assessments of existing policies and operations and improving written communication, spoken communication, and physical or virtual navigation.

5.1. Organizational Health Literacy Assessment

Organizational health literacy assessments are useful in stimulating improvement activity [40] and serve as powerful tools to:

- promote awareness and discussion of current practices,
- identify strengths and areas for improvement,
- gain consensus for prioritizing health literacy interventions, and
- stimulate health literacy strategic planning.

Organizational health literacy assessment tools have been developed for a range of health care settings. (See Table 2.) The first health literacy assessment tool, the Health Literacy Environment Review, targeted hospitals and health centers [41]. It was closely followed by the publication of an audit tool for pharmacies [42]. These assessment tools, and others that followed for primary care practices health plans, and health and social service organizations were designed to be used for *internal improvement* purposes rather than by outside auditors for *accountability* purposes [32, 43-46].

Organizations have often adapted assessment tools, mixing and matching items from different assessment tools or changing the wording of items to better suit their environment [47]. They have used frameworks (such as the ten attributes of a health literate health care organization), home grown surveys of staff or patients, chart audits, patient tracers (shadowing a patient during a visit or inpatient stay), rounding on units, sampling patient education materials, and other means to gain intelligence on how health literate the organization is [48]. Some systems have used more rigorous patient experience surveys to flag a problem, and then followed up with these less scientific methods to peer inside the black box and pinpoint its source.

While these assessment tools were all pilot-tested for overall usability, none of these tools was validated as being reliable to measure improvement. Even the American Medical Association's Communication Climate Assessment Tools, which underwent rigorous testing to determine their validity, did not establish their ability to measure change over time [49]. Nevertheless, organizations have used repeated administration of assessments to measure their progress.

Table 2. Organizational health literacy assessment tools

Tool and Publication Date	Target Audience	Domains	Assessment Methods	Features
Health Literacy Environment Review (2006)	Hospitals and Clinics	• Navigation • Print Communication • Oral Exchange • Technology • Policies and Protocols	Self ratings (Done, Needs Improvement, Done Well)	• Composite scores (not validated) • Linked to options for reducing literacy-related barriers
Pharmacy Health Literacy Assessment Tool (2007)	Pharmacies	• Promotion of Services • Print Materials • Clear Verbal Communication • Sensitivity to Literacy • Physical Environment • Care Process and Workforce • Paperwork and Written Communication • Culture	• Assessment tour by objective auditors (Not Done, Needs Improvement, Done Well) • Staff survey (Not Done, Needs Improvement, Done Well) • Patient focus Groups	• Guidance on analyzing data • Guidance on using data for quality improvement.
Organizational Communication Climate Assessment Toolkit (2008)	Hospitals and Primary Care Clinics	• Organizational Commitment • Data Collection • Workforce Development • Community Engagement • Individual Engagement • Addressing Health Literacy • Meeting Language Needs • Cross-cultural Communication • Performance Monitoring	• Set of patient, clinical and nonclinical staff, and leadership surveys • Optional focus group protocols	• Team oriented self-assessment workbook • Composite scores (validated)
Primary Care Health Literacy Assessment (2010, 2015)	Primary Care Practices Clinics	• Practice Change • Spoken Communication • Written Communication • Self-Management and Empowerment • Supportive Systems	Self ratings (Doing Well, Needs Improvement, Not Doing, Not Sure/Not Applicable)	• Links to tools from the AHRQ Health Literacy Universal Precautions Toolkit

Tool and Publication Date	Target Audience	Domains	Assessment Methods	Features
Health Plan Organizational Assessment of Health Literacy Activities (2010)	Health Plans	• Printed Member Information • Web Navigation • Member Services/Verbal Communication • Forms • Nurse Call Line • Member Case/Disease Management	Self ratings (Tailored response categories)	• Recommends separate assessments if plans/products are different • Accompanying Suggestions for Areas of Improvement
Enliven Organisational Health Literacy Self-assessment Audit Resource (2013)	Health and Social Service Organizations	Each of the 10 attributes of a health literate organization is a domain (See Table 1.)	Checklist	• Provides space for notes/future action

Health care organizations need to be mindful of the limitations on appropriate uses of assessment instruments and the complexities associated with correctly interpreting their results. For example, systems have reported a lack of consistency between numerical ratings and subjective comments on an assessment instrument, which may indicate a failure of respondents to understand the meaning of a question or a social desirability bias.[3] Declines in self-assessment scores might actually signal increased sensitization to organizational deficiencies rather than changes in practice [50]. Finally, staff perceptions of organizational health literacy could increase without an actual increase in the use of health literacy strategies [51].

Probably more important than the particular tool chosen to guide the assessment activity is the process of assessment. Features of successful health literacy assessment processes have included:

- High commitment level. Establishing a dedicated work group with senior members and regular meetings is critically important.
- Adequate time. It has taken large systems up to a year to complete both the internal and external scans.
- Hiring consultants. Organizations frequently have not had in-house health literacy expertise and have sought external specialists to guide their assessment.
- Harnessing patient's stories. Understanding how patients see the organization and move through the system is critical to both figuring out where to target improvement and gaining buy-in for health literate changes.

---

[3] Social desirability bias occurs when respondents answer questions in a way that puts them in a good light. It can take the form of exaggerating good behavior or minimizing undesirable behavior.

- Broad engagement. Systems have sent assessment tools throughout the organization, either to be completed by key individuals or collectively in various departments or facilities.
- Strategic deployment. Especially at the outset, systems have conducted assessments in a few domains that demonstrated a critical need for action.

These insights on conducting assessments are generic and could apply to any quality improvement effort. It is the assessment topics that are specific to health literacy. Common to virtually all the health literacy organizational assessment tools are domains on written communication, spoken communication and physical or virtual navigation. These are frequently the next steps on the journey to become health literate.

5.2. Focus on the Written Word

Health literacy has often been incubated in committees or offices responsible for patient education materials. This reflects both the historical concern with individuals with limited literacy and the narrow connotation people have with the term "health literacy" with reading and writing. This branch of health literacy improvement has coincided with the plain language movement, which had its antecedents in frustration first voiced during the 1950's with confusing regulations and other bureaucratic-sounding publications of the federal government [52]. The plain language movement started to get traction in agencies of the Department of Health and Human Services around the same time that health literacy came into prominence with the publication of health literacy objectives for Healthy People 2010 [53].

Guides to making written health care information easier to understand date back to the earliest days of the health literacy field [54, 55]. Over time, guidance has become more sophisticated and begun to address online written materials [56, 57]. Automated readability formulas that roughly gauge the reading demands of written materials by counting up syllables in words and words in sentences to estimate grade level are widely used to signal that reading demands may be too high. Commercial products now detect reading level and stylistic deficiencies, such as use of the passive voice, and suggest alternatives. Three new tools involve quantitative measures of the use of health literacy principles, understandability, and actionability – the Health Literacy INDEX, the Clear Communication Index (CCI), and the Patient Education Materials Assessment Tool (PEMAT) [58-60]. Many organizations use these tools as part of their strategy to ensure people understand their written materials.

No single approach has emerged as the most effective for improving written materials. Some organizations have relied on mainstream vendors that, in response to demand, promote their materials as following health literate principles. Others have turned to niche vendors who specialize in easy-to-understand, multi-lingual materials. Still others have produced their own materials in-house, having found that the patient education materials they have purchased do not meet their standards.

Even organizations that do purchase patient education materials often have to also produce many of their own documents. With input from stakeholders, large health systems have established processes for creating and approving of written materials. The processes themselves frequently involve a wide range of representatives from throughout the system, such as from legal, marketing, accreditation, and safety departments; physician groups; and facilities. The resources required to manage written materials generally exceed what systems have allocated for the task. One strategy to reduce the workload of centralized editorial staff is to increase the quality of submitted materials. Organizations have accomplished this by providing health literacy training and tools (such as plain language glossaries, commercial software products, and style manuals) to writing staff throughout the system. Nevertheless, editorial staff frequently report having to prioritize important documents and an inability to review and update materials as frequently as their policy dictates.

Many organizations have recognized the importance and value of incorporating feedback from patients and families into their review process. Approaches have included getting feedback from general Patient and Family Advisory Councils, using committees of patient and families formed specifically to review materials, holding focus groups with diverse and disadvantaged members, and testing materials for comprehension with individuals with low literacy. One key source of confusion and frustration for many patients has been the bill for services [61]. Systems have found that revamping their bills to make them more understandable to be a huge undertaking, involving designing prototypes, gathering consumer feedback, and making information technology changes in the bill production process.

Despite all these labor intensive efforts, there is a segment of the population for whom written material, however simplified, will still be incomprehensible. The most recent attempts to serve these populations involve technological alternatives. For example, some systems provide inpatients with multi-lingual, interactive edutainment systems. These systems, made available on a television screen or computer tablet, allow patients to learn about their conditions and how to take care of themselves through video and other audio-visual content, and can even test learning and allow users to ask questions. In addition to overcoming literacy and language barriers, such systems are showing potential to reduce the amount of time clinicians have to spend educating patients and even reduce the length of inpatient stays. High-tech cannot completely replace high-touch for some patients who need extra help, but interfaces designed specifically for those with limited literacy and computer skills can be easy to use and well-liked by vulnerable populations [62].

Most organizations that have worked hard to reduce the literacy demands of their materials will acknowledge that these improvements are incremental and further work is needed. Moreover, as has been said earlier, what distinguishes organizations that have embarked on the health literate journey is that they have issued policies and set up structures to standardize processes across the board. With regards to written materials, adopting a system approach has included many, if not most of the following.

- Establishing accountability and requiring consistency for written materials system-wide
- Setting standards for user-centered materials for in-house production and vendor purchase
- Instituting processes for taking inventory, prioritizing, reviewing, and updating written materials
- Establishing policies, such as prohibiting materials that have not gone through the editorial process and used professional translators to be uploaded into information systems.
- Adhering to a schedule to re-assess materials
- Making materials easily accessible by including them in electronic health records (EHRs)

5.3. Focus on Spoken Communication

Like making written materials easy to understand, effective interpersonal communication is an attribute of health literate organizations that receives early attention. Improving spoken communication is a particularly important health literacy strategy for meeting the needs of non-readers. A study reporting that people immediately forget half of what they are told, and inaccurately recall half of what they retain, has been a rallying cry for efforts to improve health literacy [63]. As a result, health literacy training has often been directed at improving the spoken communication skills of the clinical team, for example by emphasizing speaking slowly, using plain language, limiting the amount of information given at one time, and encouraging questions. Role playing is a very popular form of teaching spoken communication skills. As systems spread health literacy beyond the clinician-patient interactions, they have training to all staff who interact with patients, from registration to billing staff.

Unlike other communication enhancement efforts that might focus on building clinician-patient relationships or having difficult conversations, efforts to improve health literacy focus on improving understanding [5, 64]. Confirming understanding has become a staple of organizations' health literacy improvement strategies, and teach-back – asking people to state in their own words what they have been told – is its poster child. Teach-back and the show-me method (asking people to demonstrate how they will do something at home) are acclaimed as the only way to truly confirm understanding. As one of the few health literacy strategies with an evidence base that links it directly to self-management and outcomes [65-68], teach-back has been the subject of training programs [14, 69], deemed a safe practice with regard to informed consent by AHRQ and the National Quality Forum, and promoted by accreditation organizations [27, 70, 71].

Methods of stimulating conversation are also being used. Some organizations are using or adapting Ask Me 3®, a program to encourage patients to get answers to three questions: 1) What is my problem? 2) What do I need to do? 3) Why is it important for me to do this? While some organizations use the National Patient Safety Foundation's Ask Me campaign materials (e.g., posters, notepads), others use Ask Me 3 as a guide for providers to make sure providers give information such that patients can answer the three questions by the end of a visit.

Systems will sometimes allow for local tailoring of improvement efforts. This can spark innovation and encourage implementers to own the changes they make. An example of a creative, home grown way of promoting clear spoken communication was to use white boards to write down complex language staff caught teammates using, along with plain language alternatives. In contrast, a more regimented approach was taken by a system that wanted to ensure all patients received exactly the same education during inpatient stay; it developed a specific curriculum and required nurses to document when each segment was taught.

5.4. Navigating Facilities and Systems

Navigation was first raised as a health literacy problem out of concern over the complexity of health care facilities and their poor signage [72]. Large systems responding to this challenge have gone beyond using more recognizable terminology on their signs (e.g., x-ray instead of radiology). Creative tactics have included using color coded pathways, standardizing plain language directions, having volunteer escorts, posting directions in commonly used languages, training all staff to be on the lookout for the puzzled expressions of people who are lost, and using golf carts to transport individuals across large campuses. Navigation apps to leverage mobile technology are on the horizon. Such navigation efforts are often aligned with more general initiatives to adopt a customer service orientation.

Navigation in health care also refers to negotiating a fragmented system – coordinating among care providers and managing transitions. The professions of cancer care navigators, community health workers, care coordinators, and case managers are all dedicated to guiding people through the maze of health services that patients must access. These programs frequently target vulnerable populations such as those with limited English proficiency or high disease burden. In addition to steering patients through the health care system, navigators frequently attend to non-medical needs, link them with resources in the community, and teach them the skills to navigate for themselves. These programs guard against the neediest from falling through the cracks of the system.

Organizations whose goal is to be health literate, however, have to relieve the coordination burden for **all** patients. One method for doing so is to "close the loop" when referring patients from one provider to another. If a warm handoff (i.e., a personal introduction with a transfer of responsibility for follow-up) cannot be achieved, the referring provider will follow up with the patient to confirm that a connection was made. Other efforts to make care more seamless have included making specialized referral agreements among providers, for example for drop-in mammograms. Policies designed to lower the demands on patients are sometimes used, such as not asking patients to convey medical information from one provider to another. Most organizations, however, would acknowledge that they are not where they would like to be on this aspect of being health literate.

Finally, as penalties for excess readmissions have kicked in, systems have given particular attention to transitions from hospital to home, which are among the most fraught and challenging to navigate. For systems aiming to be health literate, the focus on the discharge process has triggered a broader examination of how inpatients are educated. This in turn fueled efforts to improve both written and spoken communication, and to formally structure the education process. Additionally, the strategies of making post-discharge phone calls and ensuring patients connect with outpatient clinicians have grown popular.

6. Maturation: Scaling Up and Institutionalizing

As was noted at the outset of this chapter, when an organization sets a goal of becoming health literate, it replaces fragmented quality improvement activities with a systematic and comprehensive approach. Health care organizations do not start the journey in a single place, and the journey is not linear. Headway is made in spurts, losing ground is not uncommon, and the journey is a lengthy one.

The move from health literacy quality improvement toward transformation into a health literate organization entails:

- the highest levels of the organization embracing health literacy,
- making strategic plans for initiating and spreading health literate practices,
- establishing a health literacy workforce and supporting structures,
- raising health literacy awareness and training staff system-wide,

- expanding patient and family input,
- establishing policies,
- leveraging information technology and monitoring policy compliance,
- addressing population health, and
- shifting the culture of the organization.

This section examines how health care organizations aspiring to become health literate have institutionalized their health literacy activities.

6.1. Organizational Leadership

When C-suite officials (e.g., Chief Executive Officer, Chief Nursing Officer, Chief Medical Officer, Chief Experience Officer) have championed health literacy, it is usually because health literacy goals are closely aligned with the organization's mission, goals, and business imperatives. They set their sights on becoming health literate because they view it as instrumental to achieving important organizational priorities such as:

- providing person-centered care and patient experience,
- engaging patients,
- ensuring patient safety (e.g., medication safety and readmission reduction),
- reducing disparity reduction (e.g., language assistance, cross-cultural communication), and
- containing cost.

A sign that health literacy has become entrenched is when it is viewed a means to an end rather than another thing to do. Even mission-driven organizations have considered the business case for health literacy, however, justifying doing the right thing by linking it to obtaining a larger market share or reducing costs. Furthermore, with systems worried about staff burnout and change fatigue, organizational leaders have to see health literacy as a new and better way of doing business.

In some organizations, there are silos of health literacy activity but a lack of leadership to integrate them into a unified force for change. Organizational leaders need to not only communicate the importance of health literacy at the launch of a holistic improvement program, but also to be stalwartly and visibly supportive and attentive throughout implementation and maintenance phases. They have done so by serving on oversight committees, reviewing metrics of success, and making resources available as needed.

6.2. Strategic Planning

Systems leading the pack have engaged in strategic planning to become health literate. Organizational assessments, discussed earlier in this chapter, are a necessary step in strategic planning. Strategic plans, however, go farther than plugging some of the gaps identified by assessments. Strategic plans include concrete goals across multiple health literacy domains and spell out precisely what actions are going to be undertaken to achieve these goals, who will undertake those actions, and how accomplishments will be measured. Inherent in the strategic plan, therefore, is a logic model for how change will happen and which outcomes will be achieved.

Systems that reached the stage of conducting health literacy strategic planning generally have had a foundation in both continuous improvement and intra-organizational spread of innovation. Varied methodologies have been used, sometimes in combination. These have included use of key driver diagrams [73], quality improvement testing cycles [74], SWOT analyses (analyzing the strengths, weaknesses, opportunities, and threats) and Lean A3 problem solving. What has mattered has not been the choice of methods, but rather the experience in improvement and change management, which has provided an infrastructure for health literacy advancement.

6.3. Health Literacy Workforce and Structures

While there is no single recipe for becoming health literate, a key ingredient in all successful efforts is the designation of staff to be responsible for health literacy as all or part of their jobs. An organization cannot, however, become health literate if a single health literacy manager or coordinator in a large system is expected to do all of the heavy lifting. Thus, systems truly committed to becoming health literate typically have established structures that assume responsibility for health literacy. These have sometimes taken the form of task forces or councils established specifically to ensure that health literate policies and practices are being followed. Often the responsibility for health literacy has been overlaid on existing quality improvement or patient safety functions. By contrast, in many not-yet-fully-health-literate organizations, health literacy staff are relatively isolated internal advocates, accumulating small victories without shifting the orientation of the organization.

The success of these important structures – and of organizational literacy efforts more generally – depends on support from health literacy champions throughout the organization. Beyond the organizational leaders mentioned earlier, these include both formal health literacy liaisons and staff who have more informally become standard bearers for health literacy in the course of doing their jobs. For example, patient experience staff may take on the responsibility of raising health literacy issues as they sit on operational committees.

6.4. Universal Awareness and Training

Training programs have ranged from across-the-board training to targeting particular facilities or professions. Large systems and hospitals sometimes start by training nursing staff, since they often have less direct control over physicians and physicians are viewed as more recalcitrant [48]. Health care systems try to strike a balance between the ability to reach a wide audience using online formats with a more intensive in-person approach. Key to such efforts is a combination of system and local leadership underscoring the importance of addressing health literacy and a boots-on-the-ground strategy with local trainers and coaching.

To achieve training goals, adult learning approaches, such as using videos and interactive content, are common. While individuals and small organizations typically use nationally available training materials [44, 75, 76], large systems frequently only consult them and then customize their own programs. Some systems have established professional competencies for attainment of health literacy knowledge, attitudes, and skills.

Systems that have reached more mature levels of health literacy are implementing health literacy training that is:

- Universal – Everyone in the organization gets awareness and skills training.
- Verifiable – Procedures are in place to record when training is completed.

- ✓ Recurrent – Training begins with new employee orientation and is refreshed on a regular schedule (e.g., annually).
- Remedial – Extra training is targeted to those who can benefit the most from it.
- Fortified – Train-the-trainer models use middle management who can reinforce the training and the importance of being health literate (e.g., staff meetings, huddles, newsletters).

6.5. Patient and Family Advisory Councils

Patient and Family Advisory Councils (PFACs) originated in the 1990s in recognition that consumer input into policy and program development was critical to implementing family-centered care [77]. By 2016, 2,000 hospitals had launched a PFAC, and PFACs have erupted in other health care settings as well. Organizations like the Institute for Patient- and Family-Centered Care and, more recently, the Beryl Institute have created resources and training to spur and prepare organizations to create and engage with PFACs [78].

PFACs are a chief avenue for including populations served in the design, implementation, and evaluation of health information and services, as called for by the ten attributes of health literate organizations. PFACs, however, tend to attract participants who, for the most part, have adequate health literacy and English proficiency. Organizations on the health literacy journey have been challenged in engaging more disadvantaged populations. Some organizations have especially reached out to these populations, providing them with training and supportive services that allow them to effectively participate in PFACs. Organizations have also supplemented PFACs by holding focus groups with these populations. This approach has the benefit of drawing out people who might not be vocal on a PFAC, but falls short of engaging these populations fully as partners in the formation of a health literate system.

6.6. Policies

Organizations have promulgated and enforced a variety of policies as a way of standardizing the delivery of care. Health literacy policies generally have reflected a universal precautions approach to delivering health literate care, one which assumes that every individual is at risk of misunderstanding and benefits from clear communication and uncomplicated care pathways. The following are illustrations of common types of health literacy policies:

- All patient education materials will go through reviews by editors and patient volunteers. Readability guidelines and health literacy principles will be followed.
- Only qualified interpreters will be used to communicate with patients with limited English proficiency.
- Patients will not be discharged until they can teach-back the signs of deterioration and what to do about them, as well as how to follow discharge instructions.
- Clinicians must ask patients to show how they will perform self-management activities, such as wound care.

- Patient education and successful knowledge checks will be documented in the EHR.
- All new employees will complete health literacy training within the first 30 days of employment.
- Clinicians will refer patients who meet specified criteria to navigators.
- Follow-up calls will be made to patients who fail to show for an appointment.
- Referring clinicians will provide all relevant information.
- All patients will be offered help with forms.

Policies are not always precise, but can give cues regarding expected behavior without detailing what that means. Lack of precision is sometimes necessary to permit flexibility that lets the policy fit into local work flow and culture. For example, a system might issue a directive to "treat patients with respect" or "encourage patients' questions" but leave open which strategy to use to achieve the stated goal. Vagueness in policy statements become problematic, however, when people are uncertain about how to comply with the policy. For example, hospitals with ambiguous informed consent policies left staff confused about their appropriate roles in the process [79].

While policies are used to drive change, systems are sometimes reluctant to issue a policy that substantially alters current practice. In part, this is out of a concern that accrediting organizations will deem them to be out of compliance with their own policies. Formalization of a policy is therefore sometimes a mark of completing change rather than triggering it.

6.7. Information Technology and Monitoring

Organizations pursuing health literacy try to hardwire it into their information technology (IT). This can be challenging and requires that top leadership prioritize changes needed to support health literacy over other changes that may be in their IT department's queue. Health literate IT changes fall into two categories: those that make it easier to deliver health literate care, and those that document that health literate care has been given.

Examples of IT fixes that make it easier to get patients the care and information they need include: purging the IT system of unauthorized documents and closing back doors used to post materials that have not gone through the approval process; creating standard order sets of health literate materials that save clinicians the trouble of searching for them; and giving prominence to actionable information, such as displaying a patient's preferred language at the top of every page.

Systems have struggled with the documentation of health literate care. To create useful data, documentation must be standardized in the EHR, which usually requires creating new data entry fields. Organizations have frequently opted for check boxes that get ticked when the activity occurred (e.g., the patient was taught something, the patient was able to teach it back), despite the danger of gaming the system. Systems think that requiring an entry with the date and time of completion and sign off by supervisors minimizes false entries. Furthermore, requiring such documentation was thought to communicate health literacy expectations to staff, and at a minimum allowed the identification of locales that did not even bother to check the box.

Systems, however, have also relied on means other than self-report to assure compliance with policies, such as using other data sources for verification (e.g., use of interpreter services) and requiring observations of the activity. For example, nurse managers in one system verified that white boards were updated and discussed using a bedside shift report with observation checklist. Observations were made twice a week unless performance is poor, in which case daily checks were made.

6.8. Population Health

Some systems have addressed health literacy by targeting particularly disadvantaged geographic areas and, in doing so, attended to broader challenges that affect population health. In these instances, the system established alliances with community organizations, sometimes taking advantage of existing coalitions. Recognizing that individuals in these communities, especially those with limited health literacy, face a host of barriers to achieving optimal health outcomes, these systems worked to make sure residents connected with help in obtaining insurance coverage, affording medicines, obtaining employment, accessing healthy food, and getting basic adult education. While such efforts fall outside of some definitions of health literacy, addressing the social determinants of health by improving supportive systems for patients is considered part of taking health literacy universal precautions [43].

6.9. Culture

Even with policy changes and significant investments in training, transformation will not occur or endure if it goes against organizational culture [80]. Systems that have had to undergo culture change to routinize new health literate practices have recognized that culture change is something that has to be shaped over time. Fortunately, health literacy found an affinity with efforts to create a more person-centered culture. More specifically, health literacy has been compatible with cultural changes aimed at patient engagement, cultural and linguistic competence, and providing a medical home.

Systems striving to be health literate have recognized that culture change requires a multi-prong approach. This has included defining unacceptable behavior (e.g., trying to "get by" without an interpreter for a patient who is not proficient in English) as well as required behavior (e.g., having a friendly, helpful demeanor), monitoring whether the changes had been made, and supplementing training with constant reinforcement from leadership [81].

It is hard to measure whether cultural change has been successful. Systems have used mixed methods, such as employee surveys and rounding, to gauge the impact of their efforts. Often progress can be seen in subtle changes in behavior that are not formally measured. For example, in one hospital that used training modules with the slogan "Make informed consent and informed choice," the change lead noted, "When we began to hear clinicians utter the words 'informed choice,' we knew we had made headway."

7. The Journey: Three Organizations' Efforts to Become Health Literate

Driven by mission as well as pragmatic considerations, an increasing number of organizations are commencing the journey to become health literate organizations. This section highlights the experiences of three organizations that have explicitly set a goal of becoming health literate: Carolinas Healthcare System, Intermountain Healthcare, Northwell Health [82-84]. These organizations are not typical. They are pioneers that approached health literacy in a systematic fashion, each exemplifying different routes along the journey to organizational health literacy. The information in each profile has been selected to highlight different aspects of each of their journeys. An approach may be described in one profile and not another even though both organizations followed a similar approach.

7.1. Carolinas HealthCare System: Health Literacy Top Down and Through and Through

Carolinas HealthCare System (CHS) is a Charlotte-based non-profit system with 60,000 employees and an annual budget of more than $7.7 billion. It is comprised of more than 900 care locations, including academic medical centers, hospitals, physician practices, surgical and rehabilitation centers, home health agencies, urgent care clinics, and other facilities.

Health literacy was ushered in as an organizational priority by the Executive Vice President/Chief Medical Officer (CMO). The CMO intuitively understood the importance of addressing health literacy to achieve patient-centered care and patient safety, and was influenced by the fact that another system (Iowa Health Systems) was working to improve health literacy.

The CMO set into motion actions that led to health literacy becoming a vital part of CHS' work:

- He asked the marketing department to conduct research into low literacy in Charlotte and how it affected patients and CHS financially.
- He obtained buy-in from the Board of Directors, which consisted of the heads of all the facilities owned by CHS, by engaging nationally-known health literacy scholar Dr. Darren DeWalt to win their hearts and minds.
- He established a system-wide Health Literacy Task Force (HLTF) with representation from all 25 CHS facilities. Co-led by the Director of Performance Enhancement of CHS' internal consulting team and the Director of CHS' Center for Advancing Pediatric Excellence who had QI expertise, the HLTF was charged with identifying ways to address health literacy at CHS.

Over a nine-month period, the HLTF educated itself and hashed out an approach to pursue organizational health literacy. The result was CHS' first health literacy initiative – a one-year learning collaborative. (See Box 1.) Results at the end of the collaborative showed improvement on most of nine measures. Participants were charged with extending health literacy strategies across the system. A year later, however, a survey revealed that health literate strategies had not yet been extensively adopted.

Health literacy efforts at CHS were reinvigorated by the arrival of a Chief Nurse Executive. She, together with the co-Chairs of the HLTF and the CHS Management Company, strategized about how to spread health literacy practices throughout CHS. Rather than try to spread the entire health literacy collaborative change package, they opted to focus on the spread of two high-leverage changes– teach-back and Ask Me 3. The initiative, called TeachWell (see Box 2), proposed to spread these changes to all facility-based nurses in CHS – over 10,000 nurses – as well as to all employees at the 25 ambulatory faculty practices that were affiliated with CHS hospitals.

Box 1. Health Literacy Learning Collaborative

- 25 facilities across the continuum of care and their affiliated ambulatory practices
- Targeted non-physician employees, chiefly nurses
- 2-day learning session
- Plan-Do-Study-Act QI cycles
- Change package (based on prototype of the AHRQ Health Literacy Universal Precautions Toolkit):
  - 30 changes, 11 mandatory
  - Mandatory monthly reporting on 9 measures

Box 2. TeachWell Features

- Focus on spoken communication: teach-back & Ask Me 3
- Playbook: implementation guide with tools that drew on already established approaches (e.g., Kaiser Permanente's Nurse Knowledge Exchange Plus program and the AHRQ Health Literacy Universal Precautions Toolkit)
- Implementation infrastructure at each facility:
  - Facility/Business Unit Champions
  - Project Advisors
  - Small Team Leaders
  - Small Teams
- Mandatory training for all nurses, who sign pledges to use health literacy skills
- Re-enforcement through staff meetings, daily huddles, and the use of communication self-assessments, teach-back observation forms, and tracking logs.
- Measures of observed use of health literacy strategies reported to CHS senior leadership

---

A 15-member TeachWell Steering Committee developed a structure for the implementation effort that included enlisting a top manager at each facility as a Facility/Business Unit Champion and one or two staff at each facility as Project Advisors to oversee facility-wide implementation. CHS encouraged each facility to assess their health literacy practices by providing a variety of assessment tools. Each small team in CHS facilities used small tests of change to refine their plans before rolling out the training to all nurses. Project Advisors were accountable for getting targeted staff trained and having them sign an e-Confirmation and Commitment Pledge, an online form in which they attested that they recognized the importance of health literacy and would use health literacy skills. To assess whether staff were actually using teach-back and Ask Me 3, small teams chose surveyors to make rounds to observe behavior. Senior leadership, including the Chief Nursing Executive, the CMO, Facility Presidents, and Executive Vice Presidents reviewed the four TeachWell metrics collected monthly at the beginning of implementation, and quarterly for the remainder of the implementation period. Graphs of metrics were also shared with staff to provide feedback. The TeachWell Steering Committee disbanded after the end of the implementation period.

Health literacy at CHS was given another huge boost when one of its senior vice presidents was asked to take on a new role and became CHS's first Senior Vice President of Patient Experience (CXO) overseeing a Patient Experience Team of 140. Among her first tasks was investigating how health literate CHS was. She and her team analyzed data from patient surveys and 197 responses to the Health Literacy Environmental Review that had been sent to all CHS facilities and practices. They determined that there was not a consistent "CHS way" for delivering health care. In response, CHS developed "the One Culture," which asserted that CHS "will achieve its vision through the development of a single unified enterprise focused on developing enduring relationships with our patients based on superior personalized service and high quality outcomes."

The Patient Experience Team now integrates health literacy throughout CHS. For example, a team member sits on each Differentiable Patient Experience Action Council, which the CXO established at each facility. These Councils, consisting of the Senior Vice President and other facility leadership – including those responsible for quality, safety, accreditation, education, and human resources – are a direct line into CHS' daily operations. Patient Experience Team members have additional opportunities to infuse patient experience principles, including health literacy, throughout the system. For example, they are members of various Quality and Safety Operations Councils (QSOCs). While the entire team carries the banner for health literacy, CHS has only a single full-time staff member who works exclusively on health literacy and there is no budget earmarked for health literacy. This Health Literacy Consultant serves as an internal adviser, following up with staff members who were trained in plain language, and overseeing the operations of the Patient and Family Health Education Governance Council.

Given that the watch words of the Patient Experience Team are "include, inform, and inspire," it is not surprising that health literacy was seen as central to delivering the type of experience that CHS wants to create. Toward that end, the CXO began by working with the Director of CHS' Center for Advancing Pediatric Excellence, a longtime health literacy champion who had been co-chair of the HLTF and led the Health Literacy Learning Collaborative, and the Senior Vice-President for Marketing. Using a key driver diagram that showed how becoming health literate would result in better outcomes, patient satisfaction, and value, the CXO and colleagues convinced the CHS Board of Directors to formally adopt a goal of becoming health literate by 2020 and include it in the 2014 CHS system-wide strategic roadmap. Since then, CHS has annually assessed progress towards this goal using the 10 attributes of health literate health care organizations and reported all health literacy accomplishments to the Board. Health literacy has become an organization-wide expectation. Table 3 provides examples that CHS has taken to address each of the 10 attributes of a health literate organization.

Table 3. Examples of Carolinas Healthcare System activities on 10 attributes of a health literate organization

Attribute	Examples of Activities

1. Leadership promotes	• Involvement in health literacy committees and activities by the highest level system and facility leadership.
	• Health literacy on strategic roadmap
	• Health literacy in leadership and physician leadership development
	• Health literacy policies established, e.g.,
	  o No materials can be published unless they've been reviewed by a PFAC or focus groups of patients
	  o All CHS employees – including grounds-keepers and custodians – must complete online health literacy training

2. Plans, evaluates and improves	• Assessments using Health Literacy Environmental Review • Differentiable Patient Experience Action Councils at every facility address health literacy • Health literacy measurement set (in development) • Patient experience team members carry health literacy principles and the voices of patients into redesigns of the electronic health record and the patient flow
3. Prepares workforce	• Health literacy incorporated into new employee orientation; within 30 days of arriving new employees sign a health literacy Confirmation and Commitment Pledge • TeachWell training • CURO Conversations: clinicians with room to improve patient experience scores and others identified as being able to benefit from extra sensitization are assigned to CURO training (Connect, Understand, Reveal and Relate, and Outcomes), which includes teach-back, plain language, and Ask Me 3 • Training writers on plain language and health literacy software
4. Includes populations served	• Expansion of Patient and Family Advisory Councils (PFACs), to 31 PFACs (for larger facilities) and 14 patient or family advisors (for smaller facilities), enlisting over 240 volunteers • Over 100 patients involved in bill redesign

5. Meets needs of all	• Universal precautions adopted in both spoken and written communication
	• Allocated resources to high need area by building a health literate facility in Anson County, a rural, very poor county, where the average literacy level is third grade
	  o Partnered with the community to replace critical access hospital with a new facility that met its needs.
	  o Created a PFAC
	  o Conducted a Health Literacy Environment Review of the old facility to identify health literacy gaps
	  o New, easy-to-navigate facility includes:
	    ▪ Physical design to promote coordination, e.g., no walls between the emergency department and primary care
	    ▪ Emergency department screening that directs non-emergent patients to primary care providers
	    ▪ Pharmacy with a payment-assistance program
	    ▪ On-site behavioral health specialist and tele-psychiatry, space for rotating specialists for better care coordination
	    ▪ Computer in waiting room for patient use
	    ▪ Patient navigator, a van service to transport patients to the facility, and a mobile unit that offers screenings, diagnostics and education

Attribute	Examples of Activities

6. Communicates effectively	• TeachWell expanded to all CHS ambulatory practices, not just those affiliated with facilities
	  o Trained all employees – those with clinical responsibilities (e.g., nurses, physicians, patient educators, social workers, certified medical assistants, nursing aides, dieticians) as well as all front and back office staff
	  o Plain language communication was added to the curriculum after noticing a great deal of medical jargon was used in the practices
	  o Each type of specialty (e.g., surgery, neurology, etc.) was trained together, as were primary care practice service lines (e.g., family medicine, OB-GYN), allowing the discussion of plain language substitutes to be customized
	  o TeachWell was reinforced in other venues, such as monthly practice manager meetings

7. Provides easy access	• Navigation assistance (e.g., guest services, transporters, volunteers/greeters, signage) • Language services • Improvements to patient portal
8. Designs easy-to-use materials	• Patient and Family Health Education Governance Council with 12 Health Education Committees, one for each service line, and six task forces: 1) infrastructure, 2) evaluation measures, 3) vendors and vendor relations, 4) content management, 5) discharge, and 6) diverse populations • Issued health literacy standards to vendors
9. Addresses high-risk situations	• Care coordination project • In-patient interactive edutainment system • Improved discharge instructions
10. Explains coverage and costs	• Patient experience team members participated in redesign CHS' bills and explanation of benefits, insisting that the new designs incorporate health literacy principles and involving 100 patients in those efforts • Improved descriptions of CHS employee benefits

CHS is an example of how leadership from the very top of an organization can drive the organization to become health literate. It also shows how fragile health literacy initiatives are: at the end of the Health Literacy Learning Collaborative and the first round of TeachWell, health literacy strategies did not get spread and health literacy activity died down. Fortunately, new committed leaders emerged and health literacy resurged as CHS concentrated on improving the patient experience. Health literacy has become infused throughout the system to the extent that it would not go away if any single individual were to leave the organization. It is not so deep-seated, however, that it does not require tending and expanding. CHS has pioneered health literacy measurement in the form of reporting on observed health literacy practices, but has only enforced it while scaling up initiatives. CHS acknowledges that the measures it has used are far from perfect, and like other systems continues to search for more and better gauges of health literate behavior. This, and the fact that CHS uses the ten attributes framework to report its health literacy progress annually to leadership, is a strong indication that CHS will continue its journey to become a health literate organization.

7.2. Intermountain Healthcare: Pursuing Health Literacy as a Prerequisite to Patient Engagement ✓

Intermountain Healthcare is a Utah-based, not-for-profit system of 22 hospitals, 185 clinics, a Medical Group with some 1,400 employed physicians, a health plan division called SelectHealth, and other health services. In the wake of the passage of the Affordable Care Act in 2010, Intermountain adopted a model of shared accountability, whereby patients are encouraged to take advantage of prevention and wellness programs, self-manage their conditions, and get more involved in decisions about their care. Three strategies were chosen as being instrumental to achieving shared accountability:

1. Redesigning care to ensure the delivery of evidence-based medicine.
2. Engaging patients in their health and care choices.
3. Aligning financial incentives for everyone who has a stake in healthcare.

A Patient Engagement Steering Committee (PESC) was formed to define the scope of patient engagement work at Intermountain. Initially, this committee was comprised of 25 representatives from around the system, led by Director of Clinical and Patient Engagement.

Over the course of a year of intense work, the PESC reviewed the research literature, conducted a SWOT analysis, and interviewed dozens of leaders within the organization as well as hundreds of patients. The PESC came to recognize the importance of health literacy as instrumental to engaging patients so that they could contribute to their health. The result was a Patient Engagement Framework, which included health education and health literacy as a foundational component. (See Figure 1.) The Framework was approved by Intermountain's highest level leaders, the Operations Council.

To move from concept to reality, the Operations Council directed that the PESC be restructured to reduce the number of members and include key senior officials and operations leaders. Two councils, reporting directly to the PESC, were convened to implement the Framework: the Patient Experience Guidance Council and the Health Education and Health Literacy Effectiveness Guidance Council (HEHLE). Although the work of both councils could be included in an expansive definition of health literacy, at Intermountain it is the work of the HEHLE that is labeled as health literacy.

HEHLE members include staff at the Assistant Vice President level throughout the system, as well as staff responsible for patient and provider publications, clinical education, communications, nursing, physicians, and employee health. The HEHLE's purpose is to develop, select, and deliver consistent, engaging, and effective education for clinical staff, providers, patients, families, communities and employees across the care continuum. HEHLE members constantly scanned the horizons, using outside resources to increase health literacy knowledge.

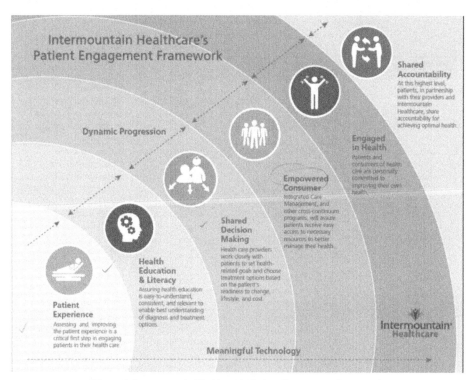

Figure 1. Intermountain Healthcare's Patient Engagement Framework
Reprinted with permission from Intermountain Healthcare

The HEHLE chose to use the "Ten Attributes of a Health Literate Health Care Organization" to gauge health literacy at Intermountain. It selected Intermountain's "go-to" medical writer to undertake an informal health literacy gaps analysis on all aspects of the health system, from pharmacy to patient safety. The result was a report on what Intermountain was doing on each attribute, and what it needed to be doing. (See Table 4.) The assessment uncovered many pockets of health literacy activity, but found that they were not coordinated. It also found that some patient experience initiatives have significant health literacy overtones, such as Intermountain's "healing commitments,"[4] bedside reporting, patient communication boards (white boards in patients' rooms), and narrating care as it is delivered.

The HEHLE decided it needed someone dedicated to promoting health literacy at Intermountain. The medical editor was chosen to be Intermountain's Health Literacy Coordinator, its only employee who works on health literacy fulltime. Her position description holds her responsible for: ensuring health information for patients and consumers is easy to access, understand, and use; ensuring system-wide processes take health literacy into account; promoting system-wide health literacy standards; and developing a system-wide strategic plan for health literacy.

While the strategic plan was being developed, the HEHLE decided to act on some of the identified opportunities for improvement and score some "quick wins" to raise

---

[4] Intermountain's healing commitments are to help patients feel safe, welcome and at ease; to listen to patients with sensitivity and respond to their needs; to treat patients with respect and compassion; to keep patients informed and involved; to ensure that care teams work with patients; and to take responsibility to help solve problems.

Table 4. Intermountain Healthcare assessment of health literacy activities
and opportunities using 10 attributes of a health literate organization

Attribute	Existing Activities	Opportunities
1. Leadership promotes	• Patient Engagement Strategic Plan • Health Education and Health Literacy Effectiveness Guidance Council (HEHLE) • Healing Commitments	• Make an explicit commitment to incorporate health literacy in policies and programs and educate leadership
2. Plans, evaluates and improves	• Health literacy vital sign pilot project • Patient satisfaction data analytics	• Use assessment, measurement, and evaluation to inform continuous health literacy improvement
3. Prepares workforce	• Teach-back training for hospital nurses	• Health literacy orientation and/or teach-back training for all employees
4. Includes populations served	• Patient and Family Advisory Council (PFAC) • Research services/focus groups • Clinical program-specific feedback	• Additional Patient and Family Advisory Councils, including one specific for education
5. Meets needs of all	• Care managers, health advocates, community care management, shared decision tools, and interpreter services	• Address health literacy universally across the care environment
6. Communicates effectively	• Teach-back training for hospital nurses	• Teach-back training for all patient-facing employees
7. Provides easy access	• Intermountainhealthcare.org • Intermountain Health Hub • MyHealth • Community Health Info Centers	• Test patient portals with low-literacy population • Test way-finding and signage with low-literacy population
8. Designs easy-to-use materials	• Strategic Patient Education Team (SPET) • Patient and provider publications • Integration of vendor content	• Update existing patient education materials for increased health literacy • Increase visual/graphic approach
9. Addresses high-risk situations	• Integrated care management • Discharge phone calls • Centralized pharmacy procedures	• Test health literacy of hospital discharge instructions and medication instructions
10. Explains coverage and costs	• Pre-registration cost estimates • Financial assistance web page • SelectHealth web pages	• Test billing procedures and web pages with low-literacy population

Reprinted with permission from Intermountain Healthcare

awareness of health literacy system-wide. One of these was the development a health literacy infographic and other health literacy content that could be dropped into presentations.

Another "quick win" was the development of an eLearning module to make health literacy more concrete to employees. Earlier Intermountain had created a training module for hospital nurses based on the teach-back tool in the AHRQ Health Literacy Universal Precautions Toolkit. The module was revised to include an introduction to health literacy and broadened to be applicable to all non-physician employees who interact with patients. Almost all of the approximately 25,000 employees across the system who were assigned to complete the module did so. Knowing that more than a one-time training is needed for staff to adopt teach-back and use it consistently, Intermountain created teach-back flash cards with conversational prompts to re-enforce the training. Subsequent communications workshops have focused on integrating teach-back into the daily workflow for specific clinical groups, including system-wide dietitians, diabetes educators, and newly hired physicians.

The HEHLE prioritized making education materials consistent across audiences (i.e., patient, provider, employee, community) while the strategic plan was being produced. Aligning patient education materials with treatment protocols ensured that patients got consistent information and instructions. The policy also served to provide clinicians with models of language to use with patients. For example, all clinician-facing materials were renamed from Hypertension to Blood Pressure in order to promote the use of plain language. Materials are scheduled to be reviewed every two years.

To ensure that all requests for new patient education materials were channeled through the Strategic Patient Education Team (SPET), a policy was set that materials not reviewed by the SPET could not be included in the EHR. The SPET assesses each new piece (using the PEMAT and other tools), vets the content with the appropriate clinical teams, and assures alignment with any related material. Because of dissatisfaction with vendor materials, Intermountain has increasingly relied on internal staff to design and write patient education materials. The health literacy review for new materials includes, whenever possible, input from the PFAC, an advisory group specifically for patient education formed with members of an adult literacy class in the community.

In January 2016 the HEHLE Guidance Council and the Patient Engagement Steering Committee approved a 3-year Health Literacy Strategic Plan. Noting the work Intermountain has completed on each of the 10 attributes of a health literate organization, the plan lays out a set of strategic initiatives as well as metrics for assessing progress. Proposed timelines for actions were flexible so that health literacy initiatives could be integrated most naturally with other initiatives.

One way that Intermountain has pushed its health literacy agenda forward is by integrating health literacy into major system-wide initiatives. For example, health literacy content was inserted into Intermountain patient safety initiative Zero Harm. Three pilot sites worked on processes to integrate teach-back into the Zero Harm workflow. They integrated it into daily safety huddle and asked the clinics to set goals around teach-back. For example, front desk staff at one clinic asked patients four questions: Did your healthcare provider ask you to repeat back any of your instructions? Do you understand what you need to do for your health when you get home? Did somebody ask you to tell you what you heard, or to repeat back what you learned? Do you feel confident knowing what you're supposed to do when you get home?

Integrating teach-back into Zero Harm was one strategy used to engage physicians. Clinicians were also exposed to health literacy more broadly through clinical education. For example, when clinicians were taught a new procedure at a Simulation Center, they were taught teach-back as part of the process of educating the patient about the procedure. Moreover, physicians applying to give a lecture to their peers are now asked whether patient education is relevant to their topic and how they will address patient understanding in their talks.

Intermountain has taken advantage of a regional infrastructure for quality improvement to further health literacy goals. Poor scores from patient experience surveys activate regional patient experience managers. When health literacy has been a factor, the Health Literacy Consultant has been brought in to share health literacy tools and provide coaching on how to implement them. Intermountain's plan is to explore which health education and health literacy practices generate the highest scores and spread those practices.

At Intermountain, the push to become a health literate organization was neither decreed from above by leadership nor driven by grass roots advocates. Rather, it was the natural consequence of organizational adoption of a model of shared accountability that necessitated patient engagement for its success. Intermountain found numerous ways to build on its previous efforts to make information easier to understand and the system easier to navigate. The approval of a 3-year Health Literacy Strategic Plan marked an acceleration of its journey. It did not, however, free up substantial new resources to address health literacy. Health literacy champions have worked to integrate health literacy into standard operating procedures. However, if enthusiasm for health literacy ebbs, it is possible that insufficiently ingrained health literate practices will fall into disuse.

7.3. Northwell Health: Linking Health Literacy to Diversity and Inclusion

Northwell Health, a health care network (formerly North Shore-LIJ Health System) has taken a different path toward becoming a health literate organization. Because Northwell is the subject of another chapter in this book (see Rosoff and Rosen), this section only highlights some of ways Northwell's trajectory is distinct from the other two systems described in this chapter.

The ascendency of health literacy at Northwell was largely due to the advocacy of a nurse turned educator. Her passion for improving patient education and other written materials, shared by a colleague who became Northwell Health's Health Literacy and Patient Education Coordinator, raised health literacy's profile, first on a regional basis and then at corporate level. Years of championing health literacy paid off when Northwell included health literacy in an office newly created to expand the delivery of culturally customized care in response to the growing diversity of the population served – the Office of Diversity, Inclusion, and Health Literacy (ODIHL).

Like other systems, Northwell undertook a health literacy gaps analysis, but it chose to use a tool that measures the effectiveness of communication policies and practices with people from diverse populations – the American Medical Association's (AMA) Communication Climate Assessment Tool (C-CAT). Northwell compared results from four of its hospitals with 20 other hospitals in the AMA's benchmarking database. The results, along with analyses of patient experience data, indicated that much work could be done to improve effective communication. Northwell's health literacy efforts were further propelled by the belief that the Affordable Care Act would usher in an era of value-based payment, which would make investments that yielded better patient outcomes pay off. ODIHL got support and guidance from Northwell Health's leadership, including members of the Board of Trustees, to move forward with a multi-year strategic plan.

Northwell's view of health literacy was colored by the recognition that a person's culture is strongly linked to the way they perceived and understood health problems and outcomes [82]. For example, training – including new employee training, a case-based interactive web-based learning module was available to all employees, and training for future system leadership – combines health literacy with cultural and linguistic competence.

The creation of ODIHL also forged a close alignment of health literacy with language assistance services. Previously distinct improvement streams, their confluence reflects the view that language assistance is a part of health literacy since it is a prerequisite to effective communication. Northwell's approach to language access provides an example of how policies, training, and infrastructure improvements combine to change the norms for patient care.

Northwell's Limited English Proficient Patients Policy states that everyone who has a preference to conduct health care interactions in a language other than English has the right to a qualified medical interpreter, and bilingual staff members who are not qualified interpreters are not permitted to interpret. Initially, it was commonplace for this policy not to be followed. ODIHL staff visited facilities to: educate staff about Northwell's language access policies, distribute the AHRQ tool on addressing language differences, alert them to legal ramifications of interpreting when not qualified to do so, and teach them how to access interpreters and enter documentation in the EHR. Through their site visits ODIHL staff became aware that their EHR did not facilitate the provision or documentation of language services.

ODIHL worked with information system staff to make changes to the EHR to support language access. Resources to make these changes were available because they were viewed as necessary to meet Joint Commission requirements. One change was to make the patient's language preference appear as a banner on top of every page of the EHR so it would be immediately apparent when an interpreter had to be called. Another change was to create a central location with specific fields to document patients' acceptance or refusal of interpreter services. ODIHL also created tools that let Language Access Coordinators easily generate audit reports to monitor compliance with language access policies. Training, combined with these EHR changes, produced a sharp increase in the use of telephone interpreters over a six-year period. ODIHL staff report a cultural shift; it is no longer acceptable to try to get by without using qualified interpreters.

Northwell Health established system-wide policies and procedures to advance effective communication across language differences, health literacy, and cultures. While perhaps not achieving the level integration of health literacy, cultural competency and language access envisaged by the National Academies Roundtable on Health Literacy, health literacy and language access were united under the expanded umbrella of effective communication [85]. Northwell provides an example of how dedicated health literacy champions can raise health literacy to the top levels on an organization. By aligning with other efforts deemed critical to providing patient-centered care, health literacy was able to achieve a firm foothold in the system's quality improvement apparatus.

8. Lessons on the Journey

To some extent, every successful quality improvement story involves a perfect storm. Elements of that storm include enthusiastic leadership; congruence with the organization's mission, values, culture and goals; champions with the requisite expertise, including skills in training and improvement methods; a readiness to make the needed structural, process, and workforce changes; and confidence that perceived benefits will be greater than the costs – including opportunity costs [80]. The three systems profiled in this chapter are no exception. Having perceived a mission-driven imperative or strategic advantage to be gained by making health information easier to understand and systems easier to navigate, they set out to become health literate and have achieved some measure of success because the elements of a perfect storm lined up.

Organizations setting out on the journey can learn from the experiences of health literacy pioneers, including but not limited to the three profiled systems. These include the following.

- Do not discount the power of committed individuals to launch the journey to become health literate. While it takes a village to transform an organization, the journey begins with fervent adherents who persuade others of the advantages of being health literate. Bringing in outside experts and pointing to other organizations that have made headway can help gain traction.

- Start with your strength. Many health literacy efforts have commenced with attention to written documents and then blossomed into full-bodied health literacy initiatives. With the increasing emphasis on the patient experience, we may see more health literacy efforts emerge with a focus on spoken communication. Regardless of where they start, health literacy efforts benefit from building a strong foundation before setting a goal of becoming health literate.

- Take the time to determine where deficiencies lie and investments will pay off. The three systems profiled in this chapter all undertook lengthy investigations of their own operations and the experience of their patients before engaging in strategic planning. Involving a range of people with different responsibilities in this phase can garner the acceptance that will make implementation easier.

- Balance the need for a locus of accountability for health literacy with the importance of everyone perceiving health literacy is part of their job. In large systems, ideally there will be a dedicated health literacy team tasked with steering health literacy improvement. It is important, however, that health literacy not be seen as a separate program instead of an imperative that affects every aspect of the organization. Creating cross-cutting work groups or councils can harness the full array of the system's resources by making health literacy improvement everyone's responsibility.

- Plan for incremental spread. The three systems profiled all embarked on ambitious health literacy plans, but had to proceed judiciously to avoid over-whelming staff. They tended to target specific health literacy practices, sometimes with a particular profession or set of facilities. After they gained experience, they spread the practices and later layered new health literacy practices on top of the first ones. Incremental spread allows for testing and improving implementation strategies and guards against burn-out of an already taxed workforce. At the same time, these systems forged ahead on multiple fronts. Because the responsibility for different aspects of health literacy rested in different parts of the organization, systems were able to make simultaneous progress in more than one health literacy domain.

The profiles of the three systems also make clear that the opportunities for health literacy improvement are vast. Health literacy champions often felt that there were limitations on what they could get done due to competing priorities. This included both limits on how much change could be pushed through the system at one time, competition for staff resources, and scarce for funding to develop training and tools.

The three systems largely focused on what they could accomplish within their systems. That meant that non-employees, even those closely partnered with the system (e.g., staff at independent specialty practices), could not be assigned health literacy training, required to follow policies, or obligated to monitor and report on their progress. Taking this next step will require not only communicating expectations for health literate care to their partners, but also using market power to compel the meeting of those expectations

We have learned that the journey is long, and that there are bumps along the road. Nonetheless, discernable progress has been made by organizations in making it easier for people to navigate, understand, and use information and services to take care of their health. While committed to transformation, organizations seeking to be health literate recognize that it is not a destination you can ever reach. A health literate organization is constantly striving, always knowing that further improvement can be made.

Acknowledgements

This chapter could not have been possible without the generosity of staff at Carolinas HealthCare, Intermountain Healthcare, and Northwell Health who spent hours on phone interviews, shared documents, and reviewed and corrected inaccuracies in the profiles. I am also in the debt of the dozens of individuals who have talked to me over the years about how their organizations address health literacy. Finally, I would like to thank my colleague Dina Moss for her encouragement and expert editorial suggestions. The opinions expressed in this chapter are the author's own and do not necessarily reflect the views of the Agency for Healthcare Research and Quality, the Department of Health and Human Services, or the United States Government.

References

[1] Institute of Medicine. How can health care organizations become more health literate?: workshop summary. Washington, DC: The National Academies Press, 2012.
[2] Brach C, Keller D, Hernandez LM, Baur C, Parker R, Dreyer B, et al. Ten attributes of a health literate health care organization. Washington, DC: Institute of Medicine, June, 2012.
[3] Abrams MA, Kurtz-Rossi S, Riffenburgh A, Savage B. Building health literate organizations: a guidebook to achieving organizational change. Wes Des Moines, Iowa: UnityPoint Health, 2014.
[4] Luxford K, Safran DG, Delbanco T. Promoting patient-centered care: a qualitative study of facilitators and barriers in healthcare organizations with a reputation for improving the patient experience. Int J Qual Health Care. 2011;23(5):510-5. DOI: 10.1093/intqhc/mzr024.
[5] Boissy A, Gilligan T, editors. Communication the Cleveland Clinic way: how to drive a relationship-centered strategy for superior patient experience. New York: McGraw Hill Education; 2016.
[6] Doak CC, Doak LG, Root JH. Teaching patients with low literacy skills. 2nd ed. Philadelphia: J. B. Lippincott Company; 1996.
[7] Berkman ND, Sheridan SL, Donahue KE, Halpern DJ, Viera A, Crotty K, et al. Health literacy interventions and outcomes: an updated systematic review. Rockville, MD: Agency for Healthcare Research and Quality, 2011.
[8] Freda MC, Damus K, Merkatz IR. Evaluation of the readability of ACOG patient education pamphlets. The American College of Obstetricians and Gynecologists. Obstet Gynecol. 1999;93(5 Pt 1):771-4. DOI: 10.1016/S0029-7844(98)00518-3

[9]   Buck ML. Providing patients with written medication information. Ann Pharmacother. 1998;32(9):962-9. DOI: 10.1345/aph.17455.
[10] Galloway G, Murphy P, Chesson AL, Martinez K. MDA and AAEM informational brochures: can patients read them? J Neurosci Nurs. 2003;35(3):171-4. DOI: 10.1097/01376517-200306000-00007.
[11] Estrada CA, Hryniewicz MM, Higgs VB, Collins C, Byrd JC. Anticoagulant patient information material is written at high readability levels. Stroke. 2000;31(12):2966-70. DOI: 10.1161/01.STR.31.12.2966.
[12] Williams MV, Parker RM, Baker DW, Parikh NS, Pitkin K, Coates WC, et al. Inadequate functional health literacy among patients at two public hospitals. JAMA. 1995;274(21):1677-82. DOI: 10.1001/jama.274.21.1677.
[13] Kutner M, Greenberg E, Jin Y, Paulsen C. The health literacy of America's adults: results from the 2003 National Assessment of Adult Literacy. Washington, DC: National Center for Educational Statistics; 2006 September.
[14] Weiss BD. Health literacy: a manual for clinicians. Chicago: American Medical Association Foundation and American Medical Association, 2003.
[15] Rudd RE, Renzulli D, Pereira A, Daltory L. Literacy demands in health care settings: the patient perspective. In: Schwartzberg JG, VanGeest JB, Wang CC, editors. Understanding health literacy: implications for medicine and public health. Chicago: AMA Press; 2005. p. 69-86.
[16] Baker DW. The meaning and the measure of health literacy. J Gen Intern Med. 2006;21(8):878-83. DOI: 10.1111/j.1525-1497.2006.00540.x.
[17] Parker R. Measuring health literacy: What? So what? Now what? Measures of health literacy; February 26; Washington, DC; 2009.
[18] U.S. Department of Health and Human Services. Communicating health: priorities and strategies for progress: Action plans to achieve the health communication objectives in Healthy People 2010. Washington, DC: July, 2003.
[19] Adams K, Corrigan JM. Priority areas for national action: transforming health care quality. Washington, DC: The National Academies Press, 2003.
[20] Institute of Medicine. To err is human: building a safer health system. Washington, DC: National Academies Press; 2000.
[21] Nielsen-Bohlman L, Panzer AM, Kindig DA, editors. Health literacy: a prescription to end confusion. Washington, DC: The National Academies Press; 2004.
[22] Institute of Medicine Committee on Quality of Health Care in America. Crossing the quality chasm: a new health system for the 21st Century. Washington, DC: National Academies Press; 2001.
[23] Paasche-Orlow MK, Schillinger D, Greene SM, Wagner EH. How health care systems can begin to address the challenge of limited literacy. J Gen Intern Med. 2006;21(8):884-7. DOI: 10.1111/j.1525-1497.2006.00544.x.
[24] Wagner EH, Bennett SM, Austin BT, Greene SM, Schaefer JK, Vonkorff M. Finding common ground: patient-centeredness and evidence-based chronic illness care. J Altern Complement Med. 2005;11 Suppl 1:S7-15. DOI: 10.1089/acm.2005.11.s-7.
[25] Koh HK, Brach C, Harris LM, Parchman ML. A proposed 'health literate care model' would constitute a systems approach to improving patients' engagement in care. Health Aff. 2013;32(2):357-67. DOI: 10.1377/hlthaff.2012.1205.
[26] Paasche-Orlow MK, Wolf MS. The causal pathways linking health literacy to health outcomes. Am J Health Behav. 2007;31 Suppl 1:S19-26. DOI: 10.5555/ajhb.2007.31.supp.S19.
[27] The Joint Commission. What did the doctor say? Improving health literacy to protect patient safety. Oakbrook Terrace, IL: The Joint Commission, 2007.
[28] U.S. Department of Health and Human Services Office of Disease Prevention and Health Promotion. National action plan to improve health literacy. Washington, DC: U.S. Department of Health and Human Services Office of Disease Prevention and Health Promotion, 2010.
[29] http://nationalacademies.org/hmd/Activities/PublicHealth/HealthLiteracy.aspx. Retrieved: September 29, 2016.
[30] U.S. Department of Health and Human Services Office of the Secretary. National standards on culturally and linguistically appropriate services (CLAS) in health care. Federal Register. 2000;65(247):80865-79.
[31   Schillinger D, Keller D. The other side of the coin: attributes of a health literate healthcare organization. November; Washington, DC; 2011.
[32] Thomacos N, Zazryn T. Enliven organisational health literacy self-assessment audit resource. Melbourne: Enliven & School of Primary Health Care, Monash University, 2013.
[33] Pelikan JM, Dietscher C. [Why should and how can hospitals improve their organizational health literacy?]. Bundesgesundheitsblatt Gesundheitsforschung Gesundheitsschutz. 2015;58(9):989-95. DOI: 10.1007/s00103-015-2206-6.

[34]   https://www.ahrq.gov/policymakers/case-studies/201615.html. Retrieved: November 17, 2016.
[35]   Somers SA, Mahadevan R. Health literacy implications of the Affordable Care Act. Health Literacy and Health Care Reform: A Workshop; Washington, DC; 2011.
[36]   Leebov W. The history of patient experience. Southlake, TX: The Beryl Institute.
[37]   https://www.ahrq.gov/sites/default/files/wysiwyg/professionals/quality-patient-safety/quality-resources/tools/literacy-toolkit/pcmh-crosswalk.pdf. Retrieved: November 22, 2016.
[38]   Centers for Medicare & Medicaid Services. Proposed rule: Medicare Program; Merit-Based Incentive Payment System (MIPS) and Alternative Payment Model (APM) incentive under the physician fee schedule, and criteria for physician-focused payment models. Federal Register. 2016;81 28161-586.
[39]   http://www.ahrq.gov/cahps/about-cahps/index.html. Retrieved: Deember 21, 2016.
[40]   Kripalani S, Wallston K, Cavanaugh KL, Osborn CY, Mulvaney S, Amanda McDougald Scott, et al. Measures to assess a health-literate organization. Washington, DC: National Academies of Medicine, 2014.
[41]   Rudd RE, Anderson JE. The health literacy environment of hospitals and health centers. Partners for action: making your healthcare facility literacy-friendly. Boston: National Center for the Study of Adult Learning and Literacy and Health and Adult Literacy and Learning Initiative, Harvard School of Public Health, 2006.
[42]   Jacobson KL, Gazmarian JA, Kripalani S, McMorris KJ, Blake SC, Brach C. Is our pharmacy meeting patients' needs? A pharmacy health literacy assessment tool. User's guide. Rockville, MD: Agency for Healthcare Research and Quality, 2007.
[43]   DeWalt DA, Callahan LF, Victoria H. Hawk, Broucksou KA, Hink A, Rudd R, et al. Health literacy universal precautions toolkit. Rockville, MD: Agency for Healthcare Research and Quality, 2010.
[44]   Brega A, Barnard J, Mabachi NM, Weiss BD, DeWalt DA, Brach C, et al. AHRQ health literacy universal precautions toolkit, 2nd edition. Rockville, MD: Agency for Healthcare Research and Quality, January, 2015. Report No.: 15-0023-EF.
[45]   Gazmararian JA, Beditz K, Pisano S, Carreon R. The development of a health literacy assessment tool for health plans. J Health Commun. 2010;15 Suppl 2:93-101. DOI: 10.1080/10810730.2010.499986.
[46]   DeWalt DA, Broucksou KA, Hawk V, Brach C, Hink A, Rudd R, et al. Developing and testing the health literacy universal precautions toolkit. Nurs Outlook. 2011;59(2):85-94. DOI: 10.1016/j.outlook.2010.12.002.
[47]   O'Neal KS, Crosby KM, Miller MJ, Murray KA, Condren ME. Assessing health literacy practices in a community pharmacy environment: experiences using the AHRQ Pharmacy Health Literacy Assessment Tool. Res Social Adm Pharm. 2013;9(5):564-96. DOI: 10.1016/j.sapharm.2012.09.005.
[48]   Institute of Medicine. Organizational change to improve health literacy: workshop summary. Washington, DC: The National Academies Press, 2013.
[49]   Wynia MK, Johnson M, McCoy TP, Griffin LP, Osborn CY. Validation of an organizational communication climate assessment toolkit. Am J Med Qual. 2010;25(6):436-43. DOI: 10.1177/1062860610368428.
[50]   Bockrath S. Nebraska's current health department efforts in health literacy. Implications of Health Literacy for Public Health; November 21; Irvine, CA; 2013
[51]   Hadden K, Prince L. Health literacy universal precautions in a primary care network: lessons learned. Health Literacy Annual Research Conference; Bethesda, MD; 2014.
[52]   http://www.plainlanguage.gov/whatisPL/history/locke.cfm. Retrieved: December 19, 2016.
[53]   U.S. Department of Health and Human Services. Healthy people 2010: understanding and improving health. 2nd ed: U.S. Government Printing Office; 2000.
[54]   National Cancer Institute. Clear & simple: developing effective print materials for low-literate readers. Washington, DC: National Cancer Institute, 1995. Report No.: NIH 95-3594.
[55]   Centers for Disease Control and Prevention. Scientific and Technical Information Simply Put. 2nd ed. Atlanta GA: Centers for Disease Control and Prevention, Office of Communication, 1999.
[56]   U.S. Department of Health and Human Services Office of Disease Prevention and Health Promotion. Health literacy online: a guide to writing and designing easy-to-use health Web sites. Washington, DC: U.S. Department of Health and Human Services Office of Disease Prevention and Health Promotion, 2010.
[57]   U.S. Department of Health and Human Services Centers for Medicare and Medicaid. Toolkit for making written material clear and effective. Baltimore: U.S. Department of Health and Human Services Centers for Medicare and Medicaid, 2011.
[58]   Shoemaker SJ, Wolf MS, Brach C. The Patient Education Materials Assessment Tool (PEMAT) and user's guide. Rockville, MD: Agency for Healthcare Research and Quality, November 2013.
[59]   Baur C, Prue C. The CDC Clear Communication Index is a new evidence-based tool to prepare and review health information. Health promotion practice. 2014;15(5):629-37. DOI: 10.1177/1524839914538969.

[60] Kaphingst KA, Kreuter MW, Casey C, Leme L, Thompson T, Cheng MR, et al. Health Literacy INDEX: development, reliability, and validity of a new tool for evaluating the health literacy demands of health information materials. J Health Commun. 2012;17 Suppl 3:203-21. DOI: 10.1080/10810730.2012.712612.

[61] Mad*Pow. A bill you can understand research report. Washington, DC: U.S. Department of Health and Human Services, 2016.

[62] Bickmore TW, Pfeifer LM, Byron D, Forsythe S, Henault LE, Jack BW, et al. Usability of conversational agents by patients with inadequate health literacy: evidence from two clinical trials. J Health Commun. 2010;15 Suppl 2:197-210. DOI: 10.1080/10810730.2010.499991.

[63] Kessels RP. Patients' memory for medical information. Journal of the Royal Society of Medicine. 2003;96(5):219-22. DOI: 10.1258/jrsm.96.5.219.

[64] Back AL, Arnold RM, Baile WF, Fryer-Edwards KA, Alexander SC, Barley GE, et al. Efficacy of communication skills training for giving bad news and discussing transitions to palliative care. Archives of internal medicine. 2007;167(5):453-60. DOI: 10.1001/archinte.167.5.453.

[65] Schillinger D, Piette J, Grumbach K, Wang F, Wilson C, Daher C, et al. Closing the loop: physician communication with diabetic patients who have low health literacy Archives of internal medicine. 2003;163(1):83-90. DOI: 10.1001/archinte.163.1.83.

[66] Dinh TTH, Bonner A, Clark R, Ramsbotham J, Hines S. The effectiveness of the teach-back method on adherence and self-management in health education for people with chronic disease: a systematic review. JBI Database of Systematic Reviews & Implementation Reports. 2016;14(1):210-47. DOI: 10.11124/jbisrir-2016-22.

[67] Peter D, Robinson P, Jordan M, Lawrence S, Casey K, Salas-Lopez D. Reducing readmissions using teach-back: enhancing patient and family education. J Nurs Adm. 2015;45(1):35-42. DOI: 10.1097/NNA.0000000000000155.

[68] Shermont H, Pignataro S, Humphrey K, Bukoye B. Reducing pediatric readmissions: using a discharge bundle combined with teach-back methodology. Journal of nursing care quality. 2016;31(3):224-32. DOI: 10.1097/NCQ.0000000000000176.

[69] http://www.teachbacktraining.org/. Retrieved: November 22, 2016.

[70] Agency for Healthcare Policy and Research. Making health care safer: a critical analysis of patient safety practices. Evidence report/technology assessment, no. 43. Rockville, MD: Agency for Health Care Policy and Research; 2001.

[71] National Quality Forum (NQF). Safe practices for better healthcare–2010 update: a consensus report. Washington, DC: NQF, 2010.

[72] Rudd R. Navigating hospitals: literacy barriers. Literacy Harvest. 2004;Fall:19-24.

[73] Knox L, Brach C. Primary care practice facilitation curriculum (module 20). Rockville, MD: Agency for Healthcare Research and Quality, September 2015. Report No.: 15-0060-EF.

[74] Langley G, Moen R, Nolan K, Nolan T, Norman C, Provost L. The improvement guide: a practical approach to enhancing organizational performance. 2nd edition. San Francisco: Jossey-Bass Publishers; 2009.

[75] U.S. Department of Health and Human Services Health Resources and Services Administration. Effective communication tools for healthcare professionals.

[76] http://cccm.thinkculturalhealth.org/. Retrieved: June 22,, 2005.

[77] Johnson BH. Family-centered care: four decades of progress. Family System and Health. 2000;18:137-56. DOI: apa.org/journals/fsh/18/2/137.pdf.

[78] Lewis B. PFACs: where's the money? The financial impact on hospitals. Southlake, TX: The Beryl Institute, December 30, 2016.

[79] Brach C, Chitavi S, Alrick Edwards, Shradley K, Shoemaker S. Using training modules to move informed consent to informed choice. Health Literacy Annual Research Conference; October 13; Bethesda, MD; 2016.

[80] Brach C, Lenfestey N, Rousel A, Amoozegar J, Sorenson A. Will it work here? A decisionmaker's guide to adopting innovations. Rockville, MD: Agency for Healthcare Research and Quality, 2008.

[81] Diamond LC, Schenker Y, Curry L, Bradley EH, Fernandez A. Getting by: underuse of interpreters by resident physicians. J Gen Intern Med. 2009;24(2):256-62. DOI: 10.1007/s11606-008-0875-7.

[82] North Shore-LIJ Health System. North Shore-LIJ health diversity, inclusion and health literacy inaugural report. Lake Success, NY: North Shore-LIJ Health System Diversity, Inclusion and Health Literacy, 2015.

[83] Intermountain Healthcare. 3-year strategic plan: health literacy. Salt Lake City, UT: Intermountain Healthcare, 2015.

[84] Noonan L. Carolina HealthCare System. Implementation of attributes of health literacy: a workshop; April 11; Washington, DC; 2013.

[85] National Academies of Sciences Engineering and Medicine. Integrating health literacy, cultural competence, and language access services: workshop summary. Washington, DC: The National Academies Press, 2016.

238

Health Literacy
R.A. Logan and E.R. Siegel (Eds.)
IOS Press, 2017
© *2017 The authors and IOS Press. All rights reserved.*
doi:10.3233/978-1-61499-790-0-238

The Role of Health Literacy in Professional Education and Training

Linda ALDOORY[a1]
[a]*Department of Communication, University of Maryland, College Park*

Abstract. This chapter marks the territory and leadership potential found in research, practice and policy related to the role of health literacy in higher education and professional training. There is limited published work that has summarized the role and scope of health literacy in higher education and professional training. This chapter will provide a review of the research in the area, a description of some of the educational practices in health literacy, and a case example of how policy might influence the role of health literacy in professional higher education.

Keywords. Health literacy education, continuing education, health literacy training

1. Introduction

There has been growing national concern toward health literacy and its leadership in policy and healthcare. In 2006, the U.S. Surgeon General devoted a workshop to improving health literacy [1]. In 2010, the U. S. Department of Health and Human Services released its *National Action Plan to Improve Health Literacy*, and concluded that "by focusing on health literacy issues and working together, we can improve the accessibility, quality, and safety of health care; reduce costs; and improve the health and quality of life of millions of people in the United States" [2]. Also, health literacy was explicitly included in the U.S. Patient Protection and Affordable Care Act. The ACA lists health literacy as a "barrier to care in underserved populations" and states that the U.S. health care workforce be trained in "cultural competency and health literacy" [3].

A large component of the current discourse about health literacy in the U.S. is the role and scope of professional education and training. Should there be health literacy curriculum provided to students and professionals in medicine, public health, nursing, dentistry and other allied health professions? The development of an engaged and empowered health consumer population begins with honed training of the practitioners who work with these consumers and improvements in their ability to communicate health information in ways that can be understood by low health literate populations.

However, professional education and training in health literacy varies significantly, ranging from a website listing health literacy resources or a single workshop on health literacy, to formal coursework and continuing experiential education focused on health literacy. Health literacy trainings are conducted by national government agencies, academic institutions and professional associations. There are blogs by individuals and portals of health literacy readings and online

---

[1] Corresponding author: Department of Communication, University of Maryland College Park, MD, 20742, USA; E-mail: laldoory@umd.edu

courses by national and local governments. Some face to face courses can be found at universities with schools of public health and medicine, but also in online formats that are free to the public.

Overall, this chapter could not possibly cover all the training and education for health professionals just in the U.S. Instead, the purpose of this chapter is to mark the boundaries of the educational territory in the U.S. that is described in the literature or reports as well as offer a broad review of the potential effects from health literacy professional education.

This chapter begins with a description of what is health literacy and an explanation for why professional training and education is so important. Then I offer examples of professional education and trainings in the U.S. and summarize the research that has evaluated effects from education and training. Finally, I describe advocacy in one U.S. state as a case example of how policy and practice can influence professional education in health literacy, and then offer recommendations for future work in professional health literacy education and training.

2. Health Literacy and Professional Education

Traditionally, health literacy encompassed reading comprehension and numeracy for understanding health information provided by healthcare entities. Today's health literacy research explores how people listen and communicate information as well as how they make informed decisions. This chapter defines health literacy as the degree to which someone has the capacity to obtain, process, and understand basic health information and services needed to make appropriate healthy decisions [4,5].

Health literacy is not just an individual's "problem" of not understanding health information. Health literacy is embedded in the health care system and affects health organizations, hospitals and health care providers. Health messages stem from health care organizations, media, government and from user-generated sources on social media and the Internet; all of these sources embody individuals who themselves have certain health literacy levels and who are attempting to communicate to certain groups of health consumers Thus, the health communication skills as well as the training of professionals and organizations provide a foundation to address low health literacy and communicate health to consumer populations.

Furthermore, many conceptualizations of health literacy rely on a skills-based perspective, albeit a skills perspective is somewhat limited in its ability to encourage multidisciplinary approaches to learning and understanding health literacy. However, the number and type of skills expected to affect health literacy have broadened over the last few years. Health literacy was traditionally only viewed as including reading and numeracy. However, today, health literacy includes a set of skills needed to navigate the health care system: reading, numeracy, critical thinking, listening, speaking, self-efficacy, and navigational skills needed to find information on the Internet and through other digitized sources [6, 7]. Functional health literacy involves "a complex, multidimensional set of dispositions, knowledge and skills that include reading, writing, numeracy, listening.., oral and visual communication, problem solving and decision making" [8]. A focus on skills that can be learned helps lay the groundwork for professional training and education that would teach the skills. The assumption undergirding most curricula is that skills can be taught and practiced in order for practitioners to become better sensitized to low health literate audiences and better able to communicate health information to these and other audiences.

There are several key players in the health care system that disseminate health messages and that play a role in the health literacy status of a community. These of course include health care providers, hospitals, and public health officials, but also government agencies, health educators, insurance companies, and commercial producers of health and safety products. Other health communicators include non-governmental advocacy organizations and media. Media can be not only national and local broadcast organizations, but also user-generated social media and bloggers.

3. The Practice of Health Literacy Education in the United States

According to the *National Action Plan*, few health care professionals in the U.S. receive formal training in communication or health literacy. Providers must learn a set of communication skills, and these would include how to convey empathy, promote trust, and encourage dialogue, how to elicit patient questions, and how to confirm comprehension and tailor education [9].

3.1 Continuing Education

There is a growing number of continuing education courses and workshops in health literacy, and several are in online formats, allowing for a global reach. Some of the U.S. agencies that have developed online health literacy training are the American Medical Association, the Health Resources and Services Administration, and the Centers for Disease Control and Prevention (CDC).

For example, the CDC created a web-based training program in 2014 for health professionals about "public health literacy" that counts as a maximum of 1.25 AMA PRA Category 1 credits for physicians and 1.0 total Category 1 contact hours for Certified Health Education Specialists; as 1.0 contact hours for nurses; and as .1 contact hours for pharmacy education. This "Health Literacy Public Health Professionals" course includes scenarios to assess, video clips, a resource list, and a self-evaluation. There are seven objectives of the online program: to define and describe public health literacy (PHL); to list the factors that influence PHL; to identify who is affected by PHL; to recognize consequences of limited PHL; to identify stakeholders in PHL; to recognize PHL's role in core public health services; and to apply lessons learned to improving PHL [11].

The American Medical Association developed a Health Literacy Educational Toolkit, and in 2009 released a 2nd edition, which included a manual for clinicians, instructional video, case discussions, and evaluation and post-test. Learning objectives for the toolkit are: to define the scope of the health literacy problem; to recognize health system barriers facing patients; to implement improved communication; and to incorporate practical strategies to create a "shame-free environment" [10]. Physicians may earn a maximum 2.5 AMA PRA Category 1 Credit for completing the health literacy training if they achieve a score of 70% on the post-test. Non-physicians can receive a certificate of participation [12].

3.2 Online Videos

In addition to the health literacy continuing education options, there are numerous training videos that can be found online. National Academies of Sciences' Institute of Medicine (now named Health and Medicine Division) borrowed clips from the

American Medical Association's video to create a video to supplement their report, *Health Literacy: A Prescription to End* Confusion [13]. The American College of Physicians has an older video about health literacy, showing patients with low health literacy attempting to navigate some health care concerns and medication questions [14].

3.3 Coursework

In terms of formal coursework in health literacy, there are limited, required courses devoted solely to health literacy in schools of medicine or public health. While there are guidelines and recommendations for courses, little is known about the extent and content of health literacy teaching within health professions' schools [15]. The more typical scenario is either a recommended course in health literacy or some health literacy curriculum incorporated in courses focused on health communication or cultural competency.

According to Coleman et al., only two published studies have reported the extent or type of health literacy teaching in U.S. training programs for health professionals [16]. Coleman and Appy conducted a survey of directors of U.S. medical schools to gain a perspective on the quantity and characteristics of health literacy teaching at U.S. medical schools [17]. Survey findings showed that 44% of respondents reported teaching about health literacy in their required curriculum, but that the median time spent teaching health literacy was only three hours. Most respondents said that health literacy teaching occurred in the first two years of school. Findings indicated that the most common health literacy teaching format was through patient role play and workshop settings. In another study, Ali conducted a survey with a convenience sample of 30 U.S. internal medicine resident programs, and found that 43% of respondents included a required health literacy curricular component [18]. A recent, updated survey was completed by Coleman and colleagues to assess the status of health literacy training for physicians in U.S. family medicine residency programs [19]. Data showed little change since the original survey. Only 42% of the directors of the schools sampled reported teaching about health literacy as part of the required curriculum, and most teaching occurred during the first year. Hours of instruction ranged from just two to five, and plain language was the predominant skill taught.

3.4 Alternative Education

One particularly interesting case example of experiential learning was found in the *National Action Plan*, where Project SHINE was described as "using college students as agents of change and as educators" [20]. The Health Literacy Initiative of Project SHINE (Students Helping in Naturalization of Elders) engaged health profession students in health literacy services for older immigrants and refugees. To address challenges with this population, Project Shine's students participated in health fairs, health education workshops, health screenings, and community needs assessments. The program also engaged adult learners and teachers of English for speakers of other languages (ESOL) to develop a health literacy curriculum designed for older immigrant adults to use in ESOL classes, tutoring sessions, and workshops. The curriculum included five topics: the doctor's office, the hospital, illness management, healthy aging, and medications.

3.5 Journalism Education

An area of health literacy training not frequently publicized is any work in journalism to educate reporters on health literacy and its role in audience understanding of news about health. One U.S. survey found that only 18 percent of journalists had any specialized training in health reporting, and 50 percent were not familiar with the term or concept of health literacy. Hinnant and Len-Rios conducted a survey of 396 newspaper and magazine journalists and completed 35 in depth interviews, to explore the role of journalists in reducing the negative effects of limited health literacy. However, journalists did respond that increasing knowledge of health literacy could help them with their reporting of medical and health news [21].

As stated in the *National Action Plan*, "The ways in which health and safety information are communicated to the public have a significant impact on health literacy." The *National Action Plan* included recommendations to engage journalists' professional associations, such as The Association of Healthcare Journalists, to raise awareness and conduct trainings on health literacy [22]. The Association of Health Care Journalists has had presentations on health literacy at its annual conferences, and it has posted summaries of research on health literacy and journalism for its members. In April, 2016, it hosted a webcast presentation of "Health Literacy: How Language, Context Affects Disparities," for its members. The Center for Health Journalism posted in 2010 a list of resources to learn more about health literacy, and the list included such sites as the Centers for Disease Control and Health Literacy Out Loud, but no journalist-specific resource was listed [23].

4. Research on U.S. Professional Education and Training

There are several studies describing pilot health literacy workshops and recommended curricula, and a few of these cite short term benefits, such as improving confidence in communicating with patients. However, there is a dearth of research on the impact of health literacy education on clinical behaviors or on patient health outcomes [24]. Coleman found in his meta-analysis that teaching techniques and tools for health literacy have not been evaluated adequately through controlled trials, and that no comparative studies were found to help recommend one teaching approach over another [25]. Toronto and Weatherford found nine research articles that met their inclusion criteria for reviewing studies of health literacy education in schools for nursing and other health professions. Their findings showed that evaluation of content was performed, but only one study measured health literacy skills in the students [26]. No published research was found on journalists' training in health literacy.

4.1 Short-term Effects

Research on one-time health literacy workshops for medical students reveal some short-term effects on knowledge of health literacy and perceived efficacy to communicate to low health literate patients [27, 28]. For example, in one pilot intervention medicine residents participated in a small group workshop that involved lecture, role play with a standardized patient and individualized feedback from video recorded encounters with real patients. Findings from pre and post test showed that knowledge of health literacy increased and familiarity with the concept of health literacy increased, and confidence in communicating with patients increased [29].

In a similar pilot study, family medicine residents participated in a one-time training that involved lecture, video and patient role play. The curriculum covered clear language, how to confirm patient understanding and how to provide reinforcement for communication. Findings from pre and post tests showed an increase in health literacy knowledge, but no increase in using the teach-back method appropriately with patients [30].

Another pilot evaluation was conducted by researchers who developed a skills-based health literacy workshop as part of an internship preparatory clerkship during the fourth year of medical school. They found that students felt more confident with patients of low health literacy than their counterparts who did not complete the workshop [31]. Hadden reported on a different type of training, one that was a semester long course and for public health students. The course trained students in plain language and how to assess written health materials for patients. Five students were in the pilot course, and results showed that students were able to reduce reading level of test documents from 10th grade to 6th grade level after editing. In post-tests, students reported high levels of confidence in assessing written materials and intention to use the new skills after graduation [32].

In a different study, Coleman and Fromer compared physicians to non-physician health professionals for short term effects from a health literacy training. For both groups, post-test results indicated a significant increase in self-perceived health literacy knowledge. Physicians with more experience (more than 3.5 years) reported higher levels of knowledge about health literacy. Physicians in this study did not show improvement on likelihood of speaking slowly or using plain non-medical language with patients, as non-physician participants did. One finding in particular was interesting in that it showed that almost half the participants from both groups overestimated their pre-training understanding of health literacy. This could be interpreted to mean that health professionals do not perceive a need to participate in trainings, if they believe that they already have the knowledge and skills to address low health literacy in patients. Coleman and Fromer concluded, "Making health literacy trainings mandatory may be an important strategy for educators and administrators to consider" (p. 389) [33].

4.2 Long-term Effects

Most recently, Coleman, Peterson-Perry and Bumsted examined whether there would be long-term effects of a health literacy lesson plan on medical students after one year and two years. They conducted pre- and post-training assessments of health literacy knowledge and planned behavior. One year after training, knowledge and expected behavior were not significantly different than pre-test levels. Authors argued that teaching health literacy should be integrated into other courses and be ongoing in order to maintain any effect on practice [34].

5. Advocacy for Health Literacy Education: One State Example

The *National Action Plan* suggests that licensing and accreditation organizations can play a critical role in creating training standards for health care professionals. "They can lead the way in changing the skills and competencies of professionals and the organizations in which they practice and provide services" (p. 26). Suggested strategies for licensing and credentialing organizations are the following: Include coursework on health literacy in curricula for health professionals; support health literacy training opportunities for students and residents; incorporate diverse patients, including new readers, in course presentations and trainings; include assessment of health literacy skills in licensure requirements; and establish minimum continuing education requirements in health literacy (p. 28). The organizations may also play a role through advocacy for requirements in continuing education [35].

Here I offer one U.S. response to the call for professional education, as I was involved in the Maryland action toward mandating health literacy education for the state's health professions' schools. The Maryland Office of Minority Health and Health Disparities, of the Maryland Department of Health and Mental Hygiene, developed a Cultural Competency and Health Literacy Initiative in 2014, to help increase cultural and linguistic competency of the State's healthcare workforce and improve their health communication with low health literacy patient audiences. In collaboration with the University of Maryland and the Herschel S. Horowitz Center for Health Literacy, the Office promoted the need for required health literacy courses in all health professions' schools in the state. To assist its efforts, it created a Primer, a document to guide development of curriculum in cultural competency and health literacy for professional schools. First year was to advocate for a bill that would recommend health literacy and cultural competency as units in medical, dental, social work and public health schools in the State. The bill passed with the help of testimony and resources provided by health literacy advocates across the state. The following year a proposed bill that would require health literacy education in professional schools did not reach enough votes to pass the State House.

6. Conclusion

Three main recommendations emerge from the review of literature and practice in health literacy professional education. One pertains to the need for additional research, a second addresses questions of standards and certification, and a third seeks to expand practice.

6.1 Areas for Research

The lack of empirical evidence on effects of health literacy education makes it challenging to argue for standards or credentials in health professions. Any moves toward mandating health literacy curriculum in professional schools would require evidence to show that effects are worth it. It also limits the ability to gain funding for trainings and for "train the trainer" initiatives, which are critical to the success of trainings. Thus, two of the most pressing needs for research are 1) evaluation of training effects, and 2) feedback from trainers and assessment of trainers.

First, studies are needed to support effects from health literacy education. The limited research that has already been done does show short term effects on knowledge and perceived communication confidence, but findings are mixed. Randomized controlled trials on curriculum interventions would offer valid data that support use of certain training modules and content. Outcomes measured can include communication confidence, cultural competency, clear language use, and behavioral outcomes, such as when to call for a medical interpreter, when to write down something versus saying something to a patient, and how to use teach-back method for measuring understanding

partner with university
to conduct research
RCT &
reports

in a patient. The health literacy levels of the students could also be measure pre and post curriculum.

Second, apart from the curriculum content, the greatest influence on learning outcomes is the trainer and his/her experience, presentation skills and knowledge. Coleman argued, "Specifically, there is urgent need for more rigorous educational outcomes studies, including studies designed to compare different teaching strategies, and to determine the optimal timing for teaching various health professionals about key health literacy principles" (p. 76) [36]. Teaching strategies may include optimum speed at which curriculum is taught, best visuals to include in lessons, and level of interactivity and student participation during classes. Other factors to examine include how to measure student pace of learning understanding of different student learning capacities, and how to best develop rubrics for measuring learning outcomes. Initial studies may include focus groups with trainers to provide feedback on feasibility, usability and preference of curriculum and modules for teaching it. Control trials could then be used that would provide trainings to the trainers and then observations during class time of performance.

Given the paucity of research in the area, there are several other topics that could be addressed through research:

- Comparison studies that look at differences between health professions. For example, studies could examine how health literacy trainings in nursing schools should be different from trainings in dental schools, social work schools or medical schools.
- Comparisons between students are also needed. Health literacy training might have different impact depending on students' race, gender, country of origin, and prior experience in the health field. All of these are factors that can be studied via cross sectional survey post curriculum, or through a controlled trial design.
- Differences in teaching modality should be studied as well. Today there are several opportunities to do online trainings, and research should be done to compare online format from in-person format.
- Continuing education training effects have to be measured. The impact of short-term, one time trainings while working as a professional are likely to be limited yet perhaps more potent in the immediate time post training. Research can detect differences over time and compare in school trainings with continuing education interventions.

6.2 Standards and Credentialing

A second recommendation is to establish some standards or principles to be used in developing health literacy education and continuing education. In order to do so, the field of health literacy education needs to foster leadership that can coordinate professional education and training efforts, support organizations that participate in education efforts, and motivate institutions to incorporate standards and principles that can be evaluated. Leadership might come in the form of a professional association that provides credentialing and accreditation to advance health literacy education and training's standing.

One case example for developing standards can be found in the forum co-hosted by the Canadian Centre for Literacy in 2008. The purpose of the forum was to develop core principles that should underpin new and adapt existing health literacy curricula. The group of health literacy scholars and practitioners used previous research as well as their own expertise to discuss certain criteria and content for health literacy trainings. The document that emerged, *Calgary Charter on Health Literacy: Rationale and Core Principles for the Development of Health Literacy Curricula,* has been signed by dozens of health literacy allies and shares seven curriculum principles, which are listed here.

First, health literacy curricula should be based on the current evidence base for health literacy interventions. Second, the use and applications of health literacy curricula should actively participate in furthering the development of the evidence base for health literacy interventions by using sound methodological approaches to evaluation. Also, development and use of health literacy curricula and evaluation/measurement tools should: use a participatory approach by involving the intended audience at all stages; be based on, and designed to advance theory about health literacy; and be based on the same underlying understanding of health literacy, regardless of health issue addressed. Sixth, a health literacy curriculum should take an integrated approach to the social, cultural, political, economic, and environmental determinants of health in order to most effectively help people and health systems address the complex paths to better health. Finally, the curriculum should attempt to take account of the skills and abilities associated with individual health literacy [37].

6.3 Innovation in Practice

The third recommendation is to offer additional opportunities for practitioners in professional education and training of health literacy. Few programs have been conducted and less has been evaluated, leaving the area wide open for innovation in practice. In particular, advocacy can be a critical component to encouraging and funding professional training. Continuing education credits provide an arena for more pilot training because it reaches the workforce outside of health professions' schools, who often have the least health literacy training. Within health professional schools, health literacy training should be mandated in order to ensure future provider exposure. It may be that this is the process to consider, given the paucity of opportunities to engage in health literacy training and study the effects of it on the student, the practitioner, and ultimately, the consumer and patient.

References

[1]   Office of the Surgeon General. Proceedings of the Surgeon General's workshop on improving health literacy. Office of Disease Prevention and Health Promotion. Bethesda, MD: National Institutes of Health; September 7, 2006.
[2]   USDHHS. National action plan to improve health literacy. Office of Disease Prevention and Health Promotion. Washington, DC: U.S. Government Printing Office; 2010. p. 2.
[3]   ACA. U.S. Patient Protection and Affordable Care Act. Washington, DC: U.S. Government Printing Office; 2010; subtitle D, sec. 5301, 3I.
[4]   Nielsen-Bohlman L, Panzer AM, Kindig DA, editors. Health literacy: a prescription to end confusion. Washington, DC: National Academies Press; 2004.
[5]   Ratzan SC, Parker RM. Introduction. In CR Selden, M Zorn, SC Ratzan, RM Parker, editors. National Library of Medicine Current Bibliographies in Medicine: health Literacy, NLM Pub. No. CBM 2000-1. Bethesda, MD: National Institutes of Health, U.S. Department of Health and Human Services; 2000.

[6]   Paasche-Orlow MK, Wolf MS. The causal pathways linking health literacy to health outcomes. Am J Health Behav. 2007;31:S19-S26. DOI: 10.5555/ajhb.2007.31.supp.S19.

[7]   Osborn CY, Paasche-Orlow MK, Bailey SC, Wolf MS. The mechanisms linking health literacy to behavior and health status. Am J Health Behav. 2011; 35:118-128. DOI: 10.5993/AJHB.35.1.11.

[8]   Helitzer D, Hollis C, Sanders, M, Roybal S. Addressing the "other" health literacy competencies-- Knowledge, dispositions, and oral/aural communication: development of TALKDOC, an intervention assessment tool. J Health Commun. 2012; 17(Supp. 3):160-175. p. 161. DOI: 10.1080/10810730.2012.712613.

[9]   Paasche-Orlow MK, Schillinger D, Greene SM, Wagner EH. How health care systems can begin to address the challenge of limited literacy. J Gen Intern Med. 2006;21:884-887. DOI: 10.1111/j.1525-1497.2006.00544.x.

[10] Weiss BD. Health literacy and patient safety: help patients understand, manual for clinicians. 2nd ed. Chicago: American Medical Association Foundation; 2009. p. 2.

[11] http://www.cdc.gov/healthliteracy/gettrainingce.html Retrieved December 1, 2016.

[12] http://med.fsu.edu/userFiles/file/ahec_health_clinicians_manual.pdf for manual, and https://www.youtube.com/watch?v=cGtTZ_vxjyA for video. Retrieved December 1, 2016.

[13] https://www.youtube.com/watch?v=iBy3I7YKCQQ. Retrieved December 1, 2016.

[14] https://www.youtube.com/watch?v=ImnlptxIMXs. Retrieved December 1, 2016.

[15] Coleman CA, Peterson-Perry S, Bumsted T. Long-term effects of a health literacy curriculum for medical students. Fam Med. 2016;48: 49-53.

[16] Coleman CA, Peterson-Perry S, Bumsted T. Long-term effects of a health literacy curriculum for medical students. Fam Med. 2016;48: 49-53.

[17] Coleman CA, Appy S. Health literacy teaching in U.S. medical schools, 2010. Fam Med. 2012;44:504-507.

[18] Ali N. Are we training residents to communicate with low health literacy patients? J Community Hosp Intern Med Perspect. 2012;2:1-6. DOI: 10.3402/jchimp.v2i4.19238.

[19] Coleman CA, Nguyen NT, Garvin R, Sou, C, Carney PA. Health literacy teaching in U.S. family medicine residency: A national survey. J Health Commun. 2016;21(sup. 1):51-57. DOI: 10.1080/10810730.2015.1131774.

[20] USDHHS. National action plan to improve health literacy. Office of Disease Prevention and Health Promotion. Washington, DC: U.S. Government Printing Office; 2010. p. 34.

[21] Hinnant A, Len-Rios ME. Tacit understandings of health literacy: Interview and survey research with health journalists. Sci Commun. 2009;31:84-115. DOI: 10.1177/1075547009335345.

[22] USDHHS. National action plan to improve health literacy. Office of Disease Prevention and Health Promotion. Washington, DC: U.S. Government Printing Office; 2010. p. 18.

[23] http://www.centerforhealthjournalism.org/blogs/health-literacy-online-resources-journalists. Retrieved December 1, 2016.

[24] Coleman CA, Nguyen NT, Garvin R, Sou, C, Carney PA. Health literacy teaching in U.S. family medicine residency: a national survey. J Health Commun. 2016;21(sup. 1):51-57. DOI: 10.1080/10810730.2015.1131774.

[25] Coleman CA. Teaching health care professionals about health literacy: a review of the literature. Nurs Outlook. 2011, April;59(2):70-78. DOI:10.1016/j.outlook.2010.12.004.

[26] Toronto CE, Weatherford B. Health literacy education in health professions schools: an integrative review. The J Nurs Educ. 2015;54:669-676. DOI: 10.3928/01484834-20151110-02.

[27] Farrell TW. Review of a geriatric health literacy workshop for medical students and residents. J Am Geriatr Soc. 2011;59:2347-2349. DOI: 10.1111/j.1532-5415.2011.03720.x.

[28] Mackert M, Ball J, Lopez N. Health literacy awareness training for healthcare workers: improving knowledge and intentions to use clear communication techniques. Patient Educ Couns. 2011;85:e225-e228. DOI: 10.1016/j.pec.2011.02.022.

[29] Green JA, Gonzaga AM, Cohen ED, Spagnoletti CL. Addressing health literacy through clear health communication: a training program for internal medicine residents. Patient Educ Couns. 2014;95:76-82. DOI: 10.1016/j.pec.2014.01.004.

[30] Pagels P, Kindratt T, Arnold D, Brandt J, Woodfin G, Gimpel N. Training family medicine residents in effective communication skills while utilizing Promotoras as standardized patients in OSCEs: a health literacy curriculum. Int J Family Med. 2015;2015:1-9. DOI: 10.1155/2015/129187.

[31] Bloom-Feshbach K, Casey D, Schulson L, Gliatto P, Giftos J, Karan, R. Health literacy in transitions of care: an innovative objective structured clinical examination for fourth-year medical students in an internship preparation course. J Gen Intern Med. 2106;31:242-6. DOI: 10.1007/s11606-015-3513-1.

[32] Hadden KB. Health literacy training for health professions students. Patient Educ Couns. 2015;98:918-920. DOI: 10.1016/j.pec.2015.03.016.

[33] Coleman CA, Fromer A. A health literacy training intervention for physicians and other health professionals. Fam Med. 2015;47:388-392.

[34] Coleman CA, Peterson-Perry S, Bumsted T. Long-term effects of a health literacy curriculum for medical students. Fam Med. 2016;48:49-53.

[35] USDHHS. National action plan to improve health literacy. Office of Disease Prevention and Health Promotion. Washington, DC: U.S. Government Printing Office; 2010. p. 2.

[36] Coleman CA. Teaching health care professionals about health literacy: a review of the literature. Nurs Outlook. 2011, April;59(2):70-78. DOI:10.1016/j.outlook.2010.12.004.

[37] http://www.centreforliteracy.qc.ca/health_literacy/calgary_charter). Retrieved December 1, 2016,

Developments and New Directions in Disciplines Similar to Health Literacy

Health Literacy
R.A. Logan and E.R. Siegel (Eds.)
IOS Press, 2017
doi:10.3233/978-1-61499-790-0-251

251

Patient Activation and Health Literacy: What's the Difference? How Do Each Contribute to Health Outcomes

Judith HIBBARD[i]
Health Policy Research Group
University of Oregon

Abstract. In this paper we define health literacy and patient activation, discuss how each construct is measured, and review the evidence linking each construct to outcomes.

Studies indicate that health literacy and patient activation are separate concepts that are only moderately correlated with each other. The studies indicate that patient activation and health literacy can each make independent contributions to outcomes. This is important, as it indicates the need to attend to both health literacy and patient activation in the design of interventions. This means that interventions that are successful in increasing health literacy will not necessarily also influence patient activation, and interventions that are successful in increasing patient activation will not necessarily also influence health literacy. Both are likely necessary.

The studies show that patient activation is often a stronger predictor of behaviors and health outcomes than is health literacy, however, health literacy is sometimes a stronger predictor of understanding and using information for choice. Some of the differences observed in these studies reflect the fact that health literacy is primarily a skills based concept, and patient activation includes skills, but also includes confidence, beliefs, and role expectations. These differences suggest different pathways for effectively intervening to improve outcomes. The implications for interventions and research directions are discussed.

Key Words. Patient activation, patient engagement, health literacy, health behaviors

1. Introduction

As delivery systems and providers bear more financial risk and accountability for health outcomes, there is growing interest in understanding and influencing patient choices and patient behaviors. Patient engagement or activation, has been identified as critical to reaching the triple aim, of improved experiences, improved health, and restrained costs [1]. Similarly, improvements in health literacy have also been identified as central to achieving gains in the quality of care [2]. With so much attention on the patient role in determining health care costs and health outcomes, the

---

[i] Corresponding author: Health Policy Research Group, University of Oregon- 1209, 119 Hendricks Hall, Eugene, Oregon, 97403-1209; E-mail: jhibbard@uoregon.edu.

question arises about how much patient activation and health literacy are the same or different, and how do each contribute to determining health outcomes.

In this paper we define health literacy and patient activation, discuss how each construct is measured, and review the evidence linking each construct to outcomes. Finally, we discuss the implications for interventions and for future research.

1.1. Definitions

Health literacy refers to an individual's ability to derive meaning from health related texts and tables. While there is no one gold standard for the definition, The Institute of Medicine Report, "Health Literacy: A Prescription to end Confusion," defines health literacy as, 'the degree to which individuals have the capacity to obtain, process, and understand basic health information and services needed to make appropriate health decisions.' This definition indicates that health literacy is a set of individual capacities that allow the person to acquire and use new information. Thus, health literacy is a skills-based concept.

Patient activation refers to an individual's knowledge, skill, motivation, and confidence for managing their health and health care [3]. Being an *activated* patient implies more than simply complying with medical regimens or seeking out health information; it means taking a proactive role in our own health. Being activated refers to the degree to which an individual understands his own role in maintaining and promoting personal health and the extent to which he possesses a sense of self-efficacy for taking on this role. It is a global construct reflecting an individual's overall knowledge, skill, and confidence for self-management. The concept of activation puts the focus on fundamental factors supporting behavior change: whether the individual possesses the necessary knowledge, skill, and confidence to manage her own health. This focus is new and suggests innovative and different ways to intervene and ultimately to improve health behaviors and health outcomes.

Patient engagement, a related concept, is also a term that is widely used. The concept of engagement has been defined in different ways, and there is considerable conceptual confusion about what patient/ consumer engagement entails [4]. Because the same term is used to denote different ideas, communication can be impeded, and efforts to develop programs in this area and to research it can become muddled [5-6]. The term patient engagement is used to denote a wide range of activities and states: patient interest or attention, a synonym for patient activation; taking actions in managing one's own health; or it is used to describe interventions intended to activate patients [7-9]. Most definitions place the emphasis on consumer involvement or taking action related to health and health care [8,9]. Other definitions broaden the scope of actions to include involvement in decisions for personal health as well as decisions that affect the health of the larger collective [8]. [ii]

[ii] Community engagement should not be confused with consumer engagement or consumer activation. Community engagement refers to the process by which community organizations and individuals build ongoing, permanent relationships for the purpose of applying a collective vision for the benefit of a community.

1.2. Measurement

There are multiple measurement tools assessing health literacy, McCormick and colleagues identify 35 different measures of health literacy [10]. Two of the most commonly used instruments include the Rapid Estimate of Adult Literacy in Medicine (REALM) [11] and the Test of Functional Health Literacy in Adults (TOFHLA) [12]. Most of the measures take a skills based approach, assessing an individual's ability to understand information, or navigate a document.

At this point there is only one validated measure assessing patient activation: The Patient Activation Measure (PAM) is a 13 or 10-item survey. The PAM was created using Rasch analysis, it is an interval level, uni-dimensional, Guttman-like scale that measures people on a 0-100 scale. The PAM measures a latent construct.

Because latent constructs are theoretical in nature and not directly observable, we use indicators that represent the underlying construct. The latent construct measured in the PAM likely reflects an individual's self-concept as a self-manager of their own health. The respondent may not be consciously aware of this "self-concept," but it is revealed in the sum of their responses.

2. How Are Two Constructs Related?

There are important conceptual as well as measurement differences between patient activation and health literacy. Several studies report a statistically significant but weak relationship between the two constructs [13-16]. One key difference is how the two constructs are related to measures of social advantage or disadvantage. It appears that health literacy is more closely linked with socio-demographic characteristics, than is patient activation. In an analysis that assessed how much age, education, income, and gender accounted for variation in health literacy, the findings showed that 25% of the variation was accounted for. The same analysis assessing how much those same socio-demographic factors account for variation in patient activation scores, showed that only 5-6% of the variation in patient activation scores was accounted for [13]. These findings indicate that health literacy deficits are more strongly related to lower education and income than are low PAM scores, where there is a significant but weak association.

2.1. Health Behaviors and Health Outcomes

There is research that shows that both health literacy and patient activation scores are predictive of health behaviors, health outcomes, clinical markers and utilization. For example, a longitudinal study following older adults, found that those with limited health literacy were more likely to experience meaningful declines in functioning over time than those with adequate health literacy [17]. At the same time, a systematic review found a statistically significant, although weak relationship between health literacy and medication adherence [18]. Another systematic review examined how low health literacy is related to many health behaviors and health outcomes. The review found that low health literacy was consistently associated with more hospitalizations; greater use of emergency care; lower receipt of mammography screening and influenza vaccine; poorer ability to interpret labels and health messages; and, among elderly persons, poorer overall health status and higher mortality rates [19]. Thus, it appears that limited health literacy impacts outcome and utilization, through individual behaviors and the choices.

The same mechanism appears to be operating with patient activation, activation seems to impact health outcomes and utilization by influencing choices and behaviors. Multiple studies from a variety of settings and different populations indicate that patient activation is correlated with a full range of health behaviors and many health outcomes. For example, the PAM score is significantly correlated with most preventive behaviors (screenings, immunizations, etc.), healthful behaviors such as diet and exercise, health-information-seeking behaviors, and disease-specific self-management behaviors, such as medication adherence and monitoring one's condition [20-25] . Higher activation is also linked with having less unmet medical need, having a regular source of care, and higher participation in physical therapy after spine surgery [26-27]. These findings remain statistically significant even after controlling for socio-demographic factors and insurance status. Further, activation scores are predictive of outcomes within condition-specific populations, such as those with a serious mental health diagnosis, heart disease, multiple sclerosis, COPD, cancer, hypertension, asthma, HIV/AIDS, and diabetes [28-32]. Finally, lower PAM scores are also predictive of the use of costly health care services, such as emergency department use, hospitalizations, and being re-hospitalized within 30 days of discharge [33-37].

2.2. Examining the Relative Contribution of Patient Activation and Health Literacy.

There are several published empirical studies that examine the relative importance of patient activation and health literacy to health behaviors and outcomes. All the studies use the Patient Activation Measure (PAM), however, four different measures of health literacy are used in these studies.

Some of the studies examine the relative contribution of health literacy and patient activation to decision-making and some examine behaviors and health outcomes. For example, one study examined how much health literacy versus patient activation contributes to making an active informed choice of a provider. Specifically, they asked if their primary care doctor referred them to specialist, would they just take that referral, or would they look for other information and make an "active" choice? They report, in a multivariate analysis, that health literacy did not contribute to 'active choices', only, gender, education level, and patient activation scores were significant predictors [14]. Another study found that patient activation was a stronger predictor of seeking out and using health information for choice than was level of health literacy [15]. Greene and Hibbard found that both health literacy and patient activation were significantly correlated with behavioral, comprehension, and decision-making outcomes. For some outcomes one factors was the stronger predictor, and for other outcomes the other factor was the stronger predictor. Health literacy was a stronger predictor among Medicare beneficiaries of understanding information about their Medicare choices than was patient activation. However, they also found that patient activation was a better predictor of healthcare related behaviors, healthy behaviors, and self-management behaviors than was health literacy. An important finding was that both patient activation and health literacy contributed independently to most of the outcomes examined, with one factor contributing more than the other, depending on the outcome.

Similarly, Sheikh and colleagues examined both patient activation and health literacy as predictors of hospital admissions though the emergency department (ED), among ED users. They found in multivariate analyses that both patient activation and health literacy were significant predictors of hospital admissions [38].

Serper and colleagues studied how much health literacy and patient activation contributed to adequate preparation for a colonoscopy. The preparation for the procedure requires patients to follow detailed instructions for bowel preparation. Their findings show that in multivariate analysis, patient activation was an independent significant predictor of the adequacy of their bowel preparation, but that health literacy was not a significant predictors [39].

A final study provides a more in-depth look at the question. This study assesses health literacy and patient activation, to determine the relative contribution of each to being able to understand and use information to make informed choices [40]. The findings showed that people with lower health literacy, not surprisingly, have lower comprehension of information. However, people who were higher activated and had lower health literacy skills compensated for their lower skills with extra effort and were able to make up any comprehension deficits. That is, higher activated/ lower health literacy participants, demonstrated the same level of comprehension as those with higher health literacy skills. Likely, this is because higher activated individuals are more motivated, they see the importance of the information, and put more effort into trying to understand. The findings also showed that, making good choices, when tradeoffs are necessary, is related to activation, separate from comprehension and health literacy. This is important as many real-life choices involve trade-offs, and making trade-offs is one of the more difficult cognitive tasks involved in making good choices [41].

The findings indicate that health literacy and patient activation are separate concepts, each potentially independently contributing to outcomes. The studies show that patient activation is often a stronger predictor of behaviors and health outcomes than is health literacy, however, health literacy is sometimes a stronger predictor of understanding and using information for choice. Some of the differences observed in these studies reflect the fact that health literacy is primarily a skills based concept, and patient activation includes skills, but also includes confidence, beliefs, and role expectations. These differences suggest different pathways for effectively intervening to improve outcomes.

The studies indicate that patient activation and health literacy can each make independent contributions to outcomes. This is important, as it indicates the need to attend to both health literacy and patient activation in the design of interventions. This means that interventions that are successful in increasing health literacy will not necessarily also influence patient activation, and interventions that are successful in increasing patient activation will not necessarily also influence health literacy. Both are likely necessary.

3. Implications for Interventions

Both heath literacy and patient activation appear to underlie health behaviors and health outcomes, however, the mechanisms though which they operate on behaviors and choices appears to be different. Health literacy appears to impact outcomes because individuals lack the skills to understand information important to informing their choices. Patient activation appears to influence behaviors because of individual beliefs about their role, or their level of motivation, or perceived efficacy in taking actions related to their health. They may also lack knowledge. The foci of the interventions are necessarily on these presumed mechanisms that result in sub-optimal outcomes. For example interventions to increase health literacy usually focus on improving patient knowledge and skill or they focus on improving communications and written materials. While interventions to increase patient activation tend to focus on increasing self-efficacy, skill, and role delineation.

There is some evidence that interventions to improve health literacy does increase health-related knowledge and comprehension [42]. A systematic review of health literacy interventions found that improving written materials can increase patient health knowledge. Further studies show that it is possible to improve behaviors including adherence when combining good written materials with brief counseling sessions [43].

As interventions to increase patient activation are relatively new, and since there is considerable research on improving health literacy, we focus most the rest of this section on interventions and strategies to increase patient activation in the clinical setting.

The most effective interventions to increase activation are tailored to the patient's level of activation. The approach is to meet patients where they are and help them more forward. PAM scores indicate where an individual falls on a continuum of activation. The PAM score can give the clinician insight into a range of behaviors and behavioral tendencies. With appropriate support, patients can gain in activation, and a number of studies have documented that these tailored interventions can increase activation and improve outcomes [44-46]. Research also shows that when PAM scores increase, multiple behaviors improve [47,48]. When patients begin to feel more "in charge" of their health, they apparently do many things different. This is important, in that it indicates why increasing activation is considered an important intermediate outcome.

Empirical evidence also suggests that there are 4 activation levels (based on PAM scores) which people go through in the process of becoming fully competent managers of their own health. At level 1, patients may not yet grasp that they must play an active role in their own health, they may believe that being a passive recipient of care is appropriate. Patients at level 1, may not have good problem-solving skills, they are more likely to believe they cannot positively influence their own health, they are often over-whelmed with the task of managing their health, and they have very little confidence in their own ability to self-manage. At level 2, patients may lack confidence or a basic understanding about their health or recommended health regimens. At level 2, patients also have difficulty handling stress and are less optimistic that they can positively influence their own health. At level 3, patients typically have the basic information and are beginning to take action but may still lack some skills and confidence for making and sustaining changes. At level 4, patients have adopted many necessary behaviors but may not be able to maintain them over time or in the face of life stressors [49]. The key value of identifying activation level is to gain insight into possible strategies for supporting self-management among patients at different points along the activation continuum. The score is important in that a change of only a few points is linked with behavioral changes [22]. That is, the level (1-4) is useful for designing effective interventions and communications that will meet patients' needs, while the score (0-100) is most useful for tracking progress.

Measuring patients' activation levels gives clinicians three key advantages in supporting patients. First, it provides an assessment to help clinicians tailor the type and amount of support that is necessary for an individual patient. It lets clinicians know where a patient is on this continuum, and allows them to meet the patient there. Second, the score provides guidance on the kind and amount of support that is likely to be helpful to the patient. Third, it provides a metric to know if progress is being made with an individual patient or a whole population of patients.

Assessing a patient's activation level can provide information on the patient's ability to take on the self-management role, but it can also give the clinician information on how best to support the patient so that they gain knowledge, skill and confidence for doing so. Clinician's currently using the PAM to assess patients, use it as an additional *vital sign*, providing them with vital information that they need to effectively work with the patient.

Four levels of Patient Activation

- Level 1 - patients tend to be passive and feel overwhelmed with managing their own health.
- Level 2 - patients may lack knowledge and confidence for managing their health.
- Level 3 - patients appear to be beginning to take action but may still lack confidence and skill to support their behaviors.
- Level 4 - people have adopted many of the behaviors to support their health but may not be able to maintain them in the face of life stressors

Tailoring Support to Activation Levels:

- At **level 1**, focus on building self-awareness and understanding behavior patterns, and begin to build confidence through small steps.
- At **level 2**, work with patients continue small steps that are "pre-behaviors," such as adding a new fruit or vegetable each week to their diet; reducing portion sizes at two meals daily; and begin to build basic knowledge. At **level 3** work with patients to adopt new behaviors and to ensure some level of condition-specific knowledge and skills. Supporting the initiation of new "full" behaviors (e.g. 30 minutes of exercise 3 times a week) and working on the development problem solving skills.
- At **level 4** the focus is on relapse prevention and handling new or challenging situations as they arise. Problem solving and planning for difficult situations help patients maintain their behaviors.

Tailoring support to a patient's activation level, means focusing on the challenges typically faced by people at their level of activation.

Acquiring the basic knowledge, beliefs, and skills to progress through the early levels of activation are likely necessary for building a sense of efficacy for the self-management tasks involved in the later levels. Focusing on a behavioral change that the patient chooses helps the individual begin to take ownership of their health, it is also the behavior they are more likely to succeed at, as they are more motivated to make the change. By experiencing a series of successes, the individual begins to feel competent to take on the next challenge. Experiencing success actually builds motivation to keep moving forward. Thus, starting with behaviors the individual chooses (and not necessarily the behaviors that the clinician views as the most important clinically), will start the process of taking ownership and building a sense of competence.

Team-based care can be ideal for supporting patient activation. For example, when a team-based approach is employed, all members of the health care team can use a patient's PAM score to be consistent and coordinated in the way they interact with and support patients. Team members would all know that a patient at level 2 should not be given reams of paper to read or a long list of behavior changes to make. By understanding the challenges faced by patients at different levels of activation, team members can all reinforce the same messages and approaches. This is a potentially much more powerful strategy than relying on one clinician to provide support for behavior change. Hearing the same message from the dietician, the nurse, and the physician is much more reinforcing than just hearing it from one clinician. It is also more efficient. If, instead of providing a one-size-fits all to all patients, resources were deployed according to the needs of different segments of the population, resources might be used more effectively. For example, because low activated patients are more passive, it may be necessary to reach out to them with a more "high touch" approach. Spending more staff time and/ or getting the right mix of support services for low activated patients is another way to more efficiently use existing resources. At the same time, because the more activated patients are more motivated and ready to use information relevant to them, pushing information, web based resources, and community referrals out to them may be effective. That is, by segmenting patient populations, it is likely possible to achieve better outcomes while using fewer resources.

Using person-mediated supports for some and electronic-mediated supports for others is another way to tailor and segment. For example, a large national health insurer used a segmentation approach to support members with a new diagnosis of cancer. They provide electronic resources to the high-activated patients, and at the same time they provide person-mediated navigation, decision support and emotional support to the less-activated enrollees, via health coaches on the telephone [50]. The assumption is that the high-activated patients are more motivated and ready to use information sources on their own. For the less activated patients, who are more passive about their health, the health coaches tailor how they interact with and support these enrollees in a way that recognizes that they are less confident and less skilled.

Tailoring to activation level is also being extended to shared decision-making. Shared decision-making is an important vehicle for improving clinical choices that reflect both evidence and patient preferences. Research indicates that individuals with high activation scores are significantly more likely to perceive benefits associated with shared decision-making [50]. Smith and colleagues examined the perceived benefits of shared decision-making across six different types of decisions. In multivariate models the results showed that higher activated respondents were more likely to see the value of shared decision-making in four of these six decision types. The authors conclude that low activation is a barrier to shared decision-making [50]. It may be that less activated patients, because they often do not understand their role in the care process, may not see that they have something to contribute in shared-decision-making. If this is the case, then these patients will need help engaging the evidence and preparing to fully participate in shared decision-making in order to derive benefit from it.

4. Implications for Evaluations

Because less activated consumers tend to be more passive about their health, it is the higher activated consumers who respond to new health opportunities to engage with health issues. Of course it is not ideal to utilize resources to primarily help the already activated and engaged. Evaluations of interventions to improve informed consumer choice and health behaviors should use a patient activation "lens," to ask, *who is the intervention reaching*? Is it reaching only the high-activated consumer, or is it also reaching the less-activated consumer? Is it reaching those with limited health literacy? To be successful, interventions may need to explicitly target less activated less literate consumers. A failure to do this may mean, that most interventions end up supporting the already activated consumer.

In addition, the evaluation should also ask: *who is the intervention helping*? Is the intervention helping the less activated consumer to become more pro-active about their health? Is it helping those with limited health literacy skills? By asking these questions in evaluations, we can have a fuller understanding of the impact of our programmatic efforts, how well our resources are being deployed, and it will help to identify where improvements are needed.

5. Future Research

Research that focuses on both patient activation and health literacy are just emerging. Most of the studies that include both health literacy and patient activation are observational designs, examining how much each factor contributes to outcomes. However, since we know that most often when each construct is contributing to outcomes, each has an independent impact, future work should be expanded to include a focus on interventions. For example, do interventions designed to increase activation have an impact on health literacy? Or, do interventions designed to improve health literacy also increase patient activation? Are there any synergistic or additive effects on outcomes when interventions are designed to impact both health literacy and patient activation? Such studies would help to illuminate approaches that may boost the efficacy of current approaches.

6. Conclusions

Meeting patients where they are and providing them with information and supports that can inform choices will be a key challenge in a value-based health care environment. The research shows that interventions to improve health literacy, as well as interventions to increase patient activation will be necessary, as both factors independently contribute to outcomes.

References

[1] D.M. Berwick, T.W. Nolan, J. Whittington, The triple aim: care, health, and cost., Health Aff. (Millwood). 2008; 27: 759–69. DOI:10.1377/hlthaff.27.3.759.

[2] Institute of Medicine, Health Literacy: A Prescription to End Confusion, (2004). http://www.nationalacademies.org/hmd/Reports/2004/Health-Literacy-A-Prescription-to-End-Confusion.aspx.

[3] Hibbard, J. Stockard, E.R. Mahoney, M. Tusler, Development of the Patient Activation Measure (PAM): Conceptualizing and Measuring Activation in Patients and Consumers, Health Serv. Res. 2004; 39(4):Pt 1,1005–1026.

[4] Noteboom M., What does "patient engagement" really mean? | Healthcare IT News, Heal. Care IT News. http://www.healthcareitnews.com/news/what-does-patient-engagement-really-mean. Retrieved March 7, 2016.

[5] Barello S, Graffigna G, Vegni E, The Challenges of Conceptualizing Patient Engagement in Health Care: A Lexicographic Literature Review. J. Particip. Med. http://www.jopm.org/evidence/reviews/2014/06/11/the-challenges-of-conceptualizing-patient-engagement-in-health-care-a-lexicographic-literature-review/. Retrieved February 2, 2016.

[6] Hurley RE, Keenan PS, Martsolf GR, Maeng D, Scanlon D, Early experiences with consumer engagement initiatives to improve chronic care., Health Aff. (Millwood). 2009; 28:277–283. DOI:10.1377/hlthaff.28.1.277.

[7] Hibbard JH,Greene J, What the evidence shows about patient activation: better health outcomes and care experiences; fewer data on costs., Health Aff. (Millwood). 2013;32:207–214. DOI:10.1377/hlthaff.2012.1061.

[8] K.L. Carman, P. Dardess, M. Maurer, S. Sofaer, K. Adams, C. Bechtel, et al., Patient and family engagement: a framework for understanding the elements and developing interventions and policies., Health Aff. (Millwood). 2013;32:223–31. DOI:10.1377/hlthaff.2012.1133.

[9] J.N. Mittler, G.R. Martsolf, S.J. Telenko, D.P. Scanlon, Making sense of "consumer engagement" initiatives to improve health and health care: a conceptual framework to guide policy and practice., Milbank Q. 2013: 91;37–77. DOI:10.1111/milq.12002.

[10] L. McCormack, J. Haun, K. Sørensen, M. Valerio, Recommendations for advancing health literacy measurement., J. Health Commun. 2013:18 Suppl 1:9–14. DOI:10.1080/10810730.2013.829892.

[11] T.C. Davis, M.A. Crouch, S.W. Long, R.H. Jackson, P. Bates, R.B. George, et al., Rapid assessment of literacy levels of adult primary care patients., Fam. Med. 1991;23:433–5. http://www.ncbi.nlm.nih.gov/pubmed/1936717 (accessed July 6, 2016).

[12] D.W. Baker, M. V Williams, R.M. Parker, J.A. Gazmararian, J. Nurss, Development of a brief test to measure functional health literacy, Patient Educ. Couns. 1999; 38:33–42.

[13] J. Greene, J.H. Hibbard, M. Tusler, How much do health literacy and patient activation contribute to older adults' ability to manage their health?, AARP Public Policy Institute, Washington, DC, 2005.

[14] J. Rademakers, J. Nijman, A.E.M. Brabers, J.D. de Jong, M. Hendriks, The relative effect of health literacy and patient activation on provider choice in the Netherlands., Health Policy. 2014; 114:200–6. DOI:10.1016/j.healthpol.2013.07.020.

[15] J. Nijman, M. Hendriks, A. Brabers, J. de Jong, J. Rademakers, Patient activation and health literacy as predictors of health information use in a general sample of Dutch health care consumers., J. Health Commun. 2014; 19: 955–69. DOI:10.1080/10810730.2013.837561.

[16] S.G. Smith, L.M. Curtis, J. Wardle, C. von Wagner, M.S. Wolf, Skill set or mind set? Associations between health literacy, patient activation and health., PLoS One. 2013;8:e74373. DOI:10.1371/journal.pone.0074373.

[17] S.G. Smith, R. O'Conor, L.M. Curtis, K. Waite, I.J. Deary, M. Paasche-Orlow, et al., Low health literacy predicts decline in physical function among older adults: findings from the LitCog cohort study., J. Epidemiol. Community Health. 2015; 69: 474–80. DOI:10.1136/jech-2014-204915.

[18] N.J. Zhang, A. Terry, C.A. McHorney, Impact of health literacy on medication adherence: a systematic review and meta-analysis., Ann. Pharmacother. 2014; 48: 741–51. DOI:10.1177/1060028014526562.

[19] N.D. Berkman, S.L. Sheridan, K.E. Donahue, D.J. Halpern, K. Crotty, Low health literacy and health outcomes: an updated systematic review., Ann. Intern. Med. 2011; 155:97–107. DOI:10.7326/0003-4819-155-2-201107190-00005.

[20] E.R. Becker, D.W. Roblin, Translating primary care practice climate into patient activation: the role of patient trust in physician. 46(8):795-805. DOI:10.1097/MLR.0b013e31817919c0. http://journals.lww.com/lww-medicalcare/Fulltext/2008/08000/Translating_Primary_Care_Practice_Climate_into.6.aspx.

[21] B.G. Druss, L. Zhao, S.A. von Esenwein, J.R. Bona, L. Fricks, S. Jenkins-Tucker, et al., The Health and Recovery Peer (HARP) Program: a peer-led intervention to improve medical self-management for persons with serious mental illness., Schizophr. Res. 2010;118:264–270. DOI:10.1016/j.schres.2010.01.026.

[22] J.B. Fowles, P. Terry, M. Xi, J. Hibbard, C.T. Bloom, L. Harvey, Measuring self-management of patients' and employees' health: further validation of the Patient Activation Measure (PAM) based on its relation to employee characteristics., Patient Educ. Couns. 2016;77:116–122. DOI:10.1016/j.pec.2009.02.018.

[23] D.M. Mosen, J. Schmittdiel, J. Hibbard, D. Sobel, C. Remmers, J. Bellows, Is patient activation associated with outcomes of care for adults with chronic conditions?, J. Ambul. Care Manage. 2007; 30: 21–29. http://www.ncbi.nlm.nih.gov/pubmed/17170635.

[24] J.H. Hibbard, E.R. Mahoney, R. Stock, M. Tusler, Do increases in patient activation result in improved self-management behaviors? Health Serv. Res. 2007;42:1443–63. DOI:10.1111/j.1475-6773.2006.00669.x.

[25] I. Willaing, S.-A. Rogvi, M. Bøgelund, T. Almdal, M. Schiøtz, Recall of HbA1c and self-management behaviours, patient activation, perception of care and diabetes distress in Type 2 diabetes., Diabet. Med. 2013: 30:e139-42. DOI:10.1111/dme.12121.

[26] J.H. Hibbard, P.J. Cunningham, How engaged are consumers in their health and health care, and why does it matter?, Center for Studying Health System Change, Washington, DC, 2008.

[27] R.L. Skolasky, E.J. Mackenzie, S.T. Wegener, L.H. Riley, Patient activation and adherence to physical therapy in persons undergoing spine surgery., Spine (Phila. Pa. 1976). 2008:33:E784--91. DOI:10.1097/BRS.0b013e31818027f1.

[28] M. Kukla, M.P. Salyers, P.H. Lysaker, Levels of patient activation among adults with schizophrenia: associations with hope, symptoms, medication adherence, and recovery attitudes., J. Nerv. Ment. Dis. 2013: 201: 339–44. DOI:10.1097/NMD.0b013e318288e253.

[29] L. Stepleman, M.-C. Rutter, J. Hibbard, L. Johns, D. Wright, M. Hughes, Validation of the patient activation measure in a multiple sclerosis clinic sample and implications for care., Disabil. Rehabil. 2010; 32:1558–67. DOI:10.3109/09638280903567885.

[30] R. Marshall, M.C. Beach, S. Saha, T. Mori, M.O. Loveless, J.H. Hibbard, et al., Patient activation and improved outcomes in HIV-infected patients., J. Gen. Intern. Med. 2013;28:668–674. DOI:10.1007/s11606-012-2307-y.

[31] K. Hollingworth, H. Müllerová, S. Landis, Z. Aisanov, K. Davis, M. Ichinose, et al., Health behaviors and their correlates among participants in the Continuing to Confront COPD International Patient Survey, Int. J. Chron. Obstruct. Pulmon. Dis. Volume 11. 2016; 881. DOI:10.2147/COPD.S102280.

[32] C. Remmers, J. Hibbard, D.M. Mosen, M. Wagenfield, R.E. Hoye, C. Jones, Is patient activation associated with future health outcomes and healthcare utilization among patients with diabetes?, J. Ambul. Care Manage. 2009; 32:320–327. DOI:10.1097/JAC.0b013e3181ba6e77.

[33] R.L. Kinney, S.C. Lemon, S.D. Person, S.L. Pagoto, J.S. Saczynski, The association between patient activation and medication adherence, hospitalization, and emergency room utilization in patients with chronic illnesses: a systematic review., Patient Educ. Couns. 2015; 98;545–52. DOI:10.1016/j.pec.2015.02.005.

[34] N. Begum, M. Donald, I.Z. Ozolins, J. Dower, Hospital admissions, emergency department utilisation and patient activation for self-management among people with diabetes., Diabetes Res. Clin. Pract. 2011; 93:260–267. DOI:10.1016/j.diabres.2011.05.031.

[35] J. Greene, J.H. Hibbard, Why does patient activation matter? An examination of the relationships between patient activation and health-related outcomes., J. Gen. Intern. Med. 2012;27:520–6. DOI:10.1007/s11606-011-1931-2.

[36] J.H. Hibbard, J. Greene, R. Sacks, V. Overton, C.D. Parrotta, Adding a measure Of patient self-management capability to risk assessment can improve prediction of high costs, Health Aff. 2016; 35:489–494. DOI:10.1377/hlthaff.2015.1031.

[37] S.E. Mitchell, P.M. Gardiner, E. Sadikova, J.M. Martin, B.W. Jack, J.H. Hibbard, et al., Patient activation and 30-day post-discharge hospital utilization., J. Gen. Intern. Med. 2014; 29:349–355. DOI:10.1007/s11606-013-2647-2.

[38] S. Sheikh, P. Hendry, C. Kalynych, B. Owensby, J. Johnson, D.F. Kraemer, et al., Assessing Patient Activation and Health Literacy in the Emergency Department, Am. J. Emerg. Med. (n.d.). DOI:10.1016/j.ajem.2015.09.045.

[39] M. Serper, A.J. Gawron, S.G. Smith, A.A. Pandit, A.R. Dahlke, E.A. Bojarski, et al., Patient factors that affect quality of colonoscopy preparation., Clin. Gastroenterol. Hepatol. 2014.12:451–7. DOI:10.1016/j.cgh.2013.07.036.

[40] J.H. Hibbard, E. Peters, A. Dixon, M. Tusler, Consumer competencies and the use of comparative quality information: it isn't just about literacy, Med. Care Res. Rev. 2007; 64:379–394.

[41] J.H. Hibbard, P. Slovic, J.J. Jewett, Informing consumer decisions in health care: implications from decision-making research, Milbank Q. 1977; 75:395–414. DOI:10.1111/1468-0009.00061.

[42] J. Taggart, A. Williams, S. Dennis, A. Newall, T. Shortus, N. Zwar, et al., A systematic review of interventions in primary care to improve health literacy for chronic disease behavioral risk factors, BMC Fam. Pract. 2012; 13. http://www.biomedcentral.com/1471-2296/13/49. Retrieved July 8, 2016.

[43] D.A. DeWalt, A. Hink, Health lteracy and child health outcomes: a systematic review of the literature, Pediatrics. 2009; 124; S265–S274. DOI:10.1542/peds.2009-1162B.

[44] L. Kidd, M. Lawrence, J. Booth, A. Rowat, S. Russell, Development and evaluation of a nurse-led, tailored stroke self-management intervention. BMC Health Serv. Res. 2015; 15:359. DOI:10.1186/s12913-015-1021-y.

[45] M.J. Shively, N.J. Gardetto, M.F. Kodiath, A. Kelly, T.L. Smith, C. Stepnowsky, et al., Effect of patient activation on self-management in patients with heart failure., J. Cardiovasc. Nurs. 2013; 28:20–34. DOI:10.1097/JCN.0b013e318239f9f9.

[46] J.H. Hibbard, J. Greene, M. Tusler, Improving the outcomes of disease-management by tailoring care to the patient's level of activation, Am. J. Manag. Care. 2009; 15:353–360.

[47] J.H. Hibbard, E.R. Mahoney, R. Stock, M. Tusler, Do increases in patient activation result in improved self-management behaviors?, Health Serv. Res. 2007;42:1443–1463. DOI:10.1111/j.1475-6773.2006.00669.x.

[48] L. Harvey, J.B. Fowles, M. Xi, P. Terry, When activation changes, what else changes? the relationship between change in patient activation measure (PAM) and employees' health status and health behaviors., Patient Educ. Couns. 2012; 88:338–43. DOI:10.1016/j.pec.2012.02.005.

[49] J.H. Hibbard, M. Tusler, Assessing activation stage and employing a "next steps" approach to supporting patient. J Ambul Care Manage. 2007;30;2-8.

[50] S.G. Smith, A. Pandit, S.R. Rush, M.S. Wolf, C.J. Simon, The role of patient activation in preferences for shared decision making: results from a national survey of U.S. adults, J. Health Commun. 2015; http://www.tandfonline.com/DOI/full/10.1080/10810730.2015.1033115#.Veg_X-k6Vp8. Retrieved September 3, 2015.

Health Literacy
R.A. Logan and E.R. Siegel (Eds.)
IOS Press, 2017
© 2017 The authors and IOS Press. All rights reserved.
doi:10.3233/978-1-61499-790-0-263

Shared Decision Making Interventions: Theoretical and Empirical Evidence with Implications for Health Literacy

Dawn STACEY [a,1], Sophie HILL [b], Kirsten MCCAFFERY [c], Laura BOLAND [a], Krystina B. LEWIS [a] and Lidia HORVAT [d]

[a] Faculty of Health Sciences, University of Ottawa and Ottawa Hospital Research Institute, Canada
[b] School of Psychology and Public Health, La Trobe University, Melbourne, Australia
[c] School of Public Health, University of Sydney, Australia
[d] Victoria State Department of Health and Human Services, Melbourne, Australia

Abstract. Basic health literacy is required for making health decisions. The aim of this chapter is to discuss the use of shared decision making interventions for supporting patient involvement in making health decisions. The chapter provides a definition of shared decision making and discusses the link between shared decision making and the three levels of health literacy: functional, communicative/interactive, and critical. The Interprofessional Shared Decision Making Model is used to identify the various players involved: the patient, the family/surrogate/ significant others, decision coach, and health care professionals. When patients are involved in shared decision making, they have better health outcomes, better healthcare experiences, and likely lower costs. Yet, their degree of involvement is influenced by their level of health literacy.
    Interventions to facilitate shared decision making are patient decision aids, decision coaching, and question prompt lists. Patient decision aids have been shown to improve knowledge, accurate risk perceptions, and chosen options congruent with patients' values. Decision coaching improves knowledge and patient satisfaction. Question prompts also improve satisfaction. When shared decision making interventions have been evaluated with patients presumed to have lower health literacy, they appeared to be more beneficial to disadvantaged groups compared to those with higher literacy or better socioeconomic status. However, special attention needs to be applied when designing these interventions for populations with lower literacy. Two case exemplars are provided to illustrate the design and choice of interventions to better support patients with varying levels of health literacy.
    Despite evidence indicating these interventions are effective for involving patients in shared decision making, few are used in routine clinical practice. To increase their uptake, implementation strategies need to overcome barriers interfering with their use. Implementation strategies include training health care professionals, adopting SDM interventions that target patients, such as patient decision aids, and monitor patients' decisional comfort using the SURE test. Integrating health literacy principles is important when developing interventions that facilitate shared decision making and essential to avoid inadvertently producing higher inequalities between patients with varying levels of health literacy.

Keywords. Interprofessional shared decision making, patient decision aids, health literacy, decision coaching, question prompts, implementation

---

[1] Corresponding author: School of Nursing, Faculty of Health Sciences, University of Ottawa, 451 Smyth Road, Ottawa, Canada, K1H 8M5; E-mail: dstacey@uottawa.ca.

1. Introduction

Fundamental in the definition of health literacy is the use of health information to make health decisions. Patients are frequently faced with making health decisions and often experience a sense of personal uncertainty about the best course of action. This personal uncertainty, also known as decisional conflict, is often triggered by the need to weigh benefits/risks across options, anticipate loss, and/or address challenge to personal life values [1]. However, only about half of patients are actually involved in decision making and the other half defer to the clinician's recommendation [2,3]. Furthermore, clinicians are poor judges of patient preferences [4]. A basic level of health literacy is required for making health decisions and can be supported with shared decision making interventions.

The overall aim of this chapter is to discuss the use of shared decision making interventions for supporting patient involvement in making health decisions. We will discuss interventions to facilitate shared decision making, strategies to increase their use in clinical practice, and implications for health literacy, research, and practice. As well, two case examples are provided to demonstrate how health literacy strategies can be considered when developing shared decision making interventions and integrating them into clinical practice.

This chapter starts by providing a definition of shared decision making and discusses the link between shared decision making and the three levels of health literacy: functional, communicative/interactive, and critical. The Interprofessional Shared Decision Making Model is used to provide a more detailed definition of shared decision making and identify the various players involved: the patient, family/surrogate/significant others, decision coach, and health care professionals. In the next section, interventions to facilitate shared decision making such as patient decision aids, decision coaching, and question prompt lists, are described with empirical evidence indicating their impact on patient outcomes and evidence supporting their use with specific populations with lower health literacy. Two case exemplars are provided to illustrate the design and choice of interventions to better support patients with varying levels of health literacy. Finally, considerations for implementing shared decision making interventions into clinical practice are discussed with emerging evidence on effective strategies to overcome barriers to their use and ways to monitor patients' level of comfort in the decision making process. Opportunities for research and implications for health literacy are highlighted.

Shared decision making is the *process* by which health decisions are made by the patient and the clinician using the best available evidence and discussion of patients' preferences. Based on a review of 161 articles providing conceptual definitions of shared decision making, essential elements of the shared decision making process include: a) making explicit the decision to address the problem; b) presenting options, pros, and cons including the communication of quantitative risk information; c) assessing patients' values, preferences, and abilities; d) verifying patients' understanding; and e) making or explicitly deferring the decision [5]. Hence for patients to participate in shared decision making, they need to understand they have a choice, be able to understand the health information and the availability of different options, clarify their personal values, and discuss the information and their values with the clinician. Quality decisions are consistently defined as choices informed by the best available evidence and patients' informed preferences [6,7].

Table 1. Shared decision making interventions for enhancing health literacy

Levels	Health literacy levels applied to shared decision making	Shared decision making interventions
Functional health literacy	- able to read basic information - able to write in response to basic questions - able to understand health information	• Patient decision aids • Values clarification exercises • Decision coaching
Interactive health literacy	- able to communicate with others - able to extract and discuss health information - able to share personal values, concerns, goals with others	• Trained health professionals • Question prompt sheets
Critical health literacy	- have advanced cognitive and social skills - critically analyze information, clarify values, - make decisions informed by information and personal preferences	

Patient engagement in the process of shared decision making requires three levels of health literacy skills according to Nutbeam [8]. The three levels are defined as functional health literacy, communicative/interactive health literacy, and critical health literacy. The intersection between health literacy and shared decision making is captured in Table 1. Nutbeam's health literacy definition has been influential and helps to scope the complexity of health literacy, encompassing information accessibility and also communication, exchange and appraisal [8]. In recent years, health literacy developments have recognized the importance of these levels by emphasizing the need to build health literacy of individuals while concurrently emphasizing the role of health professionals to communicate effectively for this to occur and for systems to support the routine use of strategies [9]. In fact, health literacy has been described as a product of good communication between the clinician and patient [10].

2. Shared Decision Making Research & Importance

On a continuum of decision making, shared decision making is situated between clinician controlled (paternalistic) to patient controlled (autonomous) [11,12]. Historically, paternalistic decision making was standard with physicians identified as knowing what is best for the patient. In fact, the American Medical Association Code of Ethics in the mid-1800's advised physicians not to consider patient perspectives in medical care [13]. However, there has been a shift to more shared or patient controlled decision making driven by the rise in the consumer movement with demands for autonomy, informed consent, and patient-centred care [14,15].

Shared decision making often occurs with interprofessional healthcare teams. Interprofessional shared decision making is defined as a process by which a healthcare choice is made between the patient and two or more healthcare professionals [16]. Interprofessional collaborations build on the strengths of each profession's approach to care delivery such that professionals work within their full scope of practice and without intentional duplication of services. According to the Interprofessional Shared Decision Making Model (Figure 1), there are four key assumptions to consider. First, involving patients in shared decision making is essential for achieving quality decisions

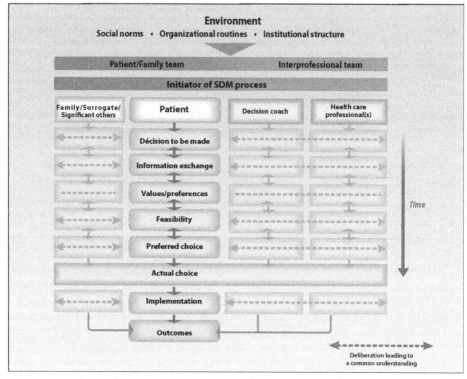

Figure 1. Interprofessional Shared Decision Making Model.

defined as informed and based on individual patient values. Second, it is more likely to reach a shared decision when the interprofessional team has a common understanding of the elements of the shared decision making process and recognizes the influence of various individuals on the process. Third, achieving an interprofessional approach to shared decision making may occur synchronously (e.g., in a family conference), but more often occurs asynchronously as patients interact separately with various members of the team. Fourth, family or significant others are important stakeholders involved or implicated by the decision and their values and preferences may not be consistent with the patient.

Patients frequently involve family members and/or significant others either informally or formally engaged in health decision making processes. Informally, when family or significant others share their opinions on a preferred option, their input may be interpreted by a patient either as supportive or a source of undue pressure to select a specific option. More formally, family members or significant others may be directly involved in a decision making process when patients have limited English language skills, exhibit different cultural beliefs about roles in decision making, or have inadequate cognitive function (e.g., adults with dementia). In the latter situations, it is important to differentiate the values/preferences of the surrogate from the surrogate's understanding of the values/preferences of the patient he or she represents [17]. When children reach competencies to participate in decision making, but are legally underage to make decisions on their own, decisions can be made by children and parents together with health professionals [18]. Consistent with patient involvement, family members or surrogate's understanding of the options, health literacy skills, and values/preferences have the potential to support or interfere with a shared decision making process. When there are differences in values/preferences among family members, there can be added conflict and disagreement in reaching a consensus, or mutually agreed upon selected health option.

Overall, activated patients experience better health outcomes, better healthcare experiences, and likely lower costs [19]. A review of 22 studies, found patients were more satisfied and less depressed when their preferred and perceived level of involvement matched. However, mismatches fostered poorer outcomes for patients such as: depression, fatigue, less satisfaction, and post-consultation anxiety [3]. Regardless of preferred role in decision making, two studies suggest patients fare better when they are actively involved in decision making processes [20,21]. However, only 34% to 80% of patients (median 60%) experienced a match between their preferred and actual role in decision making, and patients preferred more active roles when mismatches occurred [3].

There is also the potential for patient involvement in decision making to impact positively on health systems. According to Coulter, sustainability of healthcare systems "will depend on the effectiveness of efforts to eliminate the unhealthy paternalism that still characterizes patient-professional relationships" (page 5) [22]. Since 2010, several healthcare policies have integrated shared decision making into healthcare legislation [14,23–26].

Unfortunately, patients' health literacy appears to mediate their level of involvement. A review of studies reported patients with lower health literacy had less health knowledge and were less likely to want to be involved in decision making compared to those with higher health literacy [27]. Furthermore, patients having lower interactive health literacy skills were less likely to ask questions. Health literacy may also explain differences in satisfaction with the decision making process. For example, those with higher critical health literacy rated the information provided by clinicians in a consultation as inadequate and those with lower health literacy rated it as adequate. Involvement of patients with varying levels of health literacy in decision making is a modifiable behaviour when exposed to shared decision making interventions [28,29].

3. Shared Decision Making Interventions

Interventions to facilitate the process of shared decision making are patient decision aids, decision coaching, and question prompt lists [28,30–32]. In fact, when patients get more 'contact' with health professionals (e.g., they can ask questions and review the information) their health literacy needs are more likely to be addressed and their knowledge improves [33]. Although most interventions are developed and evaluated in adult populations, there have been some studies examining their effectiveness in pediatrics and with other disadvantaged groups [27].

3.1. Patient Decision Aids

Patient decision aids are evidence-based tools designed to supplement rather than replace patient-clinician interactions. Patient decision aids are printed materials, videos, and/or online interactive programs. At a minimum, these tools make explicit the decision, provide information on options, benefits and harms, and help patients clarify their

Table 2. Effect of shared decision making interventions on patient outcomes

Outcomes	Decision aids	Decision coaching	Question prompts
Improve knowledge	√	√	
More accurate risk perception of outcomes	√		
Chosen option congruent with patients' values	√		
Less decisional conflict (uninformed, unclear values)	√		
Fewer remaining undecided	√		
Higher patient participation in decision making	√	√	
Improved patient-clinician communication	√		√
Increased satisfaction		√	√

√ statistically significant improvement

values for outcomes of options to reach a preferred option [28]. They may also include probabilities indicating the chances of benefits and harms, personal stories of others who have made this decision, and guidance in the steps of decision making. Patients can use these decision aids in preparation for the consultation and some are designed specifically for use when discussing the decision within the consultation. Their development has been guided by several different decision theories, translational and risk communication frameworks from economics, psychology, and sociology [34,35].

Patient decision aids improve knowledge and patient participation in decision making (Table 2). A systematic review evaluating the effectiveness of patient decision aids for adults facing treatment or screening decisions identified 115 randomized controlled trials [28]. Compared to usual care, patients who used decision aids had improved quality of decisions as evidence by enhanced knowledge (+13%), a more accurate understanding of the chances of benefits and harms (+82%), and improved match between patients' values and the chosen option (+51%). The process of decision making was improved with patients experiencing less decisional conflict, fewer feeling undecided, and higher participation in the decision making process. As well, there was improved patient-clinician communication and no difference in the length of the consultation in minutes (e.g., 8 trials no difference, 2 longer, 1 shorter). The chosen option varied by clinical problem with significantly reduced elective surgeries, use of hormone replacement therapy, and prostate specific antigen testing. For other decisions, there was no difference or too few trials to meta-analyze the results. Overall, patient decision aids showed no difference compared to usual care on anxiety, depression, generic quality of life, or satisfaction.

3.2. Decision Coaching

Decision coaching provided by trained healthcare professionals is non-directive and facilitates progress in decision making [36,37]. Either face to face or on the telephone, decision coaches: a) assess patients' decision making needs; b) provide information on options, benefits and harms (verbally or using a patient decision aid); c) assess patients' understanding; d) clarify patients' values on features and outcomes of options; and e) screen to determine patients' needs relevant to implementing the chosen option (e.g., motivation, self-confidence, barriers, commitment). The overall aim is to develop the patient's skills in thinking about the options, prepare for discussing the decision in consultation with their clinician, and implement the chosen option. A member of the interprofessional healthcare team can assume the decision coaching role. Studies have evaluated decision coaching provided by nurses, social workers, genetic counsellors, psychologists, and pharmacists [36]. There is an example protocol and video to guide decision coaching available online [38].

Decision coaching improves knowledge and involvement in the decision making process (Table 2). In a systematic review of 10 randomized controlled trials, patients exposed to decision coaching had improved knowledge compared to usual care [36]. The improvement in knowledge for those provided decision coaching showed consistent improvement to those provided with patient decision aids. Patients also had higher perceived involvement in decision making and were more satisfied with the decision making process. Despite the potential for decision coaching to improve functional, interactive, and critical health literacy (Table 1), none of these studies have been conducted among patients with lower health literacy.

3.3. Question Prompts

Question prompts sheets and pre-consultation coaching improve patient-clinician communication. A systematic review of 33 studies showed a 27% improvement in patients asking questions and 9% improvement in overall satisfaction [32]. There was no statistically significant difference in anxiety, knowledge or consultation length. A more recent set of

> **Box 1. The AskShareKnow Intervention**
>
> What are my options?
>
> What are the possible benefits and harms of those options?
>
> How likely are each of those benefits and harms to happen to me?

studies have evaluated the AskShareKnow intervention focused on patients asking health professionals three questions specific to the decision (see Box 1) [39–41]. For example, when simulated patients asked these questions in the consultation, clinicians provided them with more information and were more likely to involve them [39]. A subsequent study had patients observe the 4-minute video-clip in the waiting room and reported 87% of those making a decision asked one or more question in the consultation [40]. However, qualitative interviews with 26 adults with low literacy and/or poor English language skills revealed difficulties with understanding some terms in the AskShareKnow intervention questions [41]. With training, adults with lower literacy were better able to recall the AskShareKnow questions and were more likely to ask at least one question in the subsequent consultation with their clinician [42]. Further research is required to determine how to use question prompts for adults with low literacy or limited English language skills.

3.4. Tailoring Interventions for Specific Populations with Lower Literacy

According to the International Patient Decision Aid Standards Collaboration (IPDAS), patient decision aids should be written at a level to be understood by the majority of patients in the target group, written at less than grade 9 readability level, and, ideally, provide ways other than reading to help patients understand the information (e.g., video, audio, decision coaching) [27]. Of 97 randomized controlled trials of patient decision aids reviewed, few met these criteria [27]. For example, only five reported the reading level as less than grade 9, two reported following IPDAS health literacy criteria, and some used media other than pure text (e.g., video, audio).

When shared decision making interventions were evaluated with patients presumed to have lower health literacy, they appeared to be more beneficial to disadvantaged groups compared to those with higher literacy or better socioeconomic status. A systematic review identified 19 studies focused on interventions to improve shared decision making among disadvantaged groups [43]. Disadvantaged groups included people living in poverty, ethnic minority, low education/literacy level, or medically underserved geographic locations. These interventions included patient decision aids, communication skills workshop, decision coaching, and small group education sessions. Of 11 studies measuring knowledge, there was significant improvement in knowledge and informed choice of disadvantaged participants compared to controls. Three of five studies compared disadvantaged to higher literacy/education groups and despite baseline knowledge being lower for disadvantaged groups, the disparities between groups disappeared post-intervention. The other two studies reported lower literacy in the disadvantaged group interfering with their understanding of the intervention content. Those exposed to the interventions in four studies also had lower decisional conflict assessed using the lower literate version of this instrument [44]. In one of these studies, decisional conflict was higher at baseline for the low literacy group but this disparity disappeared post-intervention [43]. Finally, those who used the shared decision making interventions were more involved in the consultation, more active in discussing options with their clinician, and more likely to prefer a shared decision making approach. A case exemplar in Appendix A provides details on the design of shared decision making interventions to better support adults with varying levels of health literacy who are considering whether or not to have the surgical procedure to replace the implantable cardioverter-defibrillator.

Decision making in the pediatric clinical context has several unique challenges. Children's ability to participate in decision making evolves with their maturity level, experience with the health condition, and severity of the symptoms [45]. Hence, the extent of child participation in health decisions should depend on their ability and not their chronological age. Another unique challenge is the multiple stakeholders (e.g., children, parents, grandparents, health professionals) with a vested interest in the decision and potentially different values and preferences; with varying health literacy levels [18]. In pediatrics, themes of parents' decision making needs identified in 149 studies included: a) trusted evidence-based information; b) speaking to other parents in similar situations to counterbalance information from health professionals and discuss handling pressures from various others; and c) control over the process of decision making, particularly given their emotional state [46]. In a systematic review of 54 unique shared decision making interventions, 63% targeted the parents alone, 26% focused on multiple stakeholders, 7% targeted the child, and 6% targeted the health professional [47]. These interventions decreased parents' decisional conflict and improved their knowledge. A case exemplar in Appendix B provides more details on the use of decision coaching with a patient decision aid for children with diabetes and their parents considering insulin delivery options [48].

4. Use of Shared Decision Making Interventions in Practice

Shared decision making interventions are not routinely being used in clinical practice. A review identified 33 studies assessed clinician involvement of patients in decision making using the OPTION instrument [49]. Findings revealed low levels of patient involvement and few clinicians who adjust care based on patient preferences. OPTION scores were higher when interventions were used including patient decision aids, standardized patients, and training.

To better understanding how to improve use of shared decision making interventions in practice, it is important to consider a systematic process exploring barriers interfering with their use, determining effective approaches for increasing their uptake in clinical practice, and monitoring their impact on patient outcomes. In fact, implementation is more successful when interventions are designed to overcome identified barriers [50,51].

4.1. Barriers to Shared Decision Making

Several systematic reviews have identified barriers and facilitators to shared decision making from the perspective of patients and clinicians [27,43,52,53]. Patients have identified several key barriers to their participation in shared decision making (Table 3). In a systematic review of 44 studies, patients clearly indicated their individual capacity to participate in shared decision making required having: a) knowledge of their health condition, options, and outcomes, b) knowledge of their personal values/preferences, and c) perceived influence on decision making in the consultation [52]. For patients to participate in decision making, they wanted permission to participate, feel confidence in their own knowledge, and self-efficacy in using shared decision making skills. Alternatively, they identified that nurses should explain the information, provide support by listening to their preferences, and provide the clinician with their preferences. Interestingly, their barriers to knowledge could be addressed by using patient decision aids, decision coaching, and shared decision making. The bigger challenge is addressing power-imbalances between patients and clinicians.

Patients with lower health literacy have additional barriers interfering with their participation in shared decision making. A systematic review exploring the relationship between health literacy and patient involvement in shared decision making identified 13 studies [54]. Patients with lower literacy were less likely to want to participate in shared decision making and less likely to ask questions. However, with support using shared decision making interventions designed for adults with lower health literacy, it was possible to support them to have a more active role in decision making [43].

Clinicians have also identified barriers to shared decision making. In a systematic review of barriers and facilitators to implementing shared decision making in clinical practice, 38 studies were identified [53]. The most common barriers were lack of time, patient characteristics, and inappropriate clinical situation. Facilitators were clinician motivation, observed positive impact on the clinical process, and patient outcomes. As discussed earlier, studies evaluating shared decision making interventions showed improved communication in the consultation without increasing the length of the consultation [28]. As well, patient characteristics such as those with lower literacy and higher decisional conflict have the potential for greater improvements when supported to participate in shared decision making [28,43]. Hence, most of the barriers are myths to be dispelled [55].

Table 3. Barriers mapped onto shared decision making interventions

Barriers	Interventions to support uptake of shared decision making		
	Decision aids	**Decision coaching**	**Training professionals**
Patient identified barriers			
Lack of knowledge of condition, options, outcomes	Improves knowledge	Improves knowledge	
Lack of knowledge of personal values	Improves values-choice agreement	Improves values-choice agreement	
No invitation to participate and ask questions			Training to engage patients
Lack of confidence in knowledge and self-efficacy			
Clinician identified barriers			
Lack of time			Dispel myth
Patient characteristics – a priori judging who will benefit from and/or desire to be involved in shared decision making	Improves outcomes for disadvantaged groups		Training for use with all
Inappropriate clinical situations	Wide range of situations		Training for use across settings

4.2. Effective Implementation Strategies

Strategies for increasing uptake of shared decision making in clinical practice require interventions targeting patients, health professionals, or both, within a supportive healthcare environment. A Cochrane review revealed 39 studies focused on evaluating interventions for implementing shared decision making. The most common interventions evaluated in these studies were patient decision aids and training of health professionals. Compared to usual care, there was greater uptake of shared decision making when interventions targeted both patients and healthcare professionals (standardized mean difference 2.83) or targeted the patient alone (standardized mean difference 1.42). The main intervention targeting patients in these studies was a patient decision aid. Given shared decision making occurs between the patient and the clinician, it makes sense that implementation will be more successful when targeting both the patient and clinician. Interestingly, all three studies with interventions targeting the interprofessional team (e.g. more than one health professional) showed increased uptake of shared decision making in clinical practice.

Training in shared decision making and decision coaching is an effective approach to improving knowledge and skills of healthcare professionals. A systematic review identified 54 training programs in 14 countries [56]. Effective teaching methods in these studies were case-based learning, small group sessions, role play, printed materials, audit and feedback and online tutorials. An international meeting on competencies for shared decision making training programs reached consensus on the need for, at a minimum, training focused on building relational competencies and risk communication competencies [57]. In related fields, a Cochrane review of 43 trials showed skills in being patient-centered (e.g., sharing control of consultations, decisions and management) can be transferred to health professionals with training. Removing the barrier of time, it also showed shorter training (<10 hours) is as effective as longer training [58]. Hence, health services which value the goals of shared decision making and improving health literacy will need to provide opportunities for building the skills and capacity of their staff.

Little research has been conducted on building patients' knowledge and skills in shared decision making. Emerging evidence indicates interventions building skills and confidence are effective for increasing patient activation in general [19]. A cluster-randomized controlled trial evaluated a six-hour shared decision making training program in 219 adults with lower literacy skills who were attending adult education classes [42]. The training also aimed to enhance their confidence. Trained participants (49%) were more likely to think it was important to discuss benefits and harms with their healthcare professional when making decisions about their health compared to 3% of controls. Within six months of training, 51% of trained participants reported asking at least one AskShareKnow question and they better understood how to ask clinicians questions. Another study recruited oncology patients of ethnic minorities to evaluate a communication skills workshops focused on achieving a shared understanding between clinicians and patients [59]. The workshop was based on the PACE curriculum and involved 20–30 minute workshop using Power Point presentation, video clips demonstrating skills, and discussion about the skills [60]. The 16 workshop participants self-reported having improved communication behaviours and being satisfied with the workshop content.

Easy access to patient decision aids and decision coaching tools is necessary to support implementation of these resources in clinical practice. The A to Z inventory is an online clearinghouse of publicly available patient decision aids [61]. Each decision aid in the inventory has a brief summary including: options, target audience, developer, year of last update, rating on the International Patient Decision Aid Standards (IPDAS), and automated link to access the patient decision aid. There are also the generic patient decision support tools for any health or social decision titled the "Ottawa Personal Decision Guide" and "Ottawa Personal Decision Guide for Two" [61,62]. These tools are used in training of decision coaches as it provides a step by step approach to guide patients in the process of decision making. Near the end of the guides, the SURE test is used to screen for decisional conflict and there are suggestions on next steps to address remaining decision making needs. The Ottawa Personal Decision Guide is available in multiple languages and a version has been culturally adapted for aboriginal women with lower literacy skills [62–63].

Other health system supports for encouraging use of shared decision making interventions in clinical practice include use of standards, accreditation, and health policies [26,46]. Currently, one clinical practice guideline, Patient Experience in Adult NHS Services, explicitly includes several statements focused on supporting patient involvement in shared decision making [64]. This guideline also recommends patient education programs meet the literacy needs of patients. To facilitate implementation of recommendations within this clinical practice guideline, the UK National Health Service (NHS) has established a Shared Decision Making Collaborate to promote a move away from paternalistic decision making and established a national platform on shared decision making with access to patient decision aids [65]. In the USA, there are health directorate resources to support shared decision making provided by the Washington State Health Care Authority and the Agency for Health Research and Quality. Washington State was the first to launch a process for certification of patient decision aids in

Table 4. SURE Test to screen for decisional conflict

Acronym	SURE test Item
Sure of myself	Do you feel SURE about the best choice for you?
Understand information	Do you know the benefits and risks of each option?
Risk/benefit ratio	Are you clear about which benefits and risks matter most to you?
Encouragement	Do you have enough support and advice to make a choice?

Yes response = 1; No response = 0

2016 [66]. However, these initiatives are focused more on increasing resources to support shared decision making and not directly addressing health literacy issues.

4.3. Monitoring Use

Shared decision making in clinical practice can be monitored with findings used to reinforce use. A simple tool to inform clinical practice is the SURE Test [67]. The four-item SURE test is used to screen patients for decisional conflict (see Table 4). A total score less than 4 indicates decisional conflict. It is based on the original and low literacy versions of the Decisional Conflict Scale and correlates negatively with the original scale given the SURE test was reframed positively to measure decisional comfort [68–69]. For patients considering treatment, it discriminates between those who made a choice and those who have not.

There are a number of other instruments used to measure shared decision making in the consultation [70,71]. However, these measures more likely to be used in research studies given the need to analyze taped consultation by trained raters.

5. Opportunities for Research and Implementation in Practice

There are a number of areas for further research on the intersection between health literacy, cultural competence, language services and involvement of patients in shared decision making. We proposed three areas for further research to improve shared decision making interventions for improving health literacy in clinical practice.

More research is required to test shared decision making interventions with lower literacy populations and to understand factors influencing their use in practice. As discussed earlier, findings from a recent review indicated those with lower socioeconomic status have potentially more to gain from patient decision aids compared to those with higher health literacy [43]. No known research has evaluated decision coaching among lower literacy patients. Emerging research on using question prompt lists with lower literacy patients appears to indicate better question asking after patients participated in a 6-hour training workshop on shared decision making [41,42]. Given having more face-time with clinicians improves health literacy and both of these interventions provide some structure to how time is used, it is worth determining the impact of these shared decision making interventions for improving health literacy [72].

For patient decision aids, developers need to move beyond functional health literacy (readability levels) to also support communicative and critical health literacy which are required for values clarification exercises and shared decision making in the consultation [27]. However, there is a paucity of research with patient decision aids on effective approaches to enhance communicative and critical health literacy skills. Further research is required to determine if those with low capacity to participate in shared decision making benefit from decision coaching. One study with aboriginal women indicated using the Ottawa Personal Decision Guide as the "talking stick" rather than being used as another form to complete [63]. In the absence of effective approaches to develop patient decision aids for lower literacy populations, developers may want to apply and evaluate principles from the broader literature on successful health literacy interventions such as using plain language, focus on skills building, pilot testing with lower literacy populations, using a range of visual techniques, and delivering patient decision aids by clinicians in the context of clinical practice [27].

We need to better understand how to facilitate patients' involvement in shared decision making. For example, effective approaches are required to help people understand they have a role in health decision making and in particular, better support those with lower literacy who do not understand this role [52,54]. Consistently across studies, patients are often not aware of a decision being made and this is a modifiable behaviour among clinicians. In clinical practice, clinicians need to be more explicit about the decision which is a fundamental element of shared decision making [5]. Patients also reported their ability to participate in shared decision making was negatively affected by the perceived power imbalance and their lack of confidence to be involved [52]. And these power-imbalances are even more problematic for decision making in adults with lower literacy skills and pediatrics [18,53].

6. Conclusion

Shared decision making has the potential to benefit populations with lower literacy but shared decision making interventions must be developed to meet the unique needs of these populations. Unfortunately, the vast majority of shared decision making interventions are beyond average reading level of normal populations let alone the level of those with lower literacy and are not designed using good health literacy principles. Attending to these health literacy principles is the most obvious strategy for improvement. Otherwise, there continues to be the risk of creating greater inequalities among those who are health literate accessing shared decision making interventions compared to those who are not.

Appendices

Appendix A. Shared Decision Making in Adults with Implantable Cardiac Defibrillators

Adults with cardiovascular disease are living longer, in part due to rapidly expanding indications for implantable cardiac devices such as implantable cardioverter-defibrillators (ICD) [73]. Recipients of these complex implanted devices need to be engaged in their care for optimal outcomes. This includes understanding the basic functions of the ICD, complying with hospital discharge instructions following its implantation or replacement, and knowing when and how to seek medical attention. This level of comprehension is also required for quality decision-making when considering options related to ICD therapy such as replacement or non-replacement of the device at battery depletion and consideration of deactivation of tachytherapies when nearing end-of-life. Moreover, clinicians need to explain information to patients and ensure it is tailored to their particular diagnosis and prognosis.

Amongst an ethnically diverse sample of 116 patients with implantable cardiac devices, approximately 40% had marginal or inadequate functional health literacy [74]. Patients with lower health literacy were older, had lower levels of education, and had higher rates of chronic cardiovascular conditions such as diabetes, hypertension and hyperlipidemia. Furthermore, patients with ICDs often overestimate the benefit of their device, underestimate its harms and misunderstand its purpose [74,75]. As a result, many of these patients defer to their clinicians' recommendation. Such misunderstandings can impact the quality of the decisions these patients face throughout the tenure of their ICD, whether at implantation, battery replacement, or consideration of deactivation when nearing end-of-life. To promote patient involvement in these preference-sensitive decisions, clinicians should assess their patients' health literacy levels in order to tailor their approach, and, in turn, optimize decision-making.

Every five to seven years, the ICD requires replacement to maintain normal function. Multiple factors may influence a patient's decision to replace it including the risks of the surgical procedure, changes in health status and goals since the ICD's initial implantation, and the experience of living with an ICD [76]. In a large teaching hospital, 55 of 106 (51.9%) patients were unaware of ICD replacement as a noncompulsory option [77]. Misunderstandings regarding ICD function and overestimation of device benefits were commonly reported. Yet, 83.0% of patients placed great importance on a discussion of risks and benefits of continued ICD therapy before making a decision. Shared decision making interventions for this patient population are limited to patient decision aids focused on the decision to implant an ICD [78,79]. No interventions exist to support patients when facing ICD replacement.

To better engage patients facing ICD replacement in shared decision making and to support those with lower health literacy, we created a patient decision aid to be delivered with decision coaching. In an ambulatory care clinic within a tertiary care hospital, patients with ICDs have the battery status and device function monitored by nurses every six months; thereby providing lead time for preparing patients to participate in this decision. The ICD replacement patient decision aid was developed using the best available scientific evidence, the International Patient Decision Aid Standards, and a user-centered design. We established a team including researchers with expertise in patient decision aids, health care professionals, the clinic manager, and patients who have faced ICD replacement with their spouse. Drafts were iteratively developed with feedback from the development team, as well as from interviews with the ambulatory care clinic nurses, physicians, a psychologist, a palliative care expert, patients with ICDs and their family. The readability level of the final version of the patient decision aid was Flesh-Kincaid level at 4.3. Concurrently, a decision coaching protocol was developed for the nurses guiding patients in the process of decision making. In a pilot study, the shared decision making interventions were integrated into the process of care: relevant patients were identified, nurses were trained in decision coaching, and cardiologists who would facilitate shared decision-making with undecided patients were selected to ensure consistency in the new approach.

In summary, shared decision making interventions to enhance health literacy need to be used within a supportive healthcare environment. Clinicians and decision coaches must be willing and able to screen for patients with lower health literacy, and be sufficiently skilled to embed health literacy practices, communication strategies and shared decision making interventions in their consultations to support patients to understand, communicate with others, and critically apply the information [9,80]. By using these shared decision-making interventions, patients can be meaningfully engaged in their healthcare.

Appendix B. Shared Decision Making in Children with Diabetes and Their Parents

Ensuring parent and child access to good quality information for participation in healthcare decisions is a health policy priority [81]. This requires delivery of good quality information; understandable and tailored to the family's specific needs (e.g., appropriate to age, cognitive and personal abilities, and reading levels). The following case outlines how decision coaching using a patient decision aid was used to improve child and parent health literacy and their involvement in shared decision making.

Liam is a 12-year old boy who was diagnosed with Type 1 diabetes several years ago. Since diagnosis, blood glucose management was achieved using long acting basal insulin with rapid acting insulin given at meal time. Overall, Liam's glucose management has been within the target range. Liam's parents are content with the current diabetes management approach as it is familiar and has worked well. However, Liam is becoming increasingly self-conscious about his diabetes. His concerns and challenges include carrying and storing insulin, limitations and inflexibility regarding eating with friends (e.g., eating out, parties), and fluctuating insulin levels when participating in team sports. Liam and his parents have an appointment with the pediatric endocrinologist to explore diabetes management options.

Screening for health literacy revealed Liam and his family are familiar with diabetes medical terminology and treatment goals as they are experienced in diabetes management. Liam's reading level is approximately grade 6 and his parents' is grade 8. Liam tends to be passive during consultations, leaving the discussions to occur between the clinician and his parents. This has caused difficulties at home regarding treatment adherence when Liam is not in agreement with the chosen management strategy.

During the consultation with the pediatric endocrinologist, Liam and his parents are informed on the available insulin delivery options include the status quo of daily injections or changing to an insulin pump. This decision is preference-sensitive (e.g., the best choice depends on how Liam and his parent's weigh the benefits and harms) and has implications for both Liam and his parents regarding benefits, risks and inconveniences. To make an informed decision, both Liam and his parents need to understand the options and the risks and benefits of each option.

This pediatric endocrinology clinic uses decision coaching with a patient decision aid to help facilitate child and parent preparation for shared decision making [82]. The decision coach is a trained social worker who is part of the diabetes team. The decision coach's role is non-directive and focused on guiding Liam and his parents in the process of decision making by helping them: recognize the decision being made, understand the options and the benefits and harms of those options; clarify both Liam's and his parents' values regarding benefits and harms of each option; identify Liam's and his parents' preferred option; assess the presence of pressure from others; and, screen for remaining decisional needs [82]. The patient decision aid provides a structured guide

Ottawa Family Decision Guide
For Families Facing Tough Health or Social Decisions

❶ Clarify the decision.

What decision do you face?	Youth: What is the best insulin treatment plan for me? Parent(s): What is the best insulin treatment plan for my child?

What is your reason for making this decision?

When do you need to make a choice?

How far along are you with making a choice?
- ☐ Have not thought about options
- ☐ Thinking about options
- ☐ Close to making a choice
- ☐ Made a choice

❷ Explore your decision.

Knowledge: Below, list the options and main benefits and harms you already know. Underline the benefits and harms that you think are most likely to happen.

Values: Use stars (+) to show how much each benefit and harm matters to you. 5 stars means "a lot". No stars means "not at all".

Certainty: Circle the option with the benefits that matter most to you and are most likely to happen.

	Reasons to choose this option (Benefits/Advantages/Pros)	How much it matters to you Add + s/ Child/Youth	Parent(s)	Reasons to avoid this option (Harms/Disadvantages/Cons)	How much it matters to you Add + s/ Child/Youth	Parent(s)
Option #1 Standard insulin therapy (2 or 3 injections / day)	Do not have to think about diabetes as often			Probably won't control blood sugar as well as MDI or a pump		
	Record keeping is simpler			Higher risk of overnight and severe low blood sugars than with MDI or a pump		
	Least expensive regimen			Needs consistent timing of meals/snacks and carb content		
	When not mixing insulins, can use insulin pens for injection					
Option #2 Multiple daily injections (MDI)	May improve A1c levels			More injections (with every meal and snack)		
	Least likely to have overnight or severe low blood sugar reactions			Diabetes more visible to others than with standard therapy		
	More flexibility with food and activity than with standard therapy			Need to do carb counting at every meal and snack		
	Can use insulin pens with each injection			Need to check BG 4X / day plus some post meal BGs		
Option #3 Insulin pump therapy	Offers greatest flexibility with daily activities and meals			Need to check BG 6-10 times per day including overnight		
	Least likely to have overnight or severe low blood sugar reactions			Need to do accurate carb counting at every meal and snack		
	May improve A1c			Increased risk of DKA because pump tubing can block		
	Easiest for adjusting insulin for illness, sports and other activities			Parents / caregivers need to be more involved with diabetes care		
	Fewer injections			Others more likely to notice that you have diabetes		

	Child / Youth			Parent(s)		
Which option do you prefer?	☐ #1	☐ #2	☐ #3 ☐ Unsure	☐ #1	☐ #2	☐ #3 ☐ Unsure

❸ Support

	Child / Youth				Parent(s)			
Who else is involved?	Option you think this person prefers? #1 #2 #3 Unsure				Option you think this person prefers? #1 #2 #3 Unsure			
	☐	☐	☐	☐	☐	☐	☐	☐
	☐	☐	☐	☐	☐	☐	☐	☐
	☐	☐	☐	☐	☐	☐	☐	☐
What role do you prefer in making the choice?	☐ Share with others ☐ Decide myself after hearing views of others ☐ Someone else decides Who?				☐ Share with others ☐ Decide myself after hearing views of others ☐ Someone else decides Who?			
Are you choosing without pressure from others?	☐ Yes ☐ No				☐ Yes ☐ No			

❹ Identify your decision making needs.

			Child / Youth	Parents
	Knowledge	Do you know the benefits and harms of each option?	☐ Yes ☐ No	☐ Yes ☐ No
	Values	Are you clear about which benefits and harms matter most to you?	☐ Yes ☐ No	☐ Yes ☐ No
	Support	Do you have enough support & advice to make a choice?	☐ Yes ☐ No	☐ Yes ☐ No
	Certainty	Do you feel sure about the best choice?	☐ Yes ☐ No	☐ Yes ☐ No

People who answer "No" to one or more of these questions have decision making needs. They are more likely to delay their decision, change their mind, feel regret about their choice or blame others for bad outcomes.
The SURE Test © O'Connor and Légaré, 2008

❺ Plan the next steps based on your needs.

Decision making needs	Things you would like to try...
Knowledge If you feel you do NOT have enough facts	☐ Find out more about the options and the chances of benefits and harms. ☐ List your questions and note where to find the answers (e.g. library, health professionals, counselors):
Values If you are NOT sure which benefits and harms matter most to you	☐ Review the stars in Step 2 to see what matters most to you. ☐ Find people who know what it's like to experience the benefits and harms. ☐ Talk to others who have made the decision. ☐ Read stories of what mattered most to others. ☐ Discuss with others what matters most to you.
Support If you feel you do NOT have enough support	☐ Discuss your options with a trusted person (e.g. health professional, family, friends). ☐ Find help to support your choice (e.g. funds, transport, child care).
If you feel PRESSURE from others to make a specific choice	☐ Focus on the opinions of others who matter most. ☐ Share your guide with others. ☐ Ask another person involved to fill in this guide. Find areas of agreement. When you disagree on facts, agree to get more information. When you disagree on what matters most, respect the person's opinion. Take turns to listen to what the other person says matters most to them. ☐ Find a neutral person to help you and others involved in the decision.
Certainty If you feel UNSURE about the best choice for you	☐ Work through steps 2 and 4, focusing on your needs.
Other factors making the decision DIFFICULT:	List anything else you need:

Children's Hospital of Eastern Ontario Family Decision Services www.cheo.on.ca/en/DecisionServices
Content editors: Lawson ML, Balanger E, Dolin R, Lemont S, Palard G, Richardson C.
Based on information from: 2008 Clinical Practice Guidelines Expert Committee. Canadian Diabetes Association 2008 Clinical Practice Guidelines for the Prevention and Management of Diabetes in Canada. Can J Diabetes. 32 (Suppl 1), S1-201. 2008.
Format editors: Lawson ML, Gwadinski A, Krsnoutchko J, Boland L, Pesardis S, Stacey D. Based on the Ottawa Personal Decision Guide © O'Connor, Jacobsen, Stacey, University of Ottawa, Ottawa Hospital Research Institute, Canada, 2011. © Children's Hospital of Eastern Ontario, 2015.

Figure 2. Patient decision aid for insulin delivery in pediatrics (3 pages).

for the decision coach to facilitate and document the decision making process (see Figure 2). The evidence on each option with the associated risks and benefits in the patient decision aid was based on diabetes management clinical practice guidelines [83].

To facilitate value clarification, the decision coach asks the family to rate how much each risk and benefit matters to them on a scale of 0 to 5 [82]. To engage Liam, discourage biasing his responses, and to minimize power-imbalances, the decision coach asks Liam the questions first and then the parents. Then, the decision coach helps to facilitate discussions and mediate disagreement based on child/parent responses. A copy of the decision aid is printed for the family as a reference and to facilitate communication with the pediatric endocrinologist. Another copy is included in the chart for documenting the discussion and communicating with others on the team.

This interprofessional shared decision making intervention adopts several approaches to address the family's health literacy needs. These include: plain language, appropriate reading levels, organized and user friendly material, multi-modalities to convey information (i.e., written and verbal), and increased face time with a healthcare professional (i.e., decision coach) guiding the decision making process [72]. These shared decision making interventions have been evaluated in a pre-/post-test field testing study with 7 families considering insulin delivery options for their child ages 9 to 17 years with type 1 diabetes [82]. Outcomes indicated the intervention was feasible and acceptable to the participants; particularly those early in the decision making process. A full pre/post study was subsequently conducted to evaluate the shared decision making intervention [84]. Preliminary results, from 45 families (45 youth and 66 parents), showed statistically significant reductions in parent and youth decisional conflict after the shared decision making intervention. As well, youth and parents showed improved agreement regarding the best treatment option and perceived preparation for decision making. Parents and youth were generally satisfied with the intervention.

In summary, children and parents have varying health literacy needs that must be addressed to ensure they can participate in health decision making. Interventions targeting both the child and parents have been developed and tailored to support their involvement in health decision making. As such, shared decision making interventions can play a critical role in ensuring children and their parents have the capacity to understand and utilise information to promote quality decisions.

References

[1] North American Nursing Diagnosis Association. Tenth Conference for Classification of Nursing Diagnose, The Author; 1992.
[2] Coulter A, Jenkinson C. European patients' views on the responsiveness of health systems and healthcare providers. European J Public Health. 2005;15(4):355-60. DOI: 10.1093/eurpub/cki004.
[3] Kiesler DJ, Auerbach SM. Optimal matches of patient preferences for information, decision-making and interpersonal behaviour: Evidence, models and interventions. Patient Educ Couns. 2006;61:319-41. DOI: 10.1016/j.pec.2005.08.002.
[4] Mulley AG, Trimble C, Elwyn G. Stop the silent misdiagnosis: Patients' preferences matter. BMJ. 2012;345:e6572. DOI: 10.1136/bmj.e6572.
[5] Makoul G, Clayman ML. An integrative model of shared decision making in medical encounters. Patient Educ Couns. 2006;60(3):301-12. DOI: 10.1016/j.pec.2005.06.010.
[6] Sepucha KR, Fowler FJ, Mulley AG. Policy support for patient-centered care: The need for measurable improvements in decision quality. Health Affairs. 2004;Suppl VAR:54-62. DOI: 10.1377/hlthaff.var. 54.
[7] Elwyn G, O'Connor A, Stacey D, Volk R, Edwards A, Coulter A, et al. Developing a quality criteria framework for patient decision aids: online international Delphi consensus process. BMJ. 2006; 333(7565):417-22. DOI: 10.1136/bmj.38926.629329.AE.
[8] Nutbeam D. Health literacy as a public health goal: a challenge for contemporary health education and communication strategies into the 21st century. Health Promot Int. 2000;15:259-67. DOI: 10.1093/heapro/15.3.259.
[9] Koh H, Rudd R. The arc of health literacy. JAMA. 2015;314(12):1225-6. DOI: 10.1001/jama.2015. 9978.

[10] Phillips CB. Improving health outcomes for linguistically diverse patients. Med J Aust. 2016; 204(6):209-10. DOI: 10.5694/mja16.00009.
[11] Degner LF, Sloan JA, Venkatesh P. The control preferences scale. Can J Nurs Res. 1997;29(3):21-43.
[12] Emanuel EJ, Emanuel LL. Four models of the physician-patient relationship. JAMA. 1992;267(16): 2221-6.
[13] http://www.ama-assn.org/ama/pub/about-ama/our-history/history-ama-ethics.page?, Retrieved date: October 6, 2016.
[14] Shafir A, Rosenthal J. Shared decision making: advancing patient-centered care through state and federal implementation. Washington, D.C.: National Academy for State Health Policy, 2012.
[15] Committee on Quality of Health Care in American. Crossing the Quality Chasm: A new health system for the 21st century. Washington, D.C.: Institute of Medicine, 2001.
[16] Legare F, Stacey D, Gagnon S, Dunn S, Pluye P, Frosch D, et al. Validating a conceptual model for an interprofessional approach to shared decision making: A mixed methods study. J Eval Clin Pract. 2011; 17(4):554-64. DOI: 10.1111/j.1365-2753.2010.01515.x.
[17] Legare F, Stacey D, Pouliot S, Gauvin FP, Desroches S, Kryworuchko J, et al. Interprofessionalism and shared decision-making in primary care: A stepwise approach towards a new model. J Interprof Care. 2011;25(1):18-25. DOI: 10.3109/13561820.2010.490502.
[18] Gabe J, Olumide G, Bury M. It takes three to tango: A framework for understanding patient partnership in paediatric clinics. Soc Sci Med. 2004;59(5):1071-9. DOI: 10.1016/j.socscimed.2003.09.035.
[19] Hibbard JH, Greene J. What the evidence shows about patient activation: Better health outcomes and care experiences. Health Affairs. 2013;32(2):207-14. DOI: 10.1377/hlthaff.2012.1061.
[20] Hack TF, Degner LF, Watson P, Sinha L. Do patients benefit from participating in medical decision making? Longitudinal follow-up of women with breast cancer. Psychooncology. 2006;15:9-19. DOI: 10.1002/pon.907.
[21] Gattellari M, Butow PN, Tattersall MHN. Sharing decisions in cancer care. Soc Sci Med. 2001;52: 1865-78.
[22] Coulter A. Engaging patients in their healthcare. How is the UK doing relative to other countries? Oxford, UK: Picker Institute Europe; 2006.
[23] https://www.healthcare.gov/glossary/patient-protection-and-affordable-care-act/ Retrieved October 7, 2016.
[24] http://www.washingtonvotes.org/2007-SB-5930. Retrieved October 7, 2016.
[25] Chow S, Teare G, Basky G. Shared decision making: Helping the system and patients make quality health care decisions. Saskatoon, Saskatchewan, Canada: Health Quality Council, 2009.
[26] http://www.safetyandquality.gov.au/our-work/patient-and-consumer-centred-care/health-literacy/. Retrieved October 7, 2016.
[27] McCaffery KJ, Holmes-Rovner M, Smith SK, Rovner D, Nutbeam D, Clayman ML, et al. Addressing health literacy in patient decision aids. BMC Med Inform Decis Mak. 2013;13 (Suppl 2):1-14. DOI: 10.1186/1472-6947-13-S2-S10.
[28] Stacey D, Legare F, Col NF, Bennett CL, Barry MJ, Eden KB, et al. Decision aids for people facing health treatment or screening decisions. Cochrane Database Syst Rev. 2014 (1). DOI: 10.1002/14651858.CD001431.pub4.
[29] Legare F, Turcotte S, Stacey D, Ratte S, Kryworuchko J, Graham ID. Patients' perceptions of sharing in decisions: A systematic review of interventions to enhance shared decision making in routine clinical practice. The Patient. 2012;5(1):1-19. DOI: 10.2165/11592180-000000000-00000.
[30] Legare F, Stacey D, Turcotte S, Cossi MJ, Kryworuchko J, Graham ID, et al. Interventions for improving the adoption of shared decision making by healthcare professionals (Review). Cochrane Database Syst Rev. 2014 (9):1-166. DOI: 10.1002/14651858.CD006732.pub3.
[31] Stacey D, Kryworuchko J, Belkora J, Davison BJ, Durand MA, Eden KB, et al. Coaching and guidance with patient decision aids: A review of theoretical and empirical evidence. BMC Med Inform Decis Mak. 2013;13(Suppl 2):1-11. DOI: 10.1186/1472-6947-13-S2-S11.
[32] Kinnersley P, Edwards A, Hood K, Ryan R, Prout H, Cadbury N, et al. Interventions before consultations to help patients address their information needs by encouraging question asking: systematic review. BMJ. 2008;337:a485-a94. DOI: 10.1136/bmj.a485.
[33] Bonevski BRM, Paul C, Chapman K, Twyman L, Bryant J, Brozek I, et al. Reaching the hard-to-reach: A systematic review of strategies for improving health and medical research with socially disadvantaged groups. BMC Med Res Methodol. 2014;14(42). DOI: 10.1186/1471-2288-14-42.
[34] Durand MA, Stiel M, Boivin J, Elwyn G. Where is the theory? Evaluating the theoretical frameworks described in decision support technologies. Patient Educ Couns. 2008;71(1):125-35. DOI: 10.1016/j.pec.2007.12.004.

[35] O'Connor AM, Tugwell P, Wells G, Elmslie T, Jolly E, Hollingworth G. A decision aid for women considering hormone therapy after menopause: Decision support framework and evaluation. Patient Educ Couns. 1998;33(3):267-79.

[36] Stacey D, Kryworuchko J, Bennett C, Murray MA, Mullan S, Legare F. Decision coaching to prepare patients for making health decisions: A systematic review of decision coaching in trials of patient decision aids. Med Decis Mak. 2012;32(3):E22-33. DOI: 10.1177/0272989X12443311.

[37] O'Connor AM, Stacey D, Legare F. Coaching to support patients in making decisions. BMJ. 2008;336:228-9. DOI: 10.1136/bmj.39435.643275.BE.

[38] https://decisionaid.ohri.ca/coaching.html. Retrieved October 7, 2016.

[39] Shepherd HL, Barratt A, Trevena LJ, McGeechan K, Carey K, Epstein RM, et al. Three questions that patients can ask to improve the quality of information physicians give about treatment options: A cross-over trial. Patient Educ Couns. 2011;84:379-85. DOI: 10.1016/j.pec.2011.07.022.

[40] Shepherd HL, Barratt A, Jones A, Bateson D, Carey K, Trevena LJ, et al. Can consumer learn to ask three questions to improve shared decision making? A feasibility study of the ASK (AskShareKnow) Patient-Clinician Communication Model intervention in a primary health-care setting. Health Expect. 2015:1-9. DOI: 10.1111/hex.12409.

[41] Muscat DM, Shepherd HL, Morony S, Smith SK, Dhilon HM, Trevena L, et al. Can adults with low literacy understand shared decision making questions? A qualitative investigation. Patient Educ Couns. 2016. DOI: 10.1016/j.pec.2016.05.008.

[42] Muscat D, Morony S, Smith S, Dhillon H, Shepherd H, Trevena L, et al. Shared decision-making training to promote empowerment, risk understanding and question-asking: Findings from a cluster-RCT with lower literacy adults. Annual North American Meeting of the Society for Medical Decision Making; Vancouver, British Columbia2016.

[43] Durand MA, Carpenter L, Dolan H, Bravo P, Mann M, Bunn F, et al. Do interventions designed to support shared decision-making reduce health inequalities? A systematic review and meta-analysis. PLoS One. 2014;9(4):1-14. DOI: 10.1371/journal.pone.0094670.

[44] https://decisionaid.ohri.ca/eval.html. Retrieved October 7, 2016.

[45] Martenson E, Fagerskiold A. A review of children's decision-making competence in health care. Journal of Clinical Nursing. 2008;17(23):3131-41. DOI: 10.1111/j.1365-2702.2006.01920.x.

[46] Jackson C, Cheater FM, Reid I. A systematic review of decision support needs of parents making child health decisions. Health Expect. 2008;11(3):232-51. DOI: 10.1111/j.1369-7625.2008.00496.x.

[47] Wyatt KD, List B, Brinkman WB, Prutsky G, Asi N, Erwin PJ, et al. Shared decision making in pediatrics: A systematic review and meta-analysis. Acad Pediatr. 2015. DOI: 10.1016/j.acap.2015.03.011.

[48] Feenstra B. Evaluating interventions to support child-parent involvement in health decisions: University of Ottawa; 2012.

[49] Couet N, Desroches S, Robitaille H, Vaillancourt H, LeBlanc A, Turcotte S, et al. Assessments of the extent to which health-care providers involve patients in decision making: A systematic review of studies using the OPTION instrument. Health Expect. 2013;epub Jan 2013:1-20. DOI: 10.1111/hex.12054.

[50] Baker R, Camosso-Stefinovic J, Gillies C, Shaw EJ, Cheater F, Flottorp S, et al. Tailored interventions to overcome identified barriers to change: effects on professional practice and health care outcomes. Cochrane Database Syst Rev. 2010 (3):1-80. DOI: 10.1002/14651858.CD005470.pub2.

[51] Bosch M, van der Weijden T, Wensing M, Grol R. Tailoring quality improvement interventions to identified barriers: A multiple case analysis. J Eval Clin Pract. 2007;13:161-8. DOI: 10.1111/j.1365-2753.2006.00660.x.

[52] Joseph-Williams N, Elwyn G, Edwards A. Knowledge is not power for patients: A systematic review and thematic synthesis of patient-reported barriers and facilitators to shared decision making. Patient Educ Couns. 2014;94(3):291-309. DOI: 10.1016/j.pec.2013.10.031.

[53] Legare F, Ratte S, Gravel K, Graham ID. Barriers and facilitators to implementing shared decision-making in clinical practice: Update of a systematic review of health professionals' perceptions. Patient Educ Couns. 2008;73(3):526-35. DOI: 10.1016/j.pec.2008.07.018.

[54] Smith SK, Dixon A, Trevena L, Nutbeam D, McCaffery KJ. Exploring patient involvement in healthcare decision making across different education and functional health literacy groups. Soc Sci Med. 2009;69(12):1805-12. DOI: 10.1016/j.socscimed.2009.09.056.

[55] Legare F, Thompson-Leduc P. Twelve myths about shared decision making. Patient Educ Couns. 2014. 96(3):281-6. DOI: 10.1016/j.pec.2014.06.014.

[56] Legare F, Politi M, Drolet R, Desroches S, Stacey D, Bekker H, et al. Training health professionals in shared decision making: An international environmental scan. Patient Educ Couns. 2012;88(2):159-69. DOI: 10.1016/j.pec.2012.01.002.

[57]   Legare F, Moumjid-Ferdjaoui N, Drolet R, Stacey D, Harter M, Bastian H, et al. Core competencies for shared decision making training programs: Insights from an international, interdisciplinary working group. J Contin Educ Health Prof. 2013;33(4):267-73. DOI: 10.1002/chp.21197.
[58]   Dwamena F, Holmes-Rovner M, Gaulden CM, Jorgenson S, Sadigh G, Sikorskii A, et al. Interventions for providers to promote a patient-centred approach in clinical consultations. Cochrane Database Sys Rev. 2012 (12). DOI: 10.1002/14651858.CD003267.pub2.
[59]   Bylund CL, Goytia EJ, D'Agostino TA, Bulone L, Horner J, Li Y, et al. Evaluation of a Pilot Communication Skills Training Intervention for Minority Cancer Patients. J Psychosoc Oncol. 2011; 29(4):347-58.
[60]   Cegala DJ, McClure L, Marinelli TM, Post DM. The effects of communication skills training on patients' participation during medical interviews. Patient Educ Couns. 2000;41(2):209-22. DOI: S0738-3991(00)00093-8.
[61]   Saarimaki A, Stacey D. Are you using effective tools to support patients facing tough cancer-related decisions? Can Oncol Nurs J. 2013;Spring:137-40.
[62]   https://decisionaid.ohri.ca/decguide.html. Retrieved October 7, 2016.
[63]   Jull J, Giles A, Boyer Y, Stacey D. Cultural adaptation of a shared decision making tool with Aboriginal women: a qualitative study. BMC Med Inform Decis Mak. 2015;15:1. DOI:10.1186/s12911-015-0129-7.
[64]   National Institute for Health and Care Excellence. Patient experience in adult NHS services: Improving the experience of care for people using adult NHS services. London, U.K.: National Clinical Guideline Centre, 2012.
[65]   www.nice.org.uk/about/what-we-do/our-programmes/nice-guidance/nice-guidelines/shared-decision-making. Retrieved October 6, 2016
[66]   www.hca.wa.gov/hw/Documents/sdm_cert_criteria.pdf. Retrieved October 7, 2016.
[67]   Legare F, Kearing S, Clay K, Gagnon S, D'Amour D, Rousseau M, et al. Are you SURE? Assessing patient decisional conflict with a 4-item screening test. Can Fam Physician. 2010;56(8):e308-e14.
[68]   O'Connor AM. Validation of a Decisional Conflict Scale. Med Decis Mak. 1995;15(1):25-30.
[69]   Ferron Parayre A, Labrecque M, Rousseau M, Turcotte S, Legare F. Validation of SURE, a four-item clinical checklist for detecting decisional conflict in patients. Med Decis Mak. 2013;34(1):54-62. DOI: 10.1177/0272989X13491463.
[70]   Butow P, Juraskova I, Chang S, Lopez AL, Brown R, Bernhard J. Shared decision making coding systems: How do they compare in the oncology context? Patient Educ Couns. 2010;78(2):261-8.
[71]   Kasper J, Heesen C, Kopke S, Fulcher G, Geiger F. Patients' and observers' perceptions of involvement differ. Validation study on inter-relating measures for shared decision making. PLoS One. 2011;6(10):e26255. DOI: 10.1371/journal.pone.0026255.
[72]   Betterham RW, Hawkins M, Collins PA, Buchbinder R, Osborne RH. Health literacy: applying current concepts to improve health services and reduce health inequalities. Public Health 2016;132:3-12. DOI: 10.1016/j.puhe.2016.01.001.
[73]   Epstein AE, Dimarco JP, Ellenbogen KA, Estes NA, 3rd, Freedman RA, Gettes LS, et al. ACC/AHA/HRS 2008 Guidelines for device-based therapy of cardiac rhythm abnormalities. Heart Rhythm. 2008 Jun;5(6):e1-62. DOI:10.1016/j.hrthm.2008.04.014.
[74]   Hickey KT, Sciacca RR, Gonzalez P, Castillo C, Frulla A. Assessing Health Literacy in Urban Patients With Implantable Cardioverter Defibrillators and Pacemakers. J Cardiovasc Nurs. 2015 Sep-Oct;30(5): 428-34. DOI: 10.1097/jcn.0000000000000184.
[75]   Lewis KB, Stacey D, Matlock DD. Making decisions about implantable cardioverter-defibrillators from implantation to end of life: an integrative review of patients' perspectives. Patient. 2014;7(3):243-60. DOI: 10.1007/s40271-014-0055-2.
[76]   Kramer DB, Buxton AE, Zimetbaum PJ. Time for a change – a new approach to ICD replacement. NEJM. 2012 Jan 26;366(4):291-3. DOI: 10.1056/NEJMp1111467.
[77]   Lewis KB, Nery PB, Birnie DH. Decision making at the time of ICD generator change: patients' perspectives. JAMA Intern Med. 2014 Sep;174(9):1508-11. DOI: 10.1001/jamainternmed.2014.3435.
[78]   https://decisionaid.ohri.ca/AZinvent.php. Retrieved October 7, 2016.
[79]   Carroll SL, McGillion M, Stacey D, Healey JS, Browne G, Arthur HM, et al. Development and feasibility testing of decision support for patients who are candidates for a prophylactic implantable defibrillator: a study protocol for a pilot randomized controlled trial. Trials. 2013;14:346. DOI: 10.1186/1745-6215-14-346.
[80]   Coleman CA, Hudson S, Maine LL. Health literacy practices and educational competencies for health professionals: a consensus study. J Health Commun. 2013;18 Suppl 1:82-102. DOI: 10.1080/10810730.2013.829538.
[81]   Patient- and family-centered care and the pediatrician's role. Pediatrics. 2012 Feb;129(2):394-404. DOI: 10.1542/peds.2011-3084.

[82] Feenstra B, Lawson ML, Harrison D, Boland L, Stacey D. Decision coaching using the Ottawa family decision guide with parents and their children: A field testing study. BMC Med Inform Decis Mak. 2015;15(5):1-10. DOI: 10.1186/s12911-014-0126-2.

[83] Clinical Practice Guidelines Committees. Canadian Diabetes Association 2008 Clinical Practice Guidelines for the Prevention and Management of Diabetes in Canada. Can J Diabetes. 2008;32:S1-S201.

[84] Lawson ML, Shephard AL, Feenstra B, Boland L, Sourial N, Elliott-Miller P, et al. Shared decision making in pediatric type I diabetes: Evaluation of decision coaching with a patient decision aid. Society Med Decis Mak; St. Louis, MO2015. p. IS 9051.

284

Health Literacy
R.A. Logan and E.R. Siegel (Eds.)
IOS Press, 2017
© 2017 The authors and IOS Press. All rights reserved.
doi:10.3233/978-1-61499-790-0-284

Engaging Patients in Decision-Making and Behavior Change to Promote Prevention

Alex H. KRIST,[1,a] Sebastian T. TONG,[a] Rebecca A. AYCOCK,[a] Daniel R. LONGO[a]

a Department of Family Medicine and Population Health, Virginia Commonwealth University, Richmond, VA USA

Abstract. Effectively engaging patients in their care is essential to improve health outcomes, improve satisfaction with the care experience, reduce costs, and even benefit the clinician experience. This chapter will address the topic of patient engagement directly and review the relationships between health literacy and patient engagement. While there are many ways to define patient and family engagement, this chapter will consider engagement as "patients, families, their representatives, and health professionals working in active partnership at various levels across the health care system – direct care, organizational design and governance, and policy making – to improve health and health care [1]." We will specifically focus on the patient engagement and health literacy needs for three scenarios (1) decision-making, (2) health behavior change, and (3) chronic disease management; we will include the theoretical underpinnings of engagement, the systems required to better support patient engagement, how social determinants of health influence patient engagement, and practical examples to demonstrate approaches to better engage patients in their health and wellbeing. We will close by describing the future of patient engagement, which extends beyond the traditional domains of decision-making and self-care to describe how patient engagement can influence the design of the healthcare delivery system; local, state, and national health policies; and future research relevant to the needs and experiences of patients.

Keywords. Patient engagement, patient activation, patient education, health literacy, social determinants of health, delivery of healthcare

1. Introduction

This chapter addresses the topic of patient engagement directly and reviews the relationships between health literacy and patient engagement. While there are many ways to define patient and family engagement, this chapter considers engagement as "patients, families, their representatives, and health professionals working in active partnership at various levels across the health care system – direct care, organizational design and governance, and policy making – to improve health and health care." The authors specifically focus on the patient engagement and health literacy needs for three scenarios: (1) decision-making, (2) health behavior change, and (3) chronic disease management. The chapter addresses the theoretical underpinnings of engagement, the

---

[1] Corresponding Author: Alex H. Krist, One Capital Square Room 631, 830 East Main Street, Richmond VA 23219; E-mail: alexander.krist@vcuhealth.org.

systems required to better support patient engagement, how social determinants of health influence patient engagement, and practical examples to demonstrate approaches to better engage patients in their health and wellbeing. The chapter closes by describing the future of patient engagement, which extends beyond the traditional domains of decision-making and self-care to describe how patient engagement can influence the design of the healthcare delivery system; local, state, and national health policies; and research relevant to the needs and experiences of patients. The specific subtopics covered in the chapter are: the need for patient engagement; engaging patients to better understand decisions; engaging patients to improve health behaviors; engaging patients to improve chronic disease management; the influence of health's social determinants on engagement; health information seeking behaviors and engagement; as well as future directions.

2. The Need for Patient Engagement

Several U.S. studies recently reported coordinated care trials that actively engaged patients with chronic disease resulted in significant mortality reductions compared to a control group who only took appropriate medications [2-4]. The studies suggest chronically ill patient who are engaged in their care live longer than unengaged peers who otherwise receive similar treatment [2-4]. In other words, health and wellbeing are fostered by engaged and activated patients, who collaborate with their clinician to better manage care. In summarizing the hypothetical impact of widespread patient engagement on contemporary health care, Kish described the influence would be analogous to the introduction of a once-in-a-century blockbuster drug [5].

In addition, patient engagement demarcates an increasing shift from more paternalistic models of care in which clinicians tell patients what they should do (and often ineffectively), to one in which clinicians partner with patients. The collaborative partnership is intended to: help make better medical decisions; educate patients about how to stay healthy and manage conditions; develop systems and supports to activate patients; and sustain patient interest in their ongoing care.

The U.S. Institute of Medicine's landmark report, Crossing the Quality Chasm, emphasized healthcare providers should be "respectful of and responsive to individual patient preferences, needs, and values," and ensure "patient values guide all clinical decisions [6]." In the U.S., the idea of engaging patients also has been advanced by the research funded by the Patient Centered Outcomes Research Institute (PCORI) and it is at the heart of national healthcare initiatives, such as Meaningful Use and the Medicare shared-savings program for Accountable Care Organizations [7,8].

So why is patient engagement important in health care? What additional evidence is there to support the need to engage patients? What is the effect of varied health literacy on effective engagement? To begin, the need for patient engagement is posited as foundational because most adults spend little time in health care facilities and frequently are on their own to make appropriate, daily health decisions. This means patients need to be in control and the drivers of their health. Patient engagement further has an (a) ethical basis – engagement supports patient autonomy and self-determination, (b) interpersonal basis – engagement promotes confidence and trust in the clinician-patient relationship, and (c) educational basis – engagement improves knowledge, sets reasonable expectations, and reduces decisional conflict.

There is a practical need for engaging patients in their care as well. Many medical decisions have a trade-off of benefits and harms and sometimes there is a close balance of benefit to harm. Only by including patient values and preferences can a good decision be made [9]. Chronic disease management and health behavior change both must be done by the patient. Without complete buy-in and understanding of care and needed changes, a patient will not be able to effectively manage their health. Ultimately, the patient must suffer or enjoy the outcomes associated with any medical decision, test, treatment, or health behavior change.

In an international study of patients with "complex health needs" spanning 11 industrialized countries and focusing on the relationship between engagement and health care quality, substantial differences in the level of patient engagement between countries was identified. Consistently, countries with higher levels of engagement had better quality of care, lower medical error rates, and greater satisfaction in the experience of care [10]. Four case studies in diverse countries and health care settings further show the importance of engaging patients and the resulting improvements in health care quality and outcomes [11]. Collectively these findings demonstrate how patient engagement shifts the clinical paradigm from "what is the matter?" to more meaningfully discovering "what matters to you?"

There is a growing literature on how patient engagement impacts the experience and delivery of care. Minority patients frequently receive lower rates of preventive services. They suffer delays in diagnosis of diseases such as cancer, and once identified they even suffer delays in treatment. In a recent study, Sheppard has found that medical mistrust may contribute to these problems, something that could be overcome through effective patient engagement [12]. Survey data collected by Arora from cancer survivors demonstrates that better engagement increases the perception of personal control, increases trust, and decreases uncertainty [13]. Torres demonstrated that clinician communication styles are critically important to effective patient engagement and "good" communication creates a sense of not being rushed, a feeling like the clinician understands the patient, and a partnership built on trust [14]. Effective communication to better engage a diverse spectrum of patients with varying levels health literacy needs to be learned by all clinicians.

A review of proven strategies to enhance patient engagement identified three focus areas for engagement: improving health literacy, helping patients make appropriate health decisions, and improving the quality of care processes [15]. The Health Literate Care Model is an important tool to inform how attention to health literacy can improve patient engagement [16]. This model encourages clinicians to approach "all patients with the assumption that they are at risk of not understanding their health conditions or how to deal with them, and then subsequently confirming and ensuring patients' understanding." Across the spectrum of healthcare delivery, full engagement of the patient requires the patient to be able to obtain, process and communicate health information. Strategies to ensure that engagement activities are appropriate for a patient's health literacy can include adapting and simplifying language to decrease the risk of misunderstanding, providing examples that are relevant to the individual's lifestyle and cultural context, using visual representations of data, and integrating decision aids into care [17]. In a health literate care model, information needs to be presented in a manner that is congruent with a patient's ability to understand the material and span the domains in which health care occurs – the clinical setting, home, and community.

3. Engaging Patients TO Better Understand Decisions

3.1. The Evolution of Patient Engagement for Decision-Making

Engaging patients in health care decision-making has significant benefits. Patients who participate in their decisions report higher levels of satisfaction with their care; have increased knowledge about conditions, tests, and treatment; have more realistic expectations about benefits and harms; are more likely to adhere to screening, diagnostic, or treatment plans; have reduced decisional conflict and anxiety; are less likely to receive tests or procedures which may be unnecessary; and, in some cases, even have improved health outcomes [18-20].

Engaging patients in decisions has its basic grounding in the Nuremburg code which originated, mandated, and defined informed consent as a requirement for involving participants in research. Informed consent is the concept that individuals must be aware and understand what will be asked of them if they choose to participate and the risks and benefits of participating in a study. The information must be presented in a way that facilitates complete understanding – irrespective of the person's health literacy. In the mid-1970s, informed consent was extended to clinical practice requiring clinicians to disclose the risks and benefits of a medical procedure and then obtain patient permission before the procedure rather than patients simply yielding to, or complying with proposed medical care [21]. While this represents an improvement in patient engagement, it was mainly applied to surgical procedures and most efforts focused on getting signed consent rather than ensuring patient involvement in decision-making or even ensuring full comprehension of the procedure and alternatives [22,23].

3.2. Key Components of Shared and Informed Decision-Making

In the mid-1980's, informed consent evolved in to a more collaborative relationship between patients and clinicians, where both parties shared information and came to joint decisions. The closely related concepts of informed decision-making and shared decision-making emerged. Shared decision-making has been defined as, "an approach where clinicians and patients share the best available evidence when faced with the task of making decisions, and where patients are supported to consider options, to achieve informed preferences [24]." In this model, the clinician's role is to elicit the patient's understanding, values, or reasoning and serve as a partner in decision making. According to the U.S. Preventive Services Task Force (USPSTF), shared decision-making within the patient-clinician partnership universally encompasses a process in which both the patient and clinician share information with each other, take steps to participate in the decision-making process, and agree on a course of action [9].

Braddock defined seven elements that informed decision-making: (1) discussion of the patients role in decision making, (2) discussion of the clinical issue, (3) discussion of alternatives, (4) discussion of the pros and cons of alternatives, (5) discussion of uncertainties, (6) assessment of patient understanding, and (7) exploration of patient preference [25]. Braddock acknowledged that medical decisions vary in complexity and these elements will be employed to varying degrees depending on how straight forward or complex the decision. Embedded in each element is a recognition that in order for a patient to fully engage in any discussion there is need for the patient to have some health literacy. Clinicians should approach decision steps with attention to the patient's literacy needs and assess the patient's knowledge and understanding throughout.

3.3. Implementing Patient Engagement for Decision-Making

While some medical decisions are straightforward with one clear "right" choice, most decisions have multiple options each with a different set of advantages and disadvantages for patients and clinicians to consider. For some decisions, it is important to incorporate clinical information such as individual patient risks, the specifics of the condition, comorbidities, and potential prognoses. While this may be done by clinicians without much patient engagement, often patients may be the only source that knows, or has at least experienced all their medical history. Patient engagement is critical to ensure that all the medical information is being incorporated into these decisions. For other decisions, it may be more important to include patient's values, preferences, likelihood for adherence, and life circumstances. This scenario clearly involves patient engagement as only patients know this information. Effective discussions include both clinicians sharing clinical information about the options and patients sharing information about themselves.

Common examples of medical decisions include whether and how to make a health behavior changes, when to start and how to get preventive screening, management for acute or chronic conditions, how to prioritize competing health needs, and even when to change or stop a treatment. Some decisions are routine and occur frequently in practice such as when to start screening for breast cancer or how to be tested for colorectal cancer [26-29]. In one U.S. primary care setting, nearly one in five patients seen for an office visit faced a routine decision about preventive care [30]. Other more major decisions, such as how to treat localized breast cancer or manage an abdominal aortic aneurysm, may only occur once in a patient's lifetime.

Traditionally, clinicians engage patients in decision-making during in-person visits. This may work well for major decisions, which occur infrequently, have obvious consequences, and may be amenable to clinicians and patients meeting on several occasions to make the decision. More routine decisions that are part of an office visit during which multiple issues are discussed are often overlooked by patients and clinicians. When asked, more than two thirds of patients report that they would like to share decisions with their clinician – routine and major. Sadly, this happens less than half the time [31,32]; conversations between clinicians and patients rarely include all elements of a good decision [31,33,34]; and while patients consider themselves knowledgeable about decisions, patients frequently have a poor understanding of the medical facts and often over-estimate the value of medical care [35].

One solution is to use decision aids and supports to help patients make medical decisions. These tools can ensure patients receive information in a standardized format that includes all critical content, presents information in a culturally appropriate manner, and uses language and images to ensure understanding across a range of health literacy needs. Decision aids are not routinely used in clinical care [36-40]. Key barriers include time, expense, perceived legitimacy, capacity, ability to integrate into workflow, lack of clinician training and comfort with decision aids, and an environment that has not made routine use a cultural norm [41]. Despite these barriers many good decision aids have been developed. A host of organizations have cataloged and made available a range of high quality decision aids tailored to a range of literacy levels and cultural norms as well as trainings and resources to help clinicians better implement shared decision-making (see Table 1, right).

TABLE 1. Organizations and resources that promote and support informed and shared decision-making for patients and clinicians

Supports	Organization
Decision aid standards	– International Patient Decision Aids Standards (IPAD3)
Library of decision aids and supports	– Agency for Healthcare Research and Quality – Effective Healthcare Program – Decision Aids – Healthwise (also available at WebMD by typing "decision" followed by health topic) – Mayo Clinic Shared Decision-Making National Resource Center – National Health Service – Decision Aids – Ottawa Hospital Decision Center
Medical decision-making societies	– American Academy on Communication Healthcare – Informed Medical Decisions Foundation – Society for Medical Decision Making
Tools to promote and implement shared decision-making in practice	– Agency for Healthcare Research and Quality – Healthcare Innovation Exchange – Dartmouth Center for Shared-Decision Making – Institute for Healthcare Improvement
Video decision aids	– Emmi – Foundation for Informed Decision-Making – Health Dialog

Krist proposes that to be effective, decision aids must also be integrated into the clinical workflow – realistically, patients undergo a "decision journey [30]." This journey requires support over time, allowing patients to contemplate options, gather additional information, confer with family and friends, consider individual preferences, and address their personal worries or concerns. Clinicians can serve as trusted advisors during this decision journey. One example of systematically supporting decision journeys is how a group of practices used their patient portal to promote cancer screening decisions (Figure 1, below). The system anticipated the patients' decision needs; delivered decision support prior to visits; allowed patients to tailor decision supports to their interests and needs; collected patient-reported information about where they were with their decision journey, what they wanted to discuss with their clinician, and their fears; shared the patient reported information with their clinician; set a decision-making agenda; and even provided follow-up on next steps [30]. Routine implementation of similar workflows and processes, whether technology-based or not, has great potential to improve care, address health literacy issues, and better engage patients in decision-making.

FIGURE 1. A workflow to better engage patients throughout their decision-making journeys

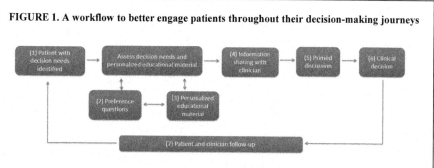

LEGEND. To better engage patients in their decisions, this workflow, which several practices programmed into their patient portal and electronic health record, guides patients and clinicians through a series of seven steps: (1) based on electronic health record data, patients with decision needs are identified, and the patient portal reaches contacts patients outside the confines of an office visit to start considering decision options; (2) the patient portal walks patients through an intake that assesses personal preferences, knowledge, needs, and readiness to make a decision; (3) the portal provides personalized educational material tailored to the patient's stated preferences and decision stage; (4) the portal allows the patient to share their preferences and decision needs with their clinician; (5) the clinician reviews the information prior to a visit, priming the discussion so the clinician is aware of the patient's needs; (6) the patient and clinicians are able to make a more informed and shared decision; and (7) the electronic health record and patient portal can follow-up with both the clinician and patient to make sure the decision is acted upon consistent with the patient's wishes (modified from Ann Fam Med 2017;in press.

4. Engaging Patients to Improve Health Behaviors

Similar to increasing patients' participation in medical decision making, clinicians need to engage patients to effect desired health behavior changes. Research has shown that incorporating patient's goals and motivations into planned behavior change increases the likelihood that a patient will be successful with behavior change. Multiple strategies have been developed to increase patient involvement in health behavior change, including the 5 As, the 5 Rs, and Motivational Interviewing. Similar to shared decision-making, each of these strategies require the clinician to elicit the patient's reasons for change and incorporate those reasons into the behavior change plan. Through this process the clinician can also ascertain a patient's understanding of their health care and address any misconceptions.

The 5As is a framework that can help guide clinician actions to better engage patients who are working towards health behavior change [42-44]. The major steps to the five As include: (1) *Ask* every patient about health behaviors, (2) *Advise* patients with an unhealthy behavior in a clear, strong, and personalized manner to modify the behavior, (3) *Assess* the patient's willingness to change the health behavior (sometimes referred to instead as seeking Agreement on the patient's willingness to change the health behavior), (4) *Assist* the patient in modifying the health behavior, and (5) *Arrange* for follow-up. For many behaviors, A1 through A3 can occur during one encounter and may take only a few moments. Conversely, A4 and A5 – assisting patients and arranging follow-up – often require intensive support extended over a period of time. For example, interventions to help patients eat right, exercise, or lose weight often take dozens of hours of face to face contact over a period of months from multiple members of a multidisciplinary team [45,46]. The exception to the intensive time and resource requirement for A4 and A5 is counseling patients to quit smoking and counseling patients against risky drinking behaviors (not treating alcoholism). A4 and A5 can be done effectively in a matter of minutes during one encounter with brief follow-up and support. While more intensive interventions to help patients quit smoking and limit risky drinking are more likely to result in lasting heath behavior changes, brief interventions for these two behaviors do have some efficacy [47,48].

For patients that are not ready to make a health behavior change, the five Rs is a tool that clinicians can use to help patients move to a stage of readiness to change their health behavior. The 5 Rs prompts the clinician to: (1) discuss the *Relevance* of the change for the patient (e.g. smoking may be contributing to your getting so many colds and missing work so often), (2) discuss the *Risks* of continuing the unhealthy behavior, (3) discuss the *Rewards* of adopting a healthy behavior, (4) identify *Roadblocks* to changing the behavior, and (5) *Repetition* of the personalized five Rs message at each visit.[49,50] The last R, Repetition, stresses the importance of reiterating the 5 Rs to help motivate patients to change behaviors whenever possible, so that when the patient is ready to make changes, the assistance and support is available.

Motivational Interviewing is a third strategy that leverages a patients' values and goals to initiate and maintain behavior change. Motivational Interviewing is defined as "a client-centered, directive method for enhancing intrinsic motivation to change by exploring and resolving ambivalence [51]." One of the key components of this definition is a patient's ability to develop intrinsic motivation which requires that he/she has a knowledge of how the behavior change directly relates to personal goals. In order to enhance intrinsic motivation, the patient must be able to relate the behavior change to their sense of self, their self in the context of family and community, and their other values and roles. Effective patient education and support tailored to the patient's needs and health literacy can increase their sense of self-efficacy. This education can help patients learn how diseases progresses and how changing behaviors can make a clear impact on their health. Making the behavior change relevant to the patient's experience may alleviate shame and guilt and instill hope that change is possible.

Sadly, unhealthy behaviors account for nearly 40% of premature deaths and substantial morbidity in the U.S. [52]. Engaging patients in health behavior change has been clearly shown to improve health and patients commonly report a clinician's advice to change an unhealthy behavior as a key motivating factor for change [53,54]. Yet few patients report being asked regularly about their health behaviors; only 10-20% of smokers report being told to quit smoking by their clinician; less than 20% of obese patients report being told by their clinician that they are overweight; and only 2-5% of patients in need of intensive diet, exercise, and weight loss counseling actually receive assistance [55,56].

There are many reasons why health behavior counseling is done poorly in practice including lack of time, competing demands, inadequate resources and support, limited training in health behavior counseling, and even lack of confidence in effecting change in patients [57-59]. Exceptional practices and health systems are increasingly trying to better address health behavior counseling by building the infrastructure support necessary for intensive assistance and follow-up, creating multidisciplinary teams that can address the range of patient needs, and having dedicated staff to follow-up and provide ongoing assistance and motivation [60,61]. To be successful all care team members must have defined roles, be effective patient communicators, understand the patient's information and social needs, and pay attention to each individual's health literacy. New payment models that reward improved outcomes and value-based care may further support and enhance these practice efforts. Alternatively, practices can form partnerships with existing community programs designed to help patients improve health behaviors. These clinical community linkages can often more effectively address patient's needs by building on the strengths of each partner – clinicians to Ask, Advise, and Assess patient's readiness to change and community programs to provide the intensive Assistance and follow-up in the places that patients live, work, and play [62-64]. One framework, proposed by Krist, depicts how clinical practices and community programs can work together to better engage patients in health behavior change and care in general (Figure 2, below).

FIGURE 2. A Framework for How Clinical Practices and Community Programs Can Partner to Better Engage Patients in Care

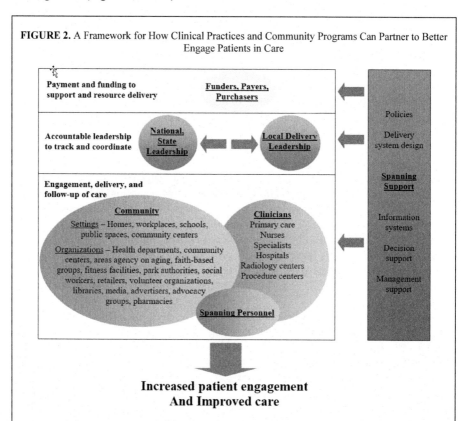

**Increased patient engagement
And Improved care**

Legend. A framework depicting how funders, policy makers, communities, and clinicians can work together with the support of personnel and infrastructure to link the care delivery systems. Funders, payers, and purchasers are tasked with financing the infrastructure needed to support integrating the clinical and community care systems. National and state leadership are empowered with the authority, resources, and responsibility to foster integrations across regions. Local leaders are the regional organizations that step forward to oversee and support local tailoring and integration activities. Community is the setting where individuals live work, and play and where the stakeholders who serve them are located. Community organizations are care providers that deliver the community elements of a clinical-community integration. Clinicians are care providers that deliver the clinical elements of a clinical-community integration. Spanning personnel are staff who specialize in helping people traverse the clinical and community settings to obtain care. Spanning support (which includes policies, delivery system design, information systems, decision support, and management support) are essential ingredients to support integrations at all levels depicted in the framework (modified from Am J Prev Med 2013;45(4):508-516).

5. Engaging Patients for Chronic Disease Care

Understanding how patients can be engaged in self-management of chronic conditions is also important given today's growing prevalence of chronic disease. For example, an estimated 70 million Americans live with hypertension and 29 million live with type 2 diabetes mellitus. Another significant proportion of the U.S. population have the precursors to these chronic diseases – 70 million have prehypertension and 86 million have prediabetes. The number and prevalence of chronic conditions that patients must live with continues to expand.

One commonly promoted model for designing systems to better address chronic conditions is the Chronic Care Model (CCM). Developed in the mid-1990s by Wagner, the CCM identifies key health system elements needed to provide effective chronic disease management and prevention [65]. These elements include (a) the community, (b) the health system, (c) self-management support, (d) delivery system design, (e) decision support, and (f) clinical information systems. When these elements function synergistically they result in a more informed, engaged, and activated patient as well as a more prepared, proactive practice team. The patient and the practice team can have more productive interactions, clinicians can better assist patients, and patients can better manage their health – all leading to improved outcomes. Use of the CCM to inform and guide the care delivery system has been evaluated extensively and is demonstrated to both improve health outcomes and cost-effectiveness [66].

When designed effectively, the healthcare and community delivery systems can provide the tools to help patients to become more informed, engaged and activated in their care. Engaged patients are more likely to practice healthy behaviors, eating right, exercising, and not smoking, mitigating any harms from their chronic condition. They seek and use more health information from a wide range of sources to learn about their condition and ways to manage it. And they better self-manage their condition by following up with their primary care clinician and specialists, getting needed tests to monitor their condition, adhering to daily medications, and participating in self-monitoring activities. Effective healthcare and community delivery systems should encourage and support these activities in a manner attentive to the patient's health literacy and health information needs.

6. The Influence of Social Determinants on Engagement and literacy

There is growing attention to the relationship between social determinants and whether clinicians can effectively engage patients in their care. It has long been known that health outcomes are affected by the social determinants of health, including socioeconomic status, education, ethnicity, race, and community of residence. The Institute of Medicine first drew attention to this problem, with a focus on racial and ethnic disparities, in their 2003 report, *Unequal Treatment: Confronting Racial and Ethnic Disparities in Health Care* [67]. The report highlighted that health outcome disparities could not be explained by merely lack of access to care, such as insurance status or availability of care. In addition, inherent stereotyping of patients and biases of clinicians contributed to poorer quality of care for minority patients. While concordance between clinician and patient in ethnicity, race, and gender have been shown to be important contributors [68], patient engagement barriers extend beyond these factors. Several studies have reported that clinicians are verbally dominant and engage less in patient centered communication in encounters with ethnic minority patients [69,70]. This lack of engagement with patients is even worse when a language barrier exists between the clinician and patient.

Clinicians are often also unable to fully comprehend the struggles with transportation, finances, housing and other economic barriers that patients of lower socioeconomic status may face. While patients with higher income may often live in the same communities as their clinicians, poorer patients either have to travel long distances to receive health care from clinics where they may be stereotyped or are served in clinics by clinicians who drive in from higher income communities. Unless directly asked, patients may often hesitate to bring up structural barriers to receipt of care and clinicians may not be aware of their barriers.

These barriers, whether created from ethnic differences, income disparities, geographic barriers, or inherent communication gaps, are often not addressed through intentional efforts to better engage patients in their care processes. In fact, special efforts need to be made since those who face barriers from social determinants have traditionally been disenfranchised within the health care system. A recent report published by the National Academies of Science, *A Framework for Educating Health Professionals to Address the Social Determinants of Health,* discusses processes in which some of these issues may be addressed. The framework includes three pillars: education, community and organization.

In terms of education, increased efforts to train clinicians in cultural competency may improve patient engagement. Defined as "a set of congruent behaviors, attitudes and policies that come together in a system, agency or among professionals and enable that system, agency or those professions to work effectively in cross-cultural situations," cultural competency may be one way clinicians can improve communication with patients and better facilitate patient engagement in care processes [71]. In 2012, the Association of American Medical Colleges and the Association of Schools of Public Health released a joint report suggesting core competencies in cultural competency for health professional students. Such curricular elements may include 1) improvement in culturally appropriate communication behavior, 2) situational awareness, 3) adaptability and 4) knowledge of core cultural issues [72].

In terms of community, joint efforts by clinicians and health systems to be involved in the communities that patients live may help facilitate better patient engagement. Through such efforts, community resources can be leveraged that may reduce social barriers that patients may face to accessing health care in a timely and appropriate fashion. Interian suggests that joint efforts by community organizations and health care organizations may help better educate patients, improve the way that structural barriers such as problems with transportation, finances and housing are addressed, and improve communication between patients and clinicians [73].

Organizational efforts may also help with patient engagement. Kauffman calls for more research is needed to address health disparities and studies need to include "hard to reach patients [74]." When including patients in outreach such as developing patient advisory councils or seeking community input, health care organizations may benefit from intentionally recruiting and including their more disenfranchised patients. From a long-term perspective, the work that health professional training schools are doing to increase minority enrolment and recruit culturally and economically diverse students may also help with future efforts to better engage patients.

While much work still needs to be done to eliminate the disparities in patient engagement, recent efforts have at least drawn attention to this issue. Attention has helped develop frameworks to understand disparities and create curricula for health professional students to learn about and start proactively addressing such disparities.

7. Patients Health Information Seeking Behaviors

Information is central to a patient being engaged in their decisions, care, and self-management. With the advent of the internet, mobile technologies, and increasingly powerful search engines, patients can now instantaneously access all kinds of information anywhere they like to help guide their health with the touch of a button.

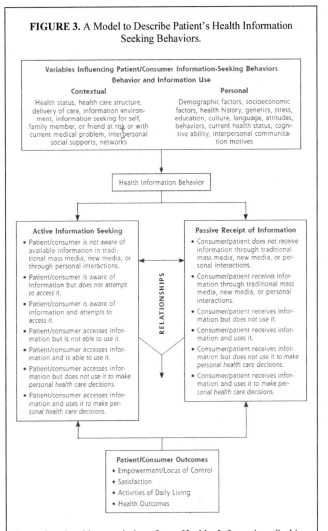

FIGURE 3. A Model to Describe Patient's Health Information Seeking Behaviors.

Some patients still rely solely on the receipt of health information from clinicians, yet many more use a combination of approaches. Receiving information from a trusted clinician can be good – it can prevent a patient from being misled by inaccurate or commercially biased information. However, not actively seeking health information can be a missed opportunity. Many local and national organizations are working to raise awareness on the power of health information by promoting the need to get informed, directing patients to health information, and even creating information, ranging from educational material about health to reports on the quality of care from hospitals and clinicians to interactive and personalized tools to manage daily activities.

There are several models that explain how, why, and where patients seek health information. One model advanced in by Longo (Figure 3, right) [75-77], identifies two axes of information seeking behaviors: active-passive and aware-unaware. Not only do patients fall into a spectrum of preferring to be active or passive seekers of health information, but patients fall into a spectrum of knowing that they need health information or knowing that health information is available. Further, there is a range of settings and sources that patients use information. Even patients involved in active searches for information are informed by passive information that they come across during usual activities of living. These passive sources include newspaper articles, television talk shows, billboards, and magazines. Passive sources can be useful or potentially misleading, particularly if commercially biased. Naturally, information needs and activities vary over time based on a multitude of patient and contextual factors. Some of these factors are modifiable and can be improved, resulting in increased health information seeking and improved health literacy. Although further research is clearly needed to identify best strategies for engaging patients in information seeking.

The information that patients can access has been continually and rapidly evolving, including the format of information, content and focus of information, and even where information is accessed. In the 1980s, a wealth of consumer information provided by professional organizations and advocacy groups emerged. Patients could access this information in lay press articles, brochures from their clinician, directly from the producer, and in community settings. This same information quickly moved to the internet and new innovative information sources emerged such as patient provided information. With the internet, individuals can reach wide audiences to share their experiences, create virtual support groups, and learn from others experiencing similar conditions; this is exemplified by tools such as *patients likeme* [78].

Now mobile devices, wearables, and the hyperconnectivity of personal health information is creating a new era of mobile health. Clinicians and health care systems are designing patient portals that can be accessed on the web or any mobile device [79-81]. Through integration of clinical information and patient reported information, these systems can anticipate patient needs and decisions, personalize educational content to better speak to the patient, reach out to patients outside of clinical encounters, and transform care from being reactive to proactive [30,82]. Asynchronous communication with clinicians and virtual visits can further facilitate information exchange between patients and clinicians. However, the impact of these clinician-provided information sources have on health outcomes is largely unknown and much research is needed about how these new approaches can better engage and activate patients in their care [83].

Similarly, smart devices have become nearly ubiquitous, with an estimated 3.5 devices per every human on earth in 2015 [84]. These devices have resulted in an explosion of applications ("apps") that can receive, collect, tailor, and transmit health information, allowing patients to self-digitize for health – often referred to now as Mobile Health or *mHealth*. *mHealth* has the potential to scale the delivery of highly personalized information directly to users and share the information with the user's clinician to better support care [85]. To date the development and dissemination of these resources has largely been driven by industry and consumer demand. There are few active, completed, or published studies that rigorously test *mHealth* interventions in randomized controlled trials to evaluate the impact on health outcomes [86], and there is less information focusing on how *mHealth* impacts patient engagement or understanding of health information [87]. In a recent systematic review, Free and colleagues only identified 42 well designed trials in North American, Europe, Asia, and Australia that showed improvements in patient self-management of diseases, clinician communication, and appointment attendance [88]. Given the potential uses of *mHealth*, much more research is needed.

Despite the proliferation of health information there is a paucity of data about the type of health information vulnerable and less health literate consumers want, particularly as it relates to newer technologies. Several studies have engaged disadvantaged populations to identify what health information would most help them with their care for a range of health topics [89,90]. Generally, two sets of desired information are commonly identified — a need for information to assist them in selecting clinicians and basic health information to assist them in self-management. Regardless of race and ethnicity, patients express a greater need for self-management information than other forms of information. Most importantly patients expressed a need for basic, straightforward information. There is some evidence for higher uptake of mobile internet technology by minorities and disadvantaged populations [91-93]. Accordingly, some disparities experts posit that *mHealth* tools have the potential to narrow disparities [94]. Yet for the most part, clinicians at safety-net practices report minimal use of even basic mobile technology in their practices [95].

Efforts are needed to both encourage and motivate patients to seek health information as well as to create high quality, patient-centered health information that is written at a basic reading level, free of jargon, culturally sensitive, non-biased, and available in multiple languages. Yet it is also important to understand where patients are with their information needs [96]. Some patients will have basic information needs, such as information about a condition, test, or treatment. Others may have more advanced needs such as information about nuanced differences between options or where to receive treatment. Some may just want information to understand and feel comfortable with care recommended by their clinician. Providing patients information mismatched to their needs is unlikely to be useful. A holistic approach is needed to providing patients information that takes into account the patient's diverse needs, desired sources, and various situations.

8. Future Directions

There is clear evidence that working to respectfully encourage patient engagement improves health outcomes and wellbeing for patients. As discussed in this chapter, engagement is critical across the lifespan and across the disease spectrum, from prevention to chronic disease control. Recent decades have seen great advances in patient engagement for clinical decision-making, promoting healthy behaviors, and self-management of chronic conditions. Understanding and addressing health literacy is a central underpinning to all of these activities.

Despite clear advances in our understanding of the value of patient engagement and effective strategies to engage patients in health, much more is needed. There are clear evidence gaps that deserve further work. Further research is needed to understand how to better inform and engage patients in decisions and self-management. Needs range from improving timely access to information for patients, ensuring that information is clear and understandable, ensuring that patients understand the importance of the information, and designing information to be actionable. As information becomes increasingly accessible from a host of venues, helping patients to navigate the morass of information and better integrating diverse sources of information could reduce patient confusion about what they need. A massive challenge will be to learn how to better redesign the healthcare delivery system to make evidence-based patient engagement part of routine care. This is especially challenging given how many decisions and health behaviors benefit from patient engagement. The health care system will also need to learn how to receive and interpret a growing expanse of patient reported information from wearables and other devices. This information may not only be able to help clinicians with decisions, but also be a mechanism in of itself to engage patients. Clinicians will also need to build and study partnerships with community resources that can extend engagement outside the clinical setting and better support patients in their daily lives. Given the diversity of patients and their needs, a host of solutions will be needed to engage patients and understanding how to match these solutions with individual patients will be critical. This challenge may be particularly important for more disadvantaged individuals and those with lower health literacy.

The future of patient engagement will need to continue to advance these activities, but also move beyond, to authentically engage patients not only in their health care, but in designing and implementing care delivery systems, developing local and national health policies, and directing health research [82]. Patient insights and lived experiences can ensure that healthcare systems and programs align with their priorities, address their needs, and are delivered in an accessible manner. Patients can help set healthcare systems' organizational priorities, participate in governance decisions, and define organizational strategies and activities. Similarly, patients can ensure that legislative, regulatory, and funding priorities reflect their needs. Patient engagement for research can help to frame research questions, select outcomes, develop study protocols, support recruitment, interpret results, translate research findings into lay language, disseminate results, and even sustain interventions.

Efforts will be needed to help patients realistically participate in these activities. Patient engagement will need to become the cultural norm. Patients will need training and support to meaningfully participate. Yet collectively, these higher levels of patient engagement can improve our very systems for promoting health.

References

[1] Carman KL, Dardess P, Maurer M, Sofaer S, Adams K, Bechtel C, et al. Patient and family engagement: a framework for understanding the elements and developing interventions and policies. Health Aff (Millwood). 2013;32(2):223-31. DOI:10.1377/hlthaff.2012.1133

[2] McCarthy D, Mueller K, Wren J. The Commonwealth Fund Case Study. Kaiser Permanente: bridging the quality divide with integrated practices, group accountability, and health information technology. 2009. Available from: http://www.commonwealthfund.org/~/media/files/publications/case-study/2009/jun/1278_mccarthy_kaiser_case_study_624_update.pdf. Retrieved September 2016.

[3] Darkins A, Ryan P, Kobb R, Foster L, Edmonson E, Wakefield B, et al. Care Coordination/Home telehealth: the systematic implementation of health informatics, home telehealth, and disease management to support the care of veteran patients with chronic conditions. Telemed J E Health. 2008;14(10):1118-26. DOI:10.1089/tmj.2008.0021

[4] Darkins A, Kendall S, Edmonson E, Young M, Stressel P. Reduced cost and mortality using home telehealth to promote self-management of complex chronic conditions: a retrospective matched cohort study of 4,999 veteran patients. Telemed J E Health. 2015;21(1):70-6. DOI:10.1089/tmj.2014.0067

[5] Kish L. The blockbuster drug of the century: an engaged patient. 2012. Available from: http://healthstandards.com/blog/2012/08/28/drug-of-the-century/. Retrieved September 2016.

[6] Committee on Quality of Health Care in America. Institute of Medicine. Crossing the Quality Chasm: A New Health system for the 21st Century. Washington, DC: National Academy Press; 2001.

[7] Electronic health records and meaningful use. The Office of the National Coordinator for Health Information Technology; 2015. Available from: http://www.healthit.gov/providers-professionals/meaningful-use-definition-objectives. Retrieved September 2016.
[8] Rittenhouse DR, Shortell SM, Fisher ES. Primary care and accountable care--two essential elements of delivery-system reform. N Engl J Med. 2009;361(24):2301-3. DOI:10.1056/NEJMp0909327
[9] Sheridan SL, Harris RP, Woolf SH. Shared decision making about screening and chemoprevention. a suggested approach from the U.S. Preventive Services Task Force. Am J Prev Med. 2004;26(1):56-66.
[10] Osborn R, Squires D. International perspectives on patient engagement: results from the 2011 Commonwealth Fund Survey. J Ambul Care Manage. 2012;35(2):118-28. DOI:10.1097/JAC.0b013e31824a579b
[11] Laurance J, Henderson S, Howitt PJ, Matar M, Al Kuwari H, Edgman-Levitan S, et al. Patient engagement: four case studies that highlight the potential for improved health outcomes and reduced costs. Health Aff (Millwood). 2014;33(9):1627-34. DOI:10.1377/hlthaff.2014.0375
[12] Sheppard VD, Mays D, LaVeist T, Tercyak KP. Medical mistrust influences black women's level of engagement in BRCA 1/2 genetic counseling and testing. J Natl Med Assoc. 2013;105(1):17-22.
[13] Arora NK, Weaver KE, Clayman ML, Oakley-Girvan I, Potosky AL. Physicians' decision-making style and psychosocial outcomes among cancer survivors. Patient Educ Couns. 2009;77(3):404-12. DOI:10.1016/j.pec.2009.10.004
[14] Torres E, Erwin DO, Trevino M, Jandorf L. Understanding factors influencing Latina women's screening behavior: a qualitative approach. Health Educ Res. 2013;28(5):772-83. DOI:10.1093/her/cys106
[15] Coulter A. Patient engagement--what works? J Ambul Care Manage. 2012;35(2):80-9. DOI:10.1097/JAC.0b013e318249e0fd
[16] Koh HK, Brach C, Harris LM, Parchman ML. A proposed 'health literate care model' would constitute a systems approach to improving patients' engagement in care. Health Aff (Millwood). 2013;32(2):357-67. DOI:10.1377/hlthaff.2012.1205
[17] Elwyn G, Laitner S, Coulter A, Walker E, Watson P, Thomson R. Implementing shared decision making in the NHS. BMJ. 2010;341:c5146. DOI:10.1136/bmj.c5146
[18] O'Connor AM, Legare F, Stacey D. Risk communication in practice: the contribution of decision aids. BMJ. 2003;327(7417):736-40.
[19] O'Connor AM, Bennett CL, Stacey D, Barry M, Col NF, Eden KB, et al. Decision aids for people facing health treatment or screening decisions. Cochrane Database Syst Rev. 2009(3):CD001431. DOI:10.1002/14651858.CD001431.pub2
[20] Stacey D, Legare F, Col NF, Bennett CL, Barry MJ, Eden KB, et al. Decision aids for people facing health treatment or screening decisions. Cochrane Database Syst Rev. 2014;1:CD001431. DOI:10.1002/14651858.CD001431.pub4
[21] Beauchamp TL, Childress JF. Principles of biomedical ethics. 7th ed. New York: Oxford University Press; 2013. xvi, 459.
[22] Annas GJ. Informed consent. Annu Rev Med. 1978;29:9-14. DOI:10.1146/annurev.me.29.020178.000301
[23] Annas GJ, Miller FH. The empire of death: how culture and economics affect informed consent in the U.S., the U.K., and Japan. Am J Law Med. 1994;20(4):357-94.
[24] Elwyn G, Frosch D, Thomson R, Joseph-Williams N, Lloyd A, Kinnersley P, et al. Shared decision making: a model for clinical practice. J Gen Intern Med. 2012;27(10):1361-7. DOI:10.1007/s11606-012-2077-6
[25] Braddock CH, 3rd, Edwards KA, Hasenberg NM, Laidley TL, Levinson W. Informed decision making in outpatient practice: time to get back to basics. JAMA Intern Med. 1999;282(24):2313-20.
[26] Siu AL. Screening for Breast Cancer: U.S. Preventive Services Task Force recommendation statement. Ann Intern Med. 2016;164(4):279-96. DOI:10.7326/M15-2886
[27] Siu AL, Bibbins-Domingo K, Grossman DC, LeFevre ML. Convergence and divergence around breast cancer screening. Ann Intern Med. 2016;164(4):301-2. DOI:10.7326/M15-3065
[28] Oeffinger KC, Fontham ET, Etzioni R, Herzig A, Michaelson JS, Shih YC, et al. Breast cancer screening for women at average risk: 2015 guideline update from the American Cancer Society. JAMA Intern Med. 2015;314(15):1599-614. DOI:10.1001/jama.2015.12783
[29] Bibbins-Domingo K, Grossman DC, Curry SJ, Davidson KW, Epling JW, Jr., Garcia FA, et al. Screening for clorectal cancer: US Preventive Services Task Force recommendation statement. JAMA Intern Med. 2016;315(23):2564-75. DOI:10.1001/jama.2016.5989
[30] Krist AH, Woolf SW, Hochheimer C, Sabo RT, Kashiri P, Jones RM, et al. Harnessing information technology to inform patients facing routine decisions. Ann Fam Med. 2017; In Press.

[31] Wunderlich T, Cooper G, Divine G, Flocke S, Oja-Tebbe N, Stange K, et al. Inconsistencies in patient perceptions and observer ratings of shared decision making: the case of colorectal cancer screening. Patient Educ Couns. 2010;80(3):358-63. DOI:10.1016/j.pec.2010.06.034

[32] Woolf SH, Krist AH, Johnson RE, Stenborg PS. Unwanted control: how patients in the primary care setting decide about screening for prostate cancer. Patient Educ Couns. 2005;56(1):116-24.

[33] Ling BS, Trauth JM, Fine MJ, Mor MK, Resnick A, Braddock CH, et al. Informed decision-making and colorectal cancer screening: is it occurring in primary care? Med Care. 2008;46(9 Suppl 1):S23-9. DOI:10.1097/MLR.0b013e31817dc496

[34] McQueen A, Bartholomew LK, Greisinger AJ, Medina GG, Hawley ST, Haidet P, et al. Behind closed doors: physician-patient discussions about colorectal cancer screening. J Gen Intern Med. 2009;24(11):1228-35. DOI:10.1007/s11606-009-1108-4

[35] Hoffman RM, Lewis CL, Pignone MP, Couper MP, Barry MJ, Elmore JG, et al. Decision-making processes for breast, colorectal, and prostate cancer screening: the DECISIONS survey. Med Decis Making. 2010;30(5 Suppl):53S-64S. DOI:10.1177/0272989X10378701

[36] Jimbo M, Rana GK, Hawley S, Holmes-Rovner M, Kelly-Blake K, Nease DE, Jr., et al. What is lacking in current decision aids on cancer screening? CA Cancer J Clin. DOI:2013;63(3):193-214. 10.3322/caac.21180

[37] Lin GA, Halley M, Rendle KA, Tietbohl C, May SG, Trujillo L, et al. An effort to spread decision aids in five California primary care practices yielded low distribution, highlighting hurdles. Health Aff (Millwood). 2013;32(2):311-20. DOI:10.1377/hlthaff.2012.1070

[38] Hill L, Mueller MR, Roussos S, Hovell M, Fontanesi J, Hill J, et al. Opportunities for the use of decision aids in primary care. Fam Med. 2009;41(5):350-5.

[39] O'Connor AM, Wennberg JE, Legare F, Llewellyn-Thomas HA, Moulton BW, Sepucha KR, et al. Toward the 'tipping point': decision aids and informed patient choice. Health Aff (Millwood). 2007;26(3):716-25. DOI:10.1377/hlthaff.26.3.716

[40] Legare F, Ratte S, Stacey D, Kryworuchko J, Gravel K, Graham ID, et al. Interventions for improving the adoption of shared decision making by healthcare professionals. Cochrane Database Syst Rev. 2010;(5):CD006732. DOI:10.1002/14651858.CD006732.pub2

[41] Shultz CG, Jimbo M. Decision aid use in primary care: an overview and theory-based framework. Fam Med. 2015;47(9):679-92.

[42] Goldstein MG, DePue J, Kazura A, Niaura R. Models for provider-patient interaction: applications to health behavior change. Handbook for Health Behavior Change. New York: Spinger; 1998. p. 85-113.

[43] Whitlock EP, Orleans CT, Pender N, Allan J. Evaluating primary care behavioral counseling interventions: an evidence-based approach. Am J Prev Med. 2002;22(4):267-84.

[44] Agency for Healthcare Research and Quality. Five major steps to intervention (The "5 A's"). 2012. Available from: http://www.ahrq.gov/professionals/clinicians-providers/guidelines-recommendations/tobacco/5steps.html. Retreived October 2016/

[45] U.S. Preventive Services Task Force. Screening for and management of obesity in adults. Available from: http://www.uspreventiveservicestaskforce.org/uspstf/uspsobes.htm. Retreived January 2013.

[46] U.S. Preventive Services Task Force. Screening for obesity in children and adolescents. 2010 . Available from: http://www.uspreventiveservicestaskforce.org/uspstf/uspschobes.htm. Retreived March 2013.

[47] Fiore M, United States. Tobacco Use and Dependence Guideline Panel. Treating tobacco use and dependence: 2008 update. Rockville, Md.: U.S. Dept. of Health and Human Services, Public Health Service; 2008. xvii, 256.

[48] Moyer VA. Screening and behavioral counseling interventions in primary care to reduce alcohol misuse: U.S. preventive services task force recommendation statement. Ann Intern Med. 2013;159(3):210-8. DOI:10.7326/0003-4819-159-3-201308060-00652

[49] Glanz K, Rimer B, Viswanath K. Health behavior and health education. 4th ed. New York City: Wiley; 2008.

[50] Glanz K, Rimer BK. Theory at a Glance. A guide for health promotion practice. U.S. Department of Health and Human Services. National Institute of Health; 2009 2nd. Available from: http://www.cancer.gov/PDF/481f5d53-63df-41bc-bfaf-5aa48ee1da4d/TAAG3.pdf. Retrevied May 2009.

[51] Miller RW, Rollnick S. Motivational interviewing: preparing people to change addictive behavior. New York, New York: The Guilford Press; 1991.

[52] Mokdad AH, Marks JS, Stroup DF, Gerberding JL. Actual causes of death in the United States, 2000. JAMA Intern Med. 2004;291(10):1238-45.

[53] Starfield B, Shi L, Macinko J. Contribution of primary care to health systems and health. Milbank Q. 2005;83(3):457-502.

[54] Goldstein MG, Whitlock EP, DePue J. Multiple behavioral risk factor interventions in primary care. Summary of research evidence. Am J Prev Med. 2004;27(2 Suppl):61-79.
[55] Rothemich SF, Woolf SH, Johnson RE, Burgett AE, Flores SK, Marsland DW, et al. Effect on cessation counseling of documenting smoking status as a routine vital sign: an ACORN study. Ann Fam Med. 2008;6(1):60-8.
[56] Leverence RR, Williams RL, Sussman A, Crabtree BF. Obesity counseling and guidelines in primary care: a qualitative study. Am J Prev Med. 2007;32(4):334-9. DOI:10.1016/j.amepre.2006.12.008
[57] Carpiano RM, Flocke SA, Frank SH, Stange KC. Tools, teamwork, and tenacity: an examination of family practice office system influences on preventive service delivery. Prev Med. 2003;36(2):131-40.
[58] Jaen CR, Stange KC, Nutting PA. Competing demands of primary care: a model for the delivery of clinical preventive services. J Fam Pract. 1994;38(2):166-71.
[59] Stange KC, Zyzanski SJ, Jaen CR, Callahan EJ, Kelly RB, Gillanders WR, et al. Illuminating the 'black box'. A description of 4454 patient visits to 138 family physicians. J Fam Pract. 1998;46(5):377-89.
[60] Rosal MC, Ockene JK, Luckmann R, Zapka J, Goins KV, Saperla G, et al. Coronary heart disease multiple risk factor reduction. Providers' perspectives. Am J Prev Med. 2004;27(2 Suppl):54-60.
[61] Bodenheimer T, Wagner EH, Grumbach K. Improving primary care for patients with chronic illness. JAMA. 2002;288(14):1775-9.
[62] Krist AH, Woolf SH, Frazier CO, Johnson RE, Rothemich SF, Wilson DB, et al. An electronic linkage system for health behavior counseling effect on delivery of the 5A's. Am J Prev Med. 2008;35(5 Suppl):S350-8.
[63] Krist AH, Shenson D, Woolf SH, Bradley C, Liaw WR, Rothemich SF, et al. Clinical and community delivery systems for preventive care: an integration framework. Am J Prev Med. 2013;45(4):508-16. DOI:10.1016/j.amepre.2013.06.008
[64] Woolf SH, Krist AH, Rothemich SF. Joining hands: partnerships between physicians and the community in the delivery of preventive care. Washington D.C.: Center for American Progress; 2006.
[65] Wagner EH, Austin BT, Davis C, Hindmarsh M, Schaefer J, Bonomi A. Improving chronic illness care: translating evidence into action. Health Aff (Millwood). 2001;20(6):64-78.
[66] Coleman K, Austin BT, Brach C, Wagner EH. Evidence on the chronic care model in the new millennium. Health Aff (Millwood). 2009;28(1):75-85.
[67] Institute of Medicine. Unequal Treatment: Confronting racial and ethnic disparities in health care. Smedley BD, Stith AY, Nelson AR, editors. Washington, DC: National Academies Press; 2003.
[68] Street Jr RL, O'Malley KJ, Cooper LA, Haidet P. Understanding concordance in patient-physician relationships: personal and ethnic dimensions of shared identity. Ann Fam Med. 2008;6(3):198-205.
[69] Johnson RL, Roter D, Powe NR, Cooper LA. Patient race/ethnicity and quality of patient–physician communication during medical visits. Am J Public Health. 2004;94(12):2084-90.
[70] Cooper LA, Roter DL, Carson KA, Beach MC, Sabin JA, Greenwald AG, et al. The Associations of Clinicians' implicit attitudes about race with medical visit communication and patient ratings of interpersonal care. Am J Public Health. 2012;102(5):979-87.
[71] Cross T, Bazron B, Dennis K, Isaacs M. Towards a culturally competent system of care. Georgetown University Child Development Center, editor. Washington, DC: CASSP Technical Assistance Center; 1989.
[72] Teal CR, Street RL. Critical elements of culturally competent communication in the medical encounter: a review and model. Soc Sci Med. 2009;68(3):533-43.
[73] Interian A, Lewis-Fernández R, Dixon LB. Improving treatment engagement of underserved US racial-ethnic groups: a review of recent interventions. Psychiatric Services. 2013;64(3):212-22.
[74] Kauffman KS, Ross M, Barnet B, Onukwugha E, Mullins CD. Engaging hard-to-reach patients in patient-centered outcomes research. 2013.
[75] Longo DR. Understanding health information, communication, and information seeking of patients and consumers: a comprehensive and integrated model. Health Expect. 2005;8(3):189-94.
[76] Longo DR, Ge B, Radina ME, Greiner A, Williams CD, Longo GS, et al. Understanding breast cancer patient's perceptions: Health information-seeking behaviour and passive information receipt. J Commun Health. 2009;2(2):184-206.
[77] Longo DR, Schubert SL, Wright BA, LeMaster J, Williams CD, Clore JN. Health information seeking, receipt, and use in diabetes self-management. Ann Fam Med. 2010;8(4):334-40. DOI:10.1370/afm.1115
[78] PatientsLikeMe. Available from: https://www.patientslikeme.com/. Retreived January 2017.
[79] Krist AH, Peele E, Woolf SH, Rothemich SF, Loomis JF, Longo DR, et al. Designing a patient-centered personal health record to promote preventive care. BMC Med Inform Decis Mak. 2011;11:73. DOI:10.1186/1472-6947-11-73
[80] Ralston JD, Coleman K, Reid RJ, Handley MR, Larson EB. Patient experience should be part of meaningful-use criteria. Health Aff (Millwood). 2010;29(4):607-13.

[81] Silvestre AL, Sue VM, Allen JY. If you build it, will they come? The Kaiser Permanente model of online health care. Health Aff (Millwood). 2009;28(2):334-44.
[82] Woolf SH, Zimmerman E, Haley A, Krist AH. Authentic engagement Of patients And communities can transform research, practice, and policy. Health Aff (Millwood). 2016;35(4):590-4. DOI:10.1377/hlthaff.2015.1512
[83] Goldzweig CL, Orshansky G, Paige NM, Towfigh AA, Haggstrom DA, Miake-Lye I, et al. Electronic patient portals: evidence on health outcomes, satisfaction, efficiency, and attitudes: a systematic review. Ann Intern Med. 2013;159(10):677-87. DOI:10.7326/0003-4819-159-10-201311190-00006
[84] Topol EJ, Steinhubl SR, Torkamani A. Digital medical tools and sensors. JAMA Intern Med. 2015;313(4):353-4. DOI:10.1001/jama.2014.17125
[85] Steinhubl SR, Muse ED, Topol EJ. Can mobile health technologies transform health care? JAMA Intern Med. 2013;310(22):2395-6. DOI:10.1001/jama.2013.281078
[86] Sutton EF, Redman LM. Smartphone applications to aid weight loss and management: current perspectives. Diabetes, metabolic syndrome and obesity: targets and therapy. DOI:2016;9:213-6. 10.2147/DMSO.S89839
[87] Barello S, Triberti S, Graffigna G, Libreri C, Serino S, Hibbard J, et al. eHealth for patient engagement: a systematic review. Frontiers in Psychology. 2015;6:2013. DOI:10.3389/fpsyg.2015.02013
[88] Free C, Phillips G, Watson L, Galli L, Felix L, Edwards P, et al. The effectiveness of mobile-health technologies to improve health care service delivery processes: a systematic review and meta-analysis. PLoS One. 2013;10(1):e1001363. DOI:10.1371/journal.pmed.1001363
[89] Longo DR, Crabtree BF, Pellerano MB, Howard J, Saver B, Hannan EL, et al. A qualitative study of vulnerable patient views of Type 2 diabetes Consumer Reports. Patient. 2016;9(3):231-40. DOI:10.1007/s40271-015-0146-8
[90] Rutten LJ, Arora NK, Bakos AD, Aziz N, Rowland J. Information needs and sources of information among cancer patients: a systematic review of research (1980-2003). Patient Educ Couns. 2005;57(3):250-61. DOI:10.1016/j.pec.2004.06.006
[91] Lustria ML, Smith SA, Hinnant CC. Exploring digital divides: an examination of eHealth technology use in health information seeking, communication and personal health information management in the USA. Health Informatics J. 2011;17(3):224-43. DOI:10.1177/1460458211414843
[92] Hesse BW, Hanna C, Massett HA, Hesse NK. Outside the box: will information technology be a viable intervention to improve the quality of cancer care? J Natl Cancer Inst Monogr. 2010;2010(40):81-9. DOI:10.1093/jncimonographs/lgq004
[93] Wakefield DS, Kruse RL, Wakefield BJ, Koopman RJ, Keplinger LE, Canfield SM, et al. Consistency of patient preferences about a secure internet-based patient communications portal: contemplating, enrolling, and using. Am J Med Qual. 2012. DOI:10.1177/1062860611436246
[94] Turner-Lee N, Smedley BD, Miller J. Minorities, mobile broadband and the management of chronic diseases. Washington DC: Joint Center for Political and Economic Studies; 2012.
[95] Broderick A, Haque F. Mobile health and patient engagement in the safety net: a survey of community health centers and clinics. Issue Brief (Commonw Fund). 2015;9:1-9.
[96] Longo DR, Woolf SH. Rethinking the information priorities of patients. JAMA Intern Med. 2014;311(18):1857-8. DOI:10.1001/jama.2014.3038

Health Literacy
R.A. Logan and E.R. Siegel (Eds.)
IOS Press, 2017
doi:10.3233/978-1-61499-790-0-303

Integrating Participatory Design and Health Literacy to Improve Research and Interventions

Linda NEUHAUSER[1]

School of Public Health, University of California, Berkeley

Abstract. Health communication is an essential health promotion strategy to convert scientific findings into actionable, empowering information for the public. Health communication interventions have shown positive outcomes, but many efforts have been disappointing. A key weakness is that expert-designed health communication is often overly generic and not adequately aligned with the abilities, preferences and life situations of specific audiences. The emergence of the field of health literacy is providing powerful theoretical guidance and practice strategies. Health literacy, in concert with other determinants of health, has greatly advanced understanding of factors that facilitate or hinder health promotion at individual, organizational and community settings. However, health literacy models are incomplete and interventions have shown only modest success to date. A challenge is to move beyond the current focus on individual comprehension and address deeper factors of motivation, self-efficacy and empowerment, as well as socio-environmental influences, and their impact to improve health outcomes and reduce health disparities.

Integrating participatory design theory and methods drawn from social sciences and design sciences can significantly improve health literacy models and interventions. Likewise, researchers and practitioners using participatory design can greatly benefit from incorporating health literacy principles into their efforts. Such interventions at multiple levels are showing positive health outcomes and reduction of health disparities, but this approach is complex and not yet widespread. This chapter focuses on research findings about health literacy and participatory design to improve health promotion, and practical guidance and case examples for researchers, practitioners and policymakers.

Keywords. Health communication, health literacy, participatory design, design sciences, health promotion, participatory action research, determinants of heath, health disparities.

1. Introduction: Determinants of Health, Health Disparities and Health Equity

People's health is thought to promoted—or hindered—by a wide range of determinants. Under the traditional "medical model," "health" was equated primarily with physical determinants and has had a strong focus on providing healthcare to identify and treat diseases. Since the last century, substantial research indicates that social, behavioral, economic, structural and environmental factors are even more predictive of people's health over the course of their lives [1–4]. Research on social determinants of health typically examines socio-economic status, age, gender, sexual orientation, disabilities,

---

[1] Corresponding author, School of Public Health, 50 University Hall MC7360, University of California, Berkeley, Berkeley, CA 94720-7360. USA. E-mail: lindan@berkeley.edu.

race and ethnicity (including discrimination and cultural beliefs and behaviors), educational levels, neighborhood conditions and many other factors. Structural determinants have been identified that impact people's health, such as access to health insurance and healthcare, provision of understandable information, quality of health care and patient-provider interactions, patient engagement in health care, medication adherence, health care costs, etc.

Determinants are hypothesized to operate within the public health "social-ecological" model at multiple individual, family, interpersonal, neighborhood, institutional, cultural and societal levels over the life course [5–7]. Individual determinants can operate within and across multiple levels, and interact with other determinants [8]. For example, the social determinant of race can interact with the structural determinant of healthcare access across individual, organizational and other levels. These interactions can be associated with multiple health outcomes such as early detection of disease and treatment. Although overall population health is improving over time, not all groups benefit equally, and among some groups, health outcomes can decline [9]. These health differences are referred to as "health disparities" (or "health inequalities") defined by the US Department of Health and Human Services [10] as:

> "A type of difference in health that is closely linked with social or economic disadvantage. Health disparities negatively affect groups of people who have systematically experienced greater social or economic obstacles to health. These obstacles stem from characteristics historically linked to discrimination or exclusion such as race or ethnicity, religion, socioeconomic status, gender, mental health, sexual orientation, or geographic location. Other characteristics include cognitive, sensory, or physical disability."

There are wide health disparities/inequalities among groups, such as birth outcomes for White vs. African American women [11]. Even though exact causal pathways are difficult to identify, research indicates that few such disparities are naturally occurring because of innate genetic, or other individual differences, or non-equal group comparisons (health of older vs younger adults), but rather by interlocking external factors related to the physical and social environments [12,13]. A disparity in health outcomes that is systematic, avoidable, and unjust is frequently referred to as a "health inequity" [14,15]. A major public health and social justice goal is to improve health, [2,3,16–19] which can be defined as a state in which people have "the opportunity to attain their full health potential and no one is disadvantaged from achieving this potential because of their social position or other socially-determined circumstances" [14].

Researchers are studying how the determinants of health interrelate and impact health positively or negatively. This is a daunting challenge, given the complex web of determinants that co-interact across many dimensions. However, studies are increasingly identifying powerful health predictors. Marmot's landmark Whitehall study of British civil servants showed that "sense of control" over work and life issues was the strongest predictor of the major differences in the health status gradient from high- to low-level workers [2]—a finding that has now been corroborated across studies worldwide. Sense of control can also be referred to as "empowerment" and is linked with "self-efficacy" [1,20]. Although socio-economic status is closely associated with empowerment—and is difficult to change—there are important public health opportunities to increase empowerment and health through health promotion interventions.

2. Health Promotion and Health Communication

Health communication is a key health promotion strategy to convert scientific findings into actionable, empowering information for the public. Health communication can be defined as "the central social process in the provision of health care delivery and the promotion of public health" [21]. Health communication is highly interdisciplinary and interacts with many disciplines, such as public health, education, medicine, mass communication, information science, sociology, engineering, etc. Health communication comprises or interacts with many areas: mass-media and tailored health information (in multiple media formats), electronic health information, bio-informatics, m-health, health campaigns, patient-provider communication, etc. [22,23]. In this chapter, "health communication" refers to health research and interventions that have a core communication component, such as most health literacy initiatives.

Health communication is critical not only to improve health for the overall population, but also for socially disadvantaged groups who face barriers due to information access, including literacy/digital literacy, language, culture, discrimination, geographic location, disability, social isolation, low healthcare access or other factors. Health communication research over the past half-century provides strong evidence that well-crafted health communication efforts can help reduce health risks, disease incidence, morbidity, and mortality, as well as improve quality of life by enabling people to make informed health decisions [15,22–24]. However, it also shows that many health communication efforts have had disappointing outcomes and that some have even shown unintended negative consequences and have been linked with widening health inequities [15,22–27].

A key weakness of traditional health communication is that it is often overly generic and not adequately aligned with the abilities, preferences and life situations of specific audiences [23,24,28–30]. These weaknesses are greatly magnified for marginalized and at-risk populations who may require significant adaptation for communication content, format, and delivery [31,32]. Unfortunately, health messages for such groups are often presented in ways that are overly technical, complex, and abstract from the experience of the intended beneficiaries. Also, much health communication focuses on rational, didactic messages that overlook emotional factors, like empathy and motivation [22,24,33–35]. Further, expert-designed. science-based messages may not be actionable, especially for people who face many barriers in their social contexts. For example, messages that encourage people to go out and exercise, may not work if they live in unsafe neighborhoods. Likewise, communication that is available only through electronic media can disadvantage groups without such access— and may increase health disparities. Taken together, these many problems can limit the overall effectiveness of health communication efforts, especially for those groups most in need. An underlying problem is the lack of intensive participation with the intended beneficiaries [22,24,30,36].

Over the past three decades, researchers and practitioners have been drawing on research findings to strengthen traditional health communication strategies, including 1) audience analyses; 2) message design and testing with the intended audiences; 3) selection of appropriate mass communication channels (especially new media) and credible mediators for messages; and 4) more rigorous evaluation of health communication interventions [31]. Logan [24] describes conceptual and methodological shifts in health campaigns moving "from a one-way expert-to-recipient model to a range of broader interactive activities for health promotion, education, engagement, and collaboration that use diverse mass media tools and services."

This chapter focuses on two other major developments during the past 20–30 years: the creation of the field of health literacy, and the increased use of participatory design, to improve health research, interventions, policy and health equity. The specific objectives of this chapter are to explore 1) associations between determinants of health, health disparities and health communication interventions; 2) definitions and dimensions of health literacy and its importance to improve health communication; 3) gaps in health literacy research and practice; 4) participatory design theory and methods and their value to improve health communication and health literacy interventions; 5) case examples about integrating participatory design and health literacy to improve health interventions and health equity; and 6) recommendations and new directions for researchers, practitioners and policymakers.

3. The Evolution of Health Literacy

During the past three decades, health literacy has emerged as a critical area to advance health research, communication interventions, population health and health equity. This new field has grown in response to accumulating research showing that people's knowledge and competencies related to accessing, understanding and using health information within their social contexts is significantly correlated with their health decisions and health outcomes. Major catalysts to the field's development began with early observations that adults' skills related to understanding and using health information seemed closely related, but distinct, from their general literacy skills [37].

In 2003, the National Assessment of Adult Literacy (NAAL), a national population-based survey, examined both adult literacy and health literacy skills and confirming that adult literacy and health-related literacy skills, although associated, were separate research constructs [38,39]. Findings showed that health literacy is significantly associated with many socio-demographic determinants of health including race, ethnicity, income, educational attainment and age. The survey also found that only 12% of US adults were estimated to have the "proficient" skills necessary to understand and use health information within the demands of health systems. Importantly, research indicated that health literacy can be an independent risk factor or determinant of health [40].

Health literacy has become an issue of national concern, prompting major research efforts to define and model this concept. Research findings have also motivated national and international "calls to action" about health literacy and interventions to address health literacy problems. Health literacy scholars have traced key events in the development of health literacy research, policy and interventions [41–44]. Research in other countries also indicates low levels of health literacy and increasing efforts to improve it [45]. Definitions, conceptual models and dimensions of health literacy have been constantly evolving and now cover a broad array of factors at individual, interpersonal, organizational, community and societal levels. Health literacy is highly interdisciplinary; it draws guidance from public health, medicine, psychology, education, communication, sociology, anthropology, architecture, and many other disciplines and their sub-fields. It operates in all societal sectors as illustrated in socio-ecological models.

3.1. Definitions

An early definition of health literacy from the World Health Organization [46] is "The cognitive and social skills which determine the motivation and ability of individuals to gain access to, understand, and use information in ways which promote and maintain good health." The American Medical Association [47] defined it as "The constellation of skills, including the ability to perform basic reading and numeral tasks required to function in the healthcare environment." In 2004, the US Institute of Medicine (IOM)—now the National Academies of Science, Engineering and Medicine—advocated for a definition that has become the most standard one in the US: "the degree to which individuals have the capacity to obtain, process, and understand basic health information needed to make appropriate health decisions" [48]. Nutbeam [49] proposed three levels of competencies related to health literacy. In the lowest basic or "functional" level, an individual has a fundamental understanding of a health problem and the ability to comply with prescribed actions to remedy the problem. At an "interactive" level, a person has more advanced knowledge and skills to function in everyday society and the ability to seek out information in order to respond to changing needs. At the highest or "critical" level, a person has a significant level of knowledge, personal skills and confidence to manage their health, and the ability to take action to change the determinants of health in the environment.

Although early definitions focused on individual skills, the importance of contextual factors has been increasingly emphasized. For example, in its 2003 action plan objectives for Healthy People 2010, the U.S. Department of Health and Human Services emphasized that the concept of health literacy not only involves patients, but also providers, and organizations [50]. Although the IOM/NAM report proposed the above definition focused on individual skills, the report also acknowledged that health literacy is an interaction between the skills of individuals and the demands of health systems, and that there is a notable mismatch between them. The trend toward more contextual definitions highlights the multiple dimensions of health literacy, including the skills of healthcare providers to present information to individuals in a way that is understandable and actionable. The Calgary Charter [51] defined health literacy as:

"• Health literacy allows the public and personnel working in all health-related contexts to find, understand, evaluate, communicate, and use information.

• Health literacy is the use of a wide range of skills that improve the ability of people to act on information in order to live healthier lives.

• These skills include reading, writing, listening, speaking, numeracy, and critical analysis, as well as communication and interaction skills."

In addition to increasing emphasis on interpersonal interactions between individuals and health educators and other providers, health literacy definitions are also highlighting the importance of healthcare and other community contexts. Kickbush and colleagues [52] proposed this definition: "The ability to make sound health decision(s) in the context of everyday life–at home, in the community, at the workplace, the healthcare system, the market place and the political arena. It is a critical empowerment strategy to increase people's control over their health, their ability to seek out information and their ability to take responsibility." This definition situates the phenomenon of health literacy within the public health social-ecological model, specifying the important associations of social and structural determinants of health. A new focus is to identify attributes of "health literate" healthcare institutions based on the degree to which they provide equal, easy, and shame-free access to and delivery of health care and health information [53,54]. Further, Freedman and colleagues [55] developed a definition for "public health literacy": "the degree to which individuals and groups can obtain process, understand, evaluate, and act upon information needed to make public health decisions that benefit the community."

In a systematic literature review, Sorensen and colleagues [45] identified 17 health literacy definitions. In their content analysis, they condensed definitions to six cluster areas: (1) competence, skills, abilities (cognitive, social, personal and communication skills, motivation, etc.); (2) actions (accessing, understanding, processing and making decisions about health information, etc.); (3) information and resources (including kinds of health information in multiple formats, and health-related services, etc.); (4) objective (promoting/maintaining health, becoming empowered, making health decisions, interacting with healthcare environments, etc.); (5) context (healthcare, home, community, workplace and political settings, etc.); and (6) time (across the life course). In a 2016 National Academy of Medicine report, Pleasant and colleagues [56] commented on the multidisciplinary and multidimensional nature of health literacy. They advocated for the development of a new definition of health literacy that provides "a description of this multidimensionality; an explanation of a variety of settings and modes and media; and the unique psychological impact of health literacy on empowerment and health decisions."

3.2. Health Literacy Models, Dimensions and New Directions

The evolution of health literacy definitions is linked to expanding conceptual health literacy models. In their 2012 systematic review, Sorensen and colleagues [45] identified 12 models and their dimensions and analyzed their similarities and differences. Models included many core health literacy factors: individual capacities related to knowledge, information access, reading, listening, speaking, numeracy, memory, healthcare navigation, and critical health decision-making. Some models incorporated behavioral factors such as health risk behaviors, use of healthcare, and medication adherence. These factors are considered important within the "medical health literacy" models that focus on individuals' abilities for self-care and interacting effectively within healthcare systems. Other "public health literacy" models take a broader view and incorporate factors that go beyond personal health literacy factors to encompass determinants of health in a variety of societal situations [57]. These models have stronger emphasis on empowerment, advocacy, and group and community factors.

The models posit a wide range of antecedents and consequences of health literacy [45]. In addition to the above-mentioned capacities, antecedents include wide range of demographic, psychosocial, cultural, media use, past health experience/knowledge, social support, and social capital factors that influence a person or groups' health literacy status. The models conceptualize that higher health literacy can result in more positive attitudes, higher motivation and self-efficacy, improved health status, improved health behaviors, lower healthcare costs, less frequent use of healthcare services, improved healthcare systems, etc. Consequences range from those at the individual level to community and societal levels, such as positive effects on social capital, intergenerational community empowerment, on (other) determinants of health, and on health equity.

The evolving definitions, conceptual models and dimensions are an impressive achievement for the relatively new field of health literacy, but important gaps remain. Sorensen and colleagues [45] suggest that these models can be improved to: 1) include more comprehensive factors related to existing knowledge about health literacy; 2) better integrate factors in "medical" and "public health" perspectives; 3) acknowledge that health literacy is not static, but rather changes over the life course; and 4) develop stronger causal pathways between antecedents and consequences [58]. They propose a new model (see their Figure 1) that conceptualizes social, environmental, situational and personal determinants of health as antecedents, and health literacy as competencies to access, understand, appraise and apply health information as a patient in healthcare, disease prevention and health promotion domains. Their model includes individual, health system and societal consequences, with additional emphasis on empowerment, and notes that consequences reflect a process over the life course, and affect health sustainability and equity.

Just as Pleasant and colleagues [56] called for a new definition of health literacy that includes its unique psychological impact on empowerment and health decisions, conceptual frameworks should also illustrate how health literacy and other determinants of health promote or hinder motivation, empowerment, self-efficacy and behavior change. Although some health literacy conceptual frameworks include these factors either as an antecedent, a health literacy "capacity," or a consequence of health literacy, the pathways are still vague, and many are still focused on cognitive, skills-based factors. Because some research shows that "patient activation" can compensate for low health literacy as an independent predictor of improved health behaviors, Hibbard [59] proposes that this factor be included in models. McCormack and colleagues [12] likewise call for expanding models to include various patient engagement factors.

As noted earlier, substantial research from the public health field of epidemiology shows that sense of control/empowerment is one of the strongest predictors of people's health [1–3]. Therefore, epidemiological research and models can greatly contribute to building out health literacy models, as can research from other disciplines, like psychology [60] and behavioral sciences. Taking an even broader view, Logan [8] cites the need for an expanded, multidimensional conceptual framework that integrates health literacy and multiple other determinants of health to posit how they overlap and how they affect health disparities and health inequities. Because health literacy is a powerful determinant of health and mediates of determinants of health, a new model could identify unique health literacy pathways for interventions that could reduce health disparities.

4. Health Literacy Interventions

The new field of health literacy field has had impressive achievements over the past two decades: a growing evidence base of theoretical and empirical research; application of research into practical interventions; and advancement of policy mandates at local, national and global levels. As discussed earlier, health literacy research has created multiple conceptual frameworks with an increasing number of dimensions, causal pathways and measurable constructs. Research has also identified a large number of existing or refined instruments that can be used to examine health literacy variables. The most comprehensive listing of these instruments is Boston University's Health Literacy Tool Shed accessible at: http://healthliteracy.bu.edu. As of 2016, the site included information on 125 tools that measure health literacy. Although the concept of health literacy emerged in the US, it has now spread globally. The ever-expanding number of scientific publications, health literacy conferences and associations, and research grants reflect the vitality of the field. Interest in the field has attracted investigators from many other disciplines who are enriching health literacy research from their perspectives.

Health literacy research has identified important relationships between health literacy levels and health knowledge, attitudes, behaviors, outcomes and disparities. According to a systematic review of the literature conducted the US Agency for Healthcare Research and Quality (AHRQ) [61], lower health literacy levels were "consistently associated with increased hospitalizations, greater emergency care use, lower use of mammography, lower receipt of influenza vaccine, poorer ability to demonstrate taking medications appropriately, poorer ability to interpret labels, health messages, and, among seniors, poorer overall health status and higher mortality." The study concluded that "health literacy level potentially mediates disparities between blacks and whites." Research is increasing indicating that health literacy can be considered as an independent predictor of health (a socially derived determinant of health) or as an intermediate variable that interacts with other social or structural determinants of health [8,40,61–64]. Most health literacy interventions to date are health communication initiatives focused in healthcare systems to provide easier-to-use health information, and to improve patient-provider communication and delivery of healthcare services.

The focus on redesigning health information was prompted by over 1,000 studies of health print materials (including medication labels) and websites showing that text readability significantly exceeded the estimated reading skills of the audiences for whom they were developed [65–68]. Strategies to design and assess "plain language" communications have been codified into health literacy principles that include reducing reading levels and improving syntax, cultural appropriateness, and format for easier comprehension. Descriptions of these recommended practices include those provided by the US Centers for Disease Control and Prevention CDC and AHRQ [69,70].

4.1. Results of Health Literacy Interventions Research

Although results are uneven, a many studies of health information using health literacy principles show improvements in patients' comprehension and/or behavioral outcomes [61,68,71–79]. Taggert and colleagues [80] found overall positive outcomes in health literacy and behavioral risk factor reduction among a wide variety of healthcare and community interventions. Another promising intervention area is applying health literacy strategies to improve medication adherence and medical device use. Some studies are showing that interventions that simplify medication labeling and instructions, combined with improved patient engagement are associated with better medication adherence and proper device use [61,71,73,81–85]. The US Food and Drug Administration and pharmaceutical companies are becoming increasingly active in health literacy research and interventions [83,86–88].

Although research about healthcare provider interactions with patients ("oral health literacy") is at an early stage, a recommended technique is "teach back" (or, "teach to goal") in which providers assess patient's comprehension of important information and clarify it as needed, is showing some positive results [73,89]. Research about "health literate" systems and is nascent, but growing [54,90]. Likewise, community-level ("public health") health literacy efforts are at an early stage, but are showing positive results [57,75,77,91,92]. Community-level interventions show promise to move health literacy efforts "upstream" to prevent disease and promote health.

The AHRQ [61] review assessed health literacy interventions among 42 interventions that met study design criteria. Among this relatively small pool of intervention studies, the review found uneven, and as yet "low" or "insufficient" evidence for efforts intended to redesign information for better comprehension. There was moderate evidence for positive effects of mixed interventions on healthcare use, intensive self-management interventions on behavior, and disease management interventions on disease prevalence/severity. Evidence was mixed and "insufficient" about the effects of health literacy interventions on knowledge, self-efficacy, and quality of life, and costs. The report suggested these priorities to advance the design features of interventions: testing novel approaches to increase motivation, techniques for delivering information orally or numerically, "work around" interventions such as patient advocates; determining the effective components of already-tested interventions; determining the cost-effectiveness of programs; and determining the effect of policy and practice interventions.

4.2. Gaps and New Directions for Health Literacy Interventions Research

Overall, health literacy intervention research shows positive, but uneven results and an updated systematic review is needed to encompass more recent efforts. Examination of basic research and interventions research in health literacy indicates important gaps. Conceptual models need to be built out to incorporate more determinants of health and their relationship to health literacy factors, including identification of mediating and moderating variables that affect health outcomes and disparities. More examination is needed of non-cognitive variables, such as motivation and self-efficacy and their relationship to health behaviors and health/quality of life outcomes. For example, it has been frustrating to learn that even with all the important health literacy principles applied to health communications, not all "health literate" information has been shown to improve people's comprehension, and evidence is still sparse about whether it significantly increases positive health behaviors. Health literacy design principles do not include all the factors that affect people's interest in, comprehension of, motivation, and ability to use health information to make changes [68,87]. Similarly, "oral health literacy" interventions to improve patient-provider communication, do not always show significant outcomes in desired behaviors. This may be related to many factors, such as the patient's anxiety in an examining room, non-verbal behavior of healthcare providers, lack of visual tools to accompany the oral communication, or lack of social support from a family member. Likewise, in these situations, a person's health concerns may be secondary to other important issues they are dealing with in their lives.

Currently, important work is underway to define attributes of "health literate" healthcare settings engage and support patients [53]. These factors include recommendations from health literacy research such as improving the design of information resources, patient-provider communication, signage, etc. However, it will be challenging to identify many other factors that are not yet clear in the literature:

What exactly is a "shame-free environment?" What colors, sounds, spaces and designs in the setting calm and engage people? How can information be presented in the setting that intrigues people to interact with it, search out their own questions, and become more "activated" to make and carry out health decisions? A deeper question is: How do researchers and practitioners even know what questions to ask? In my view, the lack of intensive participation of the users has been a major impediment to designing, implementing and evaluating more powerful health literacy interventions. The AHRQ report [61] recommends that investigators pilot test new interventions, but this is quite different from engaging users *from the start* as co-designers. Although health literacy models and principles offer helpful guidance and tools, researchers themselves cannot specifically define what helps or hinders people from making healthy changes within their multiple contexts and what actions would further health equity [64]. Fortunately, there is a growing body of research about the value of participatory design to improve health communication interventions, and some early guidance about applying these strategies to health literacy initiatives.

5. Participatory Design

In 1978, at the Alma Ata Conference on Primary Health Care [93], WHO member states signed the first international declaration about the right to health and commitment to primary healthcare. This was also the first international declaration to emphasize the importance of participation. Point 10 specifies that primary healthcare "requires and promotes maximum community and individual self-reliance and participation in the planning, organization, operation and control of primary healthcare, making fullest use of local, national and other available resources; and to this end develops through appropriate education the ability of communities to participate."

Since then, participation has been a core element of local, national and global health mandates. In the area of health communication/health literacy interventions, two decades of studies show that when users participate in designing and testing communication, outcomes are more successful, including those for vulnerable groups. Examples include: Hoy et al., Neuhauser & Kreps, Barton et al., Vaiana & McGlynn, Neuhauser, Wang, Vallance et al., Cooper et al., Gustafson et al., Minkler & Wallerstein, Logan, Hesse & Schneiderman, Neuhauser & Rothschild et al., Neuhauser & Kreps, Neuhauser & Kreps et al., Davis et al., Neuhauser, Kreps & Syme, Kreps & Sparks, Kreps & Neuhauser, Noar & Harrington, Schillinger et al., Wolf et al., Smith & Wallace, Yin et al., Arcia et al., Neuhauser & Constantine et al. [94,22,95–97,33,98–101,44,36,68,102,103,66,104,30,31,105,73,71,83,84,74,75]. An important outcome of many of these interventions is that they have been successful among groups that experience many health disparities, and thus can improve health equity. Despite the increasing evidence of the value of participatory design, *intensive* participatory processes are still not the norm in health communication/health literacy efforts. For example, in a systematic review of patient decision aids, Coulter and colleagues [106] found that only half the aids were tested with patients. Frequently, "participation" is limited to the important, but not sufficient, step of pilot testing interventions strategies initiated by researchers and/or practitioners—rather than by the users. Because many researchers and practitioners are not trained on the scientific value and specific strategies of intensive participatory design, it is useful to examine the theoretical foundation and empirical methods of participatory design.

5.1. Origin and Scientific Foundation of Participatory Design in Social Sciences

Theories and methods of participatory design have emerged over the past 60 years from multiple disciplinary roots. In the field of health promotion, participatory design is typically traced to its social science origins. Beginning in the middle of the last century, social scientists began to critique definitions and models of health as overly focused on clinical risk factors and medical treatment, rather than on broader health promotion within socio-ecological models, such as sociologist Aaron Antonovsky's model of "salutogenesis" [107]. Scholars were also concerned about the tension between investigators' agendas vs. people's needs, such as researchers' motivation to create constructs and publish papers rather than collaboratively engage in transformational actions to benefit groups. They thought the investigator-directed approach limited the theoretical understanding of conceptual models of health as well as empirical methods develop effective interventions. For example, Antonovsky criticized researcher-created health models as too focused on individual comprehension of health knowledge, rather motivational factors with social contexts.

Sociologist Kurt Lewin created the concept of "action research" in 1946 [108]. He described it as "a comparative research on the conditions and effects of various forms of social action and research leading to social action" that uses "a spiral of steps, each of which is composed of a circle of planning, action and fact-finding about the result of the action." Reason and Bradbury [109] described action research as "an interactive inquiry process that balances problem solving actions implemented in a collaborative context with data-driven collaborative analysis or research to understand underlying causes enabling future predictions about personal and organizational change." Related models that integrate highly collaborative research and action models include participatory action research and community-based participatory research [101,110,111]. These models emphasize "research for action" and "action for research, and engage researchers and community members as co-collaborators. They highlight the importance of using multiple qualitative methods in specific contexts, rather than quantitative methods to generalize research across contexts, as does traditional research. Action research, especially community-based participatory action research, generally involves long-term processes of community-researcher engagement, problem identification, reflection and intervention development, implementation and revision [101].

5.2. Origin and Scientific Foundation of Participatory Design in Design Sciences

Although researchers and practitioners in health communication/health literacy fields are more familiar with models and methods of participatory design derived from social sciences, participatory design also emerged in parallel through socio-technical sciences and offers important theoretical and methodological guidance. Architect and designer Buckminster Fuller introduced the term "design science" (the study of design) in 1963 [112]. Design science is considered one of three major categories of the systematic study of knowledge (epistemology); the others are the natural sciences and the human sciences [113]. In the natural sciences (e.g., physics, chemistry), researchers seek law-based explanations about phenomena in the natural world and assume that this knowledge can be generalized to multiple settings. This was the dominant scientific paradigm until the mid-20th century. At that time, the human, or interpretive, sciences emerged and are considered the second epistemological paradigm [114]. This research perspective includes social sciences and humanities, and acknowledges that because human phenomena are not as predictable or generalizable as are natural science laws, they should be studied using multiple methods in many settings [115].

Design sciences, or "sciences of the artificial" are concerned "not with how things are, but with how they might be" [116]. In design sciences, researchers study human-created (artificial) objects and phenomena intended to solve problems and meet goals. These artifacts can be symbols, material objects, activities, services, and learning or living environments [117]—such as health care and health literacy interventions. Design science fields include engineering, information systems, architecture, computer science and other primarily "socio-technical" fields. Because design sciences focus on things that do "not yet exist," they specifically address the so-called "wicked" nature of problems [117]. In this situation, problem understanding and problem solving should happen concurrently, and there is no end to identifying problems and refining designs. Therefore, researchers should not predict solutions or hypothesize outcomes too early, but rather conduct iterative, problem identification-problem solution processes. Because of their complexity across social-ecological contexts, most health problems, such as those related to health literacy, can be considered "wicked."

The epistemological differences between design sciences, and natural and human sciences are reflected in differences in research goals, overall research design and methods [118]. Because the goal of design science inquiry is on inductive problem solving, research is focused on studying processes to arrive at a solution. In contrast, research in both the natural and human sciences is traditionally focused on predicting and testing theories. This is an important distinction because design science research is not aligned with the traditional requirements that researchers define theories, hypotheses, interventions and analysis plans *before* a project is funded. Human and design sciences overlap in the area of participatory action research in which health and social interventions are collaboratively developed and studied iteratively [101,103]. From the design science perspective, participatory (or user-centered) design has been defined as "an approach to the assessment, design and development of technological and organizational systems that places a premium on the active involvement of . . . potential or current users of the system in design and decision-making processes" [119].

5.3. Design Science Methods

There are also methodological differences among the three research paradigms. Methods in natural sciences are primarily observational and quantitative, whereas those in human science are more mixed, qualitative and researcher-participative. Design science methods are mostly qualitative, user-intensive, and emphasize "problem and solution" and "build and evaluate" loops [120], as shown in Figure 1 [121].

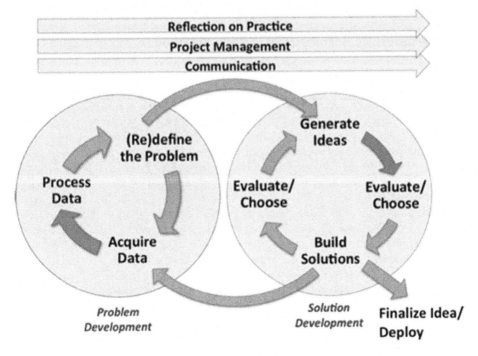

Figure 1. The general design process (Roschuni, 2012). Celeste Nicole Roschuni.
Reproduced by permission of Celeste Nicole Roschuni. Permission to reuse must be obtained from the rights holder.

In the problem development cycle in Figure 1, data are gathered from users and other sources, analyzed, and used to define problems and needs. In the solution development cycle, ideas are generated to build and test prototypes with users. Iterative feedback loops are used within and between the cycles. Although there is no theoretical end to problem identification and solution, there is a point where researchers and developers finalize and deploy a solution when it reaches the users' key specifications. For example, for a health literacy materials-based intervention, user criteria might include content and format that are attractive, navigable, comprehensible, motivating, culturally appropriate, and actionable. In addition to involving users intensively, communication with other stakeholders is also important. A health literacy intervention might require that researchers, healthcare providers, members of community organizations, policymakers or others collaborate with users on the identification of specifications, barriers to implementation, and evaluation design. Evaluation and later revisions of the "solution" (prototype) continue over time using this process. Because design methods focus equally on building and evaluating solutions, evaluation is a continuous detailed process that starts at project initiation—in contrast with traditional "before" and "after" research designs. Although this conceptual model is intricate, it can guide rapid development of viable, user-designed solutions in a more pragmatic way than traditional approaches.

Design science as a form of scientific inquiry also subsumes the area known as "human factors research" which takes into consideration the interaction between the intended users and the products, systems or processes that are being designed—such as in engineering or medical informatics. Design science approaches are frequently referred to as "user-centered," "human-centered," or "human factors" design and include many techniques from multiple fields. "Usability testing" and "design thinking" are two commonly used methods. As mentioned earlier, even though participatory action research and community-based participatory research are traditionally considered under the human sciences branch of scientific inquiry, their methods often overlap, or are synergistic with, those in the design sciences. A positive trend is that researchers and practitioners from both human and design sciences are increasingly drawing on methods—outside their traditional disciplines—that share the commonality of engaging intended users in design and implementation. The Institute of Design at the University of California, Berkeley, is developing a repository of design methods called The Design Exchange (http://www.thedesignexchange.org) that will include many design methods and cases.

Design thinking methods originated at the Stanford University Institute of Design (http://dschool.stanford.edu) and include five stages: empathize with users, define issues, generate ideas, and prototype and test solutions. Note that the requirement to reach a deep level of empathy with users *before* moving on to other steps differs from traditional research strategies that begin with identifying problems. In early design thinking exercises, users and stakeholders engage in rapid problem and solution identification. These exercises are especially effective because both experts and end users participate as equals and processes are highly visual and interactive (i.e. teams draw solutions), rather than primarily cognitive and data-oriented, as in traditional health "program planning." User-centered design is effective at individual, organizational, community and societal levels. Vechakul and colleagues [122] used these methods in a community-based project with new mothers.

Usability testing refers to a broad range of structured methods to engage users in designing communication materials [123,124]. Usability tests are often one-on-one situations that involve a tester asking a user to interact with a prototype, accomplish specific tasks related to it, and to recommend changes to it (such as to text, format, and graphics for a health communication resource). The prototype is then revised with participant input. Usability testing should continue until additional tests no longer elicit major new issues or recommendations. As participatory design becomes more widespread in health and social sciences, methods are being drawn from both the human and design sciences. One difference is that user-centered design processes are typically rapid cycles of problem identification and solution creation, whereas participatory action research emphasizes longer-term community engagement. Decisions about which approach to use and/or how to combine these approaches should be made collaboratively with participants in the specific context of a project.

6. Integrating Participatory Design and Health Literacy

As discussed earlier, two decades of research shows that participatory design strategies have improved health communication interventions, including health literacy efforts. Despite the promise of participatory design approaches in health literacy research and interventions, intensive participation is still not the norm. A problem is that health literacy researchers are typically trained in traditional research theory and methods in the human sciences. In this orientation, researchers typically build conceptual models, initiate theory-driven research, including *a priori* hypotheses, intervention design and analyses plans—as expected in the scientific community and as required by most funders. "Participation" may consist of pre-testing "health literate" information resources or patient engagement approaches, but is greatly limited by not having full user/stakeholder collaboration from the start. As a result, researchers often have less access to deep user/stakeholder input needed to build out better conceptual models and interventions.

The challenge to build out conceptual models of health literacy with better pathways related to the beliefs, habits, emotions, and motivations of intended users, and to apply these effectively to interventions is reflected in the modest and uneven results of health literacy efforts to date. Fortunately, health literacy researchers and practitioners are increasingly adopting participatory strategies and strengthening interventions, as demonstrated by the success of collaboratively designed health literacy initiatives to improve patient engagement and chronic disease management as mentioned earlier. Participatory design models and methods from both the social sciences and the design sciences provide important theoretical guidance and practical strategies for researchers and practitioners. Participatory action research, from the social sciences has begun to change how communities are engaged in research and action [101,109]. Because participatory action research is often a long-term process, it does not always align well with time constraints of many health literacy efforts. However, it is well suited to multi-year community health literacy initiatives. Design science theory and approaches are less familiar to health communication and health literacy researchers and practitioners, but offer powerful new opportunities to advance health literacy efforts relatively quickly.

In addition, health literacy models and principles can greatly improve the work of those using participatory design. Developers of electronic health communication apps generally intensely involve users during iterative design phases, but may not be familiar with guidance from health literacy research and practice that can assess and improve user comprehension and navigation. This was demonstrated at the 2011 Stanford University Artificial Intelligence and Health Communication conference. Computer science developers had created amazing health avatars and other interactive programs, but some showed disappointing results when used in interventions. Health literacy scholars at the conference pointed out problems with the high reading level (college), and lack of adherence to other important health literacy principles [103]. Nor are developers in the information sciences necessarily familiar with the many psycho-social factors that affect health. Hevner and colleagues [125] called for "synergistic efforts between behavioral science and design science researchers." Similarly, researchers and practitioners involved in community interventions can significantly benefit from incorporating health literacy guidance, as described in cases below. Although evidence is increasing about the value of integrating health literacy and participatory design strategies in health interventions, there is a lack of detailed guidance for researchers, developers and practitioners about how to do so in a way that gets to the deep personal and contextual levels needed for scientific inquiry and successful interventions.

7. Strategies to Integrate Participatory Design and Health Literacy

This section offers suggestions and case examples drawn from my 25 years of experience—and those of my colleagues—to integrate participatory design and health communication/health literacy. Most of my work has been done through the Health Research for Action center (HRA) at the University of California, Berkeley School of Public Health (http://www.healthresearchforaction.org). Center staff include multi-disciplinary researchers, communication/health literacy experts, public health practitioners, and policy scholars who have collaborated with thousands of local, national and global partners on health promotion over two decades. Staff work in interdisciplinary teams and use highly participatory methods with healthcare organizations, communities, government, and private industry. Our staff has been intensively involved in co-designing, co-implementing and co-evaluating health communication/health literacy interventions. Although participatory design processes must be selected and tailored to the specific project, we recommend the following six summary steps related to designing and testing health communication resources [104]. Each of the following steps should be documented as part of the formal evaluation.

1. Identify participants and set up an advisory committee
Participants include end-users, and subgroups of users, researchers and all relevant stakeholder groups, such as health and social service providers, community groups, government officials, policymakers, funders, media, etc. Consider establishing an advisory committee with representatives of participant groups to guide the project.

2. Conduct formative work with participants using varied participatory methods
Gather information from participant groups and research studies to co-identify problems and potential solutions. Use multiple formative methods, such as design thinking exercises, focus groups, surveys, health literacy assessments of existing resources, etc. Examine results with the advisory committee to iteratively define and refine project goals and strategies.

3. Draft health communication resources adhering to health literacy principles; develop initial dissemination plans
Co-develop new communication resources drawing on formative research, specific health literacy principles, and participant input. Begin developing plans to disseminate the resources; include advisory committee members and other relevant end-users, providers, funders, etc. in the planning. Design thinking exercises are especially useful to foster creativity.

4. Iteratively test and revise communication prototypes and implementation plans with intended users and stakeholders
Usability test and revise prototypes with subgroups of end-users over multiple rounds until participants approve them; incorporate expert review for content accuracy. Use design thinking or other strategies with users and stakeholders to refine the implementation plan.

5. Continuously evaluate and revise the health communication resource
During implementation, gather feedback from relevant users and stakeholders about the acceptance, use and effectiveness of the health communication resource and its implementation. Revise approaches as needed. Gather data using mixed qualitative and quantitative methods, such as interviews, design thinking exercises, focus groups, on-site observations, surveys, randomized trials, etc. Tailor reports to the communication

abilities and preferences of audiences (scientific publications, user-tested brief reports, etc.).

6. Sustain and extend successful programs to other populations or regions
Use participatory methods to continuously identify problems and refine the intervention. Go through the above steps to adapt the health communication intervention to new population groups, and new social and geographical contexts. *If* the initial intervention is well crafted with intense participatory design and detailed documentation, adaptation elsewhere is typically easier and less expensive [75,126].

8. Case Studies

8.1. Participatory Development of Mass Communication for Medicaid Beneficiaries

The problem: in the US, highly vulnerable populations like seniors and people with disabilities participating in Medicaid (a US program for low-income beneficiaries) are required to make complex choices to select a health plan. In California in 2008, only 25% of these beneficiaries made active choices, given the major communication barriers they faced related to literacy, language, culture and disabilities and the overly complex document about health plans that they were expected to comprehend [127]. The State of California engaged our HRA staff to work closely with Medicaid beneficiaries and stakeholders to create a guidebook that would meet their needs.

We followed all the above steps to: identify and engage user subgroups and stakeholders; establish an Advisory Group; set health literacy and cultural competency standards and iteratively test and refine prototypes of the *What Are My Medi-Cal Choices* guide; adapt the final version into 13 languages; disseminate it to hundreds of thousands of beneficiaries; and evaluate the processes and outcomes. See Neuhauser & Rothschild et al. [68] for details including the use multiple participatory methods (in-depth interviews, Advisory Group feedback, usability testing, health literacy assessments, and quantitative evaluation). The integration of health literacy principles and continuous participatory design transformed the initial ineffective state resource into a successful guide that met highly nuanced needs and preferences of intended users. In addition, the project integrated qualitative methods with a randomized-controlled trial to examine efficacy [128]. The model has now been adapted to multiple health communication interventions for people on Medicaid. Among many lessons learned, we noted that even when a prototype guide adhered to *all* currently accepted health literacy principles, users proposed making further changes to about one-third to one-half of the document to suit their needs and preferences.

8.2. Participatory Design of a Community Wellness Project with Chinese Factory Workers

The problem: China has an estimated over 250 million "migrant workers" who are moving from rural areas into industrial zones. Most of the migrants are young, have low education levels (average 7th grade) and struggle to adjust to factory jobs in urban areas. These workers one of the most vulnerable groups in China, and have little knowledge about health issues or how to access health and social services. They suffer from high rates of depression, infectious diseases and unplanned pregnancies and abortions. Taking a broader view of "health," the workers also have little knowledge about their rights at work and as non-residents of their new city, and they struggle to handle life issues (education, housing, social life, etc.). They feel they have few opportunities to change work or city policies.

Although supporting these workers is a key objective of the Chinese government, their "top down" efforts to engage workers have shown disappointing results. One reason is that the concept of health has been mostly focused on physical health and service access, rather than the broader social, structural and environmental determinants of health—especially worker empowerment. In 2011, HRA staff were invited by national and local government officials to apply our participatory design process to co-develop a project to support factory workers in Changzhou, a large industrial city with 1.5 million migrant workers. We were invited based on the success of our participatory efforts to work with Chinese Americans in California. That project created the *Chinese Wellness Guide* using the above steps.

We adapted the above six steps to the Changzhou context. Our first step was get "buy-in" about the participatory approach from key national and local government officials, health and social service providers, researchers from a local university, factory managers and others. To do that, our team conducted three participatory workshops over a one-year period to introduce the concepts of multiple determinants of health and the power of participatory design. Participants examined baseline research about workers' health and social issues and then mapped out >50 determinants of health. Surprisingly, these determinants included low health literacy—not a common concept as yet in China. After securing buy-in and enthusiasm from these decision-makers, teams of workers from two factories joined the project. Several advisory committees were established including all worker and stakeholder groups who then identified problems and solutions. Though these processes, participants defined three novel interventions: creation of an easy-to-use Changzhou Wellness Guide covering a broad range of health and social issues, service access, tips for managing life issues; a "Wellness House" in each factory where workers could socialize, solve problems, and attend trainings; and a buddy system in which established workers help new workers.

The Changzhou Wellness Guide was created using the above steps. HRA health literacy experts trained participants on health literacy principles and iterative testing and revisions of prototypes. Workers and stakeholders created guide content and formatting and conducted multiple rounds of user testing and expert feedback. Professional stakeholders were amazed at the creativity, depth and practicality of workers' ideas. After initial publication and use over one year, workers and stakeholders have revised the guide, using the same participatory methods and adhering to health literacy principles. In 2016, the project won the Institute for Healthcare Advancement's International Award for Outstanding Achievement in Health Literacy. The project has expanded to 20 factories, each of which is using participatory design to contribute to the next edition of the guide and to create other interventions and catalyze city-wide policy changes. Researchers from the local university and HRA are collaborating with all participant groups (including workers) to design and conduct research about the process and effectiveness of the project. Early research findings suggest significant increases in worker knowledge, confidence, service connections and positive health behaviors.

We learned key lessons from this project. It was important to ground the project in a social-ecological model with comprehensive determinants of health, including health literacy. This project is also a good example of why health literacy factors are essential to consider in participatory projects *and* why participatory methods are essential to consider in health literacy projects—where health literacy issues must be explored by users in their contexts. Empowerment of workers, a core goal of this project, emerged through intensive participatory methods, and the gradual development of interventions they created. The key lesson is that if end users are engaged to create and implement interventions *themselves*, they will do so in a way that incorporates many highly nuanced factors that are not codified into health literacy design principles. They will also design interventions that take into consideration many social, structural and environmental determinants of health that affect them, but may not be obvious to researchers or practitioners, or included in a health literacy model.

For example, factory workers cited the lack of summer school opportunities for their children as an overarching problem that determined whether they would have to leave the factory before the summer. For many workers, this problem greatly superseded health problems. They solved the problem by advocating for and developing summer schools in the factories. Government stakeholders, disappointed by outcomes of prior projects, are eagerly embracing the participatory approach and the value of health literacy principles. Workers in the original project factories are now engaging with those in new factories to share methods and ideas. Our HRA team was able to offer guidance about health determinants, health literacy, participatory design and research through periodic visits, without "running" the project, as happens in many researcher-controlled projects. Because this is a long-term project, it is an example of integrating participatory action research and design science methods, and it spans both "medical" and "public health" health literacy models.

8.3. ChronologyMD Mobile App

Crohn's disease is a serious, incurable inflammatory bowel disease that affects over 600,000 people in the US. Good patient-provider communication about disease symptoms and severity is critical, but it is difficult for patients to keep track of multiple symptoms accurately each day and for their physicians to make life-saving treatment decisions based on that information. The ChronologyMD project used design science methods, health literacy principles and artificial intelligence components to engage patients with Crohn's disease and their healthcare providers [103]. The project used a wide variety of participatory methods to enable patients with Crohn's disease create a mobile application that would track their detailed "observations of daily living," including symptoms and severity, mood, medication adherence, and behaviors (exercise, diet, etc.) to take more control over their health. Through artificial intelligence components, the app also passively collected biometric data, such as weight and sleep patterns, via connected wireless devices. With the participation of the patients' healthcare providers, a second app was created to display these data over time to improve shared decision-making with patients.

Intensive participatory design methods were necessary to create the highly refined features that patients and providers needed for the information to be effective in managing Crohn's disease. In addition, patients wanted and received an app that allowed them to design their own "observations of daily living" over time and assess interactions among variables such as symptoms, medication taking and behaviors. From a health literacy perspective, this highly iterative approach helped identify and address many communication barriers, such as easily inputting and understanding quantitative data (medication amounts, pain levels), and having simple displays of key information that could be understood quickly by patients and providers. Because of the iterative nature of the design, evaluation methods were also continuously revised so that interim findings could be used to constantly improve the intervention (as is done in the "build and evaluate" loops mentioned earlier). Findings from the pilot evaluation showed that the app enabled patients to greatly increase their input of symptoms and other data, better understand factors that helped or hindered their condition, and make positive changes. It also helped both patients and providers improve the quality of clinical encounters and shared decision-making. An important project lesson was that understanding of health literacy factors is at an early stage in the emerging and powerful field of artificial intelligence and health communication, and that participatory design is essential to every step of development.

8.4. Other Participatory Health Literacy Projects

• *Statewide Parenting Education Kits*
Participatory design and health literacy principles were used to create parenting education kits in five languages delivered to over 300,000 parents each year in California [75]. The project engaged many subgroups of parents with special attention to those with lower-income and/or lower-literacy. Statewide evaluation showed positive changes in knowledge and behaviors. The model has been adapted, using participatory processes, to other US states and in Australia. Participatory design activities are now underway to adapted printed information into Internet and mobile platforms.

• *Maternity Leave Resources for Pregnant Women*
English and Spanish-speaking pregnant women on Medicaid co-designed easy-to-understand resources [129]. In-person user testing uncovered and addressed many health literacy and motivational issues, even though first drafts were developed with detailed attention to health literacy principles and tested as "superior" on standardized health literacy assessments. Similar to what we found in the development of the Medicaid choices guide mentioned earlier, health literacy principles accounted for about half of what users wanted; the other half of changes covered a wide range of factors related to attractiveness, cultural appropriateness, subtleties of document "tone," types of graphics and their placement, resources for more help, etc.

• *Emergency Preparedness Communication for Deaf and Hard-of-Hearing Populations*
Because people who are Deaf tend to have especially low literacy levels, and Deaf and hard-of-hearing groups have many barriers to spoken communication, major changes are needed to adapt preparedness communication to their needs. The project used intensive participatory design and health literacy principles to recommend changes to communications, including those in American Sign Language, use of captioning, etc. [32]. There is little guidance to date about health literacy factors related to communications for people who are Deaf. For example: what determines users' comprehension of information communicated by mobile video? This area needs development through participatory design.

9. Conclusions

The emergence of the field of health literacy and the increased use of intensive participatory design are transforming theoretical guidance and empirical methods to improve health communication research and interventions. Health literacy, in association with other determinants of health, has greatly advanced our understanding of what affects people's health and intervention opportunities to address those factors. Because health literacy has been shown to mediate other determinants of health, it offers new practical pathways to positively impact people's health even without changes to intractable determinants of health, such as socio-economic status. Research on health literacy interventions has greatly advanced and shown positive, but uneven results to date. Participatory design theory and methods drawn from human/social sciences and design sciences can significantly improve health literacy models and interventions and vice versa. Participatory design is essential to understand deeper and elusive factors that impact health and specific ways to address them. If those most affected by these problems are not involved in identifying and addressing them, research models, interventions and broader policy changes will not likely improve.

Currently, most health literacy researchers and practitioners, such as those in public health, medicine, psychology, and communication, come from a social sciences perspective. However, the design sciences offer an existing, robust theoretical foundation that is currently underused. In my view, creating and studying health literacy interventions is especially well-aligned with the design sciences paradigm, given that intervention design relates to "what might be" rather than "what is." The design sciences offer powerful techniques with demonstrated success in the socio-technical fields. Combining them with our current health literacy approaches is an important direction and requires that we cultivate an active, multi-disciplinary dialogue to share new ways of thinking about health literacy, designing interventions and researching their impact. Integrating health literacy and participatory design drawn from multiple scientific paradigms and methods is complex and as much an art as a science. Multi-step models and case studies can help guide the work of researchers, practitioners, and policymakers in health communication/health literacy and those in many other fields committed to health promotion and health equity.

References

[1] Smedley BD, Syme SL. Promoting health: intervention strategies from social and behavioral research, Institute of Medicine. Washington, DC: National Academies Press; 2000.
[2] Marmot MG, Davey Smith G, Stansfield S, et al. Health inequalities among British civil servants: the Whitehall II study. Lancet. 1991; 337(8754):1387–93.
[3] Whitehead M. The concepts and principles of equity and health. Health Promot Int. 1991; 6(3): 217–28.
[4] Denton M, Prus S, Walters V. Gender differences in health: a Canadian study of the psychosocial, structural and behavioural determinants of health. Soc Sci Med. 2004; 58:2585–2600.
[5] Bronfenbrenner U. Toward an experimental ecology of human development. Am Psychol. 1977; July:513–31.
[6] Stokols D, Allen J, Bellingham RL. The social ecology of health promotion: implications for research and practice. Am J Health Promot. 1996; 10:247–51.
[7] Stokols D. The social ecological paradigm of wellness promotion. In: Jamner MS, Stokols D, editors, Promoting human wellness: new frontiers for research, practice, and policy. Berkeley: University of California Press; 2000. p. 127–46.

[8]   Logan RA. Seeking an expanded, multidimensional conceptual approach to health literacy and health disparities research. In: Logan R, Siegel E, editors. Health literacy: New directions in research, theory and practice. Stud Health Technol Inform 240, Amsterdam: IOS Press; 2017. p. 96–123. DOI: 10.3233/978-1-61499-790-0-96.

[9]   Currie J, Schwandt H. Inequality in mortality decreased among the young while increasing for older adults, 1990–2010. Science. 2016; 352(6286):708–12. DOI: 10.1126/science.aaf1437.

[10] U.S. Department of Health and Human Services. Healthy People 2020. Draft. U.S. Government Printing Office; 2009.

[11] Dominguez TP, Dunkel-Schetter C, Glynn LM, Hobel C, Sandman CA. Racial differences in birth outcomes: the role of general, pregnancy, and racism stress. Health Psychol. 2008; 27(2):194–203. DOI: 10.1037/0278-6133.27.2.194.

[12] McCormack L, Thomas V, Lewis MA, Rudd R. Improving low health literacy and patient engagement: A social ecological approach. Patient Educ Counsel. 2016. DOI: 10.1016/j.pec.2016.07.007.

[13] Phelan JC, Link BG, Tehranifar P. Social conditions as fundamental causes of health inequalities. J Health Soc Behav. 2010; 51(1 suppl):S28–S40.

[14] Braveman P, Gruskin S. Defining equity in health. J Epidemiol Community Health. 2003; 57(4): 254–58.

[15] Dutta MJ, Kreps GL, editors. Reducing health disparities: communication interventions. New York: Peter Lang Publishers; 2013.

[16] Marmot M. Social determinants of health inequalities. Lancet. 2005; 354(9464):1099–1104.

[17] Nuru-Jeter AM, Williams T, LaVeist TA. Distinguishing the race-specific effects of income inequality in US metropolitan areas. Int J Health Serv 2014; 44(3):435–56.

[18] Rawls JA. Theory of justice. Cambridge: Belknap/Harvard University Press; 1971.

[19] Krieger N, et al. Racism, sexism and social class: implications for studies of health, disease and well-being. Am J Prev Med. 1993; 9(6 Suppl):82–122.

[20] Bandura A. Exercise of personal and collective efficacy. In: Bandura A, editor. Self-efficacy in changing societies. New York: Cambridge University Press; 1995. p. 1–45.

[21] Kreps GL. The pervasive role of information in health and health care: implications for health communication policy. In: Anderson JA, editor. Communication yearbook 11. Newbury Park, CA: Sage; 1988. p. 238–76.

[22] Neuhauser L, Kreps G. Rethinking communication in the e-health era. J Health Psychol. 2003; 8:7–22.

[23] Neuhauser L, Kreps G. Ehealth communication and behavior change: promise and performance. Journal of Social Semiotics. 2010; 20:1,9–27.

[24] Logan R. Health campaign research: Enduring challenges and new developments. In: Bucchi M, Trench B, editors. Routledge handbook of public communication of science and technology. 2nd ed. New York: Routledge; 2014. p. 198–213.

[25] Snyder LB, Hamilton MA, Mitchell EW, Kiwanuka-Tondo J, Fleming-Milici F, Proctor D. A meta-analysis of the effect of mediated health communication campaigns on behavior change in the United States. J Health Commun. 2004; 9(Suppl. 1):71–96.

[26] Cho H, Salmon CT. Unintended effects of health communication campaigns. J Commun. 2007; 57:293–317.

[27] Viswanath K, Finnegan JR. The knowledge gap hypothesis: Twenty-five years later. In Burlson B, editor. Communication yearbook 19. Thousand Oaks, CA: Sage; 1995. p. 187–228.

[28] Emmons KM. Behavioral and social science contributions to the health of adults in the United States. In Smedley B, Syme SL, editors. Promoting health: Intervention strategies from social and behavioral research. Institute of Medicine, Washington, DC: National Academy Press; 2000. p. 254–321.

[29] Kreuter MW, McClure SM. The role of culture in health communication. Annual Reviews of Public Health. 2004; 25:439–55.

[30] Kreps GL, Sparks L. Meeting the health literacy needs of immigrant populations. Patient Educ Couns. 2008; 71:328–32.

[31] Kreps GL, Neuhauser L. Designing health information programs to promote the health and well-being of vulnerable populations: the benefits of evidence-based strategic communication. In: Arnott Smith C, Kesselman A, editors. Meeting health information needs outside of healthcare: opportunities and challenges. Chandos Publishing; 2015. p. 1–16.

[32] Neuhauser L, Ivey SL, Huang D, Engelman A, Tseng W, Dahrouge D, Gurung S, Kealey M. Availability and readability of emergency preparedness materials for Deaf and Hard of Hearing and older adult populations: Issues and assessments. PLoS ONE. 2013; 8(2): e55614. DOI: 10.1371/journal.pone.0055614

[33] Wang R. Critical health literacy: a case study from China in schistosomiasis control. Health Promotion International. 2000; 15(3):269–74.

[34] Deci E, Ryan R, editors. Handbook of Self-Determination Research. Rochester, NY: University of Rochester Press; 2002.

[35] Dede C, Fontana L. Transforming health education via new media. In: Harris LM, editor. Health and the new media: tTechnologies transforming personal and public health Hillsdale, NJ: Erlbaum; 1995. p. 163–83.

[36] Hesse BW, Schneiderman B. eHealth research from the user's perspective. Am J Prev Med. 2007; 32:S97–103.

[37] Doak LG, Doak CC. Lowering the silent barriers for patients with low literacy skills. Promot Health. 1987; 8(4):6–8.

[38] Kutner M, Greenberg E, Jin Y, Paulsen C. The health literacy of America's adults: results from the 2003 national assessment of adult literacy (NCES2006-483). U.S. Department of Education. Washington, DC: National Center for Education Statistics; 2006.

[39] White S. Assessing the nation's health literacy: key concepts and findings of the National Assessment of Adult Literacy (NAAL). Chicago, IL: American Medical Association Foundation; 2008.

[40] Baker DW. The associations between health literacy and health outcomes: Self-reported health, hospitalization, and mortality. In: Office of the Surgeon General. Proceedings of the Surgeon General's workshop on improving health literacy. Rockville, MD: Office of the Surgeon General (US); 2006.

[41] Parker R, Ratzan SC. Health literacy: A second decade of distinction for Americans. J Health Commun. 2010; 15(Suppl 2):20–33.

[42] Koh HK, Berwick DM, Clancy CM, Baur C, Brach C, Harris LM, Zerhusen EG. New federal policy initiatives to boost health literacy can help the nation move beyond the cycle of costly 'crisis care.' Health Affairs. 2012; 31:434–43.

[43] Paasche-Orlow MK, Wilson EAH, McCormack L. The evolving field of health literacy research. J Health Commun. 2010; 15:5–8.

[44] Logan RA. Health literacy research. In: Arnott-Smith C, Keselman A, editors. Meeting health information needs outside of healthcare: opportunities and challenges. Waltham, MA: Chandos; 2015. p. 19–38.

[45] Sorensen K, Van den Broucke S, Fullam J, Doyle G, Pelikan J, Slonska Z, Brand H, (HLS-EU) Consortium Health Literacy Project European. Health literacy and public health: A systematic review and integration of definitions and models. BMC Public Health. 2012; 12:80. DOI: 10.1186/1471-2458-12-80.

[46] World Health Organization. Health promotion glossary. Geneva: WHO; 1998.

[47] AMA Ad Hoc Committee on Health Literacy for the Council on Scientific Affairs. AMA: Health literacy: report of the council on scientific affairs. JAMA. 1999; 281(6):552–57.

[48] Institute of Medicine of the National Academies. Health literacy: a prescription to end confusion Washington, DC: The National Academies; 2004.

[49] Nutbeam D. The evolving concept of health literacy. Soc Sci Med. 2008; 67(12):2072–78.

[50] U.S. Department of Health and Human Services. Communicating health: priorities and strategies for progress. Washington, DC: U.S. Department of Health and Human Services; 2003.

[51] Centre for Health Literacy. Calgary Charter. 2008. Accessed at: http://www.centreforliteracy.qc.ca/health_literacy/calgary_charter

[52] Kickbusch I, Maag D. Health literacy. In: Kris H, Stella Q, editors. International encyclopedia of public health. Vol. 3. Academic Press; 2008. p. 204–11.

[53] Brach C, Keller D, Hernandez LM, Baur C, Parker R, Dreyer B, Schyve P, Lemerise AJ, Schillinger D. Ten attributes of health literate organizations. Institute of Medicine, National Academy of Sciences. National Academies Press; 2012.

[54] Rudd R, Renzulli D, Pereira A, Daltory L. Literacy demands in health care settings: The patient perspective. In: Schwartzberg JG, VanGeest JB, Wang CC, editors. Understanding health literacy: Implications for medicine and public health. Chicago: AMA Press; 2005.

[55] Freedman DA, Bess KD, Tucker HA, Boyd DL, Tuchman AM, Wallston KA. Public health literacy defined. Am J Prev Med. 2009; 36(5):446–51.

[56] Pleasant A, Rudd RE, O'Leary C, Paasche-Orlow MK, Allen MP, Alvarado-Little W, Myers L, Parson K, Rosen S. Considerations for a new definition of health literacy. Washington, DC: National Academy of Medicine; 2016. https://nam.edu/considerations-for-a-new-definition-of-health-literacy/

[57] Pleasant A, Cabe J, Martin L, Rikard RV. A prescription is not enough: improving public health with health literacy. In: Implications of health literacy for public health: workshop summary. Roundtable on Health Literacy, Board on Population Health and Public Health Practice. Institute of Medicine. National Academies Press; 2013.

[58] Paasche-Orlow MK, Wolf MS. The causal pathways linking health literacy to health outcomes. Am J Health Behav. 2007; 31(Suppl 1):19–26.

[59] Hibbard J. Patient activation and health literacy: what's the difference? How do each contribute to health outcomes? In: Logan R, Siegel E, editors. Health literacy: New directions in research, theory and practice. Stud Health Technol Inform 240, Amsterdam: IOS Press; 2017. p. 251–262. DOI: 10.3233/978-1-61499-790-0-251.

[60] Von Wagner C, Steptoe A, Wolf MS, Wardle J. Health literacy and health actions: a review and a framework from health psychology. Health Education & Behaviour. 2009; 36(5):860–77.

[61] Berkman ND, Sheridan SL, Donahue KE, Halpern DJ, Viera A, Crotty K, Holland A, Brasure M, Lohr KN, Harden E, Tant E, Wallace I, Viswanathan M. Health literacy interventions and outcomes: an updated systematic review. Evidence Report/Technology Assessment No. 199. Prepared by RTI International—University of North Carolina Evidence-based Practice Center under contract No. 290-2007-10056-I. AHRQ Publication Number 11-E006. Rockville, MD: Agency for Healthcare Research and Quality; 2011.

[62] Sudore RL, Yaffe K, Satterfield S, Harris TB, Mehta KM, Simonsick EM, Newman AB, Rosano C, Rooks R, Rubin SM, et al. Limited literacy and mortality in the elderly: the health, aging, and body composition study. J Gen Intern Med. 2006; 21(8):806–12.

[63] Wolf MS, Knight SJ, Lyons EA, Durazo-Arvizu R, Pickard SA, Arseven A, Arozullah A, Colella K, Ray P, Bennett CL. Literacy, race, and PSA level among low- income men newly diagnosed with prostate cancer. Urology. 2006; 68(1):89–93.

[64] Logan RA, Wong WF, Villaire M, Daus G, Parnell TA, Willis E, Paasche-Orlow MK. Health literacy: a necessary element for achieving health equity. Discussion Paper. Washington, DC: National Academy of Medicine; 2015. http://www.nam.edu/perspectives/2015/Health-literacy-a-necessary-element-for-achieving-health-equity

[65] Rudd RE, Anderson JE, Oppenheimer S, Nath C. Health literacy: an update of public health and medical literature. In: Comings JP, Garner B, Smith C, editors. Review of adult learning and literacy. Vol. 7. Mahwah, NJ: Lawrence Erlbaum Associates; 2007.

[66] Davis TC, Holcombe RF, Berkel HJ, Pramanik S, Divers SG. Informed consent for clinical trials: a comparative study of standard versus simplified forms. J Natl Cancer Inst. 1998; 90(9):668–74.

[67] Murphy PW. Reading ability of parents compared with reading level of pediatric patient education materials. Pediatrics. 1994; 93:460–68.

[68] Neuhauser L, Rothschild B, Graham C, Ivey SL, Konishi S. Participatory design of mass health communication in three languages for seniors and people with disabilities on Medicaid. Am J Public Health. 2009; 99(12):2188–95.

[69] CDC (Centers for Disease Control and Prevention). Health literacy for public health professionals. 2011. http://www.cdc.gov/healthliteracy/GetTrainingCE.html (accessed November 2016).

[70] DeWalt DA, Callahan LF, Hawk VH, Broucksou KA, Hink A, Rudd R, Brach C. Health literacy universal precautions toolkit. 2010. http://www.ahrq.gov/qual/literacy/healthliteracytoolkit.pdf. Retrieved November 2016.

[71] Wolf MS, Davis TC, Curtis LM, Webb JA, Bailey SC, Shrank WH, Lindquist L, Ruo B, Bocchini MV, Parker RM, Wood AJJ. Effect of standardized, patient-centered label instructions to improve comprehension of prescription drug use. Medical Care. 2011; 49(1):96–100. DOI: 110.1097/ MLR.1090b1013e3181f38174.

[72] Sheridan SL, Halpern DJ, Viera AJ, Berkman ND, Donahue KE, Crotty K. Interventions for individuals with low health literacy: A systematic review. J Health Commun. 2011; 16 Suppl 3:30–54.

[73] Schillinger D, Piette J, Wilson C, Daher C, Leong-Grotz K, Castro C, Bindman AB. Closing the loop: physician communication with diabetic patients who have low health literacy. Archives of Internal Medicine. 2003; 163(1):83–90.

[74] Arcia A, Suero-Tejeda N, Bales ME, Merrill JA, Yoon S, Woollen J, Bakken S. Sometimes more is more: iterative participatory design of infographics for engagement of community members with varying levels of health literacy. J Am Med Inform Assoc. 2016; 23(1):174–83. DOI: 10.1093/ jamia/ocv079.

[75] Neuhauser L, Constantine WL, Constantine NA, Sokal-Gutierrez K, Obarski SK, Clayton L, Desai M, Sumner G, Syme SL. Promoting prenatal and early childhood health: evaluation of a statewide materials-based intervention for parents. Am J Public Health. 2007; 97(10):813–19.

[76] Zite NB, Wallace LS. Use of a low-literacy informed consent form to improve women's understanding of tubal sterilization: a randomized controlled trial. Obstet Gynecol. 2011; 117:1160–66.

[77] Herman A, Jackson P. Empowering low-income parents with skills to reduce excess pediatric emergency room and clinic visits through a tailored low literacy training intervention. J Health Commun. 2010; 15(8):895–910. DOI: 10.1080/10810730.2010.522228.

[78] Sudore RL, Landefeld CS, Williams BA, Barnes DE, Lindquist K, et al. Use of a modified informed consent process among vulnerable patients: a descriptive study. J Gen Intern Med. 2006; 21:867–73.

[79] Jacobson TA, Thomas DM, Morton FJ, Offutt G, Shevlin J, Ray S. Use of a low-literacy patient education tool to enhance pneumococcal vaccination rates. A randomized controlled trial. JAMA. 1999; 282(7):646–50.

[80] Taggart J, Williams A, Dennis S, Newall A, Shortus T, Zwar N, Denney-Wilson E, Harris MF. A systematic review of interventions in primary care to improve health literacy for chronic disease behavioral risk factors. Database of Abstracts of Reviews for Effects (DARE): Quality-assessed reviews. 2012. http://www.ncbi.nlm.nih.gov/pubmedhealth/PMH0052469/ (accessed July 22, 2015).

[81] Bailey SC, Oramasion CU, Wolf MS. Rethinking adherence: A health literacy-informed model of medication self-management. J Health Commun. 2013; 18 Suppl 1:20–30. DOI: 10.1080/10810730.2013.825672.

[82] Ratanawongsa N, Karter AJ, Parker MM, Courtney RL, Heisler M, Moffett HH, Adler N, Wharton EM, Schillinger D. Communication and medication adherence: the diabetes study of Northern California. JAMA Intern Med. 2013; 173(3):210–18. DOI: 10.1001/jamainternmed.2013.1216.

[83] Smith MY, Wallace JS. Reducing drug self-injection errors: a randomized trial comparing a "standard" versus "plain language" version of patient instructions for use. Res Soc Adm Pharm. 2013 Sept–Oct; 9(5):621–25.

[84] Yin HS, Mendelsohn AL, Wolf MS, Parker RM, Fierman A, van Schaick L, Bazan IS, Kline MD, Dreyer BP. Parents' medication administration errors: role of dosing instruments and health literacy. Arch Pediatr Adolesc Med. 2010; 164(2):181–86.

[85] Smith PC, Brice JH, Lee J. The relationship between functional health literacy and adherence to emergency department discharge instructions among Spanish-speaking patients. J Natl Med Assoc. 2012; 104(11–12):521–27.

[86] Fischoff B, Brewer NT, Downs J., editors. Communicating risks and benefits: an evidence-based user's guide. Silver Spring, MD: U.S. Department of Health and Human Services. Bethesda MD: Food and Drug Administration; 2011.

[87] Neuhauser L, Paul K. Readability, comprehension and usability. In: Communicating risks and benefits: an evidence-based user's guide. Silver Spring, MD: U.S. Department of Health and Human Services. Bethesda, MD: Food and Drug Administration; 2011.

[88] Wolka A, Simpson K, Lockwood K, Neuhauser L. Focus on health literacy. Ther Innov Regul Sci. 2014; 49(3):369–76.

[89] Baker DW, DeWalt DA, Schillinger D, Hawk B, Ruo B, Bibbins-Domingo K, Weinberger M, Macabasco-O'Connell A, Pignone M. "Teach to goal": Theory and design principles of an intervention to improve heart failure self-management skills of patients with low health literacy. J Health Commun. 2011; 16(Suppl 3):73–88.

[90] Rudd R, Anderson J. The health literacy environment of hospitals and health centers. 2006. http://www.hsph.harvard.edu/healthliteracy/files/healthliteracyenvironment.pdf (accessed November, 2016).

[91] Pleasant A, Kuruvilla S. A tale of two health literacies: Public health and clinical approaches to health literacy. Health Promot Int. 2006; 23:152–59.

[92] Pleasant A. Assisting vulnerable communities: Canyon Ranch Institute's health literacy and community-based interventions. In: Logan R, Siegel E, editors. Health literacy: New directions in research, theory and practice. Stud Health Technol Inform 240, Amsterdam: IOS Press; 2017. p. 127–143. DOI: 10.3233/978-1-61499-790-0-127.

[93] WHO. International Conference on Primary Health Care. Alma-Ata, USSR, 6–12 September 1978. Report. WHO: Geneva; 1978.

[94] Hoy EW, Kenney E, Talavera AC. Engaging consumers in designing a guide to Medi-Cal managed care quality. Oakland: California HealthCare Foundation; 2004.

[95] Barton JL, Kooenig CJ, Trupin L, Anderson J, Ragouzeous D, Breslin M, Morse T, Schillinger D, Montori VM, Yelin EH. The design of a low literacy decision aid about rheumatoid arthritis medications in three languages for use during the clinical encounter. BMC Med Inform Decis Mak. 2014 Nov 25; 14:104. DOI: 10.1186/s12911-014-0104-8.

[96] Vaiana ME, McGlynn EA. What cognitive science tells us about the design of reports for consumers. Med Care Res Rev. 2002; 59(1):3–35.

[97] Neuhauser L. Participatory design for better interactive health communication: a statewide model in the USA. Electron J Commun. 2001; 11(3–4): 43.

[98] Vallance JK, Courneya KS, Plotnikoff RC, Yasui Y, Mackey JR. Randomized controlled trial of the effects of print materials and step pedometers on physical activity and quality of life in breast cancer survivors. J Clin Oncol. 2007; 25(17):2352–59.

[99] Cooper LA, Beach MC, Clever SL. Participatory decision-making in the medical encounter and its relationship to patient literacy. In: Schwartzberg J, VanGeest J, Wang C, editors. Understanding

health literacy: implications for medicine and public health. Chicago, IL: American Medical Association; 2005. p. 101–17.

[100] Gustafson DH, Hawkins R, Boberg E, et al. Impact of a patient-centered, computer-based health information/support system. Am J Prev Med. 1999; 16(1):1–9.

[101] Minkler M, Wallerstein N, editors. Community based participatory research for health: Process to outcomes. 2nd ed. San Francisco: Jossey-Bass; 2008.

[102] Neuhauser L, Kreps GL. Integrating design science theory and methods to improve the development and evaluation of health communication programs. J Health Commun. 2014; 19(12):1460–71. DOI: 10.1080/10810730.2014.954081.

[103] Neuhauser L, Kreps GL, Morrison K, Athanasoulis M, Kirienko N, Van Brunt D. Using design science and artificial intelligence to improve health communication: ChronologyMD case example. Patient Educ Counsel. 2013; 92(2): 211–17.

[104] Neuhauser L, Kreps GL, Syme SL. Community participatory design of health communication programs: Methods and case examples from Australia, China, Switzerland and the United States. In: Kim DK, Singhal A, Kreps GL, editors. Global health communication strategies in the 21st century: design, implementation and evaluation. New York: Peter Lang Publishing; 2013.

[105] Noar SM, Harrington NG, editors. eHealth applications: promising strategies for behavior change. New York: Routledge; 2012.

[106] Coulter A, Stilwell D, Kryworuchko J, Mullen PD, Ng CJ, van der Weijden T. A systematic development process for patient decision aids. BMC Med Inform Decis Mak. 2013; 13(Suppl 2):S2. DOI: 10.1186/1472-6947-13-S2-S2.

[107] Antonovsky A. Health, stress and coping. San Francisco: Jossey-Bass; 1979.

[108] Lewin K. Action research and minority problems. J Soc Issues. 1946; 2(4):34–46.

[109] Reason P, Bradbury H. Handbook of action research. 2nd ed. London: Sage; 2007.

[110] Reason P, Bradbury H, editors. The Sage handbook of action research: participative inquiry and practice. London and Thousand Oaks, CA: Sage; 2008.

[111] Chevalier JM, Buckles DJ. Participatory action research: theory and methods for engaged inquiry. London: Routledge; 2013.

[112] Fuller RB, McHale J. World design science decade, 1965–1975. Carbondale, IL: Southern Illinois University; 1963.

[113] Gregor S. Building theory in the science of the artificial. In: Proceedings of the 4th International Conference on Design Science Research in Information Systems and Technology. New York: Association for Computing Machinery; 2009.

[114] Dilthey W. Introduction to the human sciences. Detroit, MI: Wayne State University Press; 1988.

[115] Cook T. Post positivist critical multiplism. In: Shotland R, Mark M, editors. Social science and social policy. Beverly Hills, CA: Sage; 1985. p. 25–62.

[116] Simon H. The sciences of the artificial. 3rd ed. Cambridge, MA: MIT Press; 1996.

[117] Buchanan R. Wicked problems in design thinking. Design Issues. 1992; 8:5–21.

[118] March ST, Smith G. Design and natural science research on information technology. Decision Support Systems. 1995; 15:251–66.

[119] Computer Professionals for Social Responsibility. Participatory design. 2000. Retrieved from http://cpsr.org/issues/pd/

[120] Markus ML, Majchrzak A, Gasser L. A design theory for systems that support emergent knowledge processes. Management Information Systems Quarterly. 2002; 26:179–212.

[121] Roschuni CN. Communicating design research effectively. PhD dissertation, 2012. Retrieved from http://escholarship.org/uc/item/75f0z49v?query=roschuni

[122] Vechakul J, Shrimali BP, Sandhu JS. Human centered design as an approach for place-based innovation in public health: a CDC case study from Oakland, California. Matern Child Health J. 2015 Dec; 19(12):2552–59.

[123] Nielsen J. Designing web usability. Indianapolis, IN: New Riders; 2000.

[124] Rubin J, Chisnell D. Handbook of usability testing. Indianapolis, IN: Wiley Publishing; 2008.

[125] Hevner A, March S, Park J, Ram S. Design science in information systems research. Management Information Systems Quarterly. 2004; 28:75–105.

[126] Neuhauser L. Creating and implementing large-scale parenting education programs: Bridging research, decision-making and practice. In: Bammer G, Michaux A, Sanson A, editors. Bridging the "know-do" gap: knowledge brokering to improve child well-being. Australian National University Press; 2010. Available online at: http://epress.anu.edu.au/knowledge_citation.html

[127] Health Research for Action. Year two report of the Medi-Cal access project. Berkeley: University of California, Berkeley; 2008.

[128] Kurtovich E, Ivey S, Neuhauser L, Graham C. Evaluation of a multilingual mass communication intervention for seniors and people with disabilities on Medicaid: a randomized controlled trial. Health Serv Res. 2010 Apr; 45(2):397–417. DOI: 10.1111/j.1475-6773.2009.01073.

[129] Kurtovich E, Guendelman S, Neuhauser L, Edelman D, Georges M, Mason-Marti P. Development and first phase evaluation of a maternity leave educational tool for pregnant, working women in California. PLoS ONE. 10(6): e0129472. DOI: 10.1371/journal.pone.0129472.

Health Literacy
R.A. Logan and E.R. Siegel (Eds.)
IOS Press, 2017
© *2017 The authors and IOS Press. All rights reserved.*
doi:10.3233/978-1-61499-790-0-330

The Health Information National Trends Survey (HINTS): A Resource for Consumer Engagement and Health Communication Research

Bradford W. HESSE[a,1], Alexandra J. GREENBERG[b], Emily B. PETERSON[a], and
Wen-Ying Sylvia CHOU[a]

[a] *Division of Cancer Control and Population Sciences, National Cancer Institute,
Bethesda, MD USA*
[b] *Mayo Clinic College of Medicine, Rochester, MN USA*

Abstract. The contemporary healthcare system can help improve health literacy outcomes in two ways: first, by nurturing the skills and motivations needed for patients to be actively engaged in their own health and healthcare decisions; and, second, by creating a prepared and proactive healthcare system that adapts to patients' capacities and needs in efficacious ways. In 2001, the National Cancer Institute launched the Health Information National Trends Survey (HINTS) as a way for researchers and planners to understand how the public is interacting with a rapidly changing health information environment. Original iterations of the HINTS national probability sampling strategies took place on a biennial basis, but in subsequent years the protocol moved to a yearly administration. This yields a rich resource of cross-sectional, national surveillance data to evaluate for trends across and within vulnerable populations. Sixteen studies are presented from the published literature to illustrate how HINTS data were used to explore constructs of direct interest to health literacy researchers. Suggestions are given for how this ongoing public surveillance mechanism can be used: (a) to provide a sentinel view of how the public is interacting with information in the environment to address their health needs; (b) to generate research questions and hypotheses for further exploration using complementary methodologies; and (c) to explore the diffusion of new health communication channels within and between segments of the national population.

Keywords. Health Communication, Patient Engagement, Surveillance

1. Introduction

"The millions of dollars of biomedical research ... aimed at a disease that was costing tens of thousands of dollars to treat and it ultimately relied on the actions of a skinny, weak, scared 20-year old to have its impact." Jessie Gruman, Behavioral Scientist and Patient Advocate, (12/7/1953 to 7/14/2014).

---

[1] Corresponding Author: Bradford W. Hesse, National Cancer Institute, 9609 Medical Center Drive, Room 3E610, MSC 9761, Rockville, MD 20852; hesseb@mail.nih.gov.

As a behavioral scientist and a long-time Hodgkin's lymphoma patient, Jessie Gruman dedicated her life to improving health outcomes for patients. Much of her energy was focused on elevating the degree to which patients could become more actively engaged in their own health and healthcare decisions. She equally emphasized the responsibility of patients to engage directly with their health and healthcare [1] and the responsibilities of healthcare systems and researchers to create real, trustworthy support for patients struggling with disease [2]. In this chapter, we will begin by describing a behavioral science perspective on health literacy, which connects to the inception and objectives of the NCI-sponsored Health Information National Trends Survey (HINTS). We will then introduce the history, vision, and status of HINTS and summarize research contributions to the health literacy knowledge base that are based on various iterations of the HINTS instruments. We conclude with future directions that HINTS offers to health communication researchers and practitioners, particularly those charged with moving the science of health literacy forward.

1.1. Patient Activation and Prepared Systems

Per the goals for a healthier nation set by the Department of Health and Human Services' *Healthy People* initiative, health literacy refers to the degree to which individuals have the capacity to obtain, process, and understand basic health information and services needed to make appropriate health decisions [3]. Supporting health literacy, therefore, means attending to the malleable, individual characteristics of the individual as well as attending to the information environment in which the public lives and thrives. Wagner and colleagues [4] take this two-fold point of interaction further by setting goals for the healthcare system in which patients are encouraged to be fully engaged, or activated, stewards of their own care while transacting with a system that is fully prepared to offer evidence-based support for patients' personal and medical needs. On the individual side of the equation, Gruman referred to this notion of patient engagement as a critical quality encompassing the "actions people take to support their health and benefit from their health care" [5]. In a similar vein, Hibbard and Gilburt described patient activation as relating to the "knowledge, skills and confidence a person has in managing their own health and health care" [6]. Studies have demonstrated that patients who score high on measures of patient activation tend to have better care experiences [7], are less costly to the healthcare system [8], and generally experience better health outcomes than their "disengaged" counterparts [9]. Creating a public health environment that nurtures individual engagement has become a hallmark of public policy overtures in both the United Kingdom [10] and the United States [11].

Although crucial, patient motivation is only part of the formula for optimizing individual and population-level health outcomes in health service research. The other side of the equation must be considered in terms of the healthcare environment itself; that is, whether the system is built around principles of evidence-based practice in health communication and can serve as a responsive receptor site to the patient's own engaged overtures. Systems that are unprepared, or that seek to exploit transactional value from patient encounters at the expense of long-term support (as often happens within a fee-for-service vs. a value-based incentive structure), will often fail to engender the sense of response efficacy needed to sustain action over time [12]. Patients' intentional actions must work together with a supportive healthcare environment to produce sustainably productive outcomes [2, 13]. This line of thinking is delicately intertwined throughout the Institute of Medicine's (now the National Academies of Sciences, Engineering, Medicine) workshop series on quality improvement in healthcare [14-17]. The series adopts a human factors approach [18] by deconstructing sources of error within contemporary healthcare, and then offering a blueprint for how to build a more robust, higher quality healthcare system for the twenty-first century. Such a system would be patient-centric, and would focus on creating an environment that offered deep, comprehensive support for patients' medical, emotional, and information needs [12, 19]. Ideally, such a system would adopt a "universal design" [20] approach, in that it would become equitably accessible to all patients regardless of cultural backgrounds or level of personal health literacy [21]. These concepts are informing many healthcare reform efforts currently underway worldwide.

1.2. A Health Systems Perspective on Health Literacy

When considering how to support the actions individuals take to improve their health and to benefit from healthcare – that is, in considering how to support patient engagement – behavioral scientists must take into account the relationship between the individual and the environment in which they live and thrive [22]. Donald Norman, a cognitive scientist with a legacy of influence in engineering and design [23], best described this balance of interactions. When considering human behavior, he noted that it is worthwhile to recognize that there are two sources of knowledge that drive human action: one source is internal to the individual, or "knowledge in the head;" the other is external to the individual, or "knowledge in the world." The history of writing, literature, and, more recently, information technology has largely been a story of creating knowledge in the world so that it can supplement knowledge in head reliably across many stakeholders within the society. Literacy, in this context, is the ability of individuals to process and act upon information using the skills and knowledge they have acquired through experience. In a very similar sense, health literacy has been defined as "the capacity to obtain, process, and understand basic health information and services needed to make appropriate health decisions" [24]. Research on health literacy focuses generally on understanding how individuals with various levels of experience, language, and knowledge interact with the people, instructions, and tools made available to them in healthcare.

There are at least two complementary ways for intervening on behalf of patients to improve health outcomes. The first is to assess the knowledge and skills a patient might bring into the health care setting and then to supplement any deficits with education and counseling [25]. The second is to improve the availability and compatibility of information in the environment to ensure that all patients, regardless of knowledge they bring into the encounter, will fare well throughout their healthcare journeys [26]. Consider the example of a patient who presents with an early stage diagnosis of non-Hodgkin's lymphoma. The patient is likely to know very little about this disease prior to receiving this disquieting and disorienting diagnosis. After thoughtfully explaining some of the most important aspects of the disease to the patient, the treating oncologist may then elect to give the patient an "information prescription" [25] to round out their understanding of the disease and to inform future decision-making. This "prescription" might be in the form of pamphlets or other media, an informational website, or a visit with a specialized counselor. The oncologist may further explain that the patient's electronic portal will contain a secure messaging feature that can be used any time to ask a question, as well as a telephone number for use in emergencies. As treatment progresses, the oncologist may introduce the patient to a nurse navigator to help schedule appointments, arrange for tests, and report symptoms. These services provide informational support from the environment to complement the patient's evolving knowledge about their condition(s) [27].

The skilled health system designer recognizes that these two leverage points must be considered together when creating resources to support patients. A well-designed decision aid using iconographs, for example, has been shown to improve decision-making for professionals with all levels of health numeracy [28-30]. Research from medical informatics and patient education literature strongly suggests that a patient's ability to obtain, understand, and apply health information relies on much more than personal literacy skills alone [26]. Health systems can make universal improvements to improve outcomes across all types of patients equitably by creating an intelligent healthcare environment [31] that lowers the demand from patients through better informational design [23]. Such a system would reserve high-valued educational and counseling resources for those who need them the most [32]. In Figure 1, we present an enhanced version of the Chronic Care Model as developed by Gee and colleagues [33] to illustrate how the post-HITECH (i.e., the Health Information Technology for Economic and Clinical Care Act of 2009) healthcare system can be engineered to support patient engagement and to compensate for deficits in health literacy. The updated model adds in components of technology-mediated communication and support typical of today's health care settings [4, 33].

As depicted in the model, the "Informed, Activated Patient" brings with her a preexisting set of knowledge ("knowledge in the head"). In addition, she also comes in with prior experiences gathered from within and from outside of healthcare ("knowledge in the world"), which informs her decision making during the encounter. The "Prepared, Proactive Practice Team" interfaces with the knowledge of the patient by offering support in a variety of forms, ranging from traditional media (e.g., information pamphlets), clinical information systems like electronic patient portals, and eHealth education tools, to professionally trained navigators and other allied health professionals.

In sum, conceptualizing health literacy within the health care system can help inform the construction of a national communication surveillance program. In this way, construction of the Health Information National Trends Survey (HINTS) can serve to complement existing datasets and surveillance programs of relevance to health literacy researchers. For example, one of the main surveillance tools for literacy assessment is the Department of Education's National Assessment of Adult Literacy (NAAL), a performance-based national- and state-based assessments of adult literacy performance. NAAL evaluates individual competencies and deficits as a diagnostic for dedicating monetary resources or modifying curricula within educational systems. In contrast, public health surveillance programs often do not include in-depth assessments but rather gather self-reported data on knowledge, attitudes, and behaviors. As a case in point, the Behavioral Risk Factors Surveillance System (BRFSS) gathers self-reported data across states and territories on behaviors known to influence public health outcomes. These data are used to track the diffusion of beliefs, knowledge, and healthy behaviors as distributed across varying populations. Public health departments may utilize the surveillance data to inform patient outreach and education efforts, while epidemiologists may analyze the data for evidence of knowledge or belief gaps among differing populations. In what follows, we will describe how HINTS is uniquely positioned to serve as a health communication surveillance tool for health literacy researchers working within health care systems.

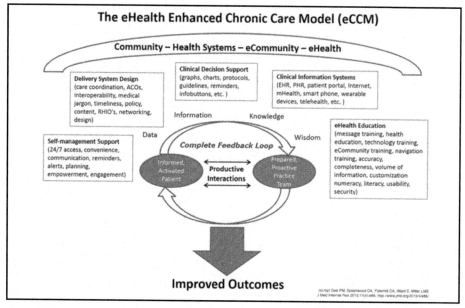

Figure 1. The eHealth Enhanced Chronic Care Model (eCCM). Created by Gee, P. M., Greenwood, D. A., Paterniti, D. A., Ward, D., and Miller, L. M. [33]

2. The Health Information National Trends Survey (HINTS)

In the late 1990s, a group of health communication experts, behavioral scientists, clinicians, and public health professionals gathered at the behest of the National Cancer Institute (NCI) to identify priorities for behavioral research related to cancer control and prevention. One priority identified by the group was to seize on the opportunities afforded by a rapidly changing health communication environment to improve support for individuals' capacities to prevent and control the disease. When recommendations from the group were published in 1999, the World Wide Web had only existed for approximately six years. Anecdotal evidence suggested that patients were already showing up at their doctors' offices with reams of paper printed from their latest foray onto Internet search engines. Some early evaluations of Internet search data suggested that the Web was becoming the first resource for many health information seekers. Recommendations from the external group of health communication experts were to monitor these changes through public surveillance of the health information environment. The recommendations were especially sensitive to the unanticipated consequences of creating a "Digital Divide" between those facile with these new communication technologies and those struggling with access, language, or technological prowess.

2.1. Establishing a Health Communication Data Program

With those recommendations in hand, the Division of Cancer Control and Population Sciences at the NCI launched the Health Information National Trends Survey (HINTS) in 2001. The program serves as the surveillance arm of a larger investment to fund research around the opportunity afforded by this larger transition to a consumer-facing, information-age economy. The purpose of the program was to monitor knowledge, attitudes, and behaviors to provide information on the ways in which people were utilizing resources and channels in the changing information environment. In this way, program administrators could gather information for communication researchers on how populations were adapting to these changes. Were people becoming more engaged as the environment shifted from a passive broadcast medium to a mixed medium facilitating both the push and pull of health information? Were some benefiting from the diffusion of technology more than others? What were the functional literacy skills that might be helping some people fare better in this new media environment than others? By trending over time, researchers could track answers to these questions across the entire diffusion of innovations curve; that is, by gathering self-reported data from early adopters, early majority adopters, late majority adopters, and laggards [34].

The survey was originally developed to provide probability-based population estimates biennially on data from non-institutionalized adults 18 years and older in the United States [12]. The first three administrations of the survey used a randomized digit dial (RDD) methodology to collect oral responses from participants through a Computer-Assisted Telephone Interview (CATI). Response rates began to plummet during the 2000s, however, as some households with caller identification avoided telephone calls with unrecognizable caller IDs and others abandoned their land-line telephones for mobile phone options. In 2007-2008, the HINTS program fielded a separate paper-and-pencil survey using a sampling technique drawn from a newly available, comprehensive list of postal addresses in parallel with the RDD administration. The dual-frame administration of both the RDD and Postal surveys allowed methodologists to evaluate the feasibility and psychometric equivalencies of the two surveillance approaches [35]. In 2011, the program switched from its biennial administration paradigm to an annual approach, with independent cycles of the survey being launched on a yearly basis using the postal frame and paper-and-pencil methodology [36]. The HINTS IV survey also included an independent cycle funded by the Food and Drug Administration containing items specially targeted towards direct-to-consumer advertising, smoking, and the use of alternative tobacco products.

2.2. Published HINTS Studies Relevant to Health Literacy Research

Shortly after publication of the first data set, communication scholars began analyzing the data to gain a better understanding of how the new communication environment might be facilitating or hindering individuals' capacities to obtain, process, and understand health information. In Table 1, we offer a synoptic list of many of the studies using HINTS to answer questions of interest to health literacy researchers.

Table 1. Articles published from HINTS data with relevance to Health Literacy researchers.

First Author, Year	Title	Journal	Health Literacy defined	HINTS Cycle: Type of Assessment
Champlin (2015)	Creating a Screening Measure of Health Literacy for the Health Information National Trends Survey	*American Journal of Health Promotion*	The Zarcadoolas' Model of health literacy	**HINTS 4, Cycle 2:** Items: E1, E2, J11, N6; *performance-based*
Chen (2014)	Numeracy, information seeking, and self-efficacy in managing health: an analysis using the 2007 Health Information National Trends Survey (HINTS).	*Health Communication*	Health Numeracy Confidence	**HINTS 3 (2007):** Items: K1/CS-02; *subjective*
Ciampa (2010)	Patient numeracy, perceptions of provider communication, and colorectal cancer screening utilization	*Journal of Health Communication*	Numeracy	**HINTS 3 (2007):** Items: K1/ CS-02, K3 [mail only]; *subjective & performance-based*
Dominick (2015)	Classification tree analysis to examine influences on colorectal cancer screening	*Cancer Causes and Control*	Numeracy	**HINTS 3 (2007):** Items: K1, CS-02; K2/CS-04; K4/CS-05; *subjective*
Ha (2011)	Determinants of consumer-driven healthcare: Self-confidence in information search, health literacy, and trust in information sources.	*International Journal of Pharmaceutical and Healthcare Marketing*	Perceived Literacy	**HINTS 3 (2007):** Items: HC-05/A5a; HC-05b/A5b; HC-05c/A5c; HC-05d/A5d; HC-06a; HC-7a; HC-20; *subjective*
Hoffman-Goetz (2009)	Literacy and cancer anxiety as predictors of health	*Journal of Cancer Education*	Literacy Levels	**HINTS 1 (2003):** Items: HC-6a; HC-7a;

	status: An exploratory study			HC-20; *subjective*
Huang (2012)	Health Numeracy Confidence among Racial/ Ethnic Minorities in HINTS 2007: Sociodemographic, Attitudinal, and Knowledge Correlates	*Literacy and Numeracy Studies*	Health numeracy confidence	**HINTS 3 (2007):** Items: K1, CS-02; *subjective*
Jiang (2016)	Health literacy and the internet: An exploratory study on the 2013 HINTS survey	*Computers in Human Behavior*	Zarcadoolas' Model	**HINTS 4, Cycle 3:** Items: G2a; F1; K1/4; I9; N1; *performance-based*
Kobayashi (2016)	Cancer Fatalism, Literacy, and Cancer Information Seeking in the American Public	*Health Education & Behavior*	Health literacy as "Newest Vital Sign"	**HINTS 4, Cycle 3:** Items: N1-N4; performance-based
Koch-Weser (2010)	The Internet as a health information source: Findings from the 2007 health information national trends survey and implications for health communication	*Journal of Health Communication*	Information Efficacy	**HINTS 3 (2007):** Items: HC-06; *subjective*
Langford (2012)	Racial and ethnic differences in direct-to-consumer genetic tests awareness in HINTS 2007: Sociodemographic and numeracy correlates	*Journal of Genetic Counseling*	Numeracy	**HINTS 3 (2007):** Items: CS-02/K1; CS-04/K2; CS-05/K4; *subjective*
Lustria (2011)	Exploring digital divides: An examination of eHealth technology use in health information	*Health Informatics Journal*	Numeracy	**HINTS 3 (2007):** Items: CS-02; CS-03; *subjective*

	seeking, communication and personal health information management in the USA			
Manganello (2011)	The association of understanding of medical statistics with health information seeking and health provider interaction in a national sample of young adults	*Journal of Health Communication*	Numeracy	**HINTS 3 (2007):** Items: CS-02; K-1; *subjective*
Nelson (2013)	Exploring objective and subjective numeracy at a population level: Findings from the 2007 health information national trends survey (HINTS)	*Journal of Health Communication*	Numeracy	**HINTS 3 (2007):** Items: K3; CS-05/K4; *subjective and performance-based*
Patel (2015)	The Role of Health Care Experience and Consumer Information Efficacy in Shaping Privacy and Security Perceptions of Medical Records: National Consumer Survey Results	*JMIR Medical Informatics*	Information efficacy	**HINTS 4, Cycle 1:** Items: A6, N6; *subjective*
Smith (2010)	Socioeconomic status, statistical confidence, and patient-provider communication: an analysis of the Health Information National Trends Survey (HINTS 2007)	*Journal of Health Communication*	Statistical confidence	**HINTS 4, Cycle 2:** Items: E1, E2, J11, N6; *performance-based*

As the table shows, several different concepts and models related to health literacy have been analyzed using HINTS items. Some of the health literacy elements studied include the components of the Zaracadoolas' Model [37] along with numeracy, health numeracy confidence, basic literacy levels, the Newest Vital Sign, and information efficacy. These health literacy items have been studied to analyze potential associations with other psychological constructs (e.g., self-efficacy), information seeking behaviors, clinical communication, and detection/preventive behaviors (e.g., colorectal cancer screening, healthy eating). While analyzing these associations, health literacy was conceptualized as the predictive variable almost twice as often as it was conceptualized as the outcome variable.

As discussed earlier, the way health literacy has been conceptualized by researchers and policymakers has varied considerably. Similarly, the ways that health literacy has been operationalized and applied using HINTS items reflect this wide range of perspectives. One major area of difference is how researchers have chosen to define health literacy or specific elements of health literacy (e.g., numeracy). This has at times resulted in a HINTS item being used to *define* health literacy in one study and at the same item being conceptualized as an *outcome* of health literacy in another study. For example, Smith and colleagues used an item assessing the participant's preference for obtaining health information by words or numbers as an *outcome* of literacy [38], while Koch-Weser and colleagues used the same item to assess the participant's health literacy level itself [39]. Similarly, Jiang and colleagues used genetic test awareness to assess the scientific literacy component of the Zarcadoolas' Model of health literacy [40], while Langford et al. conceptualized the same genetic test awareness item as an outcome of health literacy [41].

A second way that researchers have differed in their HINTS analyses is whether they measured literacy utilizing objective or subjective items. Objective items often ask participants questions designed to test numeric ability, reading comprehension skills, and knowledge of the scientific community to yield an overall literacy "score". In comparison, subjective items typically assess the participant's perceptions and confidence in his own literacy abilities during daily activities such as searching for information and interpreting statistics [42]. In this sense, objective measures may be stronger indicators of "knowledge in the head," whereas subjective measures would be more likely to assess the interaction or interface between the "knowledge in the head" to the "knowledge in the world." Consistent with the role of HINTS as a surveillance tool to assess the communication environment, most of the articles in Table 1 applied subjective items to measure health literacy at the interface between personal experience and the information environment.

2.3. Tracking Trends Over Time

One of the policy-related advantages associated with conducting routine surveillance of the general population is the ability to compare snapshots of the public's responses to literacy-related questions over time. For example, the Healthy People 2010 and 2020 initiatives represent a collective policy effort sponsored by the U.S. Department of Health and Human Services (DHHS) to identify leverage points for improving the health of the general U.S. population by targeted deadlines. The initiatives give policy makers, public health departments, intervention researchers, and local communities a set of science-based, aspirational benchmarks against which they can compare their own progress in improving the health of the nation. Targets for "Leading Health

Indicators" are central to the initiatives and include objectives related to decreasing the use of tobacco products, improving access to healthcare, improving environmental quality, improving nutrition and exercise, ameliorating the negative influence of certain social determinants of health, and more. A focus on health communication and health information technology is also included in the initiative to reflect the DHHS's concern over the role that the health information environment plays in building capacity for obtaining, processing, and utilizing health information.

HINTS is one of the national surveillance sources utilized by the DHHS to monitor progress on the Healthy People goals. The survey has been used as a check-up on policy incentives related to encouraging widespread access to the Internet, created in light of the presidential admonition stating that: "Access to high-speed broadband is no longer a luxury; it is a necessity for American families, businesses, and consumers" [43]. Data generated from the HINTS program have paralleled those of the Pew Foundation in showing that general access to the Internet has risen steadily from 63% in 2003 to over 80% in 2015. Measures related to online usage of medication ordering, emails to physicians, and access to personal medical information through online patient portals have also been incorporated into HINTS surveys since the passage of the Health Information Technology for Economic and Clinical Health (HITECH) Act of 2009. These measures have revealed a more gradual rise in the use of online tools as the culture evolves to favor patient engagement. Analyses of sociodemographic characteristics included in the HINTS surveys can help pinpoint areas of lagging adoption within certain portions of the general population. Data from those subpopulation analyses have shown a moderation in disparity over most racial/ethnic groups as general Internet adoption rises; however, they have also shown a persistent disparity related directly to respondents' education level. It is the critical thinking, English literacy, and functional problem-solving skills needed to find and interpret information from the Web that will likely be in short supply among low literacy populations [44]. Policy makers and health system administrators would do well to continue strengthening their support for low-literate populations through personal assistance from patient navigators, allied health professionals, and interpreters.

The trending capacity of repeated cross-sectional surveys of the U.S. population can also be used to assess the waxing or waning of public comprehension within the context of an increasingly multi-channel, complex, and potentially confusing media environment. In Figure 2, we track the performance of one such indicator related to the public's endorsement of a statement suggesting that there are "too many recommendations for preventing cancer to know which ones to follow." Although fewer people endorsed the "Strongly Agree" option over the last decade, their endorsement of "Somewhat Agree" has risen. From these data, confusion over health recommendations from a multi-channel media environment is a pervasive problem that is only gaining small ground over the last decade.

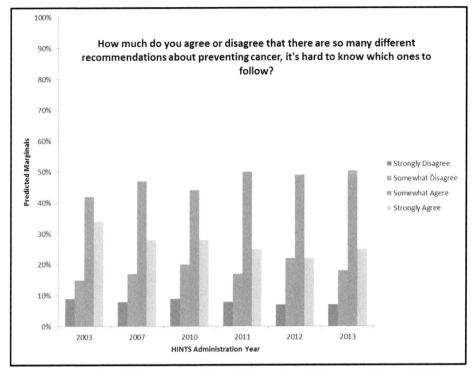

Figure 2. Tracking the public's agreement with an indicator of confusion, or cognitive overload, over a decade from 2003 to 2013.

3. Moving into the Future

Prevalent reports of emerging communication technologies and media, together with new and promising cancer prevention and treatment options underscore the need to monitor the population's capacity to obtain, process, and utilize health information for engaged decision-making. In this final section, we review the status of NCI's HINTS surveillance program and offer further suggestions for how to utilize this resource to support research on health literacy. We also look to the HINTS data and publications as a harbinger of health literacy problems that may continue, and use our understanding of technological and medical trends to forecast emerging areas of concern.

3.1. The Future of HINTS

The HINTS V survey was approved in 2015. The new phase will include the same four-cycle structure as HINTS IV and will again be collected annually using a postal-frame, paper-and-pencil modality. A timeline of the HINTS program's survey administrations is depicted in Figure 3. De-identified data from each administration of the survey have been made available at the HINTS website (hints.cancer.gov). Taken across all its iterations, the HINTS program will continue to offer a wealth of data for health communication scholars and program planners. This survey has helped cultivate a vibrant community of researchers across disciplines who access and analyze the data, publish the results, and contribute information about their published articles back to the HINTS community. A full listing of publications using HINTS can be found on the website. Several times a year, the HINTS management team selects an intriguing article to highlight in a "HINTS Brief." These briefs offer a high-level synthesis of significant trends emerging from the community presented in an engaging format designed for quick consumption by public health practitioners (see http://hints.cancer.gov/briefs.aspx).

In addition to depicting the national administrations of HINTS I, II, III, & IV above the bolded timeline, the figure also depicts two separately funded supplements aimed at gathering data at the local level. The first of these was a supplement awarded to researchers at the University of Puerto Rico to gather an assessment of the changing health information landscape in the largest of the U.S. territories in the Caribbean. The supplement funding allowed in-depth analyses of a health communication context that was different from the mainland. For instance, mobile phones gained traction earlier in the island territory as compared to mainland US, and the mix of monolingual and bilingual Spanish speakers provided insight from a distinct cultural context. The second funding opportunity was a supplement program designed to support 15 of the NCI-funded National Cancer Centers in gathering data from a variety of sources within their local catchment areas. Hospitals are increasingly being held accountable for population health outcomes among members within their service areas. They are encouraged to conduct community health needs assessments to take stock of community needs, and then to support community action in meeting public health goals. The supplement funding was awarded to participating cancer centers in 2016 as way to explore the utilization of communication variables in conjunction with other clinically relevant surveillance data to assist in local community planning. The intent of these supplements is to move beyond national surveillance to enable local action for the specific needs of each catchment area.

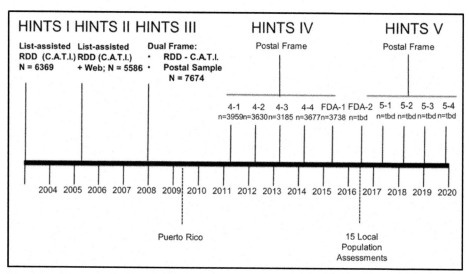

Figure 3. Health Information National Trends Survey Timeline. Dotted lines indicate supplemental studies conducted in local areas.

3.2. Future Challenges in Health Literacy

With an increasing focus on the multidisciplinary health research, the field of health literacy continues to grow and connect with other disciplines in health and communication. While HINTS serves as a valuable resource and stimulates new analytic opportunities, it is a cross-sectional survey with some inherent limitations; therefore, we believe the survey is best used when it complements other methods of inquiry. In the following, we highlight three key challenges and opportunities in health literacy research, and within each we discuss how HINTS can serve as a resource in addressing the challenges.

First, the field is gradually moving beyond assessing and "diagnosing" individuals' health literacy and numeracy levels. Scholars have developed and tested a multitude of literacy assessment tools, both objective and subjective. While no tool is perfect, many well-validated instruments and survey items have been developed for researchers and care providers. Rather than continue to develop additional assessment tools to measure individuals, more work is needed to assess the environment and broader context of public health and clinical care, including family interactions, communication with providers within and across care delivery teams, and experience with the communication environment more generally. HINTS is a useful tool to consider how individuals interact with the environment by not just including items related to static "knowledge in the head," but additionally by gauging how well the environment meets the needs of the individual. Previous HINTS work has suggested that this interaction is an important area for future research in a variety of contexts. For example, one study focused on information seeking [45] found that participants who reported difficulties finding and understanding information while searching for health information were less likely to be knowledgeable about cancer prevention and engage in healthy behaviors related to fruit/vegetable intake, smoking status and exercise. Another study that was focused on clinical communication found that young adults with lower numeracy reported more negative interactions with their health care providers [46]. Both examples illustrate the connection between one's "knowledge in the head" and the individual's environment. Beyond measurement, the development and testing of multi-level health literacy interventions are needed, whereby health literacy is addressed at the broader system's level (e.g., can aspects of the information environment be modified or improved upon to facilitate sustained patient engagement or behavior change?). Health literacy is then linked to other levels of "outcomes" including behaviors. In our review of HINTS studies that have analyzed health literacy variables, much of the work has remained on a descriptive level. While a few studies have analyzed the association between health literacy elements and health behaviors (e.g., colorectal cancer screening [47, 48]), more work should be done to connect health literacy with behavioral outcomes and health care utilization measurements. To this effect, it was interesting to observe that extant HINTS-based publications related to health literacy have conceptualized health literacy as a predictor, rather than an outcome, variable.

Second, to gain a more holistic understanding of the role of health literacy in communication and health care, there are opportunities to complement HINTS analyses with other methods of inquiry. HINTS can be used to generate and test hypotheses, and findings from the analyses can then inform the design and delivery of subsequent interventions. For example, HINTS cycles have been used to track the American public's general acceptance and reported use of emerging media, such as social media and health information technologies [49, 50] to solve health-related problems. These descriptive analyses can provide the baseline data to inform the development and testing of health literacy interventions using related platforms and technologies.

Finally, despite the proliferation of technology and new media in health, there has been limited health literacy research aimed at understanding the impact of new/novel communication strategies and channels (e.g. mobile and social media and other peer-to-peer communication platforms).   Health information and messages are quickly becoming ubiquitous through online channels, which may increase the demand on individuals and communities to process and discern the quality of the available technology-mediated information. Moreover, the intersection of health literacy and technology literacy deserves further investigation. This includes understanding how diverse populations with varying degrees of health literacy access and make use of health information technology, and how technology-mediated interactions serving specific communities can be optimized to facilitate healthy behaviors. HINTS, with its many items related to technology and new media across the iterations, offers unique opportunities to examine the impact of the emerging health communication landscape.

4. Conclusion

For the past 13 years, researchers have used HINTS as a tool to study interrelationships and interactions between health communication items, test communication theories, and address issues related to information access and usage. Literacy-related items found in HINTS iterations are uniquely situated to increase our understanding of the health systems perspective of health literacy, both by analyzing a single cycle "snapshot" and by identifying changing trends and practices over time. In this chapter, we outlined different approaches for conceptualizing health literacy, described the rationale and history behind HINTS, and detailed both how HINTS has already been used to address health literacy-related questions, as well as identified gaps and opportunities for future work in this area. New trends and constantly-emerging technologies underscore the need for researchers to utilize HINTS to monitor and assess how the population's "knowledge in the head" responds to and interacts with the constantly-evolving "knowledge in the world."

References

[1] Gruman JC. Preparing patients to care for themselves. Am J Nurs. 2014;114 (7):11. DOI: 10.1097/01.NAJ.0000451657.77642.36.
[2] Gruman JC. Making health information technology sing for people with chronic conditions. Am J Prev Med. 2011;40 (Supp 2): S238-40. DOI: 10.1016/j.amepre.2011.02.003.
[3] U.S. Department of Health and Human Services. Healthy People 2010. Washington, DC: U.S. Department of Health and Human Services; 2000.
[4] Coleman K, Austin BT, Brach C, Wagner EH. Evidence on the chronic care model in the new millennium. Health Aff (Millwood). 2009;28 (1):75-85. DOI: 10.1377/hlthaff.28.1.75.
[5] Center for Advancing Health. Here to Stay: What health care leaders say About patient engagement. Washington, DC: Center for Advancing Health; 2014. p. 169.
[6] Hibbard JH, Gilburt H. Supporting people to manage their health: an introduction to patient activation. In: Fund TKs, editor. London, UK: The King's Fund; 2014.
[7] Greene J, Hibbard JH, Sacks R, Overton V. When seeing the same physician, highly activated patients have better care experiences than less activated patients. Health Aff (Millwood). 2013;32 (7):1299-305. DOI: 10.1377/hlthaff.2012.1409.

[8] Hibbard JH, Greene J, Overton V. Patients with lower activation associated with higher costs; delivery systems should know their patients' 'scores'. Health Aff (Millwood). 2013;32 (2):216-22. DOI: 10.1377/hlthaff.2012.1064.

[9] Greene J, Hibbard JH, Sacks R, Overton V, Parrotta CD. When patient activation levels change, health outcomes and costs change, too. Health Aff (Millwood). 2015;34 (3):431-7. DOI: 10.1377/hlthaff.2014.0452

[10] Cayton H. The flat-pack patient? Creating health together. Patient Educ Couns. 2006;62 (3):288-90. DOI: 10.1016/j.pec.2006.06.016.

[11] Institute of Medicine (U.S.). Roundtable on Value & Science-Driven Health Care., Olsen L, Saunders RS, McGinnis JM. Patients charting the course: citizen engagement and the learning health system: workshop summary. Washington, D.C.: National Academies Press; 2011.

[12] Zuboff S, Maxmin J. The support economy: why corporations are failing individuals and the next episode of capitalism. New York: Viking; 2002.

[13] Clauser SB, Wagner EH, Aiello Bowles EJ, Tuzzio L, Greene SM. Improving modern cancer care through information technology. Am J Prev Med. 2011;40 (5 SUPP): S198-207. DOI: 10.1016/j.amepre.2011.01.014.

[14] Institute of Medicine (U.S.). Committee on Quality of Health Care in America. Crossing the quality chasm : a new health system for the 21st century. Washington, D.C.: National Academy Press; 2001.

[15] Berwick DM. A user's manual for the IOM's 'Quality Chasm' report. Health Aff (Millwood). 2002;21 (3):80-90. DOI: 10.1377/hlthaff.21.3.80.

[16] Kohn LT, Corrigan J, Donaldson MS. To err is human: building a safer health system. Washington, D.C.: National Academy Press; 2000.

[17] Reid PP, Compton WD, Grossman JH, Fanjiang G, National Academy of Engineering., Institute of Medicine (U.S.), et al. Building a better delivery system: a new engineering/health care partnership. Washington, D.C.: National Academies Press; 2005.

[18] Vicente KJ. The human factor: revolutionizing the way people live with technology. 1st ed. New York: Taylor and Francis Books; 2003.

[19] Epstein R, Street RJ. Patient-centered communication in cancer care: promoting healing and reducing suffering. Bethesda, MD, 2007: National Cancer Institute; 2007.

[20] Hesse BW. Curb cuts in the virtual community: telework and persons with disabilities. 28th Annual Hawaii International Conference on System Sciences. Maui, HI1995. p. 418-25.

[21] Hesse BW, Shneiderman B. eHealth research from the user's perspective. Am J Prev Med. 2007;32 (5 SUPP):S97-103. DOI: 10.1016/j.amepre.2007.01.019

[22] Stokols D, Grzywacz JG, McMahan S, Phillips K. Increasing the health promotive capacity of human environments. Am J Health Promot. 2003;18 (1):4-13.

[23] Norman DA. The design of everyday things. Revised and expanded edition. ed. New York, New York: Basic Books; 2013.

[24] Nielsen-Bohlman L, Institute of Medicine (U.S.). Committee on Health Literacy. Health literacy : a prescription to end confusion. Washington, D.C.: National Academies Press; 2004.

[25] Kemper DW, Mettler M. Information therapy: prescribed information as a reimbursable medical service. 1st ed. Boise, Idaho: Healthwise, Inc.; 2002.

[26] Ancker JS. Addressing health literacy and numeracy through systems approaches. In: Patel VL, Arocha JF, Ancker JS, editors. Cognitive Informatics in Health and Biomedicine: Understanding and Modeling Health Behaviors. London, UK: Springer; in press.

[27] Hesse BW, Suls JM. Informatics-enabled behavioral medicine in oncology. Cancer J. 2011;17:222-30. DOI: 10.1097/PPO.0b013e318227c811.

[28] Galesic M, Garcia-Retamero R, Gigerenzer G. Using icon arrays to communicate medical risks: overcoming low numeracy. Health Psychol. 2009; 28 (2):210-6. DOI: 10.1037/a0014474.

[29] Gigerenzer G. What are natural frequencies? Bmj. 2011; 343: d6386. DOI: 10.1136/bmj.d6386.

[30] Gigerenzer G, Edwards A. Simple tools for understanding risks: from innumeracy to insight. Bmj. 2003;327 (7417): 741-4. DOI: 10.1136/bmj.327.7417.741.

[31] Hesse BW. Harnessing the power of an intelligent health environment in cancer control. Stud Health Technol Inform. 2005; 118: 159-76.

[32] Hesse BW, Cole GE, Powe BD. Partnering against cancer today: a blueprint for coordinating efforts through communication science. J Natl Cancer I Mono. 2013(47):233-9. DOI: 10.1093/jncimonographs/lgt024.

[33] Gee PM, Greenwood DA, Paterniti DA, Ward D, Miller LMS. The eHealth enhanced chronic care model: a theory derivation approach. J Med Internet Res. 2015;17 (4):e86. DOI: 10.2196/jmir.4067.

[34] Rogers EM. Diffusion of innovations. 4th ed. New York, NY: The Free Press; 1995.

[35] Finney Rutten LJ, Hesse BW, Moser RP, Kreps GL. Building the evidence base in cancer communication. Cresskill, NJ: Hampton Press; 2010.

[36] Finney Rutten LJ, Davis T, Beckjord EB, Blake K, Moser RP, Hesse BW. Picking up the pace: changes in method and frame for the Health Information National Trends Survey (2011 – 2014). J Health Commun. 2012;17 (8):979-89. DOI: 10.1080/10810730.2012.700998.

[37] Zarcadoolas C, Pleasant A, Greer DS. Understanding health literacy: an expanded model. Health Promotion International. 2005;20 (2):195-203. DOI: 10.1093/heapro/dah609.

[38] Smith SG, Wolf MS, Wagner Cv. Socioeconomic status, statistical confidence, and patient–provider communication: an analysis of the Health Information National Trends Survey (HINTS 2007). J Health Commun. 2010; 15 (Supp 3):169-85. DOI: 10.1080/10810730.2010.522690.

[39] Koch-Weser S, Bradshaw YS, Gualtieri L, Gallagher SS. The internet as a health information source: findings from the 2007 Health Information National Trends Survey and implications for health communication. J Health Commun. 2010;15 (Supp 3):279-93. DOI: 10.1080/10810730.2010.522700.

[40] Jiang S, Beaudoin CE. Health literacy and the internet: An exploratory study on the 2013 HINTS survey. Comp Human Behav. 2016; 58:240-8. DOI: 10.1016/j.chb.2016.01.007.

[41] Langford AT, Resnicow K, Roberts JS, Zikmund-Fisher BJ. Racial and ethnic differences in direct-to-consumer genetic tests awareness in HINTS 2007: sociodemographic and numeracy correlates. Journal of Genetic Counseling. 2012;21 (3):440-7. DOI: 10.1007/s10897-011-9478-2.

[42] Nelson WL, Moser RP, Han PKJ. Exploring objective and subjective numeracy at a population level: findings from the 2007 Health Information National Trends Survey (HINTS). J Health Commun. 2013;18 (2):192-205. DOI: 10.1080/10810730.2012.688450.

[43] Obama B. Presidential memorandum -- expanding broadband deployment and adoption by addressing regulatory barriers and encouraging investment and training 2015.

[44] Hesse BW, Gaysynsky A, Vieux S, Ottenbacher AJ, Moser RP, Blake KD, et al. Meeting the Healthy People 2020 goals: using the Health Information National Trends Survey to monitor progress on health communication objectives. J Health Commun. 2014;19(12); 1497-509. DOI: 10.1080/10810730.2014.954084.

[45] Ha S, Lee YJ. Determinants of consumer ‑ driven healthcare: self ‑ confidence in information search, health literacy, and trust in information sources. Int J Pharmaceutical & Healthcare Marketing. 2011;5 (1):8-24. DOI: 10.1108/17506121111121550.

[46] Manganello JA, Clayman ML. The association of understanding of medical statistics with health information seeking and health provider interaction in a national sample of young adults. J Health Commun. 2011;16 (Supp 3):163-76. DOI: 10.1080/10810730.2011.604704.

[47] Dominick GM, Papas MA, Rogers ML, Rakowski W. Classification tree analysis to examine influences on colorectal cancer screening. Cancer Cause Control. 2015;26 (3):443-54. DOI: 10.1007/s10552-015-0523-6.

[48] Ciampa PJ, Osborn CY, Peterson NB, Rothman RL. Patient numeracy, perceptions of provider communication, and colorectal cancer screening utilization. J Health Commun. 2010;15 (Supp 3) :157-68. DOI: 10.1080/10810730.2010.522699.

[49] Chou W-YS, Hunt YM, Beckjord EB, Moser RP, Hesse BW. Social media use in the United States: implications for health communication. J Med Internet Res. 2009;11 (4): e48. DOI: 10.2196/jmir.1249.

[50] Jackson DN, Chou W-YS, Coa KI, Oh A, Hesse B. Implications of social media use on health information technology engagement: Data from HINTS 4 cycle 3. Transl Behav Med. 2016; 6 (4): 566-576. DOI: 10.1007/s13142-016-0437-1.

Health Literacy
R.A. Logan and E.R. Siegel (Eds.)
IOS Press, 2017
doi:10.3233/978-1-61499-790-0-347

The Relevance of Health Literacy to mHealth

Gary L. KREPS[1]

George Mason University, Center for Health and Risk Communication

Abstract. This chapter examines the importance of health literacy to the design and use of mobile digital health information technology (mHealth) applications. Over the past two decades mHealth has evolved to become a major health communication channel for delivering health care, promoting health, and tracking health behaviors. Yet, there are serious communication challenges that must be addressed concerning the best way to design and utilize mHealth application to achieve key health promotion goals, including assuring the appropriateness and effectiveness of mHealth messaging for audiences with different communication competencies, styles, and health literacy levels, to ensure that mHealth applications are truly effective tools for health promotion.

Health literacy is one of the major communication issues relevant to the effective use of mHealth. To be effective, mHealth applications need to match the messages conveyed via these mobile media to the specific health communication needs, orientations, and competencies of intended audience members. Unfortunately, current evidence suggests that many mHealth applications are difficult for audiences to utilize because they provide health information that is not easy for many consumers to understand and apply.

Health literacy refers to the ability of participants within the health care system to accurately interpret and utilize relevant health information and resources to achieve their health goals. Evidence suggests that many consumers possess limited levels of health literacy to adequately understand health information, especially when they are feeling ill, since health literacy is both a trait (limited education, language facility, etc.), and a state condition (based on how their current physical and mental states influence their abilities to communicate effectively). Therefore, it is incumbent upon mHealth developers to design and utilize message systems. Strategies for designing and implementing mHealth applications to meet the health literacy levels of different audiences are described in this chapter.

Keywords. mHealth, health literacy, health communication, applications, health promotion

1. Introduction

The use of mHealth (mobile digital information technologies designed to deliver care, track health behaviors, and promote health) has evolved over the past two decades to become a major channel for health promotion [1,2]. This increasingly popular use of mHealth channels for communication has mirrored the phenomenal international growth in public adoption of mobile phone technologies, especially the use of smart

---

[1] Corresponding author: University Distinguished Professor and Director of the Center for Health and Risk Communication, George Mason University, 4400 University Drive, MS 3D6, Fairfax, VA. USA; E-mail: gkreps@gmu.edu.

phones that enable Internet access [2]. Implementation of mHealth applications has shown tremendous promise as an important evolving communication medium for supplementing and extending the use of more traditional channels for health communication, such as in-person clinical interpersonal interactions with health care providers (and other sources of health information), use of print health education materials (such as books, articles, pamphlets, and posters), public presentations (such as school and conference lectures), and access to entertainment media programs via radio, television, and film [3].

A number of different emerging and interrelated mobile communication systems have been adopted and adapted for delivering mHealth, including the increasing use of:

- audio and video enabled telemedicine applications, such as closed circuit telephone and/or televised conferencing systems, with both data collection tools (often collecting images, or measuring body temperature, heart rate, and brain activity for diagnostic and monitoring purposes) and delivery tools (that can remotely control surgical equipment, and provide treatment instructions) can be set up in different sites to provide mediated (virtual) care to patients who may not have easy access to health care delivery systems [4];
- telephonic and internet-based message systems that can provide individuals with health information via SMS text messages, phone calls, or e-mail via mobile phones [5];
- websites and web-based portals (intranets) that are available to health care consumers via portable lap-top computers, tablets, and smart phones;
- wearable (sometimes implantable) devices such as fitness tracking wristbands and other digital monitoring devices [6];
- specialized application software programs (apps) that are typically downloaded on to smart phones, tablets, or laptop computers that provide health information and support, and are often linked to Internet delivered resources and services [7].

The added value provided by mhealth applications for health promotion is the ability to use these media to provide key audiences (health care consumers and providers) with relevant health information and support that they need exactly at the points in time when they need it and right where they need it to enhance timely and on-the-spot informed health decision making [3]. As a result, there is growing enthusiasm for using mHealth applications within health care and health promotion communities with a range of different audiences, both domestically and internationally [2,8].

Yet, there are serious communication challenges that must be addressed concerning the best uses of mHealth for health promotion, including assuring the appropriateness and effectiveness of mHealth messaging for audiences with different communication competencies, styles, and health literacy levels, to ensure that mHealth applications are truly effective tools for health promotion [9,10]. It is not merely the use of mobile communication channels that can make these applications effective, it is also the ability to match the messages conveyed via these mobile media to the specific health communication needs, orientations, and competencies of intended audience members [11]. For example, practitioners of mHealth must strategically develop and refine health messaging to match the health literacy levels of key audiences [12,13].

This chapter examines the tremendous potential of mHealth applications for providing relevant health information to diverse populations of health care providers and consumers and for enhancing health decision making. The chapter also illustrates how mHealth applications can be designed to deliver appropriate and effective messages that meet the unique communication competencies, styles, and health literacy levels of different key audiences to become effective health communication channels.

2. The Promise of mHealth

There have been a number of unique and important contributions made to the delivery of care and the promotion of health with the use of mHealth applications as supplements to traditional channels of health communication [11]. For example, mHealth applications have been shown to increase the timeliness of health care delivery and the ability to provide relevant health information to key audiences wherever they may be via their mobile phones that they carry with them [14]. Health care providers like mobile health applications and have been early adopters and users of mhealth systems to gather health information and to communicate with their colleagues and clients [15]. mHealth systems have been successfully used to address a wide variety of serious health conditions, including heart health promotion [16], infectious disease control [17], respiratory health [18], maternal and child health [19,20].

There has also been a great deal of evidence that mHealth has been used effectively to promote consumers' adoption of healthy behaviors and reduction of unhealthy behaviors [21], including the following behavioral health issues: consumer adherence with treatment recommendations and prescribed medications [22,23], reducing risky sex behaviors and adopting safer sex strategies [24,25], increasing physical activity and exercise [26,27], maintaining healthy diets [28,29], tobacco control [30,31] drug and alcohol abuse reduction [32–34], and promoting screening behaviors for early detection of serious health problems [23,35,36]. Furthermore, evidence suggests that mHealth applications have the potential to improve health care delivery performance and retention of community health workers [37].

Rapid and widespread adoption of mobile communication technologies, such as the smart phones, tablets, and wearable devices have been shown to provide health communicators with powerful new channels for disseminating health information [4,7]. Mobile communication tools have become increasingly well-liked, adopted, and frequently used channels for communication by diverse audiences, including by members of at-risk populations who often suffer from health inequities and poor access to health information [38]. mHealth application provide great opportunities to reach key audiences with health information right at the point when they are making important health decisions, providing these audiences with relevant health information exactly when they need it and where they need it [14]. Advances in mHealth technologies are making these communication tools increasingly easy to use, enable them to disseminate a variety of different message formats (text, oral, graphic, video, etc), and enable interactivity (feedback between health communicators) [7]. mHealth technologies can be integrated with other digital health tools, such as exercise trackers, telehealth monitors, and electronic health records, to provide users with rich sources of health information. Tailored information systems and the use of artificial intelligence can be used with mHealth tools to provide relevant, interactive, adaptive, and sensitive health messages to users [39].

3. Challenges to Using mHealth Technologies Effectively

There are serious communication challenges that must be addressed before mHealth technologies can reach their potential as effective tools for health promotion. These challenges include designing appropriate and effective mHealth messaging for use with audiences who possess different communication competencies, styles and health literacy levels [3,40,41]. While sophisticated and often elegant new technological media receive the bulk of attention in mHealth, the effects of these media on health promotion are highly dependent on the quality of messages that are exchanged via these advanced media.

Health literacy refers to the ability of participants within the health care system to accurately interpret and utilize relevant health information and resources to achieve their health goals [42]. Evidence suggests that many consumers possess limited levels of health literacy to adequately understand health information, especially when they are feeling ill, since health literacy is both a trait (limited education, language facility, etc.), and a state condition (based on how their current physical and mental states influence their abilities to communicate effectively) [42]. Therefore, it is incumbent upon mHealth developers to design and utilize message systems that will be easy for consumers with health literacy challenges to understand [43].

Due to the limited channel capacity on many mHealth technologies, such as the limited number of characters that can be used for SMS texting or tweeting, care must be taken to strategically design health messages that will convey full, accurate, timely health information, as well as resonate with and make sense to diverse audiences [39]. In many cases this will mean targeting, or even tailoring, health messages for specific users so the messages include appropriate language, provide meaningful examples, and suggest health options that the users can implement.

Whenever possible, it is preferable to build in feedback loops into mHealth systems, so users can pose questions and receive clarifications [39]. If possible, mHealth systems should be designed to incorporate visual, animated, and narrative messages to enhance understanding, especially for users with low health literacy and numeracy skills [39]. Narrative descriptions of health topics that imbed health information within rich, dramatic, and engaging stories has been found to be a particularly robust communication strategy for communicating health information to users with low levels of health literacy.

In addition, Weinstein et al, 2014 [4], describe three major bureaucratic challenges that challenge the widespread adoption and effective use of telemedicine and mHealth applications:

- The need for clear and standardized reimbursement strategies and business models to make it less challenging to fund the development, implementation, and maintenance of mHealth interventions;
- The need to establish interstate medical licensure for implementing domestic mHealth applications that cross state lines, as well as international licensing for applications that cross national boundaries;
- The need for hospital credentialing to implement mHealth applications as standardized tools within modern health care delivery systems.

4. Evaluating mHealth Applications

Message design processes for mHealth technologies should begin with careful audience analysis of potential system users, identifying key communication factors, including language use, health literacy levels, communication channel utilization patterns, familiarity with mHealth technologies, interest levels in different health topics, relevant health beliefs, and attitudes [9; 44]. The Centers for Disease Control and Prevention (CDC) recently introduced an excellent tool for evaluating the health literacy levels of health promotion materials, the CDC's Clear Communication Index, that can be easily applied to the evaluation of mHealth messaging [45]. Similarly, Stoyanov and colleagues (46) recently introduced and tested the Mobile App Rating Scale (MARS), demonstrating that is a simple, objective, and reliable measuring instrument for designing effective mHealth applications.

   With key background information from evaluation research mHealth developers can guide the design of appropriate, understandable, relevant, and compelling health messages to deliver via mHealth devices [47]. Message testing with targeted audiences can also provide relevant information about how well potential mHealth users can understand and accept health messages [40]. Additionally, usability testing of mHealth technologies and information programs can provide relevant information for refining mHealth systems [48].

   In addition, it is important to assess the economic viability of mHealth applications to ensure that these health promotion tools are cost-effective for different users and in different settings [49, 50]. Cost and benefit analyses can provide information needed to demonstrate the value of mHealth applications, support decision making about adoption and institutionalization of these applications, and also provide direction for developing business models for supporting the introduction and continued use of these new health promotion systems [50,51]. Bergmo provides cogent advice about conducting relevant economic analyses of ehealth systems that can be effectively applied to assessing the costs and benefits of mHealth applications [49].

5. Conclusion

Mounting evidence clearly illustrates that mHealth applications have tremendous potential for supplementing traditional channels of health communication as an important evolving communication medium for promoting health [1,2,4,8,52]. The ability of mHealth systems to provide individuals with the relevant health information they need when they need it and where they need it has great potential for enhancing health decision making. Yet, there are serious communication challenges that must be addressed, including the appropriateness and effectiveness of mHealth messaging for audiences with different communication competencies, styles and health literacy levels, before mHealth can become an effective tool for health promotion [3]. This chapter provides recommendations for the development and use of mHealth technologies to meet the unique health communication needs of diverse users for enhancing health decision making and improving health outcomes.

   A critical factor in the whether mhealth applications will reach their potential to make significant contributions to the promotion of public health depends on the ability of these systems to communicate effectively with different audiences, who have different health information needs and unique communication orientations and capacities [39,53]. There are a broad range of different potential users for mhealth systems who will want these systems to communicate effectively with them, providing them with the specific information they need and using language and examples that they can relate to [6,53]. For example, research shows that mHealth systems have been designed for older and younger health care consumers, users with different education levels, people with different sexual orientations, people with drug and alcohol addictions, people from different minority and ethnic groups, people from different countries, including those who speak different languages, all of whom are likely to have different communication preferences and skills [17,19,22,25,26,28,33,34]. It will be important for mHealth system designers to conduct audience analysis research to evaluate the literacy levels of different mHealth users to determine the best ways to communicate effectively with these groups [6,45].

Adapting to the health literacy levels of different mHealth users is one of the most critical communication factors that will influence the effectiveness of mHealth in effectively reaching and influencing system users [40,41,42,45]. Adapting to differing levels of health literacy means that the messaging used in mHealth systems will need to be designed specifically for different groups of users, assuring the utilization of appropriate language, examples, and visuals that are meaningful for these groups of users. The most current mHealth systems are now being designed to interactively assess the communication competencies, needs, expectations, and literacy levels of different system users. These modern mHealth systems are programmed with smart, adaptive, interactive learning systems that utilize artificial intelligence to learn about and adjust messages to individual users [54,55]. As these smart mHealth systems interact with users they learn through analysis of user comments and responses to system messages how to best adapt future system messages for these users, enabling the use of relationally sensitive and appropriate communication that can enhance communicative understanding, relevance, and immediacy for users of mHealth systems [55].

References

[1] Fox S, Duggan M. Mobile health 2012. Pew Internet Project. November 8, 2012. http://www.pewinternet.org/2012/11/08/mobile-health-2012/.
[2] Steinhubl SR, Muse ED, Topol EJ. The emerging field of mobile health. Sci Trans Med. 2015 Apr 15;7(283):283rv3. DOI: 10.1126/scitranslmed.aaa3487.
[3] Kreps GL. Communication technology and health: The advent of ehealth applications; Cantoni L, Danowski JA, editors. Communication and technology. Berlin, Germany: De Gruyter Mouton Publications; 2015.
[4] Weinstein RS, Lopez AM, Joseph BA, Erps KA, Holcomb M, Barker GP, Krupinski EA. Telemedicine, telehealth, and mobile health applications that work: opportunities and barriers. Am J Med. 2014;127(3):183–7. DOI: 10.1016/j.amjmed.2013.09.032.
[5] Déglise C, Suggs LS, Odermatt P. SMS for disease control in developing countries: a systematic review of mobile health applications. J Telemed Telecare. 2012;18(5):273–81. DOI: 10.1258/jtt.2012.110810.
[6] Alpert JM, Krist AH, Aycock BA, Kreps GL. Designing user-centric patient portals: clinician and patients' uses and gratifications. Telemed J E Health. 2016 ahead of print. DOI: 10.1089/tmj.2016.0096.
[7] Boudreaux E, Waring M, Hayes R, Sadasivam R, Mullen S, Pagoto S. Evaluating and selecting mobile health apps: strategies for healthcare providers and healthcare organizations. Transl Behav Med. 2014;4(4):363–71, DOI: 10.1007/s13142-014-0293-9.
[8] Fiordelli M, Diviani N, Schulz PJ. Mapping mHealth research: a decade of evolution. J Med Internet Res. 2013;15(5):e95. DOI: 10.2196/jmir.2430.
[9] Grundy QH, Wang Z, Bero LA. Challenges in assessing mobile health app quality: a systematic review of prevalent and innovative methods. Am J Prev Med. 2016;51(6):1051–59. DOI: 10.1016/j.amepre.2016.07.009.

[10] Aungst TD, Clauson KA, Misra S, Lewis TL, Husain I. How to identify, assess and utilise mobile medical applications in clinical practice. Int J Clin Pract. 2014 Feb;68(2):155–62. DOI: 10.1111/ijcp.12375.

[11] Steinhubl SR, Muse ED, Topol EJ. Can mobile health technologies transform health care? JAMA. 2013;310(22):2395–96. DOI: 10.1001/jama.2013.281078.

[12] Levy H, Janke AT, Langa KM. Health literacy and the digital divide among older Americans. J Gen Intern Med. 2015 Mar 1;30(3):284–89. DOI: 10.1007/s11606-014-3069-5.

[13] Kim H, Xie B. Health literacy and internet-and mobile app-based health services: a systematic review of the literature. Proceedings of the Association for Information Science and Technology. 2015 Jan 1;52(1):1–4, DOI: 10.1002/pra2.2015.145052010075.

[14] Klasnja P, Pratt W. Healthcare in the pocket: mapping the space of mobile-phone health interventions. J Biomed Inform. 2012 Feb 29;45(1):184–98. DOI: 10.1016/j.jbi.2011.08.017.

[15] Li J, Talaei-Khoei A, Seale H, Ray P, MacIntyre CR. Health care provider adoption of eHealth: systematic literature review. Interact J Med Res. 2013;2(1):e7. DOI: 10.2196/ijmr.2468.

[16] Burke LE, Ma J, Azar KM, Bennett GG, Peterson ED, Zheng Y, Riley W, Stephens J, Shah SH, Suffoletto B, Turan TN. Current science on consumer use of mobile health for cardiovascular disease prevention a scientific statement from the American Heart Association. Circulation. 2015 Sep 22;132(12):1157–213. DOI: 10.1161/CIR.0000000000000232.

[17] Ha YP, Tesfalul MA, Littman-Quinn R, Antwi C, Green RS, Mapila TO, Bellamy SL, Ncube RT, Mugisha K, Ho-Foster AR, Luberti AA. Evaluation of a mobile health approach to tuberculosis contact tracing in Botswana. J Health Commun. 2016 Sep 26:1–7. DOI: 10.1080/10810730.2016.1222035.

[18] Pak KJ , Seoane L, Bakker JP, Bertisch S, Pham C, McNaughton N, Park J, Severensin K, Bazzano LA. Effect of mobile health technology on positive airway pressure adherence in patients with sleep apnea. In B63. My Way: OSA Outpatient Models of Care. 2016 May (pp. A4185). American Thoracic Society. DOI: 10.1164/ajrccm-conference.2016.193.1_MeetingAbstracts.A4185.

[19] Sondaal SF, Browne JL, Amoakoh-Coleman M, Borgstein A, Miltenburg AS, Verwijs M, Klipstein-Grobusch K. Assessing the effect of mHealth interventions in improving maternal and neonatal care in low- and middle-income countries: a systematic review. PLoS One. 2016;11(5):e0154664. DOI: 10.1371/journal.pone.0154664.

[20] Amoakoh-Coleman M, Borgstein AB, Sondaal SF, Grobbee DE, Miltenburg AS, Verwijs M, Ansah EK, Browne JL, Klipstein-Grobusch K. Effectiveness of mHealth interventions targeting health care workers to improve pregnancy outcomes in low-and middle-income countries: a systematic review. J Med Internet Res. 2016 Aug;18(8). DOI: 10.2196/jmir.5533.

[21] Buller DB, Floyd AHL. Internet-based interventions for health behavior change. In: Noar S, Harrington NW, editors. eHealth applications: promising strategies for behavior change. New York: Routledge; 2012. p.59–78.

[22] Chi BH, Stringer JS. Effects of a mobile short message service on antiretroviral treatment adherence in Kenya (WelTel Kenya1): A randomized trial. Lancet. 2010;376(9755):1807–8. DOI: 10.1016/S0140-6736(10)62046-6.

[23] Free C, Phillips G, Galli L, Watson L, Felix L, Edwards P, Patel V, Haines A. The effectiveness of mobile-health technology-based health behaviour change or disease management interventions for health care consumers: a systematic review. PLoS Med. 2013 Jan 15;10(1):e1001362. DOI: 10.1371/journal.pmed.1001362.

[24] Miller LC, Appleby PR, Christensen JL, Godoy C, Si M, Corsbie-Massay C, Read SJ, Marsella S, Anderson AN, Klatt J. Virtual interactive interventions for reducing risky sex: adaptations, integrations, and innovations. In: Noar S, Harrington NW, editors. eHealth applications: promising strategies for behavior change. New York: Routledge; 2012. p.79–95.

[25] Holloway IW, Rice E, Gibbs J, Winetrobe H, Dunlap S, Rhoades H. Acceptability of smartphone application-based HIV prevention among young men who have sex with men. AIDS Behav. 2014 Feb 1;18(2):285–96. DOI: 10.1007/s10461-013-0671-1.

[26] Kreps GL, Joy S, Cary M, Wolf H, Villagran M, Cai X, Zhao X. Evaluating the use of mobile health information technology to promote physical activity and weight management for addressing the obesity epidemic. Presented to the MHealth Summit, Washington, DC, November, 2010.

[27] Blackman KC, Zoellner J, Berrey LM, Alexander R, Fanning J, Hill JL, Estabrooks PA. Assessing the internal and external validity of mobile health physical activity promotion interventions: a systematic literature review using the RE-AIM framework. J Med Internet Res. 2013;15(10):e224. DOI: 10.2196/jmir.2745.

[28] Hebden L, Cook A, Ploeg HP, King L, Bauman A, Allman-Farinelli M. A mobile health intervention for weight management among young adults: a pilot randomised controlled trial. J Hum Nutr Diet. 2014 Aug 1;27(4):322–32. DOI: 10.1111/jhn.12155.

[29] Silva BM, Rodrigues JJ, de la Torre Díez I, López-Coronado M, Saleem K. Mobile-health: a review of current state in 2015. J Biomed Inform. 2015 Aug 31;56:265–72. DOI: 10.1016/j.jbi.2015.06.003.

[30] Abroms LC, Ahuja M, Kodl Y, Thaweethai L, Sims J, Winickoff JP, Windsor RA. Text2Quit: results from a pilot test of a personalized, interactive mobile health smoking cessation program. J Health Commun. 2012 May 2;17(sup1):44-53. DOI: 10.1080/10810730.2011.649159.

[31] Whittaker R, McRobbie H, Bullen C, Borland R, Rodgers A, Gu Y. Mobile phone-based interventions for smoking cessation. The Cochrane Library. 2012 Jan 1. DOI: 10.1002/14651858.CD006611.pub3.

[32] Mares ML, Gustafson DH, Glass JE, Quanbeck A, McDowell H, McTavish F, Atwood AK, Marsch LA, Thomas C, Shah D, Brown R. Implementing an mHealth system for substance use disorders in primary care: a mixed methods study of clinicians' initial expectations and first year experiences. BMC Med Inform Decis Mak. 2016 Sep 29;16(1):126. DOI: 10.1186/s12911-016-0365-5.

[33] Gustafson DH, McTavish FM, Chih MY, Atwood AK, Johnson RA, Boyle MG, Levy MS, Driscoll H, Chisholm SM, Dillenburg L, Isham A. A smartphone application to support recovery from alcoholism: a randomized clinical trial. JAMA Psychiatry. 2014 May 1;71(5):566–72. DOI: 10.1001/jamapsychiatry.2013.4642.

[34] Schulte M, Liang D, Wu F, Lan YC, Tsay W, Du J, Zhao M, Li X, Hser YI. A smartphone application supporting recovery from heroin addiction: perspectives of patients and providers in China, Taiwan, and the USA. J Neuroimmune Pharmacol. 2016 Feb 4:1–2. DOI: 10.1007/s11481-016-9653-1.

[35] Lee HY, Koopmeiners JS, Rhee TG, Raveis VH, Ahluwalia JS. Mobile phone text messaging intervention for cervical cancer screening. Obstetrical & Gynecological Survey. 2015 Jan 1;70(1):26–27. DOI: 10.1097/OGX.0000000000000142.

[36] Catalani C, Philbrick W, Fraser H, Mechael P, Israelski DM. mHealth for HIV treatment & prevention: a systematic review of the literature. Open AIDS J. 2013 Aug 13;7:17–41. DOI: 10.2174/1874613620130812003.

[37] Källander K, Tibenderana JK, Akpogheneta OJ, et al. Mobile health (mHealth) approaches and lessons for increased performance and retention of community health workers in low- and middle-income countries: a review. J Med Internet Res. 2013;15(1):e17. DOI: 10.2196/jmir.2130.

[38] Fiordelli M, Diviani N, Schulz PJ. Mapping mHealth research: a decade of evolution. J Med Internet Res. 2013;15(5):e95. DOI: 10.2196/jmir.2430.

[39] Kreps GL, Neuhauser L. Artificial intelligence and immediacy: designing health communication to personally engage consumers and providers. Patient Educ Counsel. 2013 Aug 31;92(2):205–10. DOI: 10.1016/j.pec.2013.04.014.

[40] Levy H, Janke AT, Langa KM. Health literacy and the digital divide among older Americans. J Gen Intern Med. 2015 Mar 1;30(3):284–89. DOI: 10.1007/s11606-014-3069-5.

[41] Levy H, Janke A. Health literacy and access to care. J Health Commun. 2016 Mar 28;21(sup1):43–50. DOI: 10.1080/10810730.2015.1131776.

[42] Amann J, Rubinelli S, Kreps GL. Revisiting the concept of health literacy. The patient as information seeker and provider. European Health Psychologist. 2015;17(6):286–90.

[43] McNiel P, McArthur EC. Evaluating health mobile apps: information literacy in undergraduate and graduate nursing courses. J Nurs Educ. 2016 Jul 28;55(8):480. DOI: 10.3928/01484834-20160715-12.

[44] Neuhauser L, Kreps GL. Integrating design science theory and methods to improve the development and evaluation of health communication programs. J Health Commun. 2014 Dec 2;19(12):1460–71. DOI: 10.1080/10810730.2014.954081.

[45] Alpert JM, Desens L, Krist AH, Aycock RA, Kreps GL. Measuring health literacy levels of a patient portal using the CDC's Clear Communication Index. Health Promot Pract. 2016 May 17:1524839916643703. DOI: 10.1177/1524839916643703.

[46] Stoyanov SR, Hides L, Kavanagh DJ, Zelenko O, Tjondronegoro D, Mani M. Mobile app rating scale: a new tool for assessing the quality of health mobile apps. JMIR Mhealth and Uhealth. 2015;3(1):e27. DOI: 10.2196/mhealth.3422.

[47] Alpert JM, Krist AH, Aycock RA, Kreps GL. Applying multiple methods to comprehensively evaluate a patient portal's effectiveness to convey information to patients. J Med Internet Res. 2016;18(5):e112. DOI: 10.2196/jmir.5451

[48] Ma X, Yan B, Chen G, Zhang C, Huang K, Drury J, Wang L. Design and implementation of a toolkit for usability testing of mobile apps. Mobile Networks and Applications. 2013 Feb 1;18(1):81–97. DOI: 10.1007/s11036-012-0421-z.

[49] Bergmo TS. How to measure costs and benefits of eHealth interventions: an overview of methods and frameworks. J Med Internet Res. 2015 Nov;17(11). DOI: 10.2196/jmir.4521.

[50] Schweitzer J, Synowiec C. The economics of ehealth and mhealth. J Health Commun. 2012;17 Suppl 1:73–81. DOI: 10.1080/10810730.2011.649158.

[51] Kreps GL. Evaluating health communication programs to enhance health care and health promotion. J Health Commun. 2014 Dec 2;19(12):1449–59. DOI: 10.1080/10810730.2014.954080.

[52] Zhao J, Freeman B, Li M. Can mobile phone apps influence people's health behavior change? An evidence review. J Med Internet Res. 2016 Nov 2;18(11):e287. DOI: 10.2196/jmir.5692.

[53] Kreps GL. One size does not fit all: adapting communication to the needs and literacy levels of individuals. Annals of Family Medicine, 2006. http://www.annfammed.org/cgi/eletters/4/3/205.

[54] Neuhauser L, Kreps GL, Morrison K, Athanasoulis M, Kirienko N, Van Brunt D. Using design science and artificial intelligence to improve health communication: ChronologyMD case example. Patient Educ Couns. 2013;92(2):211–17. DOI: 10.1016/j.pec.2013.04.006.

[55] Kreps GL, Neuhauser L. Artificial intelligence and immediacy: designing health communication to personally engage consumers and providers. Patient Educ Couns. 2013;92(2):205–10. DOI: 10.1016/j.pec.2013.04.014.

Developments and New Directions in Health Literacy Practice

Health Literacy
R.A. Logan and E.R. Siegel (Eds.)
IOS Press, 2017
doi:10.3233/978-1-61499-790-0-359

Global Health Systems and Policy Development: Implications for Health Literacy Research, Theory and Practice

Gillian ROWLANDS[a,b,1], Sarity DODSON [c,d], Angela LEUNG[e], and Diane LEVIN-ZAMIR[f,g]

Additional contributions from
Dr Jyoshma DESOUZA[h]
Ms Kelly KIDD[i]
Dr Sanjay PATTANSHETTY[h]
Dr Frederico PERES[j]
Ms Nadege UWUMAHORO[b]
Ms Anita TREZONA[d]
Mag.Dr. Christina DIETSCHER[k]
Ms Janet SOLLA[l]
Ms Helen BAKER[l]

[a]*Institute of Health and Society, University of Newcastle, UK*
[b]*Institute of Public Health, Aarhus University, Denmark*
[c]*The Fred Hollows Foundation, Australia*
[d]*School of Population Health, Deakin University, Australia*
[e]*School of Nursing, The Hong Kong Polytechnic University, Hong Kong*
[f]*Clalit Health Services, Tel Aviv, Israel*
[g]*Israel and School of Public Health, University of Haifa, Israel*
[h]*Department of Public Health, Manipal University, India*
[i]*Philadelphia, US*
[j]*Brazilian National School of Public Health, Brazil*
[k]*Bundesministerium fur Gesundheit und Frauen, Vienna, Austria*
[l]*Community Health and Learning Foundation, UK*

Abstract. Accessible and responsive health systems are critical to population health and human development. While progress has been made toward global health and development targets, significant inequities remain within and between countries. Expanding health inequities suggest a widespread and systemic neglect of vulnerable citizens, and a failure to enshrine within policies a responsibility to tailor care to the variable capabilities of citizens. Implementation of health and social policies that drive the design of accessible health systems, services, products and infrastructure represents the next frontier for health reform.

Within this chapter we argue the need to consider health and health literacy across policy domains, to operationalize the intent to address inequities in health in meaningful and pragmatic ways, and to actively monitor progress and impact within the context of the Sustainable Development Goals (SDGs). We contend that viewing and developing policies and systems within a health literacy framework will assist in placing citizens and equity considerations at the center of development efforts.

---

[1] Corresponding author: Institute of Health and Society, Newcastle University, Baddiley-Clark Bldg, Newcastle upon Tyne NE2 4AX, UK. E-mail: gill.rowlands@newcastle.ac.uk

In this chapter, we explore the relationship between health literacy and equitable access to health care, and the role of health system and policy reform. We first explore international policies, health literacy, and the SDGs. We then explore national policies and the role that national and local services and systems play in building health literacy, and responding to the health literacy challenges of citizens. We discuss the World Health Organization's (WHO) Framework for Integrated People-Centered Health Services and the way in which health services are being encouraged to understand and respond to citizen health literacy needs. Each section of the chapter ends with a summary and a review of health literacy research and practice. Throughout, we illustrate our points through 'vignettes' from around the world.

Keywords. Health literacy; policy; health and education systems; disparities; health reform; access to care; organisation and delivery of care

1.   Introduction

Accessible and responsive health systems are critical to population health and human development. While progress has been made toward global health and development targets, significant inequities remain within and between countries. Emerging health challenges, such as the Zika virus, and ongoing complex, multi-faceted public health problems, such as diabetes, require strategic, coordinated and sustained responses. In this chapter, we explore the role of health literacy theory and practice in strengthening global and national policies and systems of importance to health, and in promoting and improving equity. Further, we identify opportunities to undertake research to promote ongoing systems development.

People make decisions about their health within personal, social and environmental constraints. The availability and accessibility of health and social services interact with the health literacy of individuals, families and communities to influence health decisions (see Figure 1). In another chapter, Levin-Zamir et. al.

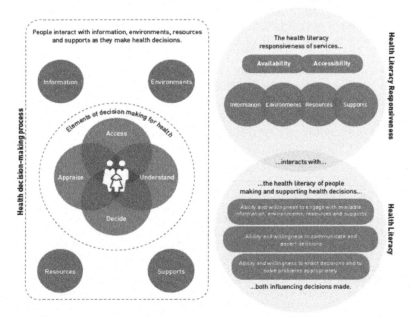

Figure 1. The interaction between health literacy and the health literacy responsiveness of services. Reproduced from: Dodson, Beauchamp, Batterham and Osborne, 2015 [2]

describe the influence of cultural context upon the health literacy of individuals, families, and communities [1]. In this chapter, we focus on the national and international policies and systems that influence health decisions and behaviors.

1.1 Why national and international policies are important to health literacy research, policy and practice

Health decisions and actions, at their core, emerge from an interaction between the capacities of individuals, and the contexts within which they 'live, learn, work, play and love' [3,4]. Since these contexts are shaped by policy, it can be argued that policy is a central influence upon the health literacy of a society. Expanding health inequities in many developing and developed countries suggest a widespread and systemic neglect of vulnerable citizens [5], and a failure to enshrine within policies a responsibility to tailor care to the variable health capabilities of citizens. Implementation of health and social policies that drive the development of systems, services, products and infrastructure that are accessible to all represents the next frontier for health reform. Viewing policies and systems with a health literacy lens will assist to place citizens and equity considerations at the center of development.

Policies can be international, national or local. International policies establish global or regional objectives and expectations. They enable collective action to be taken and inequities between countries to be addressed, and they facilitate sharing of knowledge in relation to system and human developments. National policies set out national priorities, goals, objectives, targets and resourcing, and drive national and local development. Local policies, not explored in this chapter, often sit within national or regional frameworks, and respond to the needs of their local populations and communities.

1.2 Structure of this chapter

In this chapter, we first explore international policies and health literacy, using the example of the Sustainable Development Goals (SDGs). We then explore national policies, using the example of the WHO Framework for Integrated People-Centered Health Services. We then examine services and systems, both those that develop health literacy (e.g. education systems through the life course) and those that respond to the health literacy needs of a population to promote health, prevent illness and support citizen management of diseases, illness and frailty (e.g. the health, public health, and social care systems).

Each section of the chapter ends with a summary and a review of health literacy research and practice. Throughout the chapter, we illustrate our points through 'vignettes' (case studies) from around the world.

2.   International policy and health literacy research, theory and practice

The year 2016 marked the introduction of the United Nations Sustainable Development Goals (SDGs), a new global agenda for human development [6]. The 17 SDGs are accompanied by targets and indicators that guide local and global efforts to end poverty, fight inequalities and tackle climate change. The SDG agenda pledges to 'leave no one behind' and acknowledges the interconnectedness of efforts across development domains and the need to ensure that 'development' does not take place at the expense of health and social equity [5,6]. The SDGs call for an unprecedented coordination effort across sectors, countries and regions.

With the launch of the SDGs, analyses have explored lessons learned from the Millennium Development Goal (MDG) experiment. The global MDG targets for HIV, TB and malaria were met, and child and maternal mortality have seen a sharp decline [7]. While many targets were not achieved, significant global progress was made. The success of the MDGs have been widely attributed to several key drivers: 1) the use of a limited number of time-bound, measurable and easy to communicate goals as a mechanism for targeting and motivating action and partnerships; 2) the intensity of focus and investment as a driver of innovation; 3) measurement and the development of monitoring systems; and 4) national public commitments to achieving specific targets and the associated political pressure and accountability. The SDGs redouble the efforts associated with the MDGs and set an ambitious global agenda.

In this section, we apply SDGs #3 'Ensure healthy lives and promote well-being for all at all ages', #4 'Ensure inclusive and equitable quality education and promote lifelong learning opportunities for all' and #6 'Ensure availability and sustainable management of waste and sanitation for all' as exemplars of the role and influence of international policy in shaping national priorities, and to highlight the relationship between health literacy and development progress. They also provide exemplars of approaches to system strengthening, and the potential of the SDGs to focus attention upon issues of inequity. We then explore the role of cross border collaborations, focusing on the movement of people and disease across borders. We then explore the role of research in supporting the development and evaluation of international policy.

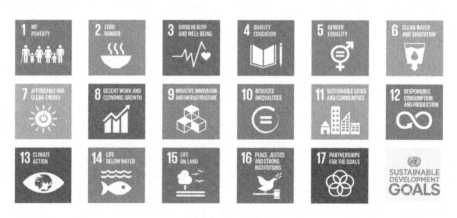

Figure 2. The United Nations 2030 Sustainable Development Goals [6]

2.1. Health literacy and Sustainable Development Goals 3 and 4

The two goals that most clearly highlight the relationship between development and health literacy are SDG 3 'Ensure healthy lives and promote well-being for all at all ages' and SDG 4 'Ensure inclusive and equitable quality education and promote lifelong learning opportunities for all'. Goal 3 highlights the need to strengthen the quality, coverage and accessibility of disease control and prevention programs, medicines and vaccines, healthcare services, and mental health care. Empowered, health literate citizens and communities can act as key drivers of the needed reform and support effective engagement with developed systems and services. Goal 4 highlights the importance of education across the life course, with emphasis on the education of children (both boys and girls) and women. Reforms in education provide significant opportunities to develop health literacy capabilities.

An example from Ethiopia (Box 1) shows how the realization of SDG 4 supports development of health literacy, and how health literacy is fundamental to the achievement of SDG 3. Ethiopia is blighted by trachoma; an infectious blinding eye disease, which is spread through contact with linen, hands and flies carrying the infection. Those that develop blinding trachoma, predominantly women/mothers, are often unable to carry out productive work and are reliant on the care of family members. In these households, additional duties often fall to girls/daughters, who then miss out on education and other opportunities. Ending the epidemic of trachoma requires improved health services, particularly improved access to surgical services and antibiotics, and enhanced engagement of the community in facial cleaning and environmental sanitation behaviors. Engagement of community members with services and effective hygiene practices requires development of awareness, an understanding of how trachoma transmission can be interrupted, and the skills, resources and motivation to persistently act to minimize the risk of transmission.

Box 1. Developing health literacy and achieving Sustainable Development Goals 3 (Good health and well-being) and 4 (Quality education): An example from Ethiopia.

Mrs E is a 35-year old married woman with five children, aged between one and fourteen years. She lives in a remote Kebele (village) in the Oromia region of Ethiopia. Oromia has the highest prevalence of blinding trachoma in the world.

Mrs E has been experiencing eye pain, vision loss and severe headaches now for two years. These symptoms are common in her community and she believes it is hereditary and nothing can be done. The nearest primary health service is 150 km away, but Mrs E has no knowledge of this service and no way to reach it as her only means of transport is by foot. Mrs E and her husband make a living growing Teff (a local grain) and selling it at the local market. They earn enough money to feed their family and purchase basic supplies. Public transport is not affordable, nor is soap, clothing, towels, bedding or linen. In anticipation of losing her sight completely, Mrs E has removed her ten-year-old daughter from school to teach her household management skills and to receive support with childcare and other chores.

Mrs E and her family live in a compound with four single room mud structures – one to live and sleep in, one to house the large livestock, one for smaller livestock, and a kitchen. The eight household members share a single room, two mattresses, and three blankets. There is no source of electricity and the nearest water source is 30 minute's walk. There are restrictions on the amount of water Mrs E's family can take from the local water pump, and they prioritise this for drinking. They use the river for bathing and laundry once per week. Last year Mrs E's husband constructed a latrine for the family after receiving some donated supplies and education from an international NGO. Mrs E and her husband use the latrine occasionally, but Mrs E feels she is too busy to encourage the children to use it, and so they continue to defecate around the periphery of the mud structures. The flies breed readily in the human excrement.

Childhood education that empowers and supports development of literacy and language skills can be seen here as fundamental in enabling access to the required information and to social interactions that assist to shape attitudes and encourage adoption of positive health behaviors. Effective basic childhood education may therefore be an important prerequisite for public health programs requiring significant changes in citizen behavior. Upon a foundation of basic childhood education, interventions targeting development of specific health literacy capabilities are likely to enable the generation of community led solutions to local health problems that are more likely to be enacted, relevant, and sustainable than those conceived and imposed upon communities from the outside.

This dual health literacy and SDG focus assists to ensure that, globally, population health is being improved, while locally the freedoms, capabilities and health literacy of individuals are being developed. This approach also acts to bridge the actions taken to progress health related targets, and efforts to progress the interconnected environmental, education, legal, economic and social welfare targets.

2.2. Other Sustainable Development Goals and health literacy

While the SDGs most closely linked with health literacy are 3 and 4, many other goals can also be closely related. As examples, our Ethiopian story shows that SDG 6 'Ensure availability and sustainable management of waste and sanitation for all' could also be promoted through the development of health literacy. It is only through community understanding of the health risks of poor water quality and sanitation, and the benefits to be gained from addressing those risks, that such policies will be effective. Box 2 gives another example, this time from India.

These examples demonstrate the need to develop coordinated approaches across policies, as espoused in WHO's 'Health in All Policies' (HiAP) [8]. HiAP is discussed in more depth in the context of national policies in the next section, where it

---

Box 2: Developing health literacy to promote Sustainable Development Goal 6 (Clean Water and sanitation)

Mrs Chaudhari is a 22-year old mother who lives with her three sons and her parents-in-law in a rural village. She knows that vomiting and diarrhoea is a big problem; all her children have had severe diarrhoea at some points in their lives, and her younger sister died of this when she was a child.

When listening to the radio with her family she heard about the 'Nirmal Bharat Abhiyan' (or 'Clean India') campaign to help reduce the risk of diarrhoea through building toilets, and persuading people to use them. Mrs C has heard about the new toilets coming to the village, but does not know why they are needed or why she and her family should use them. The nurse on the radio talks about how open defecation causes illness, and how using the new toilets will make it far less likely that she and her family will get diarrhoea. Her local Panchayat (local administrator) talks about how everyone can benefit, and the whole village will work together. The Panchayat says that there will be a Swechhata Doot (cleanliness ambassador) in every village and that half of them will be women. Each Swechhata Doot will earn RS 22,000 ($330) a year.

After listening to the radio show, Mrs Chaudhari understands about how the new toilets will help, and wonders whether she could become the Swechhata Doot for her village.

is evident that coordination across health, education, economic, infrastructure development and environmental policies (amongst others), is vital for effective and sustainable development. Again, ensuring that health literacy is a central consideration assists co-ordination, a focus on equity, and consideration of the needs of individuals, families and communities.

2.3. Cross border collaborations

In this subsection, we explore the movement of people across borders, the related health risks and their management. We examine both the way that health literacy is currently conceptualized and operationalized in cross border health issues, and the role it potentially can play in the future.

2.4. Movement of people across borders

The increasing global mass movement of people across borders creates several policy challenges for host governments, and the need for international collaboration and coordination. Countries receiving migrants and refugees have responsibilities to develop and implement policies that promote equitable access to care, issues that have implementation implications for health literacy, human rights and medical economics.

Current evidence reveals a 'migrant health decline' [9-11], which appears to result from the disconnect that emerges, following migration, between the social, economic, and healthcare opportunities available in the host country, and the skills, knowledge and beliefs (health literacy) of migrants. The cumulative impacts associated with the erosion of pre-migration lifestyles, and barriers to healthcare access due to language and cultural factors, appear to be substantive and observable two years following migration [12]. The burden that poor migrant health may pose to host countries because of global inaction, and failure to collaborate on global health issues, is likely to emerge as a significant issue of public debate in coming years.

While there is a growing tendency within immigration debates for developed countries to favor a closed-door solution, migration and temporary movements between borders is likely an irreversible phenomenon, especially in the context of globalization, and ongoing within and across border conflicts. Health systems will need to find a way to respond to, and overcome migration related challenges over the coming decades. Such a response is illustrated by the example from Israel shown below in Box 3, reproduced from Levin-Zamir et al. [1].

This example, which can also be contributing to SDG 3 'Ensure healthy lives and promote well-being for all at all ages', illustrates that rather than expecting migrants to fit with current systems, adaptations can be made to support migrants to learn to navigate their new environment. Both linguistic and cultural liaison between the individual and those providing his/her care appear important to ensure new migrants can effectively access healthcare. The expense of providing such liaison is likely to be offset by the health savings arising from more effective and streamlined care, with fewer wasted health appointments, and the longer-term benefits arising from improved illness self-management. In addition to the potential benefits of specialized liaison roles to support new migrants, health providers within host countries would benefit from education that enhances their understanding of the health systems, cultural practices and norms, and common health beliefs and conceptualizations held within countries of origin.

Box 3. The impacts of migration upon health literacy and the challenges created for health systems in host countries.

Asmara and his six children and their families immigrated from Ethiopia to Israel 10 years ago. He came expecting to encounter the perfect health support system. Feeling tired all the time, he sought help from the local community clinic. He quickly realized that the health providers not only speak a different language from the one he speaks, but they also arrange the way they provide health and medical treatment to people very differently from what he knew in Ethiopia.

When Asmara approached the family doctor in the community clinic, he was first sent to have a blood test, on a completely different day, and still received no treatment. He was expected to return to the physician to receive the test results, however this time he understood from neighbors that he was to make an appointment through the telephone or an online system, which he was unsure how to do. He finally decided to return to the clinic and just wait until the doctor could see him. He sat in the waiting room for a long time and watched how other people who arrived after he did, could see the doctor before him. He finally decided to go home. Concurrently, the clinic office had been trying to reach him by phone to make an appointment, as his test results reflected why he was feeling so exhausted.

A week later Asmara heard from his neighbors that a new service is offered in the community clinic, called "Refuah Shlema". Casia, a specially trained health liaison and cultural mediator, now greets Asmara each time he comes to the clinic, seeks to understand what Asmara is feeling, and helps him to communicate his needs and experiences to the clinic staff. She also helps to interpret the recommendations, in culturally appropriate terms, and sits with Asmara to explain to him more in depth his condition, one that he never heard about in Ethiopia – diabetes

---

2.5. Movement of disease across borders

There is now wide recognition of international influences on health. Increasing globalization, growth in international travel, migration and displacement have implications for the way both communicable and non-communicable diseases (NCDs) are managed. The example from Israel discussed above highlights some of the issues for NCDs. Increasingly, though, infectious diseases are presenting new challenges. This is complicated by the fact that while it is inevitable that new acute infectious disease crises will occur, such as the recent Ebola and Zika virus outbreaks, the nature and site of the outbreaks cannot always be predicted. In its recent review of the Ebola epidemic, the US Center for Disease Control (CDC) highlighted the need for international collaborations, and the development of strong partnerships and systems to provide personnel and skills, and contribute to research and development (such as developing new vaccines [13]). Such partnerships between high-income countries and their middle- and low-income neighbors are critical to generating speedy identification of, and responses to, incipient epidemics. Consideration of health literacy within the development and operationalisation of policies assists in ensuring that responses are citizen focused. Further discussion of this, illustrated with an example from Brazil on the response to the Zika virus epidemic, is provided below (Box 7).

2.6. Health literacy research and international policies

Robust data are needed for making a case for policy changes, and to monitor the impact of such changes. In recognition of the power of data, significant work is being directed by the WHO towards establishing indicators of SDG progress. Equity data feature prominently as critical to ensuring within-and-across-country initiatives 'leave no-one behind'. Effective indicators, high quality data collection approaches, central data registries, and coordinated dissemination efforts, in combination, act to support policy initiatives, and keep governments accountable [14]. Health literacy capabilities do not feature in the SDGs, their targets or indicators. However, complementary thematic indicators are being developed by experts in the field, and encouraged as a means of collecting the input and process data required to make meaning of any observed change. There is an opportunity to advocate that health literacy capabilities be represented effectively within these thematic indicators as they evolve over the next two years. Development of health literacy indicators across thematic areas of global significance, and effective advocacy at national, regional and global levels, is required to build awareness of the role of health literacy in the attainment of the health-related SDGs, and of the critical role that effective policy plays in ensuring community engagement and health care access. The importance of international metrics as drivers for change at a national level can be seen through recent policy and system changes in Austria (see Box 4).

Box 4: Using health literacy data to make the case for changing policy: an example from Austria.

The Austrian government was surprised and disappointed by the results from the 2011 European Health Literacy survey, which found that a high proportion of Austrians had 'problematic' or 'inadequate' health literacy. On reflection and after discussions with the survey leads, the government concluded that part of the problem was that it is difficult for Austrian patients and citizens to gain information and meaning from the complex health system.

The key stakeholders in designing and running the system – the federal government, the nine Austrian states (Länder), and the social insurance companies – agreed to develop and then implement a strategy to improve communication. Talks with the major health care providers – the hospitals – and those training health care professionals – the universities – are ongoing to develop and implement concrete interventions to improve health care communication practice. The main pillars will be training and improvements to the healthcare culture, that encourage communication to be understood as an important clinical skill. Improvements in organizational practice driven by self-assessments and toolkits are expected to enable organizations to improve.

The strategy was launched in Autumn 2016 and will be implemented from 2017. Interventions to implement the strategy will be selected and designed together with key stakeholders, and there will be an accompanying monitoring system.

Health literacy researchers and advocates have important roles to play in identifying robust indicators that support collection of meaningful data to both drive SDG progress, and to lobby for their incorporation into monitoring frameworks. The choice of indicators is crucial; they should capture both the capacities of individuals, families and communities, and the capacities of the health, social care and education systems to work with citizens and communities to promote health. These connections (between the capabilities of citizens, and global and national health policies and population health targets) are easy to lose sight of. However, effective operationalization of policies requires an understanding of the mechanisms of change, at personal and interpersonal levels.

Collective change is the culmination of individual change and the social momentum that can be created once a tipping point is reached [15]. It is the health literacy capabilities of citizens and communities, and the extent to which healthcare services respond effectively to their needs, that represent the key focal points of interventions geared towards the attainment of the SDGs. The SDG targets form the more distal population level outcomes that will signal medium to long-term progress. Once robust health literacy indicators are successfully included in monitoring frameworks, associations between health literacy, health and social outcomes, and economic progress may be explored. Techniques such as Social Return on Investment, a method that enables the capture of extra-financial value (such as environmental and social value) not captured well in more conventional cost-benefit analyses, [16] are useful in this regard. Qualitative work should be a key component of any evaluation research undertaken, and include gathering insights from those developing or implementing policies, and those experiencing the impacts of policies.

Work is also required to analyse policies with regards to the extent to which they facilitate development of health capabilities and optimise ease of choice and access to health services, products and environments. Comparison and critical analysis of policies can facilitate information exchange, and shorten the development process if countries can adapt policies known to work elsewhere. For example, Trezona et al. (under review) propose a framework that supports assessment of the degree to which a policy effectively prioritises and resources health literacy. Policy can be assessed across three categories: the extent to which health literacy or related concepts are mentioned or defined within the policy; the extent to which health literacy is prioritised within the policy; and the extent to which health literacy is operationalized through specific actions and whether these actions are supported through the allocation of resources and establishment of monitoring mechanisms (see Table 1). Policy analyses across a range of sectors and settings will enable policy makers to improve the effectiveness of their policies, and will support advocacy efforts and raise awareness of the role of public policy in addressing the issues contributing to inequities.

2.7. International policy and health literacy research and practice - Summary

In this section, we have described how international policy can promote health literacy, using the example of the United Nations Sustainable Development Goals (SDGs). Of the 17 goals, the two most closely related to health literacy are goal 3 'Ensure healthy lives and promote well-being for all at all ages' and goal 4 'Ensure inclusive and equitable quality education and promote lifelong learning opportunities for all'. Using the example of trachoma in Ethiopia, we explored the relationship between health literacy and achievement of the goals. We also discussed how health literacy, with its placement of people and communities at the center of development activities, can shape development of policies that promote equity and ensure 'no-one is left behind'.

Table 1. Framework for analysing health literacy in public policy documents

	Prominence of health literacy	**Rating**
Category 1	Health literacy is not explicitly mentioned, nor is a related concept	*0*
	A concept related to health literacy is mentioned, but health literacy is not explicitly mentioned	*1*
	Health literacy is mentioned, but not defined or explained	*2*
	Health literacy is defined or explained	*3*
Category 2	Prioritisation of health literacy	
	Health literacy is mentioned, but its relationship to health outcomes is not explained	*1*
	Health literacy is discussed as a concept related to health outcomes, but is not noted as a strategic priority	*2*
	Health literacy is noted as a strategic priority	*3*
Category 3	Health literacy actions, resourcing and monitoring	
	No specific actions are identified to address health literacy	*0*
	Health literacy actions are identified, but no resources are provided to support implementation and no monitoring of outcomes is proposed	*1*
	Health literacy actions are identified. Resources are allocated to support implementation, OR monitoring of outcomes is proposed (but both are not evident).	*2*
	Health literacy actions are identified, resources are allocated to support implementation, and monitoring of outcomes is proposed.	*3*

In relation to the needs for future research, we explored the opportunity for development of health literacy indicators and of monitoring frameworks that effectively communicate the link between health literacy and the SDGs. In addition to this we highlight the opportunity for analysis of existing health policy and the extent to which health literacy is considered and strategies for responding to health literacy issues operationalized.

International policies are thus crucial in setting frameworks for international collaboration and joint action, and for the development of coherent national policies with complementary foci. It is, however, national governments, and the policy decisions they make that will determine the systems within which people 'live, learn, work, play and love' [3]. That is the focus of the next section in this chapter.

3. National policy and health literacy research, theory and practice

National policy plays a critical role in not only endorsing principles of equity and quality, but also in driving the establishment and maintenance of the many prerequisites of an integrated, people-centered health system. A key challenge for national health departments, and other bodies responsible for driving health policy, is developing and implementing policies that enable strengthening of health systems such that they deliver responsive local care, while also ensuring consistency of standards and ease of navigation across jurisdictions [17].

To complement its guidance role in relation to health systems, WHO recently released a Framework for Integrated People-Centered Health Services (See Figure 3) [17]. This organizational level guidance provides policy makers with support to understand how to approach the task of service design and reorientation. The Framework seeks to ensure that "all people have equal access to quality health services that are co-produced in a way that meets their life course needs, are coordinated across the continuum of care, and are comprehensive, safe, effective, timely, efficient and acceptable; and all carers are motivated, skilled and operate in a supportive environment". Five interdependent strategies are proposed: in the following section each of these is explored in turn. We then explore the need for a 'Health in All Polices' (HiAP) approach to ensue effective co-ordination. We end this section with a discussion of the role of health literacy research in developing and monitoring national policies.

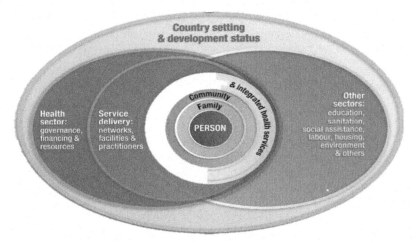

Figure 3. Conceptual framework for people-centered and integrated health services. *Reproduced from [17]*

3.1 Empowering and engaging people and communities

The earlier example from India (Box 2 above) provides an example of the benefits of empowering and engaging people and communities. In some ways, the situation in India in regard to sanitation is similar to that in Ethiopia (Box 1 above). In both cases, there is a public health problem arising from transmission of infectious diseases due to lack of safe sanitation facilities and access to water. It is reasonable to hypothesize that the issues continue in these countries, in large part due to limited health literacy regarding opportunities to minimize the risk of infection and illness. The Indian case study describes the potential benefits of developing health literacy on the issue within the community; Mrs. Chaudhari comes to understand how open defecation causes disease, and can share that information with her family and friends. In parallel, issues such as poverty, gender equality, and community engagement may potentially be addressed, at least in part, through the Indian approach.

3.2 Strengthening governance and accountability

Rwanda provides an example of how having strong, accountable systems, which place the citizen and community at the center, can have remarkable impacts on health (Box 5, information gathered from [18-21]). While Rwanda's health system has its share of

---

Box 5: Strong governance and accountability leading to effective, health literate, systems.

The 1994 genocide in Rwanda devastated the country's health infrastructure and substantively depleted the health workforce. The government established in the aftermath of the genocide commenced reconstruction of Rwanda's health system and has continued to develop and implement health system reform since this time. Rwanda now has a largely decentralized health system with district health offices responsible for oversight or administration of public and private health services in the localized areas. National programs and policies act to ensure consistency of services across districts. Centrally, policies, strategies and technical frameworks are developed, monitored and reviewed. A minimum package of activities has been defined for common health conditions and the ten most important causes of morbidity and mortality.

At the health center level, the minimum package of activities includes health literacy promotion activities, preventative care services, and curative activities relevant to each target disease. Health committees have been established in all health centers and district health offices, which act to oversee the financial management of health centers, ensure the health concerns and communities are represented, and to mobilize the community to participate in activities and projects. Since 2000, the committees have included health promoters elected by the population, to ensure better representation of community concerns. The system is financed by a combination of state funds, insurance contributions and direct fees for service. The Community-Based Health Insurance Scheme sees members pay annual premiums of approximately USD$6 per family member with a 10% service fee paid for visits to services. 91% of Rwandans were insured through this scheme in 2010.

Rwandan national life expectancy at birth for both genders increased by 19 years over the period of 2000 to 2012, in contrast to an average increase of 7 years across the Central / Eastern Africa region. Deaths from malaria decreased by 85% between 2005 and 2011, HIV by 78% between 2000 and 2009, and TB by 77% between 2000 and 2010.

---

ongoing challenges, including poor workforce distribution, poor service integration, and ongoing reliance on international aid, it sits in stark contrast to the health systems of many of its regional counterparts. National leadership and effective policy implementation have played a key role in the health system development and achievement of Universal Coverage (UC) observed in Rwanda. UC is defined as 'all people receiving the health services they need, including health initiatives designed to promote better health (such as anti-tobacco policies), prevent illness (such as vaccinations), and to provide treatment, rehabilitation, and palliative care (such as end-of-life care) of sufficient quality to be effective, while at the same time ensuring that the use of these services does not expose the user to financial hardship' [22]. Efforts to provide UC, involvement of the community in the development process and ongoing management of the health system, successful public health campaigns to address communicable diseases, and inclusion of health literacy development activities as core components of minimum packages of care delivered by district health services, are key features of the Rwandan success story. The Rwandan case example highlights what can be achieved when health policy that seeks to address access inequities and build citizen capacity and engagement is effectively implemented.

3.3. Re-orientating the model of care

Historically, in Western societies, health care systems have been bio-medically focused and hierarchical. A powerful, informed doctor instructs and treats disempowered, uninformed patients who are expected to do what the medical system advises them to. Over the last 20 years, huge strides have been made in re-orientating the model of care to be person-centered, and in empowering patients to control their health and health

---

Box 6. Re-orientating health care to become health literate' and patient-centered

The community health and learning foundation is a UK Non-Government Organisation that works to create a more Health Literate Health and Social Care system. It has developed a training course for General Practitioners (Family Physicians) and their practices, with a face-to-face half- or full-day training course. The course includes practical information about what health literacy is, why it is important, and how it can impact on patients in everyday life, and on patients and doctors in clinical encounters. Those attending the course are also given practical tools to use in the consultation, such as 'Teach-back' and using clear language and communication techniques. Feedback from doctors at the end of the course indicated a previous lack of awareness of the issue of health literacy; "Thought provoking – very disturbed by the huge number of people who struggle to read/write/count" and a recognition that improving their health literacy skills will improve their patient care "If I am able to communicate better with clients then their experiences will be better". The course is now undergoing an evaluation to better capture the impact of the course on patients and the care they receive.

---

care. Implementing health literacy focused strategies is one way to promote this change, either through building patient and citizen skills, and/or through building physician knowledge, skills and understanding. See Box 6 for an example (information about teach back from [23]).

3.4 Co-coordinating services within and across sectors

The 2016 Zika epidemic, centered in Brazil, has highlighted the problems that arise when services are not coordinated. The epidemic had all the features of a 'perfect public health storm'; the evolution of the virus to a more virulent form with sexual as well as vector-transmission [24], its emergence in a country facing severe social, economic, and infrastructure issues, and the potential for global spread through the very high international travel linked with the 2016 Olympic Games. The following example from Brazil illustrates some of the key factors in that situation.

Box 7. The impact of poorly coordinated services within and across sectors.
Mrs A is a 34-year old married woman living in Rio de Janeiro (Brazil) with three children. She and her husband live with their extended family in cramped conditions without running water or sanitation. Her husband is unemployed; she is the family earner, working shift hours as a cleaner. She is worried about the Zika virus, and what might happen to her and her baby if she were to become pregnant again, particularly as she will not use contraception on religious grounds, and abortion is illegal. She has talked with her friends and family – they are all very concerned but don't know what to do. The government messages talk about citizens' responsibilities for cleaning and avoiding having standing water, but Mrs A's family have to collect water and store it for use for cooking, drinking and washing, and there are no local plumbed-in toilet facilities. Also, Mrs A cannot follow the government instructions to clean every Saturday as she often must work on Saturdays, and anyway feels that the main issue is not how clean her home is, but the piles of trash and discarded tires and household goods (which often contain stagnant water) in the locality, and urine and faeces in the street and the road.

The public health messages referred to in this example were well distributed and easy to understand, but could not be applied by those targeted by the campaign. An alternative approach that considered the local context, was community led, and that developed the Zika virus-specific health literacy of individuals, families and communities might have had a greater chance of addressing public sanitation issues, reducing mosquito breeding, and reducing the risk of maternal: fetal viral transmission.

3.5. Creating an enabling environment

Health will not be fully achieved unless people are living in health promoting environments. In many countries, culture and stigma inhibit well-being and maintenance of health. HIV is a specific example. Given that, initially, the main means of transmission was sexual contact, being HIV positive carries huge stigma. This has multiple negative effects; Many children and young people with HIV, have contracted the virus pre- intra- or post-partum, and are unaware they have the condition. Even when they are aware, the stigma associated with it makes it very difficult to be open about their HIV status, resulting in adverse effects on attendance at clinics, medication compliance, and disclosure to friends, family, and sexual contacts. Tiwonde's story (see Box 8, reproduced from Levin-Zamir et al. [1]), from Malawi, is a common one.

Box 8. The case of young people living with HIV in Malawi.

Tiwonde is a 19-year old girl who lives with her aunt ever since her parents died of AIDS when she was three years old. She was born with HIV, but she discovered that she was HIV-positive when she was 13 years old. Before that, she was taking medication without knowing why, but with time, she has come to understand that if she takes her medication, she can be healthy. Life is not easy for someone with HIV because there is a lot of fear and stigma and discrimination!

Tiwonde often finds it difficult to take her medication because her aunt's husband and children do not know that she is HIV-positive. She and her aunt fear that her aunt's husband will throw her out of the house if he finds out, so she must hide her medication very well and make sure that no one sees her taking her medication. She goes to a boarding school where she has problems with attending classes when she must go for check-ups and to collect her medication.

Tiwonde has been nicknamed "the sick one" because she always gives random excuses for going to the hospital. Like at home, she hides her medication, and she unintentionally misses taking medication when she fails to find an opportunity to take it discretely. There is a boy a little older than her who has been showing interest in dating her, but she is afraid to start a relationship because she does not know how to tell him she is HIV-positive, and that he will abandon her and tell people at school about her status. Moreover, her aunt has told her that she can only be together with someone who is also HIV-positive.

Tiwonde has tried to talk to doctors and nurses about relationship issues, but they have shouted at her and accused her of wanting to spread the virus. She has heard rumors about a pastor who cures HIV through prayer, and she is considering going to see him. Her aunt once took her to a village doctor who gave her some herbs, but they never worked. She wants to meet other young people living with HIV but is afraid that people will find out about her status if she joins a support group.

Changing attitudes is difficult, and may at first glance be beyond the scope of a health system or program – however it is only by challenging myths, misconceptions and stigma, and encouraging openness and discussion, that people with stigmatized illnesses will receive equitable access to health care, be able to effectively control their own health, and future transmission will be reduced. Research with young people with HIV in Malawi (Uwamahoro, in progress) shows high awareness and a desire for empowerment and freedom, in other words the critical health literacy skills [25] to talk openly about their condition to address and reduce associated stigma.

3.6. Health in All Policies

National policies set the contexts within which people live. They will influence the opportunities, capabilities and environments of the population, and the capacity of the health system to adapt to the health literacy of the people it serves. The Health in All Policies (HiAP) approach [8] emerged out of the recognition that, in order to achieve health, the Social Determinants of Health (SDH) must be addressed. It encourages governments to identify and respond to opportunities across ministries, and to develop or reform services, environments and products in ways that enhance citizen access to information and support. Development of citizen health capabilities and the removal of restrictions upon freedoms to exercise health capabilities requires effort across sectors.

An initial step in operationalizing HiAP is understanding local and national needs and priorities, including the ways in which cultural norms and stigma may be reducing health or causing illness, as in the example of HIV in Malawi highlighted above. Thorough assessment of local health, health system and equity issues, and their relationship to policy and country context, is critical. Addressing complex health issues, particularly those with significant health behavioral components, requires a detailed and contextualized understanding of the personal, interpersonal, societal, cultural political, economic and environmental determinants. Amongst these considerations is the health capabilities (i.e. health literacy) of citizens, families and communities and how these interact with local contexts to influence health decisions, behaviors and outcomes.

National tobacco control in Brazil provides a case example (see Box 9: data from [26]) of inter-sectoral cooperation and strong political will to achieve health change. The multi-pronged, multi-level, cross-sectoral approach adopted by the Brazilian government promoted the health literacy of Brazilian citizens with regards to smoking, and constructed environmental, economic and social arrangements that made smoking more difficult, costlier and less attractive to engage in.

Box 9. National tobacco control in Brazil

In 2003 Brazil established the inter-ministerial National Commission for Implementation of the Framework Convention on Tobacco Control. The commission convened representatives from 18 government sectors, and had a broad set of responsibilities to advance tobacco control across Brazil. Some of the cross sectorial actions taken toward tobacco control in Brazil have included the Ministry of Finance raising taxes on cigarettes, changes to legislation that include a ban on smoking in public spaces and on advertising at the point of sale, the Ministry of Agrarian development taking steps to support tobacco growers to diversify their activities, and The National Cancer Institute supporting smoking cessation program development and delivery. Smoking prevalence decreased to 17% in 2009 from 32% in 1989 due to collective action.

3.7. Health literacy research and national policies

Health literacy has much to add in development, implementation, and evaluation of national policy, much the same as with international policy. Pre-implementation assessment of policies can be used to improve policies before implementation, to maximise benefits for citizens and their health literacy. Timely descriptions and evaluations of a policy's impacts support future planning, both within the country concerned but also across sister countries facing similar issues and challenges. Health literacy thematic indictors that may be developed to monitor the progress of the SDGs (see section 2.3 above) could also be applied to the evaluation of national policies. International evaluation frameworks enable direct comparison between countries, and allow assessments to be made about which policies are the most effective in promoting health literacy and associated SDG progress indicators. Inclusion of economic indicators, in particular, will provide countries with information that enables them to effectively decide how best to spend limited national resources. As described in section 2.3, techniques such as social return on investment (SROI) can capture costs and benefits not only within, but also beyond, the health field i.e. increased employment and productivity, and reduced sickness benefits. Finally, qualitative research will bring unique insights into how new policies affect those who receive, as well as those who deliver, services.

3.8 Summary

In this section we explored the value of frameworks (such as the Framework for Integrated People-Centered Health Services) and international policy approaches (such as Health in All Policies) in guiding the development of effective policies and approaches to health systems strengthening that incorporate consideration of health literacy issues and contributors to inequity. We also highlight the importance of strong leadership, effective governance structures, effective inter-sector coordination, and consistent effort in influencing how effectively policy acts to reform health systems, respond to health crises, and improve health and citizen capacity.

National policies focused on health, education and social care, have a significant influence upon the nature and qualities of services, structures and systems, and upon how effectively they respond to the health literacy of individuals, families and communities. It is these services, structures and systems that are explored in the following sections of this chapter.

4. Services, structures and systems to develop health literacy

The development and maintenance of health literacy is a lifelong process. The importance of education in enabling all to achieve their capacities and capabilities, including health, is highlighted by its prominence within the Sustainable Development Goals (SDG 4). In this section we describe what is known about education, both general and health literacy-specific, and cognitive skills and health literacy, including research into these areas. We follow this with a call for more research to inform the development of health literacy through the life course.

4.1 Developing health literacy through the life-course

Cognitive development capacities start to develop in utero, a fact recognized by the WHO Commission on the Social Determinants of Health, resulting in their focus on ante-natal and early years provision as key to promoting health and reducing health inequity [5]. Learning then takes place throughout childhood, adolescence and adulthood. As societies age, more people will face the challenges of cognitive decline in parallel with the development of multiple health conditions. Education, for both children and adults, is key to developing and maintaining health literacy, as well as for promoting social equity and justice [27]. A fuller description and discussion of the place of education in health literacy is given elsewhere in this book by Levin-Zamir et al [1]; here we discuss issues in relation to developing coordinated education systems that develop and maintain health literacy through the life course.

Of key importance is building health literacy competencies that recognize and complement cognitive development. Graham and Power describe a model whereby parental background and environment influence childhood cognition, education and health behavior, with ongoing influences in childhood and later adult health [28]. Cognitive development starts before birth and develops most rapidly in early years. Good nutrition and a health promoting environment antenatally and in early years are vital [5], have been shown to improve cognitive performance [29], and are likely to increase capacities for health literacy. High level cognitive abilities, as evidenced by high qualification levels and employment status, are associated with higher health literacy skills [30], and while not everyone with high cognitive abilities will have high health literacy, it is reasonable to hypothesise that they have latent capacities to develop health literacy given the right circumstances.

Building health literacy in childhood and adolescence should link with cognitive developmental stages [31], and can start very early with activities such as hand- and oral-hygiene. As children develop into adolescents, cognitive development enables the capacity to develop critical health literacy. In addition to simply understanding, and being able to discuss, health messages from a wide range of sources, adolescents can be supported to develop critical analysis and decision making skills as relevant for health. They can learn to ask questions such as Where does the information come from? How trustworthy is the source? Are there hidden messages? How do I know that this information is right for me? How do I take the actions that are best for me? [32-33]. Adolescence is a time when people make lifestyle and sexual health decisions that will influence their future health, so investment in building skills in this period will be valuable. In addition, the qualifications that come with a good general education greatly increase employment opportunities and lifestyle chances, all of which are associated with health and health literacy [5,34].

The development of health literacy in adulthood, described in more detail by Levin-Zamir et al [1] can be immensely valuable both for building skills for health, particularly in mental health and in knowledge about lifestyles and health, but also as a vehicle for developing more general literacy and numeracy skills [35]. A currently underexplored area in health literacy is the 'teachable moment'; where major life changes, both positive (such as having a baby) or negative (such as a diagnosis of a serious health condition) bring opportunities for health-related learning [36]. Cross-generational learning such as family learning, and development of skills within communities, again described by Levin-Zamir et al in this book [1] are also of proven value.

An area where little health literacy teaching or research has been undertaken to date is in older people, particularly during cognitive decline. Wolf et al have shown that much of the loss of health literacy in older people is due to cognitive impairment [37]. However, what is not known is whether health literacy training could benefit this group, or indeed whether effective assessment of health literacy challenges and provision of tailored care is an appropriate way to support older people experiencing these challenges.

There is therefore a need to have 'Health literacy in all *Education* policies'. Extant policies for pre-school, school, and adult learning often are mutually exclusive. Having health literacy taught at all life stages, tailored to cognitive development and life stage, could do much to promote healthier societies.

4.2 Health literacy education and health literacy research

While there is some research on education in health literacy in adolescents and adults, described above, there is much work still to be done. In particular, there appears to be little or no research into the impact of health literacy training at the extremes of life and cognitive capacities, i.e. early years and during old age with and without cognitive decline. More research is needed on the impacts of health literacy interventions through the life course. This evidence can then be used to make the case for routine incorporation of health literacy into education systems.

4.3 Lifelong learning and health literacy research and practice - Summary

Learning health literacy should be seen as a lifelong activity. A coordinated health literate education system would build health literacy throughout the life course, with the optimal life stages and learning styles identified for different people at different times. There is, as yet, little research into the health benefits of building health literacy at different life stages. Exploration of the benefits of teaching health literacy in pre-school, junior, and high schools would be very valuable, as children and adolescents develop the knowledge and skills to move into adulthood. There is some evidence that building adult health literacy, at least at functional and interactive levels, improves health and health behaviors; more research in this area, including the impacts of developing critical and distributed health literacy (in other words, health literacy distributed within networks and social groups [38]), would be very valuable. Finally, more research is needed about the benefits of health literacy training at the extremes of life, both early years and older age, including exploring the extent to which health literacy helps to protect from deterioration of physical and mental health seen with cognitive decline, and whether interventions to build health literacy in these groups are beneficial.

5. Services, structures and systems to promote health, prevent illness, and manage disease, illness and frailty

Citizens within societies will have a range of health capabilities [39,40]. There will certain challenges and barriers they experience, but also skills and attributes they possess that support them to effectively manage their health and engage with health care interactions. Services that seek to promote health, prevent illness, and manage disease, illness and frailty need to be responsive to the health literacy of the citizens they serve. As discussed above, viewing systems through a health literacy lens facilitates the placement of the citizen/patient/client and their family at the center of care, and supports them to design programs that act to reduce inequity. We seek to demonstrate how services and systems that respond effectively to the health literacy of local populations, and work to develop competencies for health, are of key importance in promoting health, and reducing and managing illness. We argue that responsive systems are also more resilient and able to act appropriately and effectively.

In this section, therefore, we discuss those systems of most relevance to health literacy; health, public health, and social services. We then discuss the health literacy research and evaluation opportunities in relation to these systems.

5.1 Health systems

It is only through building and strengthening health systems that it will be possible to secure better health outcomes. To promote the development of strong health systems, the WHO has proposed a framework [41] that describes six key building blocks for strong, resilient services, all of which require attention for maximum benefit for patients. We explore each of these building blocks through a health literacy 'lens', and describe how the health literacy concept may strengthen these building blocks.

This section focuses on health services provided to individuals and families. Systems that focus on populations (public health) are explored in the next section.

5.1.1 Health Services

Examining health literacy is a sensitive way to explore the extent to which citizens feel they are receiving the services they need. The European health literacy survey, in addition to highlighting the prevalence and impact of low health literacy across eight countries, highlighted some interesting international differences in health literacy (Figure 4).

In Box 4 above, we describe how these data stimulated the Austrian Government to develop a policy to reduce the complexity of the system, focus on centering care around the patient, and improve communication and service responsiveness to patients' capacities and needs. This shift in focus was stimulated through high quality international comparative research, which highlighted not only the problem, but also indicated where to focus service reform. The Austrian example also illustrates the need for a planned and coordinated approach across many levels in policy and service. There needed to be a recognition of the problem and willingness to change at three levels – policy (government), organizations (hospitals) and health professionals. This involved recognition of the benefits that could be achieved at these three levels; for the government, there was the potential for increased health of citizens and increased cost-effectiveness of services, for hospitals there was the potential for better patient health outcomes, improved cost-effectiveness due to, for example, fewer missed appointments and unplanned hospital readmissions, fewer patient complaints, and a reduced risk of lawsuits. Health professionals valued the potential for greater patient satisfaction, fewer patient complaints, and better work satisfaction. Finally, for the system to improve there needed to be tools to enable hospitals to assess their 'health literacy' and to take action to improve.

Austria is a high-income country with many resources to improve systems; however Box 5 above describes the development of health literate friendly/focused services in the very different setting of Rwanda. What these system developments have is common, however, is a 'health literacy' focus that prioritizes communication with the patients and communities served. These two examples show how understanding health literacy capabilities, needs and barriers, and making communication with service users central to the service, can inform health system redesign. Future quantitative and qualitative research should be undertaken to assess the impact of the changed services on patients and the public, and 'open the black box' to identify the key barriers to, and facilitators of change, and the extent to which a health literacy focus promotes equity as well as quality in health services.

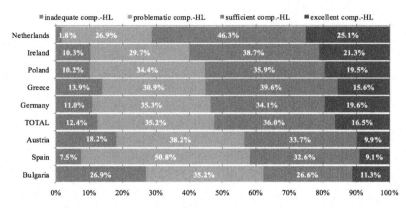

AT [N=996] BG [N=955] DE (NRW) [N=1041] EL[N=998] ES[N=981] IE[N=972] NL[N=993] PL[N=946] TOTAL [N=7883]

Figure 4. Health literacy levels in the 2011 European health literacy survey. Reproduced from the HLS-EU Consortium

5.1.2 The health workforce

For the health workforce to be responsive to patients, particularly those with lower health literacy, they need to have health literacy appropriate skills, knowledge and supportive attitudes [42]. In many countries, such awareness and skills are low. For example, in a study involving junior doctors training to be family physicians in the UK, Groene found that health literacy skills, knowledge and attitudes were low, and reflected low levels of inclusion of health literacy in undergraduate and postgraduate medical training [43]. Initiatives to build health literacy skills in the health workforce are emerging, as shown in Box 6 above.

Techniques such as 'teach back' have been shown to improve patient understanding in the doctor-patient consultation and improved self-management [44,45]. What is not known is what other benefits health practitioner understanding of, and adoption of best practice in, health literacy, might have in terms of efficiency and fairness. It is reasonable to hypothesise that a health literate workforce would lead to better quality of care and better health service efficiency. There is evidence that people with lower health literacy are costlier to health providers, and use a less efficient mix of health services [30,46]. It is worth examining what impact a more skilled workforce in health literacy would have in these areas.

5.1.3 Health information

Within the WHO health systems strengthening framework, this building block focuses solely on the production of high quality and timely health and health system statistics. While important, this fails to articulate the key importance that health information has for patients as enshrined in definitions of health literacy; individuals and communities need to be able to access, understand, appraise and use information and services to make decisions about health [2], and only by providing information at times, and in ways, that citizens can 'understand appraise and use' can health services be truly person-centered. The US has provided international leadership in this area through the promotion of a universal precautions approach, which advocates that services, including health information, are provided in ways that can be accessed and understood by all service users regardless of their health literacy levels [42]. Furthermore, tools have been developed to help hospitals and health centers audit the extent to which their information and systems are health literate, enabling them to plan and implement service improvements [47]. The adult education literature and basic skills surveys have much to teach us about the importance of developing and offering information for health in multiple formats. Preferred learning styles are individual, for example some people prefer learning through specific media (written / audio / visual). Different people have different levels of comfort in understanding and manipulating numbers. For people at the lower end of the skills spectrum, these 'spiky profiles' are more pronounced [34], meaning that information must be tailored to individual preferences in order to be understood, and hence acted upon. In practical terms, this means developing information in a range of formats (written, pictorial, audio or video clips, mobile phone apps) so that patients and the public can choose the modality that best suits them.

Digital technology offers exciting possibilities. In developing societies with poor health systems and infrastructure, and often low literacy and numeracy levels, mobile health (m-health), such as the use of cell phone, offers great opportunities for disseminating health information using formats suitable for patient skills. Such technologies also offer potential benefits for populations in more developed countries who face issues of poor health care access (usually societal rather than geographical access issues) and low health literacy. A systematic review of public health cell phone interventions in developing countries found 34 interventions, mostly focusing on reducing the risk of contracting or transmitting infectious diseases. Of note is that only five of the interventions were evaluated, and none were part of randomized controlled trials [48]. One paper from China has described a randomized controlled trial to evaluate an intervention to develop health literacy using SMS. The study found high acceptability (nearly 90%), and a significant increase in health literacy in the intervention group [49]. Making better use of the health literacy opportunities of cell phone technology thus brings rich possibilities for partnership between experienced triallists in developed countries and researchers in developing countries, with outcomes that may be applicable to socially disadvantaged and immigrant populations globally. Furthermore, in cultures where there is stigma attached to certain illnesses or health promotion activities (such as the HIV in Malawi example, Box 8 above), access to online or m-health information can enable people to access the information they need confidentially, empowering them to make the decisions that are right for them. Such interventions could be of use not only in developing countries, but for immigrant populations in transition in new countries. However, in countries with limited resources, funding such an infrastructure would take resources away from other health care provision. Research into the impact of mobile technologies should therefore include cost: benefit analyses that include the costs of the infrastructure and well as the health benefits accrued.

5.1.4. Equitable access to essential products and technologies

We argue that health literacy is an important driver in promoting equitable access to essential products and technologies. Promotion of health literacy in groups and communities in society means that citizens can become involved in discussions about which products, vaccines and technologies should be available, and how they should be prioritized and funded. In combination with a 'proportionate universalism' approach [50], equitable distribution and access can be ensured. It may be that 'public health literacy' i.e. 'the degree to which individuals and groups can obtain, process, understand, evaluate, and act on information needed to make public health decisions that benefit the community' [51] will emerge as important here. Examples might be public discussions about whether anti-retroviral therapies, which reduce HIV transmission and improve economic productivity, should be prioritized over high-technology diagnostic equipment for diagnosis and management of non-communicable diseases? Or whether investment should be directed towards low-technology but effective products such as mosquito nets, and systems for clean drinking water? Involvement of citizens and communities in such discussion, promotes critical health literacy, can inform government policies, and promote truly person-centered health systems.

5.1.5. Health financing

A central tenet of the global health systems strengthening agenda is Universal Coverage (UC). UC is, to a large extent determined by national health system financing structures, and the need, or otherwise, for patients to pay directly for health care rather than payment through national taxation. The degree to which health care is available and accessible interacts with health literacy capacities to contribute to the degree to which inequities in health are observed within and across countries. Individuals that are both under-resourced and most limited in relation to opportunities to develop health literacy, and exposed to significant barriers to health service access, often fare poorly in both developed and developing country settings.

It is likely that in a health system without UC, those with the lowest health literacy levels are also the most likely to be excluded from health care. Studies comparing the association between capacities, including health literacy, and levels of UC, would provide insights into the cost-benefit of universal coverage and inform decisions about whether, and to what extent, countries should move towards it. It may also be useful to explore in more depth, the impact of health literacy interventions on the health literacy of health service users. It may be that such interventions have less impact on service users within a system that provides better coverage and minimizes barriers to health care. Examples of stark comparisons in levels of UC, and therefore logical natural experiments, would be to compare systems such as in the US where, until recently, a significant proportion of the population had no access to health care, with a health system such as that in Denmark, where a significant proportion of national revenue from a high-tax system are fed into a health system with UC that is free at the point of delivery.

In the US, the 2010 introduction of the Patient Protection and Affordable Care Act, providing access to health care for people previously without such care, brings opportunities to explore the impact of policy on the health of people with low health literacy [52]. Ideally such an evaluation should include quantitative measures such as the numbers of citizens affected, their socio-demographic characteristics and health literacy, and the impact on health outcomes and health care costs, as well as qualitative research to understand from citizens themselves what the impact on their life and health has been. Such endeavors will be of great benefit to other countries exploring the costs and benefits of moving towards UC.

Health systems vary in their level of complexity, which is in part due to funding mechanisms for health care. The main health care funding mechanisms are; 1) directly from national tax revenue (such as Denmark and the UK) and 2) from health insurance systems (such as the Netherlands and the US). Interestingly the type of funding mechanism is not associated with the levels of spending on health. A Commonwealth Fund report showed that the US is an outlier in terms of national Gross Domestic Product (GDP) spent on health care, due largely to high spending on high-technology [53]. However, health spending within the other 12 countries studied was not associated with the system of health service funding [53-54].

In those systems where funding is based on health insurance, such insurance may be mandatory or optional and may or may not be automatically linked with employment. There may be multiple competing options for insurance, varying levels of cover, for current and previous health conditions, and there may or may not be a 'safety net' for those with pre-existing conditions or those unable to afford health insurance [55]. People with low health literacy may have difficulties dealing with the complexities of such systems [56]; they may have insufficient financial resources to afford insurance, they are more likely to be unemployed [40,57], and are more likely to suffer from chronic/longstanding health conditions. [30,58], which may make insurance cover unobtainable. In a report comparing the health care systems and costs for nine countries, the US had the highest proportion of the population (37%) reporting cost-related barriers to accessing needed health care, while the UK National Health Service had the lowest proportion (4%) [55]. In the example from the US described below, the system required college-level literacy and numeracy skills, well above the mean skill levels of US adults [57]. This means that in settings with complex systems, basic literacy and numeracy skills are essential pre-requisites for health literacy. Without these basic skills, citizens are unable to independently access the health care they need.

In such situations, community support systems, including non-government organizations, can provide invaluable help, in particular ensuring that those with

---

Box 10. Accessing health care in a complex health system.

Chris W is a 40-year old man living with HIV. He graduated from high school with basic literacy and numeracy levels, and has a good understanding of his condition and the importance of Anti-retroviral therapy (ART) to keep himself well. In his last job, he had low health insurance cover, so used the federal AIDS Drug Assistance Program (ADAP) to help meet the costs of his ART. He has now moved to a higher-paid job with better health insurance cover, but finds that the new scheme will not cover maintenance therapy from his local pharmacy, and that the mail-order alternative does not accept the secondary insurance provided by ADAP, leaving him with an expensive monthly payment he cannot afford. He finds that, despite reading the website and trying to read the information sent to him by the insurance company (reading age of material: 18 years) he cannot understand the new system, and cannot find out who to talk with about this at the insurance company. He is unable to discuss this with his employer as he does not wish to disclose his HIV status.

Chris has now found a community advisor, employed by a local not-for profit organisation, who is experienced in US health insurance systems, and can help. The advisor arranged for a co-payment system directly with the pharmaceutical company providing the ART, which has reduced the monthly payments to a manageable level.

knowledge of the complex systems are available to help support those whose lack of skills is impeding access to health resources and services. Complex systems, such as in the US, require integrated health and social systems in which community and non-government organizations have a role in ensuring health related services are available and accessible. The cost of providing assistance in such settings may be high, and may not be covered by health insurance payments. Systems to monitor the costs of different systems should capture these, and wider societal, costs such as loss of economic productivity due to chronic illness.

5.1.6 Leadership and governance

The experience from Austria (see Box 4 above) illustrates the critical role that leadership can play; first at a policy level where it can enable a health literate system to develop, and second at an operational level -- to build the coalitions required for meaningful engagement of stakeholders, and tools for providers to audit and improve performance. Australia provides another useful example; the Australian Commission on Safety and Quality in Healthcare has written a report on health literacy that identified professional and organizational legal accreditation requirements of which health literacy is an essential component [59-60]. This approach ensures that action is swiftly taken, without need to introduce new accreditation processes and requirements.

5.1.7. Health systems and health literacy research and practice

The HLS-EU survey has shown how comparative research on health literacy can be a stimulus for system improvement and change. Further comparisons involving more countries will provide great opportunities for stimulating improvements in other countries and settings. In addition, evaluation research has much to add. If service improvement programmes routinely explored the impact of system changes on patients and their health literacy and health, not only would the impact of their changes be known, but also others could benefit from implementing such evidence-based changes in different settings.

As mentioned, the impact of practitioner skills training on patient health literacy and health outcomes is another important area. More research would greatly add to our understanding of which practitioner skills have the most impact, and in which settings they are best applied. Findings from such research could then be fed into practitioner training.

Finally, further research into mHealth and eHealth, and integration of these into the more 'classic' health systems, could bring a wide range of additional benefits to those with low health literacy, or with difficulties accessing health care.

5.2 Public health systems

Public health is 'The science and art of promoting and protecting health and well-being, preventing ill-health and prolonging life through the organised efforts of society'. It is population based, and emphasises collective responsibility for health, its protection and disease prevention [61]. This emphasis on making decisions that are best for population, rather than individual, health requires different capacities and approaches i.e. 'public health literacy' [51]. Because of this fundamental difference from other health services, we look at public health systems separately in this chapter.

As with health-delivery systems, public health systems vary widely around the world. There is variation in levels of funding made available to public health, with some public health systems underfunded in absolute terms or relative to the funding for other health services. In most countries, public health is part of the health system. However in England, public health services are part of local government authorities, and are thus aligned more closely to education and social services than to health services. Public health services also vary in the extent to which they focus on prevention of infectious diseases, support reduction in substance abuse (smoking reduction services and harmful alcohol drinking services) and/or promote health through support for healthy lifestyles (such as healthy diet and physical exercise promotion), early detection of health problems, and self-care.

We discussed above the importance of international and national policy to develop resilience and the ability to respond to public health emergencies, both acute emergencies (e.g. infectious disease epidemics such as the Ebola virus and the Zika virus) and more 'slow-burn' emergencies such non-communicable diseases such (i.e. diabetes and cardio-vascular disease) and the challenges of HIV. The reason policy is important is because it determines the public health and health-delivery systems. If there is failure to develop resilient systems, there is a risk of failure of the systems themselves when faced with acute and more chronic emergencies. When a health system fails under such burdens, it is the people with low health literacy who are likely to be the most severely affected, both through increased likelihood of illness, but also due to reduced health care access. In its review of its response to the Ebola epidemic, the US Centers for Disease Control and Prevention (CDC) highlighted the importance of not only the resilience of local health services, and the need for ongoing international partnerships to respond to such emergencies, but also the importance of health literacy within communities -- where misconceptions about the disease and the responders facilitated the spread of the Ebola epidemic and hampered treatment and prevention of transmission [13]. Health literacy research within communities can add much to our knowledge of how individuals, communities and families understand health and illness, and develop health literacy to develop effective and healthy responses to such challenges. As a result, it can be argued that health literacy should be integral to building both resilient systems, and resilient communities.

The example from Malawi, earlier described by Levin-Zamir et al [1], and repeated in Box 8 above, illustrates some of these issues. People living with HIV in many countries, and their families, face great stigma, exacerbated by public misunderstandings about HIV and its transmission, and the fact that, with treatment, HIV is now a manageable long-term condition rather than the 'death sentence' it once was. Public health campaigns to increase public understanding and promote openness and public dialogue could do much to break this cycle of stigma, sub-optimal treatment and unnecessary transmission of HIV. Such campaigns would aim to build distributed health literacy skills i.e. 'the skills to draw on the health literacy abilities, skills and practices of others as a resource to help seek, understand and use health information to help manage health and make informed choices' [38]. A focus on building such distributed health literacy skills in schools and families would be of particular help, as Tiwonde's story suggests that HIV-positive children and young people who are living with the virus are unaware of their condition. In addition, many school children must attend boarding school due to the distance to school from home, therefore informed and engaged teachers can make a real difference both to children's and young people's understanding, but also to ensuring that antiretroviral treatment is taken optimally to maintain control of the condition.

5.2.1 Public health systems and health literacy research and practice

Public health systems are thus key to developing resilience and the ability to respond to public health challenges, and thus protect the most vulnerable in societies, including those with low health literacy. Research to help policy makers and practitioners to understand citizens' views on health and illness, and the approaches that public health should then take to build understanding and action to combat threats to health. Public health literacy requires an understanding of the importance of the health of the wider population. In addition, there are times when public health literacy may come into conflict with individual health literacy. What is best for an individual or their family may not be best for society; examples might be decisions about immunization or taking antibiotics for mild infections. Qualitative research is needed to understand current views of citizens and communities on issues of public health importance, and to develop ways in which public health literacy can be developed. This links with distributed health literacy; such skills may be best developed at a community level. Understanding more about these complex and often challenging areas of health literacy would be valuable.

5.3 Social care systems

Social Care concerns itself with helping people live their lives comfortably, particularly those people who require a certain degree of extra practical and physical help [62]. It is therefore of importance to health and autonomy for the more vulnerable in society; those with congenital or acquired physical, mental, or cognitive disability, and those vulnerable through unemployment, severe financial stress, or homelessness. As with the other systems described in this chapter, social care systems vary in their levels of complexity, and also the extent to which they are funded by the state [55]. In addition, in most countries, health and social care systems are separate, with particular impacts on older people, those with multiple health conditions, and those with unemployment and / or low incomes, all groups known to have lower health literacy [30,40,58]. An extreme example of this is the UK where, in contrast to the health service, social care is expensive and disjointed, while at the other end of the spectrum, countries like Japan and Sweden have social systems that are co-funded and coordinated with the health system [55].

An important aspect of the social care system is the extent to which families and communities expect to provide care for the older and more frail in their communities. These cultural aspects to social care will impact on the extent to which the social care system needs to provide a social care 'safety net'. This issue is also of importance in migration between different settings within a country, such as migration from rural to urban areas, and also migration between different countries and different cultural settings. People who migrate may well bring with them deeply embedded notions of what care and support should be provided by the family or community as opposed to the state. Health literacy is needed to learn about and navigate social care systems in new settings.

To date, no studies have been published exploring the issues around health literacy and social care. As with health, such exploration could approach the issues of health literacy and social care systems from complementary approaches. First, to what extent do people have the health literacy skills to use social care information and systems to access, understand, appraise and use information and services to make decisions about health? Second, given that people in receipt of social care are likely to have lower health literacy, to what extent is the social care system responsive to the health literacy of the people it serves? Such studies are urgently required in national settings, and, as with health research, international comparative studies will be very informative about which systems and settings work best from a health literacy perspective.

5.3.1 Summary

Social care systems are of vital importance in supporting the most vulnerable in societies, and their families and carers. As with health, the provision of such systems, and the ways in which they are funded, vary widely between countries. It is likely that health literacy is significant in determining the extent to which people needing care can lead healthy and fulfilling lives. Conversely, the health literacy capabilities of the system will also be important. Health literacy research, both qualitative and quantitative, is vitally important in starting to understand where we are now, and how social care systems need to develop to promote wellbeing and mitigate frailty.

6.   National and international policy and systems: implications for health literacy research, policy and practice

In this chapter, we have explored international, and national policies and the systems that arise from those policies through the 'lens' of health literacy, looking to see both how policies and systems can develop health literacy, and how health literacy can aid in the development of coherent person-centered policies and systems that will promote equity. We have illuminated these using examples from around the world.

Several key messages arise throughout this chapter. First, there is a need to co-ordinate policies across the multiple areas of importance to health -- health, public health, social services and education to name just some. We argue that policies should be the first area of focus, as policy determines systems -- coordinated Health in All Policies means that there will be coordinated well-functioning systems. Second, we argue that health literacy theory has much to bring to the development of policies and systems, as situating policy within a health literacy paradigm will place empowered patients, citizens and communities at the center of systems. Person centered policies are more likely to promote equity and reduce inequalities.

Third, we argue that embedding health literacy within policies requires more than simply referring to the concept and its role in health outcomes. Operationalization of the intent to ensure equitable access for all requires policy driven change across all aspects of the health systems, and beyond the health system into other policy domains. Better understanding of the policy frameworks and pragmatic solutions that prove to be effective, and that governments can adopt, can do much to support speedy development of health literacy and health literate systems.

Finally, we identify health literacy policy and systems research as a vital – and yet under-developed – area. The European health literacy survey has shown the power of comparative studies to identify the problem, and act as a driver for change. Incorporation of health literacy into monitoring systems for policies would provide a wealth of information, on which countries can act, singly or collaboratively. Other systems of importance to health, such as social care systems, currently have little or no health literacy research, and citizens have much to gain from a better understanding of the problems, and potential solutions, for the most vulnerable in society. It is reasonable to hypothesize that more responsive systems and services are more effective, more appropriate, and more cost effective. However, these hypotheses are yet to be empirically tested and as such caution is required.

Health literacy theory and practice have much to add to global health systems and policy, through providing a coherent framework for development and promoting citizen empowerment and equity. Embedding health literacy into research and evaluation of systems and policy will not only broaden the field of health literacy enquiry, but also provide opportunities to feed back into, and further improve, policies and systems for health.

References

[1] Levin-Zamir D, Leung AYM, Dodson S, Rowlands G. Health literacy in selected populations: individuals, families, and communities from the international and cultural perspective. In: Logan RA, editor. Health literacy: new directions in research, theory, and practice. Amsterdam: IOS Press; 2017. p.xx-yy.

[2] Dodson S, Good S, Osborne RH. Health literacy toolkit for low and middle-income countries: a series of information sheets to empower communities and strengthen health systems. New Delhi: World Health Organization, Regional Office for South-East Asia; 2015. http://www.searo.who.int/entity/healthpromotion/documents/hl_tookit/en/

[3] World Health Organization. The Ottowa charter for health promotion. Geneva. 1986. http://www.who.int/healthpromotion/conferences/previous/ottawa/en/

[4] Parker R. Measuring health literacy: what? So what? Now what? In: Hernandez L, editor. Washington DC.: The National Academies Press; 2009. p.91-98.

[5] Commission of Social Determinants of Health (CSDH). Closing the gap in a generation: health equity through action on the social determinants of health. Geneva. World Health Organization; 2008. http://apps.who.int/iris/bitstream/10665/43943/1/9789241563703_eng.pdf

[6] United Nations. Transforming our world: the 2030 Agenda for Sustainable Development. New York. United Nations; 2015.

[7] United Nations. The Millennium Development Goals Report. New York. United Nations; 2015.

[8] World Health Organization. Health in all policies: Helsinki Statement, framework for country action. 8th Global Conference on Health Promotion. Helsinki. 2013. http://www.healthpromotion2013.org/health-promotion/health-in-all-policies

[9] Antecol H, Bedard K. Unhealthy assimilation: why do immigrants converge to American health status levels? Demography. 2006;43:337-360. DOI:10.1353/ dem.2006.0011

[10] Jatrana S, Pasupuleti SSR, Richardson K. Nativity, duration of residence and chronic health conditions in Australia: do trends converge towards the native-born population? Soc Sci Med. 2014;119:53-63. DOI: 10.1016/j.socscimed.2014.08.008.

[11] Vandenheede H, Willaert D, De Grande H, Simoens S, Vanroelen C. Mortality in adult immigrants in the 2000s in Belgium: a test of the 'healthy-migrant' and the 'migration-as-rapid-health-transition' hypotheses. Trop Med Int Health. 2015;20(12):1832-1845. DOI:10.1111/tmi.12610.

[12] Kim IH, Carrasco C, Muntaner C, McKenzie K, Noh S. Ethnicity and postmigration health trajectory in new immigrants to Canada. Am J Public Health. 2013;103(4):e96-104. DOI:10.2105/AJPH.2012.301185.

[13] Dahl BA, Kinzer MH, Raghunathan PL, Christie A, De Cock KM, Mahoney F, Bennett SD, Hersey S, Morgan OW. CDC's Response to the 2014–2016 Ebola Epidemic — Guinea, Liberia, and Sierra Leone. Centers for Disease Control and Prevention; 2016. p.12–20. https://www.cdc.gov/mmwr/volumes/65/su/su6503a3.htm

[14] Sustainable Development Solutions Network: A global initative for the United Nations. Indicators and a monitoring framework for the Sustainable Development Goals: launching a data

revolution for the SDGs. Leadership Council of the Sustainable Development Solutions Network; 2015. http://unsdsn.org/resources/publications/indicators/

[15] Gladwell M. The tipping point: how little things can make a big difference. United States: Little Brown; 2000.

[16] A Guide to Social Return on Investment. Social value UK. http://www.socialvalueuk.org/resources/sroi-guide/

[17] World Health Organization. WHO global strategy on integrated people-centred health services 2016-2026. Geneva: World Health Organization; 2015. http://www.who.int/servicedeliverysafety/areas/people-centred-care/en/

[18] National Institute of Statistics (NIS) [Rwanda]. Rwanda Service Provision Assessment Survey 2007. http://www.statistics.gov.rw/datasource/47

[19] Rwanda Community Based Health Insurance Policy. Ministry of Health, Republic of Rwanda. Kigali; 2010. http://www.moh.gov.rw/fileadmin/templates/Docs/Mutual_policy_document_final1.pdf

[20] Nyandekwe M, Nzayirambaho M, Baptiste Kakoma J. Universal health coverage in Rwanda: dream or reality. Pan Afr Med J. 2014;17:232. DOI:10.11604/pamj.2014.17.232.3471.

[21] National Institute of Statistics of Rwanda, Ministry of Health. Rwanda Demographic and Health Survey, 2014-2015 Final Report. Kigali: Rwanda; 2016. https://dhsprogram.com/pubs/pdf/FR316/FR316.pdf

[22] World Health Organisation and The World Bank. Tracking universal health coverage. First Global Monitoring Report. France; 2015. p.1. http://www.who.int/healthinfo/universal_health_coverage/report/2015/en/

[23] http://www.nchealthliteracy.org/toolkit/tool5.pdf. Retrieved April 11, 2017.

[24] Faye O, Freire CC, Iamarino A, Faye O, de Oliveira JV, Diallo M, Zanotto PM, Sall AA. Molecular evolution of Zika virus during its emergence in the 20th Century. PLoS Negl Trop Dis. 2014;8(1):e2636. DOI:10.1371/journal.pntd.0002636.

[25] Nutbeam D. Health literacy as a public health goal: a challenge for contemporary health education and communication strategies into the 21st century. Health Promot Int. 2000;15(3):259-267. DOI:10.1093/heapro/15.3.259.

[26] Pan American Health Organisation. Report on tobacco control for the region of the Americas. WHO Framework Convention on Tobacco Control: 10 Years Later. Washington, DC: Pan American Health Organisation; 2016.

[27] Freire P. Pedagogy of the oppressed: 30th anniversery edition, New York: Continuum; 2000.

[28] Graham H, Power C. Childhood disadvantage and health inequalities: a framework for policy based on lifecourse research. Child Care Health Dev. 2004;30(6):671-678. DOI: 10.1111/j.1365-2214.2004.00457.

[29] Grantham-McGregor SM, Powell CA, Walker SP, Himes JH. Nutritional supplementation, psychosocial stimulation, and mental development of stunted children: the Jamaican Study. Lancet. 1991;338(8758):1-5.

[30] HLS-EU Consortium (2012): Comparative report of health literacy in eight EU member states. The European health literacy survey HLS-EU; 2012. online publication: http://www.health-literacy.eu.

[31] Inhelder B, Piaget J. The growth of logical thinking from childhood to adolescence. An essay on the construction of formal operational structures. London and New York: Routledge; 1985.

[32] Levin-Zamir D, Lemish D, Gofin R. Media Health Literacy (MHL): development and measurement of the concept among adolescents. Health Educ Res. 2011;26(2):323-335. DOI:10.1093/her/cyr007.

[33] Begoray D, Wharf Higgins J, Harrison J, Collins-Emery. Adolescent reading/viewing of advertisements. J Adolesc Adult Lit. 2013;57(2):121-130. DOI: 10.1002/JAAL.202.

[34] Department for Business Innovation and Skills. The 2011 Skills for Life Survey: a survey of literacy, numeracy and ICT levels in England. London: Department for Business Innovation and Skills; 2012. https://www.gov.uk/government/publications/2011-skills-for-life-survey

[35] The Tavistock Institute and Shared Intelligence. Evaluation of the second phase of the Skilled for Health Programme. London: The Tavistock Institute and Shared Intelligence; 2009. http://www.tavinstitute.org/projects/report-evaluation-of-phase-two-of-the-skilled-for-health-programme/

[36] McBride CM, Emmons KM, Lipkus IM. Understanding the potential of teachable moments: the case of smoking cessation. Health Educ Res. 2003;18(2):156-170.

[37] Wolf MS, Curtis LM, Wilson EA, Revelle W, Waite KR, Smith SG, Weintraub S, Borosh B, Rapp DN, Park DC, Deary IC, Baker DW. Literacy, cognitive function, and health: results of the LitCog Study. J Gen Intern Med. 2012;27(10):1300-1307. DOI:10.1007/s11606-012-2079-4.

[38] Edwards M, Wood F, Davies M, Edwards A. 'Distributed health literacy': longitudinal qualitative analysis of the roles of health literacy mediators and social networks of people living with a long-term health condition. Health Expect. 2015;18(5):1180-1193. DOI:10.1111/hex.12093.

[39] Rudd RE. Health literacy skills of U.S. adults. Am J Health Behav. 2007;31 Suppl 1:S8-18.

[40] Rowlands G, Protheroe J, Winkley J, Richardson M, Seed PT, Rudd R. A. A mismatch between population health literacy and the complexity of health information: an observational study. Br J Gen Pract. 2015;65(635):e379-386. DOI:10.3399/bjgp15X685285.

[41] World Health Organization. Everybody's business: strengthening health systems to improve health outcome: WHO's framework for action. Geneva: World Health Organization; 2007. http://www.who.int/healthsystems/strategy/everybodys_business.pdf

[42] DeWalt DA, Callahan LF, Hawk VH, Broucksou KA, Hink A, Rudd R, Brach C. Health literacy universal precautions toolkit. Rockville MD: Agency for Healthcare Research and Quality; 2010. https://www.ahrq.gov/sites/default/files/wysiwyg/professionals/quality-patient-safety/quality-resources/tools/literacy-toolkit/healthliteracytoolkit.pdf

[43] Groene O. Health literacy in the undergraduate and postgraduate medical education of general P\practitioners, PhD. London South Bank University; 2016.

[44] Peter D, Robinson P, Jordan M, Lawrence S, Casey K, Salas-Lopez D. Reducing readmissions using teach-back: enhancing patient and family education. J Nurs Adm. 2015;45(1):35-42. DOI:10.1097/NNA.0000000000000155.

[45] Schillinger D, Piette J, Grumbach K, Wang F, Wilson C, Daher C, Leong-Grotz K, Castro C, Bindman AB. Closing the loop: physician communication with diabetic patients who have low health literacy. Arch Intern Med. 2003;163(1):83-90.

[46] Eichler K, Wieser S, Brugger U. The costs of limited health literacy: a systematic review. Int J Public Health. 2009;54(5)313-324. DOI: 10.1007/s00038-009-0058-2.

[47] Rudd RE, Anderson J. The health literacy environment of hospitals and health centers. Partners for action: making your healthcar facility literacy-friendly. Boston, MA: Harvard School of Public Health; 2006. https://cdn1.sph.harvard.edu/wp-content/uploads/sites/135/2012/09/healthliteracyenvironment.pdf

[48] Deglise C, Suggs LS, Odermatt P. SMS for disease control in developing countries: a systematic review of mobile health applications. J Telemed Telecare. 2012;18(5):273-281. DOI:10.1258/jtt.2012.110810.

[49] Zhuang R, Xiang Y, Han T, Yang GA, Zhang Y. Cell phone-based health education messaging improves health literacy. Afr Health Sci. 2016;16(1):311-318. DOI:10.4314/ahs.v16i1.41.

[50] Fair Society, Healthy lives. Strategic review of health inequalities in England. London: Department of Health (England); 2010. http://www.instituteofhealthequity.org/projects/fair-society-healthy-lives-the-marmot-review

[51] Freedman DA, Bess KD, Tucker HA, Boyd DL, Tuchman AM, Wallston KA. Public health literacy defined. Am J Prev Med. 2009;36(5):446-451. DOI:10.1016/j.amepre.2009.02.001.

[52] Baur C. United States: Health literacy and recent federal initiatives. Washington, DC: Health Literacy: Improving Health, Health Systems, and Health Policy Around the World: Workshop Summary; 2013. p.20-23. https://www.nap.edu/catalog/18325/health-literacy-improving-health-health-systems-and-health-policy-around

[53] Squires D, Anderson C. U.S. Health care from a global perspective: spending, use of services, prices, and health in 13 countries. The Commonwealth Fund. Washington DC: 2015. http://www.commonwealthfund.org/publications/issue-briefs/2015/oct/us-health-care-from-a-global-perspective

[54] Health expenditure, total (% of GDP). World Bank. http://data.worldbank.org/indicator/SH.XPD.TOTL.ZS

[55] Robertson R, Gregory S, Jabbal J. The social care and health systems of nine countries. Commission on the Future of Health and Social Care in England. London; 2014. https://www.kingsfund.org.uk/sites/files/kf/media/commission-background-paper-social-care-health-system-other-countries.pdf

[56] Berkman ND, DeWalt DA, Pignone MP, Sheridan SL, Lohr KN, Lux L, Sutton SF, Swinson T, Bonito AJ. Literacy and health outcomes. Evidence Report/Technology. Assessment No. 87. Prepared by RTI International–University of North Carolina Evidence-based Practice Center under Contract No. 290-02-0016; 2004. http://citeseerx.ist.psu.edu/viewdoc/download?doi=10.1.1.210.2733&rep=rep1&type=pdf

[57] Time for the U.S. to reskill?: what the survey of adult skills says. OECD Skills Studies, OECD; 2013. http://www.oecd-ilibrary.org/education/time-for-the-u-s-to-reskill_9789264204904-en

[58] Berkman ND, Sheridan SL, Donahue KE, Halpern DJ, Viera A, Crotty K, Viswanathan M. Health literacy interventions and outcomes: an updated systematic review. Rockville, MD:

G. Rowlands et al. / Global Health Systems and Policy Development   391

Evidence Report/Technology Assessment, Agency for Healthcare Research and Quality; 2011.
https://www.ncbi.nlm.nih.gov/pubmed/23126607

[59] Australian Commission on Safety and Quality in Health Care. Health literacy: Taking action to improve safety and quality. Sydney; 2014. https://www.safetyandquality.gov.au/wp-content/uploads/2014/08/Health-Literacy-Taking-action-to-improve-safety-and-quality.pdf

[60] Australian Commission on Safety and Quality in Health Care. Tip sheet 8: Health literacy and the NSQHS standards. https://www.safetyandquality.gov.au/wp-content/uploads/2015/06/Standard-2-Tip-Sheet-8-Health-literacy-and-the-NSQHS-Standards.pdf.

[61] http://www.fph.org.uk/what_is_public_health. Retrieved April 9, 2017.

[62] http://www.nisw.org.uk/socialcare. Retrieved April 9, 2017.

Health Literacy
R.A. Logan and E.R. Siegel (Eds.)
IOS Press, 2017
doi:10.3233/978-1-61499-790-0-392

Health Literacy in Selected Populations: Individuals, Families, and Communities from the International and Cultural Perspective

Diane LEVIN-ZAMIR[a,b,1], Angela Yee Man LEUNG[c], Sarity DODSON[d,e], and Gillian ROWLANDS[f,g]

Additional contributions from:
Frederico Peres[g]
Nadege Uwumahoro[f]
Jyoshma Desouza[h]
Sanjay Pattanshetty[i]
Helen Baker[j]

[a] *Clalit Health Services, Tel Aviv, Israel*
[b] *School of Public Health, University of Haifa, Israel*
[c] *Centre for Gerontological Nursing, School of Nursing, The Hong Kong Polytechnic University, Hong Kong*
[d] *The Fred Hollows Foundation, Melbourne, Australia*
[e] *School of Population Health, Deakin University, Australia*
[f] *Institute of Health and Society, University of Newcastle, UK*
[g] *Institute of Public Health, Aarhus University, Denmark*
[h] *Brazilian National School of Public Health, Brazil*
[i] *Department of Public Health, Manipal University, India*
[j] *Community Health and Learning Foundation, UK*

Abstract. International and cultural perspectives of health literacy help deepen the understanding of the global context within which health literacy plays an important role. Throughout this chapter, we explore the significance of health literacy initiatives, interventions, practices, and research for addressing health challenges on a variety of levels in the international and global context. More specifically, in this chapter, the notion of health literacy as a dynamic construct is introduced, after which we examine health literacy throughout the life course, emphasizing the impact of health literacy among children and the elderly in their families and in the community. Cultural norms and family interpersonal relations, and values influence health literacy and need to be considered when closing the health literacy disparities. Global trends of migration and immigration bring to the forefront the need for unravelling the complexity of health systems, for which health literacy plays a central role; health literacy initiatives address cultural differences between providers and patients to help narrow the communication gap. The importance of cultural competency among health care providers exemplifies how capacity building in health literacy is critical for maximizing the benefits to

---

[1] Corresponding author: Clalit Health Services, Tel Aviv, Israel; E-mail: diamos@zahav.net.il.

the public of the health care system. Health literacy provides a conceptual foundation for community participatory research, involving members of the public to take part in the planning, execution and evaluation of health education interventions. Throughout the chapter, selected case studies and picture boxes from around the globe, exemplify aforementioned topics of interest, showcased in the chapter. Practical recommendations for policy makers, practitioners and research are offered based on the studies conducted in the international context.

Keywords. Health literacy; cultural competency; patient-provider communication; digital health literacy; media health literacy

1. Introduction

This chapter will focus on the health literacy of individuals and families, then expand to discuss interpersonal considerations and cultural issues including those relating to transition and change. Much valuable work has been undertaken in the US to explore these complex issues. This chapter aims to widen the lens and examine the global and intercultural aspects of health literacy across a broad range of countries and settings. The intention is not to provide a summary of research being conducted globally, but rather to examine the global body of research for broad theoretical, methodological and practice trends and implications. More specifically we intend to show how health literacy initiatives, interventions, practices, research or perspectives impact or address specific public health issues through the more specific sections of the chapter. Following this introduction, section two demonstrates how health literacy is a conceptually dynamic construct. We then continue on to show in the third section how health literacy can be developed across the life course and the impact this might have upon health outcomes for children, adults, families, and communities. The fourth section focuses on how health literacy initiatives contribute to addressing differences in cultural norms, family interpersonal relations, and family values. The fifth section follows to show how health literacy initiatives and efforts contribute to addressing ongoing challenges from immigration and migration patterns. The sixth section addresses the role of health literacy initiatives helping to bridge gaps when conflict arises between traditional and Western cultural beliefs. The seventh section exemplifies how health literacy initiatives focusing on cultural competence impact issues associated with provider-patient relations. The eighth section covers how health literacy provides a conceptual foundation for community based participatory research. In the ninth section we offer recommendations for practitioners, researchers, and policy makers for new directions in health literacy research, theory, and practice and providing some suggested areas for applied health literacy research and exploration. Finally, in the last section we summarize the chapter's overall conclusions. We finish by drawing together all these elements to identify some key messages including implications for future health literacy research.

We will identify selected US research and service development initiatives with resonance for health literacy research in other national, cultural and linguistic settings, while also identifying where some of the global health literacy work could inspire and inform research in the US.

Throughout the chapter we illustrate our points with 'vignettes' from different settings across the globe.

2. Health Literacy is a Dynamic Construct

While concrete definitions of health literacy exist, in this section, we emphasize the importance of understanding that health literacy is a dynamic construct. Individual health literacy is the cumulative outcome of a combination of cognitive capacities, life experiences, knowledge, and opportunities. For families and communities, it arises from shared history and experiences (particularly in relation to health), the pooled health literacy of individual members, and societal influences. Health literacy thus is constantly evolving and changing. Importantly for both individuals and groups, health behaviors and engagement with health services reflect the balance between individual or group skills and ability, and the demands and complexities of societal systems. As those demands change, so must the skills and abilities of individuals, families and communities if the same health outcomes are to be achieved, as shown in Figure 1 [1].

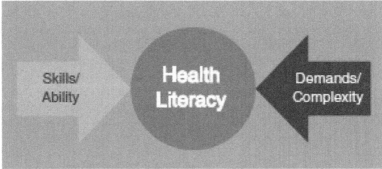

Figure 1. *Reproduced from: Parker R. Measuring health literacy: what? So what? Now what? In: Hernandez L, editor. Measures of health literacy: workshop summary, Roundtable on Health Literacy. Washington, DC: National Academies Press; 2009. p. 91–8 [1]*

2.1 The Multiple Stakeholders in Health Literacy

There are multiple stakeholders in health literacy, as shown in Figure 2 [2]. Health literacy thus is influenced by the demands and complexities of health systems, as well as social systems, workplaces, the environment, and the corporate world, particularly food and drink producers and markets.

Health literacy is key to not only health, but to human development at a population level, and to realising human potential. This is exemplified by how health literacy is integral to the Sustainable Development Goals (SDGs), particularly goal number three: "Ensure healthy lives and promote well-being for all at all ages" and goal number four: "Ensure inclusive and equitable quality education and promote life-long learning opportunities for all [3]. For example, improved health literacy may be achieved through efforts to advance the goal to achieve universal primary education. Similarly, improved health literacy and increased community participation in health and healthcare, in parallel with developments to improve health systems and widening access to Health Care (Universal Coverage or UC) [4], represent a key to achieve a reduction in child mortality, improve maternal health, and combat infectious diseases such as HIV/AIDS, and malaria. For additional discussion of health literacy and the SDGs see Rowlands et al [5].

This chapter will examine both elements in the 'Health Literacy Equation' shown in Figure 1.

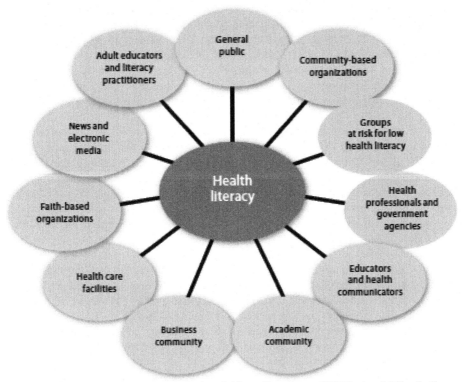

Figure 2. *Reproduced from Health literacy. The solid facts. Copenhagen: WHO Regional Office for Europe; 2013 [2]*

3. The Impact of Health Literacy across the Life Course – From Childhood to Adulthood

In this section we will focus on how health literacy can influence health outcomes for children, adults, families, and communities.

3.1. Health Literacy's Impact on Children and Adolescents

Efforts to enhance a child's health literacy, especially functional health literacy (sufficient basic skills in reading and writing to function effectively in everyday health situations) are significantly associated with improvements in basic literacy and numeracy skills [6]. Health literacy initiatives also address (or seek to counter) enduring social determinants of health (SDH); and enable children, teens, and future adults to 'achieve their goals, to develop their knowledge and potential, and to participate fully in their community and wider society' [7, 8].

The WHO links health literacy initiatives to improved global literacy, which is one of the organization's international sustainable development goals [3]. The WHO adds language, literacy, and numeracy (LLN), represent a trio of desirable sustainable development goals, which in turn foster self-development [6]. Overall, the development of critical health literacy skills promotes the participation of young persons in external activities, and cultivates their abilities to extract information and derive meaning from different forms of communication, which augments cognitive adaptation [6].

The WHO also hypothesizes that building LLN skills and health literacy in childhood and adolescence effectively provides the tools teens need to make informed decisions about lifestyle and sexual health. The U.S. Centers for Disease Control and Prevention (CDC) recognizes the need to cultivate health literacy based decision making tools, and has a collection of online resources for parents, educators, and child health professionals [7].

An example of an innovative health literacy initiative is the Bigger Picture Campaign, a youth-led diabetes prevention social media campaign co-created by the University of California, San Francisco with participating area adolescents in 2013 (http://thebiggerpicture.org/). Using social media, are adolescents were encouraged to speak to peers regarding how teen lifestyle norms (such as a high ingestion of sugar) is linked to obesity and diabetes. Such health literacy training uses a preferred mode of mass communication among the intervention's intended audience and involves teen stakeholders appropriately to self-represent the social and environmental factors that impact their health.

While there is a dearth of research about how improved literacy impacts future decision making, a measure for Media Health Literacy has been developed [8]. Also, a recent Canadian study found school children developed a better awareness of 'hidden', often health-damaging messages in popular advertising following media-health literacy training [9]. Moreover, the development of health literacy and ensuing literacy and decision-making skills among children and adolescents represent a ripe area for future research, especially regarding the effectiveness and impact of health literacy interventions on teen health and lifestyle decisions. Lifestyle decisions made in adolescence influence both current and future health, and there is evidence that lifestyle choices adopted in adolescence persist into later life [10, 11].

3.2. The Importance of Developing Health literacy Skills in Adults

Health literacy skills can also be developed in adults. The UK Skilled for Health Program, which delivered health literacy skills training to individuals and community / workplace groups, showed an increase in health knowledge (diet, exercise, smoking, and alcohol intake, and mental health). Lifestyle behaviors became healthier in the areas of diet, exercise, and mental health. In addition, participants described more confidence in interactive health literacy skills [6], particularly in discussing their health with health professionals, and also skills in navigating the, often complex, UK health system [12]. The program has since been replicated in Canada [13].

In Australia, evaluation of a community education program for adults with low basic skills, developed from the Skilled for Health program, showed improvements in participants' health literacy skills and confidence, positive student and teacher engagement with course content and self-reported improvements in health knowledge, attitudes, and communication with healthcare professionals [14].

In summary, there is a need for research to assist in identifying which skills and knowledge are needed to more effectively engage with health and healthcare and cope better when health issues arise (e.g. navigation related skills, communication and problem solving skills) – and when and how we develop these capacities in people. In addition, a better understanding is needed as to how to support people when health issues arise, to develop the condition specific skills and knowledge needed to effectively manage their health.

3.3. The Impact of Developing Health Literacy Skills in Families for Promoting Health

In developed countries, nuclear families are usually the social context within which people live. Families tend to be small (one or two parents with or without children), and often have little social networks and support. Low parental health literacy can result in unhealthy lifestyles and poorer health. In the UK, family health literacy initiatives have shown potential benefit for participants, although evaluations have been small and no large trials have been undertaken.

In both developing and developed settings, health decisions are often not made by individuals – often decisions are made collectively, often by parents or families. Culturally there are significant differences in relation to how decisions are made, but there are equally differences within cultures. Depending on the particular issue, the family and the culture, a decision might be made by an individual (about their own health or that of another family member – for example, a husband making a decision on behalf of his wife) or individuals might come together to discuss and make collective decisions. In some recent research undertaken in Pakistan, male heads of household are usually responsible for making any health related decisions that have financial implications [15].

This complexity brings to light the question of 'whose health literacy' is the most important and relevant to actions? In the case of Pakistan, there might be a very health literate wife, but if her husband is the one making the decisions, it is his health literacy that ultimately influences how she engages with health actions and services.

Health literacy programs have been noted to impact not only health decisions, but also family relations. The HEY! (Healthy Eating for Young Children) is an early childhood health improvement program which aims to improve the health literacy of parents who attend. The focus of the health education program is healthy eating within the framework of a healthy lifestyle. The course aims to improve parents' ability to make more informed and healthier choices for themselves and their toddlers [16]. Anecdotal evidence from participants on the impact of the intervention is striking. One participant describes the health benefits from healthier eating; she also describes improving family cohesion (**Box 1**).

Another family health learning initiative from the UK was the Healthy Families, Health Literacy Project. This was developed by an education team with family learning education expertise. It aimed to empower parents living is a socio-economically deprived area of London to improve their functional, interactive and critical health literacy. The learning topics were chosen by the parents and included understanding food labels, dealing with food allergies, and exercising as a family. The course included practical sessions to develop and share food recipes, cook together, and walk together. Participants found the course stimulating and exciting, with a direct and healthy impact on 'the way they lived their lives'. Participants developed functional and interactive health literacy skills [17].

> *"HEY! has changed my eating habits. My key worker got me on HEY! and it helped it coming just before Christmas so I could make a fresh start, a new year's resolution. We still have some treats but we feel much better in ourselves"*
>
> Ashley had recently moved to Leicestershire with her husband and two small children and felt isolated away from family and friends. She was introduced to the HEY! course – as well as a parenting group – at the children's center near where she lives. Ashley says HEY! made her really examine what she ate and make a lot of changes such as reducing sugar and salt – not easy as she works in a fast food café with burgers and fizzy drinks freely available. *"Before HEY! I used to have three or four coffees a day and three or four Red Bulls and full sugar Cokes. Now I have one coffee three times a week and water with sugar free squash. At work I have cup-a-soups and savoury crackers and bottled water – not burgers and chips. I'm not bloated now and have lost two stone"*.
>
> Ashley explains that she eats less and more slowly since HEY! and knows when she's full. Her husband does most of the cooking and has changed to making healthier – and smaller – meals following HEY! Ashley has started to do more cooking and now buys less ready-made and processed food. *"We make wraps now using 50/50 bread as we like Mexican food. We cook chicken breasts and haddock fillet and add vegetables and seasoning – then you know what's in it"*.
>
> Not only has Ashley moved to healthier options for food and drinks and started cooking more, she and her family have changed their eating habits, which has brought them closer together. A big change was buying a dining table and chairs so they could eat together in the kitchen instead of on their laps in the living room, which means their toddler doesn't play with his food or wander off any more. *"We have breakfast with the kids now – and enjoy each other's company"*. This led to cooking for special occasions – like Christmas and the Chinese New Year, which their toddler was learning about at pre-school. *"It's better for our marriage – doing things together. We've done a Valentine's Day meal and Pancake Day for the first time in 3 years"*.
>
> Ashley has learnt that healthy eating helps mental as well as physical health and sees eating as part of a healthy lifestyle. She's made other changes to her lifestyle including reducing her hours at work to shorter shifts and feels much better for it. *"I'm sleeping much better now – there's less stress but it's the diet as well – less coffee and so on"*.

Box 1. A Picture from the UK

4. Health Literacy Initiatives Address the Differences in Interpersonal Communication, Family Values, Community and Cultural Norms

In this section, we explore cultural influences and emphasize the role of health literacy in the interpersonal, family, and wider community contexts. When exploring the relationship between interpersonal communication and health literacy, both with regard to cultures in transition and more established cultures, a dilemma emerges regarding which approach to health literacy should be taken – the functional one or the more complex one. This differentiation has been described by Martensson [18], characterizing the more polarized approach focusing on the extremes of high and low literacy, as opposed to the complex approach acknowledging that health literacy represents a broadness of skills that includes interaction in the social and cultural context. This approach acknowledges that the individual's health literacy may fluctuate with context and is also dynamic, changing with time and with changing circumstance. In this regard, an individual may be considered health literate in one culture or context, while not in another. Furthermore, this more complex approach includes interactive and critical health literacy in addition to functional health literacy to facilitate taking health decisions, an approach which is important for the individual and society.

Two specific aspects of interpersonal relationships and health literacy are of particular significance – that of the relationships within families in the context of culture change, as well as health literacy as a vehicle for promoting social capital in disadvantaged groups

4.1. Family Relationships, Communication and Health Literacy in the Cultural Context

Cultural norms influence the way in which families communicate with regard to health. Cultures in transition, either due to geographic migration or to societal trends dictating a move from more traditional to Western paradigms, present families with challenges regarding the discourse of health and well- being within the family. Firstly, if in the more traditional model the extended family played a significant role in the individual's health and well-being, the more Western model emphasizes the dominance of the nuclear family [19]. This transition has not only narrowed the base for support, in many cases it changed the role of family members, particularly with regard to gender. Furthermore, it created challenges regarding the formerly accepted role of the younger and older generations, often creating conflict between generations. An example of this situation is described in the word picture from Malawi (**Box 2**). Malawi's story shows the challenges in promoting health literacy in light of societal contexts prohibiting individual empowerment.

The ramifications for health literacy are quite significant as exemplified in situations such as reproductive health, where in the traditional paradigm, discourse is forbidden and taboo. While the younger generation in an acculturating family may be embracing the behavioral norms of the more liberal mainstream, with respect to sexual norms, they often still lack access to health information and support from the family. The health outcomes are marked, including the younger generation's need to cope with sensitive health issues such as unplanned pregnancy and even a high rate of abortions [20]. Difficulties in initiating and maintaining discourse in families related to conditions with high levels of stigma such as mental illness or to communicable diseases such as HIV, are often exacerbated in the context of the stress of culture changes such as acculturation.

It should be noted that family acculturation is a dynamic process, with different levels of acculturation. This process supports the previous mentioned definition of health literacy as a complex phenomenon that changes with changing and variable contexts [21].

The case of young people living with HIV

Tiwonde is a 19-year old girl who lives with her aunt since her parents died of AIDS when she was three years old. She was born with HIV, but she found out that she is HIV-positive when she was 13 years old. Before that, she was taking medication without knowing why, but with time, she has come to understand that as long as she takes her medication, she can be healthy. But life is not easy for someone with HIV because there is a lot of fear and stigma and discrimination! Tiwonde often finds it difficult to take her medication because her aunt's husband and children do not know that she is HIV-positive. They fear that her aunt's husband will throw her out of the house if he finds out so she has to hide her medication very well and she takes care that no one sees her taking her medication. She goes to a boarding school where she is having problems with attending classes when she has to go for check-ups and to collect her medication. Tiwonde has been nicknamed "the sick one" because she always gives random excuses for going to the hospital. Like at home, she hides her medication, and she unintentionally misses to take her medication when she fails to find an opportunity to take it without onlookers. There is a boy a little older than her who has been showing interest in dating her, but she is afraid to start a relationship because she does not know how to tell him she is HIV-positive, and that he will abandon her and tell people at school about her status. Moreover, her aunt has told her that she can only be together with someone who is also HIV-positive. She has tried to talk to doctors and nurses about relationship issues, but they have shouted at her and accused her of wanting to spread the virus. She has heard rumors about a pastor who cures HIV through prayer, and she has been thinking about going to see him. Her aunt once took her to a village doctor who gave her some herbs, but they never worked. She wants to meet other young people living with HIV but is afraid that people will find out about her status if she joins a support group.

Box 2. A Picture from Malawi

4.2. Health Literacy as a Vehicle for Promoting Social Capital in Disadvantaged Groups

There is evidence showing that, in a diversified society, the more disadvantaged groups tend to use more online sources of health information than the mainstream population, compensating for the lack of social capital that supports more health promoting health information [22]. According to this hypothesis, it would be expected that people from cultures in transition, when families play less of a role as sources of useful health information than in the past, might be using more online tools, particularly in their native languages. If so, this phenomenon may change the assumption about the Digital Divide, however more research is needed to explore this avenue of study.

As critical as interpersonal relations in the family are with regard to health and health literacy, especially in a culturally transitional context, research is still lacking, regarding the role families play, and the most optimal strategies for intervention. Likewise, future research could explore how family role changes that often occur during cultural transitions influence family's collective health literacy and individual family members capacities and outcomes.

5. Health Literacy Initiatives Address Challenges due to Globalization or Migration

In this section, we reflect on the impact and role of health literacy in cultures and societies in light of global trends and migration.

5.1. Challenges to Immigrants: The Importance of Health Literacy in Inter-culture Encounters with the Health System

Immigrants encounter many challenges upon their arrival to a new country, one which is communication with health authorities. Some who come from authoritarian regimes or one-party states believe, for example, that health screening is a process of scrutiny to assess suitability for remaining in the country, bringing negative attitudes towards health screening [23]. In cultures where screening for diseases is not usual practice, it may be seen as an unnecessary 'secondary issue'; immigrants from such cultures often do not believe that they should undergo health screening because they perceived themselves as healthy [23]. Some believe that they have no choice about whether or not to attend health screening; the 'invitation' may be interpreted as a 'requirement' from the authorities to all the newcomers, for the benefits of society as a whole, rather than individuals themselves [24].

In addition to such misunderstandings, more practical barriers arise, such as not arriving for health appointments due to inability to read the invitation letter, not understanding the reason for invitation, and not knowing when and where the health screening would take place [23]. Such language barriers negatively affect communication between immigrants and health care professionals, reducing the accuracy and willingness of symptoms reporting [25]. Such difficulties cannot always be resolved by the presence of interpreters; often, immigrants' political or psychosocial reasons hinder the communication [23]. Cultural beliefs about an illness and health care is another determining factor influencing people's participation in health screening tests. For example, how comfortable one feels to discuss their body with a physician (physical modesty), whether one visits a physician only when there is a presenting symptom, such as pain, (crisis intervention approach) or alternatively for regular symptom-free visits, as would be the case for one to seek Eastern medicine. In a study of American Korean men [26], their cultural beliefs about cancer were found to significantly determine their recent uptake of prostate cancer screening tests. The men who used crisis intervention were less likely to seek cancer screening than those who used preventive approach; those who preferred to use Eastern medicine for health care were more likely to seek for prostate cancer screening. The use of Eastern medicine may indicate that these immigrants misunderstand and/or mistrust Westernized health care and medicine, reducing their engagement and participation in treatment [27]. This is evidence that cultural beliefs play a part in health screening decisions.

Culturally influenced preventive behaviors vary across different age groups. The older American Koreans (aged 70 or more) that preferred to use Eastern medicine were more likely to take cancer screening tests; however, the younger American Koreans (aged 50 to 60) were less likely to undergo health screening tests in spite of the fact that they also preferred to use Eastern medicine. Another immigrant group, Chinese Americans, demonstrated similar behavior. This finding suggests that in addition to culture, age also influences health screening and preventive behaviors [26].

5.2. Health Literacy as a Protective Factor for Acculturation Challenges

Migration in later life can be a stressful event; for example for older Chinese Australian immigrants, migration is associated with depression and anxiety due to language difficulty, knowledge and literacy, and the change of role and status within the family and society [28]. Loss of job, loss of physical health and loss of friends in the original country, and the changed roles in families, can produce feelings of hopeless and can lead to depression. Because mental health has stigma in many societies, some immigrants refuse to admit the clinical manifestations of anxiety or depression, and have limited knowledge about mental health symptoms and services (poor mental health literacy) [29]. As an example, acculturative stress - the stresses experienced due to migration to a country or a place in which people encounter practices that are significantly different from their own cultural practices or practices in their home countries - and depression was experienced by Filipino migrants when they migrated to Australia [29]. Acculturative stress negatively affected health-seeking behavior, with depression as a major modifying factor [28]. Health literacy and social support could be the protective factors to acculturative stress. For those migrants with higher health literacy or higher level of social support, they were more likely to have less acculturative stress [29]. In Maneze and team's study, reverse relationships (i.e. from acculturative stress to health literacy or to social support) were not tested. More effective and culturally appropriate health system responses could help migrants overcome the stress of migration and perhaps prevent resulting health challenges.

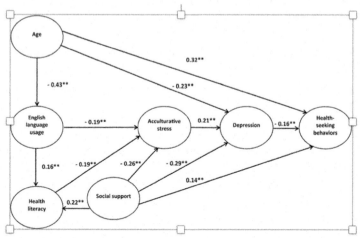

Figure 3. *Reproduced from Maneze et al., 2016 [29]*

Further research is needed to understand the complex inter-relationships between culture, language, social support and networks, use of health services, and mental and physical health. This can then lead to the development of effective interventions, culturally appropriate and based in communities, to better promote health and effective use of health services in immigrant populations. Because of the wide variety of different cultures, such interventions should be tailored to, and developed in partnership with, the communities they are designed to support. In addition, future research on the global level is needed to explore the possibility of universal stressors and challenges related to migration, that services should be mindful and responsive to, what are the culture influences, and what might be anticipated as different challenges experienced on the individual level.

6. Health Literacy Initiatives Address Enduring Conflicts between Traditional vs Western Cultural Beliefs

In this section, we demonstrate how health literacy places an important role in the bridge between traditional cultures meet Western culture.

6.1. Traditional vs. Western Cultures: Dissimilarities in Health Decision Making

Cultural values and practices affect health behaviors and health decisions. Many cultures are hierarchical in nature, with health practitioners having elevated, respected positions. For example, Chinese people will often refrain from asking health practitioners questions, believing that asking questions is impolite as it is perceived as "challenging doctors and nurses" or "putting burden on these professionals" [30]. A similar phenomenon was observed in many Chinese societies including Hong Kong, Taiwan and Chinese communities in Los Angeles, USA [30]. Cultural preferences and lack of understanding of Western medicine can lead to delays in the diagnosis of important health conditions. Estacion found that South Asian men with diabetes in UK preferred to seek the help of a religious leader/community leader, or ignore symptoms for an extended duration before referring to formal Western health services in UK [31]. Future research can help to better understand what drives these observed practices and preferences and how interventions might be developed to support health decision making in the contexts of cultures in transition. More research should be carried out to explore the impact of culture on health decision making and health behaviors. The American Diabetes Association advocates actions to be taken to address health disparities and develop structured interventions that are tailored to ethnic populations' culture, language, religion and literacy skills [32].

6.2. Cultural Change between Generations: Coping with Cultural Changes in Society

Immigration results in generational effects, with different levels of acculturalization in different generations. First-generation immigrants are less likely to report disability, as compared to the third generation [33]. Yet no significant difference in disability reporting was found between the second- and the third-plus generations. Among the first-generation immigrants in Canada, those who had not immigrated from Europe or the US were less likely to report disability than their counterparts. This is likely to be partly related to the use of language. Health literacy was found to be significantly negatively associated with disability reporting only of the first-generation immigrants. This may be due to the low functional health literacy among first-generation immigrants, while better education, employment and higher income in the new country, providing paths for the second- and third-plus generations to develop better health literacy competencies for accessing and navigating the health system [33]. Some programs have even targeted young immigrants, as a means to improve access to care for entire migrant families. Picture Boxes 3 and 4 offer real-life examples of how these concerns surface in the daily lives of immigrants, presenting challenges for improving health, even when individuals have awareness of the need for adopting health promoting behavior.

Mr. D was a Chinese immigrant in Los Angeles, serving as a cook in a Chinese restaurant. One day, while he was cooking, he looked pale, sweated tremendously and his hands were shaking. His boss noted that Mr. D was not feeling well, but Mr. D denied. His boss asked, "Are you diabetic? You look as if you are having hypoglycaemia. I had such experience as well. Go and see the doctor." Mr. D was shocked to hear this. He did have diabetes but he had never told his boss. Mr. D believed that his illness would be an excuse for his boss to fire him. As he is the breadwinner, he was desperate to keep the job and bring money home. This was his duty and he was so panicked about letting his boss know he was a diabetes. To Mr. D, family is important. He would not care about his health, but he cares about whether he could support his family in a new place like Los Angeles.

Box 3. A Picture from the US health, even when individuals have awareness of the need for adopting health promoting behavior.

Mr. E was a Chinese old man with diabetes, living with his spouse and adult children. He had poor control in blood glucose but he admitted that he did not bother with diet control. He said, "I would not let my family know that I have diabetes. I always have dinner with my family. It is the happy moment to have meals together. Why do I bother what I eat? If I let them know that I have diabetes, they will change the recipe, and reduce sugar in cooking. That is not good. We, Shanghainese, always have sweet and sour food. This is our habit. I don't want my family members to upset their eating habit for me. I like to eat with them, and like to see they enjoy the meal. So, forget about it…forget about changing the food!" Collective ideology is prominent in this story; Chinese people care about others rather than themselves.

Box 4. A Picture from China

7. Health Literacy Initiatives Affect Providers-and-individuals Communication

In this section, the importance of health literacy in enhancing effective communication between health providers and the people they serve will be explored.

7.1. The Needs for Enhancing Effective Interpersonal and Inter-cultural Communication for Health Literacy

A myriad of research has been conducted exploring a vast scope of needs and vantage points with regard to ways in which health literacy is influenced by, and influences the relationship between the individual and the health care provider. The continuing trends of massive migration and globalization have most recently amplified the need for this exploration more than ever.

The needs are particularly rooted in the fact that so many health care professionals have different ethnic/cultural backgrounds than their patients, many of them migrants and immigrants. Not only do communication barriers exist [34], many of the communities in cultural transition are, on the one hand, coping with life in a new and strange culture, while encountering new and unfamiliar health problems, some due to migration. Research suggests that immigrants coming from a more traditional, low-technology lifestyle adjusting to a Western culture, suffer from higher rates of chronic conditions and morbidity than previously experienced, and more prevalent even than the non-immigrant populations. Diabetes and depression are examples of the latter conditions [35]. This situation can be a source of misunderstanding between well-intentioned physicians and patients, fueling distrust, and resulting in mutual disappointment and eventually health disparities.

Migration, particularly migration to a country or region with different cultural beliefs and societal structures, is highly stressful, often leading to migrant health decline [36]. Generally migrants arrive in host countries in better health usually, than those from the host country. Trajectory decline in self-rated health was observed in the initial four years upon arrival, and it was particularly obvious in women and minority ethnic groups. Language partially contributes to this decline, but does not solely address the aforementioned deeper issues; merely providing oral and written translation services will not solve problems that immigrants face in a new society. Often, immigrants will have deeply-held beliefs about different systems of medicine, such as acupuncture or Ayurvedic medicine, which are based on totally different philosophical beliefs about the body, mind, health and illness. Health literacy has the potential to add significantly to our understanding of this, and to help bridge the gap between the contrasting understanding of health systems.

7.2. The Inter-cultural Context between Provider and Health Service Consumer

Many traditional cultures view health problems in the context of whole life experience, as opposed to isolated health problems, as is often the approach adopted by Western health systems. Moreover, the holistic perception of health may not differentiate between physical, emotional and mental well-being, as is often perceived among Western health providers. The opportunity to promote health literacy through interpersonal communication, is often impeded, even when there is a common language, due to the differentiated perception of what needs to be explained and expressed by the person seeking health services. Warfa et al. [37] determined that immigrant patients often attributed one reason to an illness, while healthcare providers often provided a different explanation for the same illness.

The health service professional often has never had specific training nor has been provided with tools to tackle the abovementioned issues, that are as basic as understanding health data with regard to ethnicity [35, 38]. In particular, very few academic curricula include training future providers about migrant health decline. More research needs to be conducted regarding the role that the healthcare provider can play in slowing or preventing the inevitability of health decline due to the stress, the adjustment, and the lack of concordance of existing services and systems between culture beliefs, norm and language.

7.3. Interpersonal, Community and Cultural Influences and Health Literacy Skills – Supportive Action

Cultural competency is the set of skills which enables the health care provider to function effectively within the cultural context of the people that he/she serves, whether on the individual, family or community levels. In this way, health literacy can either be promoted and improved or alternatively communication can be adapted to the individual according to his/her to health literacy needs [15]. For example, it is important to learn of the cultural perception of chronic disease in order to best communicate on chronic disease prevention, early detection or self-care. In many traditional societies the concept of a chronic/asymptomatic health problem does not exist. Rather, the individual may expect the healthcare provider to solve the cause of the problem and thus to remove it at its root. This gap in expectation can be bridged through promotion of cultural competence among the health professionals to learn of ways in which their patients understand and conceptualize health, and thus to adapt the communication [20]. Likewise, culturally sensitive interventions can be carried out that helps immigrants understand the context within which the health system can be accessed including appointment making, receiving treatment and other points of contact with the health care system.

Areas that should be addressed in health literacy and cultural competence training include involving community stakeholders for training, to help reflect upon the needs of the individuals and families that they treat [39]. Evaluation of the impact of such training could include patient satisfaction with encounters with health professionals. Since health literacy can be viewed as the balance between the capacities of patients and the demands and complexities of the health system [1] (see Figure 1), such an intervention should result in improved health literacy.

Shim [40] has expanded the concept of cultural competence to "cultural health capital" defined as the "repertoire of cultural skills, verbal and nonverbal competencies, attitudes and behaviors, and interactional styles, cultivated by patients and clinicians alike, that, when deployed, may result in more optimal health care relationships." The concept is framed within the discourse of unequitable care, due to health disparities. Such cultural health capital thus moves from physician understanding of cultural issues to two-way patient: physician partnerships. It can be hypothesized that the benefits to be expected from such interventions would be even more effective than the simpler cultural competence interventions at improving patient satisfaction, improving health literacy, and improving patient outcomes. Involving patients and families in service planning, implementation and evaluation, and adjusting the services to meet the needs of the individual, should increase critical health literacy skills i.e. 'more advanced cognitive skills which, together with social skills, can be applied to critically analyze information and to use this information to exert greater control over life events and situations' [6].

The use of cultural liaisons in primary care has proven successful [41] and as exemplified in Box 5. Rather than perpetuating a system of disconnect stemming from cultural gaps, bringing a cultural liaison (a member the cultural community being served) into the health care team helps communicate with the provider, on behalf of the person receiving care. In addition, the liaisons help narrow the gap between patients/ families and health providers by communicating and instructing the individual with regard to the treatment recommended, using culturally appropriate tools. Incorporating cultural liaisons in the community health care team helps to promote interactive health literacy, and to develop and reinforce skills that support the individual's independence in expressing his or her need to the health care providers, and thus to develop a trusting relationship. The research conducted on this shows that the program positively influenced the ability of new immigrants to navigate the health system, without increasing public or individual expenditure on services. The evidence showed that in clinics where the program was not implemented, a large number of unnecessary medical tests and referrals were performed. However, in spite of the evidence, many decision makers still place the burden on immigrants to adapt themselves, after so many years living in the country, preventing the program to be expanded to all clinics serving the Ethiopian community. Policy is being established in coordination with the Israel Ministry of Health which will place this special initiative under regulation requiring all clinics serving populations in need, to employ health liaisons through cultural mediation. Box 5 offers an example of inter-cultural perceptions of health service navigation, and offers an example of how this can be identified and addressed in the primary care system.

Asmara and his six children and their families moved from Ethiopia to Israel 10 years ago. He came expecting to encounter the perfect health support system. Feeling tired all the time, he sought help from the local community clinic. He quickly realized that the health providers not only speak a different language, and not his language, but they also arrange the way they treat people very differently from what he knew in Ethiopia. When he approached the family doctor in the community clinic, he was first sent to have a blood test, on a completely different day, and still received no treatment. He was expected to return to the physician to receive the results, however this time he understood from neighbors that he was to make an appointment through the telephone or even an online system, which he knew was beyond his capacity. He finally decided to go back to the clinic and just wait until the doctor could see him. He sat in the waiting room for a very long while and watched how other people who arrived after he did, were able to see the doctor before him. He finally decided to go home. Concurrently, the clinic office had been trying to reach him by phone to make an appointment, as his test results reflected why he was feeling so exhausted.

Box 5: A Picture from Israel

Future research should aim to study health literacy in the cultural context. Acknowledging that health literacy is a complex phenomenon, improving health literacy, is the responsibility to be shared between society and individuals/groups. Thus, interventions aimed at improving health literacy need to be directed to the individual, families, the general population, health care professionals and policy makers to increase awareness of health literacy. This can increase their awareness of the phenomenon to change attitudes, such awareness may inspire to stakeholders to develop action items that guarantee the access to relevant, health-related information, presented in ways that promote the health of individuals and groups with various life situations and with different ethnic, educational or social background. Health care professionals should be more aware of their important role as agents for improving health literacy. Through more appropriate professional training we can shed more light on health literacy in its different facets promoting a person and family centered approach in accordance with deep-rooted cultural values.

8. Health Literacy Provides a Conceptual Foundation for Community-based Participatory Research (CBPR)

In order to more fully understand the needs of the individuals in the community for developing better methods of communication and treatment, it is critical that the public itself be updated, aware and involved. The Participatory Action Research (PAR), or also referred to as the Community-Based Participatory Research (CBPR) model focuses on how the relationship between providers in the health care system can involve the public at large, or specific groups, in order to engage participation and full partnership in the needs assessment, planning, piloting of intervention, implementation and evaluation [42].

The development and refinement of the Vietnamese Dementia resource book is a good example of how the PAR model can be used [43]. The stakeholders (individuals with low health literacy, family members and carers) were invited to participate and co-design the contents of the resource book and give comments on the appropriateness of language level used to express content. Stakeholders are asked to read aloud the draft of the resource book and tell the designer how they interpret what was read. If the wordings are too complicated to understand, the stakeholders will provide suggestions how to revise the content [44]. Such participatory actions enhanced the acceptability of knowledge about dementia among the participants, and assisted health professionals with developing relationships with clients, family members and carers in a culturally appropriate manner.

The Sisters Together program is a US initiative that aims to encourage Afro-American women 18 years and older to maintain a healthy weight by being more physically active and eating healthy foods. It is a project of the National Institute of Diabetes and Digestive and Kidney Diseases (NIDDK), part of the National Institutes of Health (NIH), through the Weight-control Information Network (WIN) [45, 46] As a community health education intervention, Sisters Together is notable for its participatory, community-based approach, and it's focus on building health and empowerment skills in communities.

A critical further area of research in this domain includes identifying ways in which to engage lay stakeholders non-formal opinion leaders, citizens and non-citizens residents to take active part in assessing needs, planning action, implementing and evaluating action and intervention in health literacy, for the benefit of more positive health outcomes.

9. Innovative Opportunities for Improving Health Literacy and for Health Literacy Appropriate Interventions

This section offers a brief overview of innovative opportunities for emerging methods for improving health literacy and for adapting the communication of the health system with people of all health literacy levels.

9.1. The Contribution of Health Literacy to Digital Health Services and Systems

New strategies are emerging in light of the tremendous challenges mentioned for individual, families and communities rooted in cultures in transition vis-à-vis accessing empowering health information and even navigating the health system. New frontiers are being forged through eHealth, mHealth, and other health technologies. The broad range of applications include not only online information websites, but also interactive electronic records in various languages, health decision support programs, mobile health, and online communities that the individuals can access. An increasing body of knowledge is based in the dynamic research, showing how online sources of health information have and can be adapted to cultures, language and to groups with a particular status in society [47]. While there is concern regarding the "digital divide" great potential exists for promoting functional health literacy [6], interactive, and even critical health literacy. The vast potential for use of mobile phones to promote health literacy is beginning to unfold and must be seriously considered and utilized where appropriate for promoting health among individuals and in communities [5].

In spite of the assumption that digital tools are utilized mainly by younger populations, older adults are not exempt from reaping the potential benefits of digital development. Health literacy training that addresses the unique characteristics of older adults should be encouraged, as this age group can be the most disadvantaged group. For example: older adults in Hong Kong with no or minimal education have poor health outcomes, and frequently visit public health services. Initiatives were launched in Hong Kong in 2006 to develop community-dwelling older adults' skills and capacity to get reliable health information from the web [48]. Interestingly, participants of this study clearly indicated that having online searching skills did not replace the importance and preference of having face-to-face communication with health professionals and receiving health information through reading books or watching television [48]. This reinforces the notion that multiple channels would be needed to develop and support older adults' health literacy. It was worth noting that only one-third of older adults or soon-to-be adults preferred to seek health information from the Internet [49].

MHealth provides new opportunities for offering essential health information and support to the general public, however the criteria for increasing individuals' capacity to understand and interpret e-health information (e-health literacy) need to be met. Mobile apps have been developed to support patients in the various aspects of their involvement in promoting, maintaining and improving health, such as disease prevention, medication adherence, illness management, lifestyle modification and in navigating the health care system including making appointments in health services [51-55]. The most common disease-specific apps aim to provide education on diabetes, hypertension and hepatitis [55]. Most apps are provided on both iOS and Android platform free of charge [55].

An increasing number of studies investigating the effects of digital health interventions have suggested innovative digital tools are useful. A Cochrane review, comprised of four randomized controlled trials with 182 participants, analyzed the impact of mHealth (using mobile phone messaging) on self-management of long-term illnesses (including diabetes, hypertension, and asthma) [56]. Moderate evidence suggests some benefits mobile phone messaging interventions can: increase diabetic patients' self-management capacity including self-efficacy improve hypertensive patients' rate of medication compliance; and impact the peak expiratory flow variability for asthma patients [56]. There evidence was less pronounced regarding the impact of eHealth on health service utilization, and no evidence suggested long-term effects on health outcomes and cost-effectiveness form mobile phone messaging interventions [56]. The small number of studies and the limited number of participants in this review support the need for continued research and review of the evidence on health outcomes and service utilization.

While digital tools for promoting health are readily available as mentioned above, their appropriateness, particularly for people with low health literacy should be of concern. On the one hand, there is an increasing body of knowledge that suggests online sources of health information have and can be adapted to cultures, language and to groups with a particular status in society [47]. Additionally, a recent systematic review of 74 studies, suggests five relevant areas of future inquiry include: online health related content; features of eHealth services; interventions to improve eHealth literacy; health literacy measurement tools; and online health information seeking behavior [57]. The review suggests most online health content is not well-matched to user readability levels and therefore inaccessible. The review also suggests text-to-speech apps may help people with low health literacy access important online health information, that touch screen computers are helpful when surveying health literacy levels [57]. The review added even adults with high levels of health literacy sometimes evidenced low levels of self-efficacy, which deters finding reliable online information to inform health behaviors [57]. The review included was based on studies published in English [57]. Although cultural appropriateness was not investigated, the conclusions of the review have obvious implications regarding the extent to which digital tools can currently be considered a panacea for solving health literacy challenges across cultures. The importance of continued research and reviews cannot be overstated due to the significant investment in innovative tools and their sweeping uptake by health systems.

10. Cultural Norms and Global and Local Trends in Society: Recommendations for Practitioners, Researchers, Policy Makers for New Directions in Research, Theory, and Practice

Interventions aimed at improving health literacy need to be directed to the individual and to the families and those influencing the individual, the general population, health care professionals and policy makers to increase awareness of health literacy. Accordingly, the influences may vary depending upon the health problem of concern. Such awareness should result in the development of measures that promote:

- the access of culturally appropriate health-related information, presented in ways that have been developed through public participation, for use in various life situations and with different ethnic, educational or social background.

- the understanding of health literacy as an issue for the whole of society instead of a view in which the responsibilities for increasing health literacy lie solely on the individual and the health care system [58].

- the understanding on the part of health care professionals, of their importance as agents to improve health literacy by encouraging and supporting individuals, families and communities in accordance with their health literacy needs, empowering them to make and apply the most appropriate health decisions within the cultural context.

- the realization that the more appropriate and culturally sensitive health systems and health information are, the more it can be claimed that health literacy contributes to social justice.

11. Future Areas for Applied Research and Exploration

The answers to the following questions are essential for appropriate action and can be investigated through collaborative research:

- How can communities promote lifelong skills and knowledge building, given changing needs and circumstances and the often very contextualized nature of skills/knowledge needed for health management?
- How can health systems be prepared to effectively offer information to the right people at the appropriate opportunities in the most effective way?
- What is the best way to support community members need to develop their capacity to effectively engage/learn/adapt as their needs change over time?
- How can immigrant populations be supported to develop health literacy skills enabling and empowering them to understand the health system in their new country, understand Western medicine approaches to mind, body, health and illness, and understand the shared decision making approaches to health seen in Western medicine, where patients are seen as key stakeholders and partners in their own health?
- What is the best way to train health providers to function effectively and sensitively in a cross cultural setting? Is a generic approach more effective or is cultural specificity preferred?
- To what extent do health practitioners understand these issues from the perspective of the populations they serve, and how can they best treat their patient community in the most appropriate way?
- How can health services be structured and managed such that they are approachable, accessible, and safe for people from different cultures?
- Interpreters are often used in medical consultations with immigrants unable to speak the national language of their new home. What is the health literacy of the interpreters? How do they mediate the messages between practitioner and patient?

These are all key questions that the health literacy research, practice and policy community can help to answer; the results of such research can then lead to informed and improved practice to promote health and reduce and manage illness in immigrant populations.

12. Conclusion and Summary

In this chapter we emphasize the role of health literacy internationally across cultures, mainly from the perspectives of individuals, families and communities. We highlighted key areas where we can build on already completed research. Importantly, we have also identified some areas of focus, for the international health literacy research community, where there is little or no research, and great potential for a health literacy approach to offer people new opportunities for promoting health. We have highlighted some areas where interventions and developments are recognized and evaluated and can be implemented and re-evaluated in other countries and settings. Finally, we have emphasized some important areas where little is known, and invite the international community to consider, develop and apply new avenues for practice, research and policy.

References

[1]   Parker R. Measuring health literacy: what? So what? Now what? In: Hernandez L, editor. Measures of health literacy: workshop summary, Roundtable on Health Literacy. Washington, DC: National Academies Press; 2009. p. 91–8.
[2]   World Health Organization. Health literacy. The solid facts. Copenhagen: WHO Regional Office for Europe; 2013.
[3]   The Millennium Development Goals Report 2015. New York: United Nations; 2015.
[4]   Tracking Universal Health Coverage. First global monitoring report. France: World Health Organisation and The World Bank; 2015. p. 1.
[5]   Rowlands G, Dodson S, Leung A, Levin-Zamir D. Global health systems and policy development: implications for health literacy research, theory and practice. In: Logan R, Siegel E, editors. Health literacy: new directions in research, theory, and practice. Amsterdam: IOS Press; 2017.
[6]   Nutbeam D. Health literacy as a public health goal: a challenge for contemporary health education and communication strategies into the 21st century. Health Promot Int. 2000; 15(3):259-67.
[7]   Education and Community Support for Health Literacy: Centers for Disease Control and Prevention (CDC); Available from: http://www.cdc.gov/healthliteracy/education-support/index.html.
[8]   Levin-Zamir D, Lemish D, Gofin R. Media Health Literacy (MHL): Development and measurement of the concept among adolescents. Health Educ Res. 2011;26(2):323-35.
[9]   Begoray D, Wharf Higgins J, Harrison J, Collins-Emery A. Adolescent reading/viewing of advertisements. Understandings from transactional and positioning theory. J Adolesc Adult Lit. 2013;57(2):121-30. DOI:10.1002/jaal.202.
[10] Telama R, Yang X, Laakso L, Viikari J. Physical activity in childhood and adolescence as predictor of physical activity in young adulthood. Am J Prev Med. 1997;13(4):317-23.
[11] Degenhardt L, O'Loughlin C, Swift W, Romaniuk H, Carlin J, Coffey C, et al. The persistence of adolescent binge drinking into adulthood: findings from a 15-year prospective cohort study. BMJ Open. 2013;3(8):e003015.
[12] Evaluation of the second phase of the Skilled for Health Programme. London: The Tavistock Institute and Shared Intelligence; 2009.
[13] Health literacy: improving health, health systems, and health policy around the world, Workshop Summary. Washington DC; 2013.
[14] Muscat DM, Smith S, Dhillon HM, Morony S, Davis EL, Luxford K, et al. Incorporating health literacy in education for socially disadvantaged adults: an Australian feasibility study. Int J Equity Health. 2016;15(1):84. DOI:10.1186/s12939-016-0373-1.
[15] Qureshi RN, Sheikh S, Khowaja AR, Hoodbhoy Z, Zaidi S, Sawchuck D, et al. Health care seeking behaviours in pregnancy in rural Sindh, Pakistan: a qualitative study. Reprod Health. 2016;13 Suppl 1:34.
[16] Evaluation of the HEY! programme: A report for Danone Nutricia early life nutrition. London: Shared Intelligence; 2015.
[17] Lie DA, Lee-Rey E, Gomez A, Bereknyei S, Braddock CH, 3rd. Does cultural competency training of health professionals improve patient outcomes? A systematic review and proposed algorithm for future research. J Gen Intern Med. 2011;26(3):317-25.
[18] Mårtensson L, Hensing G. Health literacy–a heterogeneous phenomenon: a literature review. Scand J Caring Sci. 2012;26(1):151-60.
[19] Purnell L. The Purnell model for cultural competence. J Transcult Nurs. 2002;13(3):193-6; discussion 200-1. DOI:10.1177/10459602013003006.
[20] Pavlish CL, Noor S, Brandt J. Somali immigrant women and the American health care system: discordant beliefs, divergent expectations, and silent worries. Soc Sci Med. 2010;71(2):353-61. DOI:10.1016/j.socscimed.2010.04.010.

[21] Hackenthal V, Spiegel S, Lewis-Fernandez R, Kealey E, Salerno A, Finnerty M. Towards a cultural adaptation of family psychoeducation: findings from three Latino focus groups. Community Ment Health J. 2013;49:587-98.

[22] Mescha G, Manob R, Tsamirc J. Minority status and health information search: a test of the social diversification hypothesis. Soc Sci Med. 2012;58(5):854–8.

[23] Kalengayi FK, Hurtig AK, Nordstrand A, Ahlm C, Ahlberg BM. 'It is a dilemma': perspectives of nurse practitioners on health screening of newly arrived migrants. Glob Health Action. 2015;8:27903. DOI:10.3402/gha.v8.27903.

[24] Nkulu Kalengayi FK, Hurtig AK, Nordstrand A, Ahlm C, Ahlberg BM. Perspectives and experiences of new migrants on health screening in Sweden. BMC Health Serv Res. 2016;16:14.

[25] Bischoff A, Bovier PA, Rrustemi I, Gariazzo F, Eytan A, Loutan L. Language barriers between nurses and asylum seekers: their impact on symptom reporting and referral. Soc Sci Med. 2003;57(3):503-12.

[26] Lee HY, Jung Y. Older Korean American men's prostate cancer screening behavior: the prime role of culture. J Immigr Minor Health. 2013;15(6):1030-7. DOI:10.1007/s10903-013-9804-x.

[27] Liang W, Yuan E, Mandelblatt JS, Pasick RJ. How do older Chinese women view health and cancer screening? Results from focus groups and implications for interventions. Ethn Health. 2004;9(3):283-304. DOI:10.1080/1355785042000250111.

[28] Haralambous B, Dow B, Goh A, Pachana NA, Bryant C, LoGiudice D, et al. 'Depression is not an illness. It's up to you to make yourself happy': Perceptions of Chinese health professionals and community workers about older Chinese immigrants' experiences of depression and anxiety. Australas J Ageing. 2016; 35(4), 249-254. DOI:10.1111/ajag.12306.

[29] Maneze D, Salamonson Y, Poudel C, DiGiacomo M, Everett B, Davidson PM. Health-seeking behaviors of Filipino migrants in Australia: the influence of persisting acculturative stress and depression. J Immigr Minor Health. 2016;18(4):779-86. DOI:10.1007/s10903-015-0233-x.

[30] Leung AY, Bo A, Hsiao HY, Wang SS, Chi I. Health literacy issues in the care of Chinese American immigrants with diabetes: a qualitative study. BMJ Open. 2014;4(11):e005294. DOI:10.1136/bmjopen-2014-005294.

[31] Vida Estacio E, McKinley RK, Saidy-Khan S, Karic T, Clark L, Kurth J. Health literacy: Why it matters to South Asian men with diabetes. Prim Health Care Res Dev. 2015;16(2):214-8. DOI:10.1017/S1463423614000152.

[32] Diabetes care – strategies for improving care: American Diabetes Association (ADA). http://care.diabetesjournals.org/content/39/Supplement_1/S6.

[33] Omariba DW, Ng E. Health literacy and disability: differences between generations of Canadian immigrants. Int J Public Health. 2015;60(3):389-97. DOI:10.1007/s00038-014-0640-0.

[34] Betancourt JR, Green AR. Cultural competence: healthcare disparities and political issues. In, Immigrant Medicine. Saunders Elsevier; 2007.

[35] Meng Z, Molyneaux L, McGill M, Shen X, Yue DK. Impact of sociodemographic and diabetes-related factors on the presence and severity of depression in immigrant Chinese Australian people with diabetes. Clin Diabetes. 2014;32(4):163-9. DOI:10.1007/s10903-015-0233-x.

[36] Kim IH, Carrasco C, Muntaner C, McKenzie K, Noh S. Ethnicity and postmigration health trajectory in new immigrants to Canada. Am J Public Health. 2013;103(4):e96-104.

[37] Warfa N, Bhui K, Craig T, Curtis S, Mohamud S, Stansfield.S., et al. Post-migration geographical mobility, mental health and health service utilization among Somali refugees in the UK: a qualitative study. Health Place. 2006;12:503–15.

[38] Kandula NR, Kersey M, Lurie N. Assuring the health of immigrants: what the leading health indicators tell us. Annu Rev Public Health. 2004;25:357-76. DOI:10.1146/annurev.publhealth.25.101802.123107.

[39] Lie D, Carter-Pokras O, Braun B, Coleman C. What do health literacy and cultural competence have in common? Calling for a collaborative health professional pedagogy. J Health Commun. 2012;17:13-22.

[40] Shim JK. Cultural health capital: a theoretical approach to understanding health care interactions and the dynamics of unequal treatment. Journal Health Soc Behav. 2010;51(1):1-15. DOI:10.1177/0022146509361185.

[41] Levin-Zamir D, Keret S, Yaakovson O, Lev B, Kay C, Verber G, et al. Refuah Shlema: a cross-cultural programme for promoting communication and health among Ethiopian immigrants in the primary health care setting in Israel: evidence and lessons learned from over a decade of implementation. Glob Health Promot. 2011;18(1):51-4.

[42] Israel BA, Schulz AJ, Parker EA, Becker AB. Review of community-based research: assessing partnership approaches to improve public health. Annu Rev Public Health. 1998;19:173-202. DOI:10.1146/annurev.publhealth.19.1.173.

[43] Goeman D, Michael J, King J, Luu H, Emmanuel C, Koch S. Partnering with consumers to develop and evaluate a Vietnamese Dementia Talking-Book to support low health literacy: a qualitative study incorporating codesign and participatory action research. BMJ Open. 2016;6(9):e011451. DOI:10.1136/bmjopen-2016-011451.
[44] Leung A. Older adults' involvement in the development of health literacy materials: findings from cognitive interviews. Poster presented at The 62nd Annual Scientific Meeting of the Gerontological Society of America. Atlanta, USA; 2009.
[45] National eHealth Strategy Toolkit. Geneva: WHO and the International Telecommunications Union; 2012.
[46] Curtis L, Brown ZG, Gill JE. Sisters Together: Move More, Eat Better: a community-based health awareness program for African-American women. J Natl Black Nurses Assoc. 2008;19(2):59-64.
[47] Kreps GL, Neuhauser L. New directions in eHealth communication: opportunities and challenges. Patient Educ Couns. 2010;78(3):329-36. DOI:10.1016/j.pec.2010.01.013.
[48] Leung A, Ko P, Chan KS, Chi I, Chow N. Searching health information via the web: Hong Kong Chinese older adults' experience. Public Health Nurs. 2007;24(2):169-75. DOI:10.1111/j.1525-1446.2007.00621.x.
[49] Leung AYM, Leung DYP, Cheung MKT. Preference for online health information among Chinese. J Health Mass Commun. 2011;3(1-4):46.
[50] Coughlin S, Thind H, Liu B, Champagne N, Jacobs M, Massey RI. Mobile phone apps for preventing cancer through educational and behavioral interventions: state of the art and remaining challenges. JMIR Mhealth Uhealth. 2016;4(2):e69.
[51] Santo K, Richtering SS, Chalmers J, Thiagalingam A, Chow CK, Redfern J. Mobile phone apps to improve medication adherence: a systematic stepwise process to identify high-quality apps. JMIR Mhealth Uhealth. 2016;4(4):e132.
[52] Horvath KJ, Alemu D, Danh T, Baker JV, Carrico AW. Creating effective mobile phone apps to optimize antiretroviral therapy adherence: perspectives from stimulant-using HIV-positive men who have sex with men. JMIR Mhealth Uhealth. 2016;4(2):e48.
[53] Mirkovic J, Kaufman DR, Ruland CM. Supporting cancer patients in illness management: usability evaluation of a mobile app. JMIR Mhealth Uhealth. 2014;2(3):e33.
[54] Dute DJ, Bemelmans WJ, Breda J. Using mobile apps to promote a healthy lifestyle among adolescents and students: a review of the theoretical basis and lessons learned. JMIR Mhealth Uhealth. 2016;4(2):e39.
[55] Hsu J, Liu D, Yu YM, Zhao HT, Chen ZR, Li J, et al. The top Chinese mobile health apps: a systematic investigation. J Med Internet Res. 2016;18(8):e222.
[56] de Jongh T, Gurol-Urganci I, Vodopivec-Jamsek V, Car J, Atun R. Mobile phone messaging for facilitating self-management of long-term illnesses. Cochrane Database Syst Rev. 2012;12:Cd007459.
[57] Kim H, Xie B. Health literacy in the eHealth era: a systematic review of the literature. Patient Educ Couns. 2017.
[58] Health literacy: a prescription to end confusion. Washington DC: Institute of Medicine; 2004.

Health Literacy
R.A. Logan and E.R. Siegel (Eds.)
IOS Press, 2017
doi:10.3233/978-1-61499-790-0-415

Libraries and Librarians: Key Partners for Progress in Health Literacy Research and Practice

Wanda WHITNEY[a,1], Alla KESELMAN[a] and Betsy HUMPHREYS[a]

[a] *National Library of Medicine, National Institutes of Health, Bethesda, MD USA*

Abstract. The field of librarianship has a history of involvement in patient education, general literacy and information literacy efforts. This history and prominent placement in communities make libraries and librarians an excellent resource in advancing health literacy practice and research. This chapter provides an overview of health literacy and health information literacy efforts in US libraries over the past two decades.

The chapter begins with the description of the role of the US National Library of Medicine in developing resources, programs, and partnerships serving health information needs of the public. It then overviews special training programs for increasing librarians' expertise with health information and health literacy support. The narrative also presents different models of health information outreach programs in diverse communities, focusing on serving special populations that may suffer from health disparities.

The second half of the chapter describes libraries' and librarians' health information response to continuously evolving contexts, mediums, and requirements. One subsection describes librarians' outreach effort with cutting-edge technologies, such as virtual worlds and gaming. Another focuses on supporting patients' information needs in clinical settings. Two more describe how libraries meet patrons' health information needs in the context of disaster preparedness and health insurance market place sign-up.

While presenting the information, to the extent possible, the chapter draws upon research and evaluation of the effectiveness of different types of programs. It also discusses enablers of successes, limitations of the existing data, and directions for future research.

Keywords. Health information literacy, Health literacy, Patient education, Libraries, Health information outreach

1. Introduction

Libraries and librarians are excellent resources for advancing research and practice in health literacy. They are nearly ubiquitous, generally perceived as trustworthy and helpful, and collectively experienced in general health and patient education. Different types of libraries, e.g., public, hospital, academic health center, have different strengths to bring to health literacy interventions. Programs that involve multiple types of libraries may have a better chance of being sustainable and successful.

---

[1] Corresponding author: Public Services Division, U.S. National Library of Medicine, 8600 Rockville Pike, Building 38, Room 1W22C, Bethesda, Maryland 20894; E-mail: whitneyw@mail.nlm.nih.gov.

Two-thirds of the population of the United States live near a public library [1]. Many also have access to physical libraries in schools, community centers, colleges or universities, health care institutions, and places of employment. High quality digital libraries are available to anyone with access to a web-capable device and an Internet connection. This includes anyone who is willing and able to visit a public library, as well as the many millions who have their own devices and Internet access.

Relying on libraries to identify, organize, and provide easy public access to high quality, understandable health information can make health literacy interventions more scalable and sustainable. For individuals who are self-motivated to improve their understanding of health topics, organized libraries of high quality health information, whether digital or physical, greatly simplify the search for relevant information.

Long before "health literacy" became a named topic of interest or the Web browser was invented, libraries and librarians of various types were engaged in patient education and in providing health information written for consumers or the general public, often in cooperation with other organizations and institutions [2]. For more than a century, public libraries and librarians have also been deeply involved in programs to advance general literacy in children and adults, sometimes using easy-to-read health information as source material.

In the 1990s, however, an increasing focus on health literacy as a concept and as an area of research and practice, the spread of the Internet and the World Wide Web, concern about the "Wild West" of electronic health information, and the doubling of the National Institutes of Health (NIH) budget came together in ways that greatly expanded the involvement of U.S. libraries in health information literacy and health literacy activities. This chapter describes the role of the U.S. National Library of Medicine (NLM), a component of NIH, in initiating this expansion; efforts to prepare librarians to assist the public in obtaining high quality health information; and the roles librarians play in health information outreach, use of innovative technologies, providing health insurance information, health literacy interventions in clinical settings, and access to information in disasters and emergencies. The chapter concludes with thoughts about the important contributions libraries and librarians can make to health literacy research and practice.

2. The Role of the U.S. National Library of Medicine

The NLM, the world's largest medical library, builds and provides electronic information resources used billions of times each year by millions of scientists, health professionals, and members of the public around the world. Through its information systems, an informatics research portfolio, extensive training programs, and many partnerships, the NLM plays an essential role in catalyzing and supporting the translation of basic science into new treatments, new products, improved practice, useful decision support for health professionals and patients, and effective disaster and emergency preparedness and response. The NLM coordinates a 6,500 member National Network of Libraries of Medicine (NN/LM) that provides a field force for improving access to high quality health information in communities across the U.S., with an emphasis on populations with health disparities.

Prior to 1997, the NLM's involvement with health literacy was restricted to acquiring, describing, and providing access to pertinent research literature, as well as funding some relevant research and resource development projects. NLM also provided a few free databases and outreach programs designed for patients and the general public in specialized areas, such as HIV/AIDS, for which targeted funding was available.

In 1997, the NLM was able to eliminate fees for searching MEDLINE, a database of indexed citations and abstracts from biomedical journals, and its other databases due to the expansion of the Internet and the World Wide Web. As users obtained their own Internet connections, they no longer needed commercial telecommunications services to reach NLM databases, and the Library no longer needed to charge users their fair share of a large central telecommunications bill. When NLM's MEDLINE became freely searchable via the relatively simple PubMed Web interface, use skyrocketed. The general public became a major user group, although MEDLINE did not provide the basic explanations of health and disease topics that many of them were seeking [3].

The Web provided a cost-effective platform for NLM to deliver health information services to the public, and the doubling of the NIH budget gave NLM the additional funding necessary to develop new services targeted toward the general population. In this propitious environment, the NLM Board of Regents revised a previous policy against development of services for patients and the public that had been dictated by budget limitations. In 1999, the NLM Board stated that the Library should "…improve the national infrastructure that supports the public's access to electronic health information… so that all people in the U.S. have a known, accessible, understandable, and affordable source of current, authoritative health information" [4]. In 1998, the NLM had released the MedlinePlus consumer health information website [5], the first of an array of new services for the general public. NLM also expanded its outreach programs, previously directed primarily to underserved health professionals, to involve public libraries and other community-based organizations, often in partnership with the NN/LM, in improving the public's awareness of, and access to, health information services in minority, rural, frontier, inner city and other underserved communities [6,7,8].

In this same period, the NLM examined published evidence on health communication and health literacy to identify best practices applicable to consumer health information services. Scott Ratzan, editor of the Journal of Health Communication, and Ruth Parker, a pioneering health literacy researcher and advocate, were engaged to assist NLM staff in compiling an initial bibliography "… to help define and describe the evidence base for advancing health literacy programs by examining theories, strategies, and tactics in the published literature" [9]. Released in early 2000, the bibliography contained a novel definition of health literacy, "the degree to which individuals have the capacity to obtain, process, and understand basic health information and services needed to make appropriate health decisions" [10]. As of 1999, there was limited evidence about which learning strategies and tactics were most viable. However, the new definition of health literacy was widely cited and adopted by the Institute of Medicine [11], and the bibliography provided a foundation for further research.

Since 2000, the NLM has continued to expand and enhance its suite of information services and outreach programs designed to provide patients, families, and the general public with easy access to high quality health information where and when needed. The development of trusted information services that promote health literacy was identified as a major goal in the NLM Long Range Plan for 2006-2016 [12]. NLM staff members have been active participants in the programs of the Roundtable on Health Literacy, initially of the Institute of Medicine, and now of the National Academies of Sciences, Engineering, and Medicine. The Library's heavily used services for the general public now include extensive information in Spanish, as well as resources in more than 40 other languages; spoken, interactive, and "easy to read" information; websites designed to display effectively on devices of all sizes, including smartphones; application programming interfaces (APIs) so that access to patient education information can be embedded in external information systems, including electronic health records (EHRs) and patient portals; K-12 educational materials; and the NIH MedlinePlus magazine, in English and Spanish, produced in cooperation with the Friends of the National Library of Medicine and other NIH Institutes and Centers. By providing enhanced, integrated access to electronic consumer health and patient information produced by authoritative sources, NLM has facilitated Web discovery of high quality information written for the general public, both for those seeking information for themselves and those seeking materials for use in health literacy research and interventions.

In addition to expanding the universe of credible, readily available health information written for the public, the NLM has been a very significant supporter of health information outreach projects and initiatives via the NN/LM, which now incorporates many public libraries and community information centers as well as hospital and academic health sciences libraries, and in partnerships with minority serving institutions, public health departments, schools, churches, and other community-based organizations. Through the NN/LM and in cooperation with the Medical Library Association (MLA), the NLM has developed training programs and materials to assist librarians and information specialists in providing consumer health information services and designing and evaluating health information interventions [13]. In addition to the health literacy activities involving libraries that are discussed in this chapter, NLM has also supported and conducted a wide range of related research and development, including informatics research on personal health records, integration of patient education information in EHRs, and consumer health language.

Projects supported by the NLM have produced a substantial portion of the published evidence about health literacy research and practice involving libraries and librarians that is discussed in the next sections of this chapter.

3. Preparing Librarians to Assist the Public in Obtaining High Quality Health Information

In 1998-1999, with assistance from the Friends of the National Library of Medicine and the Kellogg Foundation, the NLM and the NN/LM undertook a pilot program involving 41 public libraries or library systems (more than 200 facilities) in nine states and the District of Columbia. The objectives were to learn about the current role of public libraries in providing health information and to determine how NLM and its network might help public libraries enhance the public's access to health information. Each public library received a grant to provide computers, Internet access, or health information materials to their patrons and was partnered with a NN/LM network library which provided staff training, including in the use of MedlinePlus and other NLM information services, and advice about handling health questions.

The results of the evaluation component of this project revealed that few public libraries had health information centers, but that health information ranked among the top 5 or 10 topics of interest to their patrons. Many of the public librarians involved in the pilot were inexperienced, and therefore uncomfortable, in providing health reference assistance to patrons. The training provided to an estimated 1,150 library staff and volunteers was therefore enthusiastically received and highly valued. The pilot project did not generate significant numbers of public library requests for documents from medical libraries, as some had expected [14].

Following up on this pilot, NLM increased funding for the NN/LM to support work to improve the public's access to health information. In 2000, NLM and the Regional Medical Libraries in the NN/LM set a goal to ensure that by 2005 every public library in the nation would be aware of NLM's free Web-based information resources and able to provide access to them. In addition to supporting individual projects involving public librarians in specific locations [15,16], the Regional Medical Libraries collaborated on the development of a consumer health information course available to public librarians across the country. The training modules they developed provided the basis for the MLA Consumer Health Information Specialization, which "offers basic and advanced training opportunities for individuals whose work roles demand they provide information services to the public, patients, and families" [17].

Later, in 2008, MLA sponsored a two-day Health Information Literacy Research Project conference. "Health information literacy" is a form of "information literacy" [18], defined as the ability to find and assess the relevance, validity, and utility of information for a particular purpose.

Librarians in academic settings have long provided formal and informal instruction in information literacy. For health sciences librarians, this has often involved teaching students and practitioners of medicine and other health professions to search online databases and to evaluate the quality of the clinical research evidence in journal articles [19]. Health information literacy is a prerequisite for effective selection of health information for any purpose, whether it be a library service or a health literacy intervention or a family medical question Health information literacy may be viewed as a component of health literacy pertaining to the ability to obtain health information. However, unlike health literacy, health information literacy is not essential for understanding and making use of pre-selected health information, such as signs in health facilities, written instructions provided by health professionals, or web services organized by health literate librarians. The 2008 MLA conference led to the development of a health information literacy toolkit with resources such as health literacy curricula. Librarians and others wishing to provide training can adapt the curricula to their individual communities [20]. MLA also published the Medical Library Association Guide to Health Literacy in 2008 with the goal of helping librarians to "...be better able to understand the issues that comprise health literacy, learning how to help others become health literate, and how to become change agents within their organizations" [21].

Other health information training opportunities targeted toward public librarians include those offered by the American Library Association's (ALA) and WebJunction, a division of OCLC Research. Last offered in 2015, the ALA's six-week Health Information 101 web-based course includes an introduction to the concepts of health literacy and provides guidance for providing health information to low literacy populations [22]. WebJunction offers online training and hour-long webinars on consumer health topics for librarians, as part of a series called Health Happens in Libraries with topics such as: Health Information Resources for Library Staff, Public Health and Public Libraries: Librarians as Health Literacy First Responders, and Public and Health Sciences Library Collaboration for Community Impact [23]. These and other training resources developed for librarians can be very useful to others, including anyone interested in identifying materials appropriate for health literacy interventions or research.

The last decade has definitely seen an increase in the number of librarians who have received specific training in meeting health information needs of the public and in health literacy concepts. Of course, this does not mean that all public libraries are equally well-equipped to help those seeking understandable health information or that all library workers in a given library have relevant knowledge and training [24].

4. Librarians and Health Information Outreach

The capabilities of public and medical libraries to provide consumer health information have increased as a response to consumer demand and the availability of consumer health information training [25]. Librarians field consumer questions at the information desk, taking advantage of a number of credible information resources freely available on the Internet, pamphlets and other print materials from local public health agencies, or through subscriptions to medical databases or journals. Libraries hold health fairs and other community events, inviting other community organizations with additional health information expertise to participate [26]. Here, we explore the various ways that libraries provide health information outreach, specifically through train-the-trainer models, to general and special populations, such as ethnic minorities, older adults, and children.

Although librarians in different settings are prepared to provide health information outreach within their own facilities, this model may not be the most desirable or efficacious method for populations with special needs and concerns [27]. Health literacy advocates call for more participatory methods, especially when providing outreach to diverse populations, such as communities of color, older adults, and teens. Community involvement in train-the-trainer health information programs helps libraries overcome neighborhood suspicions about the remote management of health related programs and interventions [27]. Libraries now are more likely to implement health information outreach programs that employ variations of the train-the-trainer approach by partnering with community-based organizations.

There are important advantages to train-the-trainer models of outreach. First, training community members increases libraries' reach exponentially as community members teach their peers who then go on to teach others. This method also has the potential to empower disenfranchised communities since health information is provided by the community for the community. Last, community train-the-trainer models can be adapted to fit the community being targeted based on its particular characteristics and needs. Such targeting aligns with recognition, by the NLM and many other organizations, of the need to provide health information outreach to underserved populations and communities [12].

Successful models of community engagement take on different forms. Some successful train-the-trainer programs have focused on intergenerational training. For example, in one intergenerational program, librarians demonstrated health information resources to university students in a six-month period so they could, in turn, help older adults use the Internet to locate health information [28]. There are also successful examples of peer-to-peer training. Librarians at the University of Texas Health Science Center at San Antonio worked with high school librarians to teach teens about MedlinePlus and MedlinePlus en español so that they could share that information with their friends and, later, with the broader community [29]. These peer tutors not only learned about health information, they also received training in recognizing personal situations that would require librarian support or intervention. Tutors gave presentations that increased their reach to 350 students and teachers in their school and the surrounding counties, as well as parents and other family members. The program was so successful that it expanded to other schools in the district and still continues today [30].

In another program along the Texas border region, medical librarians from the University of Texas Health Science Center at San Antonio partnered with the Texas A & M University Center for Housing and Urban Development (TAM-CHUD) to train lay community health workers, known as "promotores" in Spanish, to find consumer health information for fellow residents using MedlinePlus and MedlinePlus en español [31]. Fifteen "promotoras" provided weekly examples of how they had used health information found on MedlinePlus to learn more about a condition, make better decisions about treatment, or commit to healthier behavior. In evaluating the project, investigators determined that training the "promotoras" to use MedlinePlus resulted in increased usage of this resource within the community [31]. Although lost funding contributed to the end of this program in several community centers, the investigators found that the program had promise and could be adapted for health information outreach for any population.

Whatever approach to health information provision librarians choose, they need to keep in mind important considerations that, if unheeded, may hinder the success of such programs when working with diverse community populations. Many times a great need exists to teach basic computer and information literacy skills, especially among older adults; so many programs offer these services as well. For example, Strong, Guillot, and Badeau [32] describe the Senior CHAT project in Louisiana that taught older adults basic computer skills so that they could then move on to Internet skills that would allow them to search for health information using NIHSeniorHealth and MedlinePlus. In another example, Xie and Bugg [33], partnered with multiple agencies and public libraries to provide computer and information literacy training to senior adults so they could navigate the same sites for authoritative consumer health information. Choosing public libraries to deliver the training, they hypothesized that older adults would experience less anxiety and increased computer interest and efficacy after participating in the training.

Chu et. al. [34] completed a similar project with low-income older adults enrolled in a meal program in their local YWCA with seniors reporting higher confidence and self-efficacy using computers to search the Internet for health information. Overall, evaluations of programs with older adults, such as the ones described here, show they continue to use the consumer health web sites to learn more about their conditions and help them make better-informed health decisions. Some participants report these changes several weeks after the program has ended [32].

Other project developers focus on elementary or middle school-aged children who have unique needs and concerns that call for programs adapted to their reading level, attention span, and overall developmental readiness. For example, in Caddo Parish, Louisiana librarians sought to use story time to teach children about healthy living [35]. They also created a Web portal and other educational materials to provide children with access to up-to-date authoritative health information. Because of a relatively large increase in overweight and obese children in the state, librarians chose to focus on encouraging young children to adopt an active lifestyle. Resources also included materials related to nutrition and basic hygiene. While the project sponsors didn't complete a formal evaluation of the project, they noted nearly 800 students took part in the health-themed story hours; and the project developers received additional funding to develop new activities and reach out to more libraries requesting to participate in the project [35].

In summary, the published literature suggests successful health information outreach by librarians can take many different forms. Train-the-trainer models can be particularly effective in providing health information outreach to special populations that may suffer from health disparities and that require different approaches to satisfy different health information needs. These target populations include minority communities, such as African Americans and Hispanics. The information projects mentioned above and other research studies have shown that introducing people to new information resources works best when the providers are similar to them [27] and when special needs are considered and planned for from the beginning.

5. Using Innovative Technologies

Libraries have led the way in providing health information training and outreach via traditional approaches described above. In addition, they also have broken new ground in providing outreach via different media such as virtual worlds and gaming. These approaches, often first applied in programs for health professionals, proved adaptable to serving the public. For example, in 2006–2008, NLM funded the development of HealthInfo Island in a 3D virtual world, Second Life, managed by librarians and health professionals. Resources and programs for the island were developed in partnership with library systems in Illinois and the Netherlands [36].

Presenting health information in a virtual world draws upon an existing popular culture, encourages innovative information visualization, and may reduce accessibility barriers for people with chronic illnesses or disabilities who may be homebound. HealthInfo Island hosted a medical library and a consumer health library that linked visitors to quality interactive health and wellness information. It was also the site of "Health Information Research Lab" created by NLM that piloted providing quality consumer health information through podcasts, automated tours, and chatbots [36]. Providing individualized support, volunteer consumer health librarians developed personalized reading lists that addressed visitors' queries [37].

However, the maintenance and sustainability of virtual reality sites present a unique challenge. In part, this is due to high cost and the fact that the virtual reality environment (in this case, Second Life) is owned by an independent company with its changing rules, policies, and priorities. While we don't know how viable HealthInfo Island, now owned by Virtual Ability, Inc., will be in future years, it does offer a creative way to access consumer health information.

Gaming provides another innovative technology often used in education and training alongside virtual world simulations. One gaming employment approach is the serious games movement, which promotes the development of games with other-than-entertainment primary objectives. Serious games have been used in a number of fields, including education, emergency management, and healthcare. While published literature provides no examples of libraries using serious games in consumer health information programming, they have discovered that gaming devices such as the Wii may provide a creative way to connect the general public with authoritative health information. For example, NLM also funded a project entitled One, Two, Wii: Get Fit and Health Savvy @ Your Library [38]. The project investigators partnered with school and public libraries to offer the game consoles for the public during health fairs, meetings, or other events where library staff would also introduce them to health information resources such as MedlinePlus [38].

The success of this project led to additional NLM funding for a second project, Engage Your Health Information Seekers: Wii Health Information Resources Kit. The kit offers libraries two Wii systems and games with a manual of suggestions for health fairs or other wellness events and resources for quality health information [38]. Project leaders find that both projects have increased awareness of the outreach assistance provided by the medical library, as well as health information resources from NLM.

Libraries differ with respect to the sophistication of the technology available to them. Similarly, patrons differ in their interest and comfort level when it comes to technologies like virtual worlds and gaming. More information is needed to establish best practices of employing cutting-edge technologies in libraries. It is clear, however, that many librarians have the interest and skills needed for adapting creative technologies for health information outreach.

6. Libraries, Health Literacy, and the U.S. Patient Protection and Affordable Care Act

U.S. libraries and librarians serve the public's information needs with regard to health insurance enrollment in the context of state and federal law and regulation, currently including the Patient Protection and Affordable Care Act (ACA). In most cases, libraries respond to the public's health information needs with approaches and resources that have evolved gradually. However, there are also times when the field has to react to a time-sensitive emergent need.

For example, on June 30, 2013, in a special message to ALA conference attendees, U.S. President Barack Obama called on libraries to support the public's information needs concerning ACA. The effort was to commence during health insurance market place sign-up, scheduled to open on October 1 of that year. Asking libraries to provide such guidance placed the needed support within an easy reach of potential enrollees. The ACA provides health insurance access to populations often characterized by lower health literacy and reduced access to information technology. These populations also often have less advanced computer skills, and libraries are places that traditionally provide computer access and support to the disadvantaged. Involving libraries also built upon their support of other government services, such as information provision on the topics of income tax, citizenship, patents, and disaster relief [39]. Studies of health insurance literacy provide additional evidence in favor of engaging librarians in ACA information support. These studies suggest that most health insurance materials place too-high numeracy and literacy demands on the enrollees [40,41]. The complexity deters individuals from health insurance enrollment, while providing sign-up support increases enrollment [41]. At the same time, political controversy around the ACA, complexity of the information, and short timeframe posed challenges for libraries and librarians.

As a professional field, librarianship had an established professional development model, used by the NLM, NN/LM, and major national organizations to provide resources and training for local libraries. In response to the U.S. President's call, ALA hosted a number of events during its 2013 annual conference to address ACA support preparedness. Following the conference, ALA formed a partnership with several organizations, including NN/LM and WebJunction, in order to prepare public libraries for the task [42]. NN/LM regional libraries (e.g., the Mid-Atlantic NN/LM Region) offered webinars and built websites to support public librarians in their efforts. WebJunction offered training workshops through its Health Happens in Libraries program. At the request of NN/LM consumer health coordinators, NLM's MedlinePlus Health Insurance page became a central repository of updated ACA information from NLM and NN/LM.

Despite organizational effort at all levels, pre-rollout anxiety remained [42]. Many public librarians did not know what to expect. Their uncertainty spanned many areas, from the anticipated amount of visitors with ACA queries to the likely nature of those queries. Public librarians had to learn about ACA, as well as allocate staff time and arrange computer space in order to provide support. Due to the novelty of the situation, NN/LM, ALA, and WebJunction could not always provide the information needed, nor could they reach every single public library in the country with the information. According to one informal study, only 57% of the 88 survey responders in Massachusetts reported having received ACA information links and training prior to the ACA sign-up [39].

As ACA information provision to the public takes place in the trenches of public libraries, not much published information exists about the preparedness and reaction of first responders, as well as about the process itself. At this time, our insight has to come from small-scale informal surveys and case studies. For example, Kara Kohn [43] informally surveyed "82 libraries" in Illinois and Margot Malachowski [39] surveyed 88 Massachusetts librarians about their experience with ACA information provision. Both surveys are reported in a format that makes assessing representativeness of their sampling impossible; and the authors, both librarians, readily acknowledge the tentative (in Kohn's words, "(very) quick and dirty") nature of their data.

According to both sources, very few librarians (e.g., 5% of those surveyed by Kohn [43]) felt that libraries should not be involved in ACA information provision in any capacity. What varied was the desired and anticipated level of involvement. At a minimum, libraries felt it was their duty to provide Internet access to online forms or help enrollees with print forms and refer patrons to additional resources [39,43]. Some felt uncomfortable with providing more, out of a concern for appearing biased in regard to a controversial political issue, as well as because of the challenging nature of the information.

Others, however, conducted workshops and trainings, partnered with navigators and certified counselors from outside organizations, invited speakers, and created web pages with local ACA information resources on their websites [39,42,44]. For example, the Waukegan Public Library became a 2013 IMLS National Medal Winner for its effort to support the ACA's rollout in Lake County, IL. The Waukegan library provided extensive training to its staff and offering bilingual signup support sessions. Building upon this success, Waukegan library also continued conducting its bilingual health literacy skills classes past the rollout period [45].

The Waukegan library experience provides a small-scale example of how information support of a specific need can stimulate larger health literacy support efforts. The opportunity also was noticed by the ALA. In 2015, ALA published Libraries and the Affordable Care Act: Helping the community understand health-care options. (ALA) As a professional development resource, the book helps librarians understand the basics of the ACA and provide support to enrollees. In addition, it calls upon librarians to use the process for "engaging adults in the expansion of their functional understanding of health literacy and financial literacy as they relate to both insurance and healthy living" [46].

The emergent story of ACA information support in libraries exemplifies the potential and the challenge of libraries' response to a novel, fast-developing issue. A number of questions need to be answered in order to evaluate the response. The field needs detailed data about the nature of the public's information needs in the context of ACA; librarians' readiness to support them, including specific challenges and concerns; and actual utilization of libraries for ACA information inquiries. Fitting the three pieces of information together will bring into focus the current state of affairs and highlight future directions. To obtain data about public librarians' preparedness and practices in support of ACA, NLM is currently conducting a nationwide survey of library workers in 20 states, ten with a federal health insurance exchange and ten with state-run health insurance exchanges, in collaboration with the School of Library and Information Studies at the University of Wisconsin - Madison [47]. At the present, it is clear that the complexity of ACA information underscores the need for improving American public's health literacy [48], an endeavor in which libraries will continue playing a significant role.

7. Librarians' Role in Health Literacy Support in the Clinical Setting

Librarians also support patients' health literacy and health information needs in clinical settings. Librarians can be effective leaders or participants in efforts to make health care organizations "health literate" [49]. In outpatient and inpatient clinical settings, however, their contribution to promoting health literacy most frequently occurs via their support of information prescription initiatives. Information prescription programs, often denoted as Information Rx, involve physicians supplying patients with "prescriptions" for quality evidence-based health information that is specifically selected to address the patient's condition. Prescribed materials may also be tailored to match the patient's other characteristics, such as preferred learning style and reading level [50,51]. These programs are more targeted to the general patient education or consumer health information services.

Librarians participate in information prescription initiatives in two ways. In one model, librarians educate clinicians about quality patient education resources. Many such efforts involve promoting the NLM MedlinePlus consumer health information portal and "Information prescription toolkit" that makes use of it. The toolkit is a box that contains several information prescription pads and some promotional materials featuring MedlinePlus. A large-scale example of such initiative is the Information Prescription Program, spearheaded by NLM in 2004 in collaboration with the NIH and the American College of Physicians and implemented and evaluated in a number of institutions [52,53].

Another model involves librarians filling the prescription by selecting and packaging information materials for each individual patient. For example, the Eskind Biomedical Library at Vanderbilt University Medical Center developed Patient Informatics Consult Services (PICS) dedicated to filling information prescriptions [54]. Eskind librarians created an "information prescription" referral form for clinicians to use with their patients. After clinicians complete the form, noting, in addition to the topic, any special factors that need to be considered, patients take it to the patient section of the library to fill. There, librarians put together a packet of targeted authoritative information and discuss quality information evaluation criteria with the patient. They also send a copy of the packet to the referring clinician. In addition to implementing PICS, librarians at Eskind also demonstrated feasibility of tailoring presentation of prescription materials to patients' learning style preferences, although the impact of this tailoring on patients' satisfaction and learning was mixed [50,51].

The University of Medicine and Dentistry of New Jersey's (UMDNJ) university hospital also has a successful information prescription program [55]. There, nurses send information prescriptions for inpatients to the school's Cooper Library via the hospital's clinical information system, indicating desired readability level of the materials. Librarians respond by using patient transport to deliver two copies of the information packet (for the patient and for the chart) to the nursing station. In yet another successful hospital implementation example, health sciences librarians at Englewood Hospital and Medical Center make rounds of clinical floors, asking nurses whether any of their patients need patient education information. Frequently, nurses either request specific information, or direct librarians to speak with patients about their information needs [56].

While librarians working with information prescription programs do not always come into direct contact with patients, such interactions have the added benefit of teaching patients to recognize health information quality criteria and navigating specific websites [54,57]. Going beyond this, Leisey [58] describes a unique project that involved an NLM-funded social work information specialist position at Virginia Commonwealth University Library. The goal of the project was to help cancer patients understand their condition and the healthcare system, manage information from multiple sources, and deal with emotional issues. Social work information specialists approached patients at VCU Massey Cancer Center offering on-site sessions that provided information and basic counseling. Some participants also received project-tailored notebooks that helped them record and organize information about their providers, treatment, appointments, labs, medications, and expenses.

Several potential enablers of information prescription success stand out in the literature. One is a close collaborative connection between the library and the clinical setting that it supports. For example, at the time of its highly successful information prescription implementation, the director of the UMDNJ Cooper Library was a member of Cooper University Hospital Patient Education Committee that included clinicians and hospital administrators. At UMDNJ, the impetus for the effort came from the top because a visit from the Joint Commission on the Accreditation of Health Care Organizations (JCAHO) recommended improving documentation of patient education activities in patients' charts. In contrast, at Englewood the initiative came from the library and its collaboration with the patient education oriented Meland Foundation. There, librarians' proactive visits to clinical floors to offer their services greatly improved nurses' utilization of the library for patient education [56]. As mentioned in an earlier example, integrating information prescription with electronic hospital records is another powerful way to embed the connection between the clinic and the library into the clinic's work flow [55].

Most research into the impact of information prescription programs focuses on clinician and patient satisfaction as outcome variables, often finding increase in satisfaction in both groups [59]. There is evidence that patients who receive information prescriptions are likely to fill them and develop positive attitudes towards the resources they promote [60]. These patients also intend to continue using prescribed resources in the future [61]. Siegel et al. [62] and D'Allesandro et al. [57] also found that information prescription initiatives decrease patients' visits to poor quality sites and increase utilization of the prescribed sites. Information prescription programs may also help foster a dialogue during clinical visits and improve provider-patient communication [62]. While studies point to a number of positive outcomes of information prescription projects, with a rare exception [50], they do not assess changes in patients' knowledge, health behaviors and outcomes. Factors limiting success of information prescription programs involve low levels of clinicians' buy-in or patients' trust in librarians' expertise. For example, Leisey [58] describes a patient who preferred to receive information from her doctor directly, without librarians' mediation. In addition, patients' high initial levels of health literacy and knowledge may limit effectiveness of information prescription [50,63].

8. Providing Health Information Relevant to Disasters and Emergencies

While disaster preparedness and emergency response has long been an established field, librarians' involvement is a relatively recent development. The involvement of libraries followed the realization that librarians often provide information support to professionals and the general public. At the same time, the disaster-related information needs of professionals and lay people vary according to a disaster's type and phase. For example, information needs during the preparedness phase differ from those during the acute response phase in the immediate aftermath of a disaster. Similarly, information needs in response to a flood or an earthquake differ from those that pertain to a public health epidemic. Yet, as the goal is always to minimize the impact on human life and well-being, health information is usually a prominent component of disaster information.

In the U.S., the period between 2001 and 2005 was marked by disasters of the magnitude that brought disaster preparedness and response to the top of the national agenda. The way libraries responded to these disasters, particularly the Gulf hurricanes, including the 2005 Hurricane Katrina, brought realization of their significant potential in providing support to the public and response agencies. As known, trusted, always welcoming community centers, libraries were natural physical places to which displaced residents gravitated. In the wake of Katrina, Louisiana libraries stepped up to the task by providing the public with shelter, phone charging stations, and Internet connectivity [64]. Librarians held children's programs, distributed water, and provided emotional support to evacuees.

In addition to providing general relief, librarians also used their professional information provision skills. Librarians assisted evacuees with information-literacy-related tasks, such as completing FEMA assistance forms and job applications, creating email accounts necessary for applying for assistance, and using databases to search for friends and family [65]. In addition, librarians provided information for emergency responders, including medical professionals. In recognition of their role, in 2010 FEMA designated public libraries as essential disaster response organizations, thus making them eligible for temporary relocation funding during disasters [64]. Two years later, public libraries of New York and New Jersey played a similar safe haven and support role when Hurricane Sandy struck the East Coast in October 2012 [66].

Growing recognition of the value of applying librarians' skillset to disaster preparedness and response led to a number of initiatives. In 2008 NLM established the Disaster Information Management Research Center and implemented a Disaster Information Specialist Program, which offers special training courses and information resources [67]. The program, as well as other efforts emerging throughout the country, led to increased librarians' participation in emergency preparedness teams at different levels, from hospitals to cities and counties. While the primary emphasis involves supporting professionals, some efforts also aim to support the public's information needs with regard to different kinds of disasters, including extreme weather events and public health epidemics.

One example of such effort is an NN/LM sponsored collaboration between the University of Miami Miller School of Medicine Louis Calder Memorial Library and Miami-Dade County Public Library in South Florida [68]. The area where the libraries are located is home to a medically underserved diverse population; it is also character-ized by frequent hurricane threats. In order to conduct health information outreach, librarians from the two libraries organized community fairs, raising emergency prepar-edness awareness and distributing preparedness resources, as well as more generalized consumer health resources. As part of the collaboration, public librarians used their community connections to promote the fairs, while medical librarians prepared infor-mation items. As the aftermath of hurricanes comes with a slew of environmental health concerns, from water pollution to mold growth in homes, Miami-Dade librarians promoted a number of NLM environmental health resources, such as Tox Town, a site addressing environmental health concerns in everyday places.

While librarians' engagement with disaster health information is gaining momen-tum, response to events with complex causes and courses may seem more professional-ly challenging for public librarians. One area of the public's concern and need for reli-able health information involves epidemics of infectious diseases (e.g., the 2002-2003 SARS outbreak, the 2009 H1N1 infections). In an article about Ontario public libraries' response to SARS information inquiries, Harris et al. [69] suggest that many public library staff may be unprepared to provide such information. Similarly, in a review of public libraries' responses to the 2009 H1N1 epidemic, Zach [70] notes that about a month after the first case of H1N1 was diagnosed in the US, only 15 out of 50 public library systems in the most populated US cities linked to CDC or other e-government information about H1N1. Overall, Zach [70] concluded that, despite some notable efforts, issuing risk alerts and providing epidemics preparedness information was not a priority for public libraries. On the other hand, while comfort level with specialized information provision will always differ by setting and topic, there are also responses of active engagement. According to the same author, some libraries not only linked to e-government information about H1N1, but also posted risk alerts and related messages via their social media channels.

9. Conclusion

Libraries have been involved in efforts to improve general literacy, information litera-cy, health education, and patient education for more than a century. During the past two decades, libraries and librarians have increased their focus on improving the public's access to high quality health information, expanded their participation in research and interventions designed to address variations in health literacy, and produced related training programs and evaluation tools that are relevant to broader audiences. This increased activity in the U.S. is due in part to the development of consumer health information services by the NLM and to training and outreach programs sponsored by NLM via the NN/LM and via partnerships with minority serving educational institutions and community based organizations.

Ensuring that the public has ready access to accurate and understandable health information and that health care institutions and public health agencies make themselves understood to those they serve are never-ending challenges. People are always confronting new personal health issues, new interactions with the health care system, and new imperatives to understand environmental factors affecting community health. Advances in information technology and changes in user preferences are continually affecting the ways in which people seek and obtain understandable health information, interact with health care providers, and engage in community efforts designed to promote health.

Libraries and librarians can be effective partners in conducting research in health literacy and in building sustainable health literacy programs within organizations and communities. Libraries are natural participants and important resources for community-wide health promotion interventions [e.g., 71] that aim to present their message via multiple channels in multiple formats and different locations throughout a community. With regard to research, librarians are well-positioned to conduct investigations into how patrons and members of the public select and evaluate health information resources and integrate information from multiple sources. They can also contribute to bridging research and practice by conducting systematic evaluations of their health information outreach projects and determining what factors enable or hinder their success [72]. Finally, when it comes to research, librarians can apply their expertise in comprehensive literature searches to conducting meta-analyses of the literature on the connection between health information literacy and behavior.

Although their capabilities will vary, librarians are likely to have knowledge and experience in locating and assessing the quality of health information; networks of contacts and relationships that span organizational divisions, disciplines, and stakeholders; and access to unique, although usually modest, sources of external funding. Involving libraries in community-wide health literacy programs takes advantage of libraries' position as a shared organizational and community resource, while simultaneously increasing the value of libraries to other health organizations and surrounding communities.

References

[1]   Donnelly FP. The geographic distribution of United States public libraries: an analysis of locations and service areas. J Libr Inf Sci. 2014;46(22):110-129. DOI: 10.1177/0961000612470762.

[2]   Smith CA. "The easier-to-use version": Public librarian awareness of consumer health resources from the National Library of Medicine. J Consum Health Internet. 2011;15(2):149-163. DOI: 10.1080/15398285.2011.573339.

[3]   Lindberg DA, Humphreys BL. A time of change for medical informatics in the USA. Yearb Med Inform. 1999;(1):53-57.

[4]   National Library of Medicine (US). Board of Regents. National Library of Medicine long range plan, 2000-2005/report of the Board of Regents. Bethesda, MD: National Library of Medicine; 2000. 39 p.

[5]   Miller N, Lacroix EM, Backus JE. MEDLINEplus: Building and maintaining the National Library of Medicine's consumer health Web service. Bull Med Libr Assoc. 2000;88(1):11-7.

[6]   Wood FB, Siegel ER, Dutcher GA, Ruffin A, Logan RA, Scott JC. The National Library of Medicine's Native American outreach portfolio: a descriptive overview. J Med Libr Assoc. 2005;93(4 Suppl):S21-34.

[7]   Bowden VM, Wood FB, Warner DG, Olney CA, Olivier ER, Siegel ER. Health information Hispanic outreach in the Texas Lower Rio Grande Valley. J Med Libr Assoc. 2006;94(2):180-9.

[8]   Dancy-Scott N, Rockoff ML, Dutcher GA, Keselman A, Schnall R, Siegel ER, Bakken S. Empowering Patients and Community Online: evaluation of the AIDS community information outreach program. Inf Serv Use. 2014;34(1-2):109-148. DOI: 10.3233/ISU-140720.

[9]   Selden CR, Zorn M, Ratzan SC, Parker RM, editors. Current bibliographies in medicine No. 2000-1- Health literacy. Bethesda, MD: National Library of Medicine, National Institutes of Health, U.S. Department of Health and Human Services; 2000. 33 p. https://www.nlm.nih.gov/archive/20061214/pubs/cbm/hliteracy.pdf.

[10]   Ratzan SC, Parker RM. Introduction. In: Selden CR, Zorn M, Ratzan SC, Parker RM, editors. Health literacy. Current bibliographies in medicine No. 2000-1. Bethesda, MD: National Library of Medicine, National Institutes of Health, U.S.   Department   of   Health   and   Human   Services;   2000. https://www.nlm.nih.gov/archive/20061214/pubs/cbm/hliteracy.pdf.

[11]   Institute of Medicine of the National Academies. Committee on Health Literacy; Nielsen-Bohlman L, Panzer AM, Kindig DA, editors. Health literacy: a prescription to end confusion. Washington: National Academies Press; 2004.

[12]   National Library of Medicine (US). Board of Regents. Charting the course for the 21st century: NLM's long range plan 2006-2016/NLM Board of Regents. NIH publication no.: 07-4890. Bethesda, MD: US Department of Health and Human Services, Public Health Service, National Institutes of Health, National Library of Medicine; 2006. 66 p. https://collections.nlm.nih.gov/ext/kirtasbse/101290062/PDF/101290062.pdf.

[13]   Burroughs CM, Wood FB. Measuring the difference: guide to planning and evaluating health information outreach. Seattle, WA: National Network of Libraries of Medicine, Pacific Northwest Region; 2000.

[14]   Wood FB, Lyon B, Schell MB, Kitendaugh P, Cid VH, Siege ER. Public library consumer health information pilot project: results of a National Library of Medicine evaluation. Bull Med Libr Assoc. 2000;88(4):314–322.

[15]   Snyder M, Huber JT, Wegmann D. Education for consumer health: a train the trainer collaboration. Health Care Internet. 2002;6(4):49-62. DOI: 10.1300/J138v06n04_05.

[16]   Wessel CB, Wozar JA, Epstein BA. The role of the academic medical center library in training public librarians. J Med Libr Assoc. 2003;91(3):352-60.

[17]   http://www.mlanet.org/p/cm/ld/fid=42. Retrieved October 17, 2016.

[18]   http://www.ala.org/acrl/. Retrieved October 17. 2016.

[19]   Swanberg SM, Dennison CC, Farrell A, Machel V, Marton C, O'Brien KK, et al. Instructional methods used by health sciences librarians to teach evidence-based practice (EBP): a systematic review. J Med Libr Assoc. 2016;104(3):197-208. DOI: 10.3163/1536-5050.104.3.004.

[20]   Medical Library Association. Health information literacy curriculum-toolkit cover ideas. Chicago: Medical Library Association; 2016. http://www.mlanet.org/p/do/sd/sid=461. Retrieved October 17, 2016.

[21]   Kars M, Baker LM, Wilson FL, editors. The Medical Library Association guide to health literacy. New York: Neal-Schuman Publishers; 2008. 314 p.

[22]   American Library Association. Health information 101. Chicago: American Library Association. https://web.archive.org/web/20151016072548/http://www.ala.org/rusa/development/healthinfo. 2015. Retrieved October 17, 2016.

[23]   http://learn.webjunction.org/course/search.php?search=health. Retrieved October 17, 2016.

[24]   Smith CA. "The easier-to-use version": Public librarian awareness of consumer health resources from the National Library of Medicine. J Consum Health Internet. 2008;15(2):149-163. DOI: 10.1080/15398285.2011.573339.

[25]   Eakin D, Jackson SJ, Hannigan GG. Consumer health information: libraries as partners. Bull Med Libr Assoc. 1980;68(2):220-229.

[26]   Cooper ID, Crum JA. New activities and changing roles of health sciences librarians: a systematic review, 1990-2012. J Med Libr Assoc. 2013;101(4):268-77. DOI: 10.3163/1536-5050.101.4.008.

[27]   Dervin B. Libraries reaching out with health information to vulnerable populations: guidance from research on information seeking and use. J Med Libr Assoc. 2005;93(4 Suppl):S74-80.

[28]   Henner T. An intergenerational approach to Internet training: student-led outreach to promote seniors' use of Internet health resources. J Consum Health Internet. 2009;13(4):334-346. DOI: 10.1080/15398280903340822.

[29]   Warner DG, Olney CA, Wood FB, Hansen L, Bowden VM. High school peer tutors teach MedlinePlus: a model for Hispanic outreach. J Med Libr Assoc. 2005;93(2):243-52.

[30]   Olney CA, Hansen L, Vickman A, Reibman S, Wood FB, Siegel E. Long-term outcomes of the ¡VI-VA! Peer Tutor Project: use of MedlinePlus by former peer tutors and the adults they taught. J Med Libr Assoc. 2011;99(4):317-20. DOI: 10.3163/1536-5050.99.4.012.

[31]   Olney CA, Warner DG, Reyna G, Wood FB, Siegel ER. MedlinePlus and the challenge of low health literacy: findings from the Colonias project. J Med Libr Assoc. 2007;95(1):31-9.

[32] Strong ML, Guillot L, Badeau J. Senior CHAT: a model for health literacy instruction. New Libr World. 2012;113(5/6):249-261. DOI: 10.1108/03074801211226337.

[33] Xie B, Bugg JM. Public library computer training for older adults to access high-quality Internet health information. Libr Inf Sci Res. 2009;31(3):155. DOI: 10.1016/j.lisr.2009.03.004.

[34] Chu A, Huber J, Mastel-Smith B, Cesario S. "Partnering with seniors for better health": computer use and Internet health information retrieval among older adults in a low socioeconomic community. J Med Libr Assoc. 2009;97:12–20. DOI: 10.3163/1536-5050.97.1.003.

[35] Woodson DE, Timm DF, Jones D. Teaching kids about healthy lifestyles through stories and games: partnering with public libraries to reach local children. J Hosp Libr. 2011;11(1):59-69. DOI: 10.1080/15323269.2011.538619.

[36] Boulos MN, Hetherington L, Wheeler S. Second Life: an overview of the potential of 3-D virtual worlds in medical and health education. Health Info Libr J. 2007;24(4):233-45. DOI: 10.1111/j.1471-1842.2007.00733.x.

[37] http://www.virtualability.org/virtual-world-locations/. Retrieved October 17, 2016.

[38] Clifton S, Jo P, Jackson S, Incorporating Wiis into health information outreach activities. J Hosp Libr. 2012;12(3):258-65. DOI: 10.1080/15323269.2012.692270.

[39] Malachowski M. Obamacare and the proper role of public libraries in health literacy. Computers in Libraries. 2014;34(1):4-9. http://pqasb.pqarchiver.com/infotoday/doc/1496060324.html.

[40] Pati S, Kavanagh JE, Bhatt SK, Wong AT, Noonan K, Cnaan A. Reading level of Medicaid renewal applications. Acad Pediatr. 2012;12(4):297-301. DOI: 10.1016/j.acap.2012.04.008.

[41] Vardell E. Health insurance literacy: implications for librarian involvement. In: Vardell E, editor. The Medical Library Association guide to answering questions about the Affordable Care Act. Lanham, MD: Rowman & Littlefield; 2015. p. 23-35.

[42] Collins LN. Healthy libraries develop healthy communities: public libraries and their tremendous efforts to support the Affordable Care Act. J Consum Health Internet. 2015;19(1):68–76. DOI: 10.1080/15398285.2014.988467.

[43] Kohn K. Taking our pulse: reactions to ACA from Illinois libraries. ILA Reporter. 2013 Dec;31(6):8-11. https://www.ila.org/content/documents/Reporter_1213.pdf. Retrieved October 17, 2016.

[44] https://americanlibrariesmagazine.org/2013/12/03/studying-up-on-health-care-literacy/.   Retrieved October 17, 2016.

[45] http://www.webjunction.org/news/webjunction/no-wrong-door-at-waukegan-public-library.html. Retrieved October 17, 2016.

[46] Goldsmith F. Libraries and the Affordable Care Act: helping the community understand health-care options. Chicago, IL: ALA; 2015. 112 p.

[47] Arnott Smith C, Keselman A. Consumer health information in public libraries: user needs survey. 2016. National Library of Medicine. In progress.

[48] Hessler KE. Health literacy and law: Empowering libraries to improve access to consumer health information and ACA compliance. Serials Librarian. 2015;69(3/4):334-346. DOI: 10.1080/0361526X.2015.1105767.

[49] Brach C, Keller D, Hernandez LM, Baur C, Parker R, Dreyer B, et al. Ten attributes of health literate health care organizations, discussion paper. Washington: National Academy of Sciences; 2012. https://nam.edu/wp-content/uploads/2015/06/BPH_Ten_HLit_Attributes.pdf.

[50] Koonce TY, Giuse NB, Kusnoor SV, Hurley S, Ye F. A personalized approach to deliver health care information to diabetic patients in community care clinics. J Med Libr Assoc. 2015;103(3):123-130. DOI: 10.3163/1536-5050.103.3.004.

[51] Koonce TY, Giuse NB, Storrow AB. A pilot study to evaluate learning style–tailored information prescriptions for hypertensive emergency department patients. J Med Libr Assoc. 2011;99(4):280–289. DOI: 10.3163/1536-5050.99.4.0.

[52] Jones S, Shipman J. Health information retrieval project: librarians and physicians collaborate to empower patients with quality health information. Va Lib. 2004;50(2):11–6.

[53] Jones SD. "Information Rx" project launched in Virginia. Nat Netw. 2005;29(3):20–21.

[54] Williams MD, Gish KW, Giuse NB, Sathe NA, Carrell DL. The Patient Informatics Consult Service (PICS): an approach for a patient-centered service. Bull Med Libr Assoc. 2001;89(2):185–193.

[55] Calabretta N, Cavanaugh SK. Education for inpatients: working with nurses through the clinical information system. Med Ref Serv Q. 2004;23(2):73-79. DOI: 10.1300/J115v23n02_07.

[56] Lindner KL, Sabbagh L. In a new element: medical librarians making patient education rounds. J Med Libr Assoc. 2004;92(1):94–97.

[57] D'Alessandro DM, Kreiter CD, Kinzer SL, Peterson MW. A randomized controlled trial of an information prescription for pediatric patient education on the Internet. Arch Pediatr Adolesc Med. 2004;158(9):857-62. DOI:10.1001/archpedi.158.9.857.

[58] Leisey M. The Journey Project: A case study in providing health information to mitigate health disparities. J Med Libr Assoc. 2009;97(1):30–33. DOI: 10.3163/1536-5050.97.1.005.

[59] McKnight M. Information prescriptions, 1930-2013: an international history and comprehensive review. J Med Libr Assoc. 2014;102(4):271–280. DOI: 10.3163/1536-5050.102.4.008.

[60] Beaudoin DE, Longo N, Logan RA, Jones JP, Mitchell JA. Using information prescriptions to refer patients with metabolic conditions to the Genetics Home Reference website. J Med Libr Assoc. 2011;99(1):70-76. DOI: 10.3163/1536-5050.99.1.012.

[61] Coberly E, Boren SA, Davis JW, McConnell AL, Chitima-Matsiga, R., Ge, B., et al. Linking clinic patients to Internet-based, condition-specific information prescriptions. J Med Libr Assoc. 2010;98(2):160-164. DOI:10.3163/1536-5050.98.2.009.

[62] Siegel ER, Logan RA, Harnsberger RL, Cravedi K, Krause JA, Lyon B, et al. Information Rx: evaluation of a new informatics tool for physicians, patients, and libraries. Inf Serv Use. 2006;26(1):1–10.

[63] Oliver KB, Lehmann HP, Wolff AC, Davidson LW, Donohue P K, Gilmore MM, et al. Evaluating information prescriptions in two clinical environments. J Med Libr Assoc. 2011;99(3):237–246. DOI:10.3163/1536-5050.99.3.011.

[64] Veil S, Bishop B. Opportunities and challenges for public libraries to enhance community resilience. Risk Analysis. 2014;34(4):721-732. DOI:10.1111/risa.12130.

[65] Albanese A, Blumenstein L, Oder N, Rogers M. Libraries damaged, librarians respond, after hurricane's fury. Library Journal. 2005;130(15):16-17. http://lj.libraryjournal.com/2005/09/ljarchives/libraries-damaged-librarians-respond-after-hurricanes-fury/.

[66] Rose J. For disaster preparedness: pack a library card? Morning Edition on National Public Radio; 2013. http://www.npr.org/2013/08/12/210541233/for-disasters-pack-a-first-aid-kit-bottled-water-and-a-library-card. Retrieved October 17, 2016.

[67] Featherstone RM, Lyon BJ, Ruffin AB. Library roles in disaster response: an oral history project by the National Library of Medicine. J Med Libr Assoc. 2008;96(4):343-50. DOI: 10.3163/1536-5050.96.4.009.

[68] Paulaitis G, Vardell E, Shipley J. Collaborating with public librarians to promote emergency preparedness and safety awareness. J Consum Health Internet. 2011;15(4):313-321. DOI: 10.1080/15398285.2011.623556.

[69] Harris R, Wathen CN, Chan D. Public library responses to a consumer health inquiry in a public health crisis. Ref User Serv Q. 2005;45(2):146-154.

[70] Zach L. What do I do in an emergency? The role of public libraries in providing information during times of crisis. Sci Tech Libr. 2011;30(4):404-413. DOI: 10.1080/0194262X.2011.626341.

[71] Smith M, Mateo KF, Morita H, Hutchinson, C Cohall AT. Effectiveness of a multifaceted community-based promotion strategy on use of GetHealthyHarlem.org, a local community health education website. Health Promot Pract. 2015:16(4):480-91. DOI: 10.1177/1524839915571632.

[72] Whitney W, Dutcher GA, Keselman A. Evaluation of health information outreach: theory, practice, and future. J Med Libr Assoc. 2013;101(2):138–146. DOI: 10.3163/1536-5050.101.2.009.

Health Literacy
R.A. Logan and E.R. Siegel (Eds.)
IOS Press, 2017
doi:10.3233/978-1-61499-790-0-433

Innovative Approaches in Chronic Disease Management: Health Literacy Solutions and Opportunities for Research Validation

Michael VILLAIRE[1], Diana Peña GONZALEZ and Kirby L. JOHNSON
Institute for Healthcare Advancement, U.S.A.

Abstract. This chapter discusses the need for innovative health literacy solutions to combat extensive chronic disease prevalence and costs. The authors explore the intersection of chronic disease management and health literacy. They provide specific examples of successful health literacy interventions for managing several highly prevalent chronic diseases. This is followed by suggestions on pairing research and practice to support effective disease management programs. In addition, the authors discuss strategies for collection and dissemination of knowledge gained from collaborations between researchers and practitioners. They identify current challenges specific to disseminating information from the health literacy field and offer potential solutions. The chapter concludes with a brief look at future directions and organizational opportunities to integrate health literacy practices to address the need for effective chronic disease management.

Keywords. Chronic disease management, health literacy interventions, collaborative approach, research in practice

1. Introduction

Having one or more chronic diseases along with limited health literacy skills poses challenges for individuals' ability to manage their condition(s). It is also a challenge for the health care system overall. These challenges include:

- Onerous requirements of chronic disease management,
- Cost of chronic disease care (to the individual and the healthcare system) [1],
- Cultural differences between individuals and their primary care providers, and
- Facilitating effective communication between these groups.

These overarching issues support the consideration and inclusion of health literacy concepts in supporting effective disease management among this population.

Health literacy plays a pivotal role in overcoming the challenges of chronic disease management, achieving health equity, and eliminating disparities [2]. Skills in health literacy mediate feelings of self-efficacy in chronic disease management [[3]-[5]], especially among minority and vulnerable populations [6] and those with low educational attainment [7]. Incorporating health literacy concepts in chronic disease interventions helps ease the burden of disease management and improve health

---

[1] Corresponding author: Institute for Healthcare Advancement, 501 South Idaho Street, Suite 300, La Habra, CA 90631; E-mail: mvillaire@iha4health.org.

outcomes. Opportunities exist to collaboratively create, disseminate, and validate these practices across a wider base.

Numerous studies have shown success in achieving goals of greater self-efficacy, disease management, and self-care behaviors. Combined with health literacy principles, these studies have increased knowledge of target population characteristics and health disparities within those populations. [[3], [8]].

This chapter will explore the successes of these innovative studies, identify opportunities for the intersection of research and practice, and discuss opportunities for dissemination. The chapter will start with a review of the scope and financial impact of chronic disease management, globally as well as in the U.S., and review linkages among chronic disease management, vulnerable populations, health-seeking behaviors, and limited health literacy.

Next, specific interventions are discussed within two chronic disease domains: diabetes and pulmonary-related conditions—specifically, asthma and chronic obstructive pulmonary disease (COPD). These interventions directly address challenges within the health disparities/health equity domain and show how innovative, tailored approaches can make a difference.

Opportunities for stronger collaboration between the domains of research and practice are explored. These include innovative approaches such as embedded researchers, exemplified by the researcher-in-residence and participatory research models. Benefits of these collaborative approaches are discussed, and examples provided where these collaborations can take place.

Strategies for collecting and disseminating results of such collaborations are provided, as well as additional tools for enhancing this work. The chapter concludes with suggestions for implementing these approaches, both within the U.S. and internationally.

2. Chronic Disease Management: A Short Overview

In 2012, chronic diseases—including cardiovascular diseases, cancer, diabetes, and respiratory diseases (namely asthma and COPD)—accounted for 68% of all non-communicable disease deaths globally [9]. Furthermore, chronic disease management is a costly expense that is directly correlated with health literacy. In 2015, the United States spent $3.2 trillion on health care [8], with the largest proportion allocated to chronic disease management at 86% of all healthcare expenses [10]. While the associations between chronic disease prevalence and high costs are robust, health literacy has been identified as an intermediate variable that influences the strength of (and potentially moderates) a deleterious relationship. In the U.S., wasted dollars directly attributable to limited health literacy are as much as $238 billion annually [11]; left unchecked, these costs could increase as much as tenfold [12].

The National Assessment of Adult Literacy (NAAL) found that 36% of U.S. adults have basic or below basic health literacy skills [13]. Further, only 12% of U.S. adults are considered proficient in health literacy, meaning that only about 1 in 10 have the skills needed to successfully navigate the healthcare system. Minorities and those with lower education and economic status are more likely to have inadequate health literacy [14]. Further, a vicious cycle emerges amongst seniors, who tend to suffer from multiple chronic diseases and often lack both health literacy skills as well as remedial self-efficacy [15].

Diverse studies demonstrate links between these vulnerable populations, health-seeking behaviors, and limited literacy/health literacy, particularly in the case of chronic disease management. Those with limited health literacy are:

- Less likely to seek medical treatment [16],
- Five times more likely to misinterpret their prescription bottle label instructions [17], and
- More likely to skip preventive and screening measures [18].

These individuals also:

- Enter the healthcare system later and sicker [19],
- Have a higher rate of hospitalization and emergency department utilization [15],
- Have less knowledge of their chronic disease [20], and
- Have poorer chronic disease management skills [20].

3. Health Literacy Interventions by Disease Category

This section provides a short overview of programs, projects, and interventions that utilize health literacy innovations. Target populations, specifics on interventions, challenges, outcomes, and recommendations for future research are included.

3.1 Diabetes

The World Health Organization projects that by 2030, diabetes will be the 7th leading cause of death in the world and 4th in high income countries [21]. Diabetes ranked as the 7th leading cause of death for American adults in 2014 [22]. The year prior, diabetes had the highest personal health care cost in the United States of $101.4 billion [23]. Studies suggest that mitigating these issues requires interventions that consider patients' perceived ability to manage their disease.

Among the challenges for providers and diabetic patients is the issue of control, or more appropriately, the *perception* of control. Findings in a recent study suggest patients with limited health literacy have higher perceived ability to control their disease. Patients with limited health literacy believed that they controlled their diabetes "well" or "very well," despite contrary test results [24]. This misplaced belief decreases the likelihood that these patients will make behavioral changes to improve their HgA1C, thereby impeding the path to patient self-efficacy.

Numeracy, or quantitative literacy, can further complicate patient self-efficacy. Patients with limited numeracy and low health literacy scores are less likely to correctly identify when their test results fall within prescribed ranges [25]. Quantitative literacy mediates a patient's ability to understand and utilize numerical data commonly found in patient portals with electronic health records (EHR). Limited numeracy and health literacy abilities are significant barriers to meaningful use of EHR-type data. Primary care providers need to take into account patients' quantitative literacy level when requiring their patients to understand, use, and act upon such data.

3.1.1 Successful Diabetes Management Programs

In the U.S., innovative programs created to address patient self-efficacy and low health literacy span a number of diabetes management domains. A review of successful U.S.

interventions suggests that when programs seek to move toward patients' comfort zones—teaching where they live, so to speak—more positive results are achieved. Disparities within specific populations can be identified and addressed through such targeted interventions. Example programs are discussed in the following paragraphs.

Targeted training for specific daily management skills can have a positive impact on specific skill sets [26]. For example, mothers given a targeted training on how to read nutrition labels on juice containers showed significant improvement in moderating their child's juice intake. This targeted training provided instructions on specific nutrition label components, including serving size, calories, sugar, and vitamin C. At a one-month follow-up assessment, participants retained knowledge of the daily juice servings recommended by the American Academy of Pediatrics.

Interventions that take into account one's socioeconomic and cultural background also have a high rate of success. An intervention deployed in Chicago's South Side showed positive results among African-American diabetic patients with low scores on the Literacy Assessment for Diabetes (LAD). All participants scored at or below the 4th grade reading level on the LAD. More than half of the participants were low income (less than $15,000 annual household income) and had less than a high school education. The 10-week course tailored educational content to limited literacy levels and socio-cultural aspects of the attendees. As a result, 86% of participants attended at least 7 out of 10 classes. Participants improved their diabetes self-efficacy scores, self-care behaviors, and clinical outcomes [27].

Evidence based practices within a goal-setting model is effective to reduce disparities. An intervention aimed to improve health outcomes among African Americans, utilized conversation maps, guides, group interaction, facilitation, and individual action plans [28]. Program participants were more likely to create a list of questions regarding their diabetes and speak with their primary care provider about possible complications. They also reported greater trust in their healthcare provider and showed increases in diabetes self-efficacy and self-care behaviors.

Culturally appropriate interventions are key to help those with chronic diseases successfully learn management skills and achieve self-efficacy. Interventions that seek to address cultural, psychological, socioeconomic, and social factors on the front end have a greater potential for short- and long-term success. One example is *Latinos en Control*, a diabetes intervention delivered through 12 weekly sessions, followed by 8 monthly sessions. This course addressed literacy challenges by using picture book food guides and limited didactic training. *Latinos en Control* favored interactive learning approaches and educational games, such as *loteria* (a bingo-type game). Sessions included hands-on, experiential education in food preparation and meal-sharing. Key concepts were communicated using storytelling modeled after *telenovelas*, or soap operas, which are popular in the Latino culture. Participants showed significant improvements in HgA1C at 4 months, though a significant difference was not maintained at 12 months. At the 12-month interval, the intervention group showed statistically significant improvements in diabetes knowledge, self-efficacy, blood glucose self-monitoring, and dietary quality [29].

Critical health literacy, or one's ability to evaluate and assess health information, also impacts self-care behavior. In a study of 249 elderly patients, those with limited health literacy had poorer knowledge and self-care behavior than those with high health literacy. The findings suggested critical health literacy was an independent determinant of improved self-care behaviors [30].

Many studies suggest those with inadequate health literacy know significantly less about their disease than those with adequate literacy [3-7]. Further, information-seeking behavior tendencies and proficiency are related to appropriate self-care, management of symptoms, and knowing when to contact a healthcare provider. In contrast, limited health literacy is associated with poor medication recall, non-adherence to treatment plans, poor self-care behaviors, poor physical and mental health, increased hospitalizations, and greater mortality. Those with limited literacy skills are up to 3 times more likely to have adverse health outcomes than those with higher reading levels. They also have higher HgA1c levels and are less likely to be physically active or to perform glucose self-control [24].

3.2 Asthma / Chronic Obstructive Pulmonary Disease (COPD)

Asthma and COPD are the third leading cause of death in the United States and the world [22]. The World Health Organization estimates that in 2015, more than 3 million deaths worldwide can be attributed to COPD [30]. In 2010, the United States healthcare system spent an estimated $32.1 billion in direct and indirect costs associated with COPD [32]. To combat these alarming statistics, innovative strategies are needed.

3.2.1 Successful Respiratory Disease Management Programs

Cultural awareness is critical in targeting efforts to help patients successfully navigate their chronic illness management. Ensuring successful collaboration between providers and their patients requires understanding of the unique needs of a specific population. This strategy helps build trust and often does not impose a burden on providers to implement.

Program efficacy may be improved by providing training and information in the patient's preferred language. It is also important to consider the parent's language preferences when treating their children. Many Vietnamese-speaking adults have English-speaking children. However, providing English-only asthma training and information to English-speaking children limited their parent's ability to assist with the child's asthma action plan. Incorporating the preferred language of the child and caregiver resulted in increased asthma knowledge, decreased symptom frequency, and improved asthma control, with no concomitant increase in operational cost [33].

Social media tools also have proven useful in communicating self-management tips from peers and creating a triad of parties interested in improving self-efficacy. Using tools with which specific populations are most familiar and experienced can support knowledge acquisition. A review of visual website bookmarks ("pins") posted about COPD on the social media platform Pinterest revealed several commonalities between users [34]. The study suggests that users tended to:

- Pin (post) more pictures of patients than providers,
- Pin (post) information related to self-management, rather than general information,
- Re-pin (re-post) useful infographics, and
- Incorporate verbal persuasion and social modeling in their self-management postings.

Increasing the availability and use of electronic personal health records (PHRs) provides another example of leveraging technology to assist with chronic disease management. Patient portals can often pose navigational challenges for patients, particularly those with limited computer literacy. Mitchell and Begoray (2010) provide an evaluation framework to assess the match between PHR software and several health literacy domains, including functional, interactive, and critical health literacy [35]. Using this framework, providers can leverage the capacity and promise of PHR to create a seamless care continuum for those with COPD.

The aforementioned programs require commitment and collaboration between providers and health system administrators. Integrating health principles on a systemic level (addressed later in this chapter) can provide a solid foundation for such endeavors and can lead to broad-based successes in chronic disease management populations.

4. Opportunities for Collaborative Effort: Intersection of Research and Practice

This section makes connections between the aforementioned programs and research conducted in chronic disease management. Opportunities for researchers and practitioners to collaborate on research to practice (or practice to research) projects are also discussed. Examples include, but are not limited to, the annual Health Literacy Research Conference, the Institute for Healthcare Advancement's (IHA) annual Health Literacy Conference, and the Health Literacy Listserv.

Bridging the gap between research and practice is a worthy goal for many reasons. Each of these domains has its own power and serves its own purpose, but the results can be exponentially better when practice and research join efforts. Forming such a partnership in program design and pilot testing allows researchers and practitioners to determine whether an intervention is successful at creating change within a population. Similarly, when a rigorously designed study can show significant outcomes, diffusing these practices into popular usage can only be achieved through awareness and partnerships with engaged stakeholders.

In a recent discussion "Communicating Clearly About Medicine: A Workshop," at the Roundtable on Health Literacy, National Academies of Sciences, Engineering and Medicine, suggested the need for researchers to be embedded in the chronic disease management processes. This provides an intriguing idea on how to simultaneously implement practices and gather data in (nearly) real time.

One such idea is the Researcher-in-Residence model. While traditional methods of bridging the gap between research and practice have met with limited success [36], the researcher-in-residence model provides, in essence, a real-time opportunity to identify and address barriers and challenges as they arise in practice [39]. Using this model in a participatory research framework, researchers and practitioners can collaborate on targeted interventions within specific patient communities. Researchers can help design and evaluate interventions, controlling for health literacy to create the most effective approaches. The researcher-in-residence approach enables the inclusion of a variety of professionals as resident experts to offer their unique knowledge and expertise [39]. A successful researcher-in-residence is someone who understands the rationale for particular approaches and can help problem-solve from this shared base of understanding.

This is particularly important for vulnerable populations, where traditional approaches may not be appropriate for the community. Program areas in need of tailoring may include literacy levels, cultural considerations, and addressing trust issues with clinicians or providers.

Integrating the participatory research approach into chronic disease management interventions similarly closes the gap between traditional randomized research approaches and practice. When researchers interact with members of the intervention's target population, valuable information regarding inherent barriers, biases, challenges, and limitations can be identified and addressed. Particularly when these researchers are members of the community, factors such as trust are enhanced, thus increasing the likelihood of success.

The questions to ask are: Who benefits from a collaborative relationship between research and practice in chronic disease management? Who benefits when this activity has a health literacy aspect? One place to begin is to look is at organizations with an interest in learning more about such collaborations. Universities or any academic program with researchers in public health, medicine, nursing, or related field naturally gravitate to these or similar questions. Those considering work for their thesis or dissertation, or related fellowship type program, also might have parallel interests. Faculty mentorship provides an opportunity to ensure rigor in research design. Although there are limitations in the scope of such academic programs, they provide an excellent opportunity for early career researchers to get exposure to meaningful, community-based research efforts.

Such programs can reach out to primary care entities in communities, as well as organizations and groups serving disadvantaged or vulnerable populations. Often these include, but are not limited to:

- Community health centers (e.g., Federally Qualified Health Centers [FQHCs] and Look-Alike entities in the U.S.)
- Hospitals / health systems / outpatient facilities
- Chronic disease support groups
- Faith-based groups providing support services for disadvantaged populations (e.g., homeless, single mothers, teen mothers, elderly populations, etc.)
- Social services agencies (e.g., Family Resource Centers in the U.S.)
- Public health associations and groups (e.g., American Public Health Association, the Society for Public Health Education, the European Public Health Association, etc.)
- Chronic disease educators (e.g., diabetes educators, kidney disease educators, etc.)

In the U.S., nonprofit hospitals often have longstanding connections in the communities they serve as a result of the U.S. Internal Revenue Services' requirements to provide Community Needs Assessments and Community Benefits. Regardless of tax status or nationality, nonprofit hospitals also can serve as a vital resource by connecting agencies with community efforts and vice versa.

A growing number of U.S. hospitals and health systems also are implementing evidence-based approaches to improve health literacy and benefit their patients with limited health literacy skills. By partnering with community efforts to roll out interventions, nonprofit hospitals can learn about existing efforts and provide guidance on testing the reliability and validity of an intervention. This approach minimizes the possibility of confounding variables and provides data that may be more suitable for study replication or secondary data analysis. Participant interviews on the quality, effectiveness, and appropriateness of health literacy and community-based initiatives additionally yield qualitative data to appraise and enhance an intervention.

5. Strategies for Collection and Dissemination

One major challenge for the health literacy field is to identify a central location to bring together the work done within the field. A comprehensive catalogue of health literacy research is needed to allow health professionals to efficiently review completed research and identify opportunities and potential collaborators for future work. Among these directions are a new and innovative portal for the health literacy (and broader) community, called the IHA Center for Health Literacy Solutions, as well as encouraging broader use of MeSH health literacy search term strategies in PubMed. Regarding the latter strategy, librarians are an excellent (and largely underutilized) resource for making suggestions and providing connections to resources. The website for the U.S. National Network of Libraries of Medicine (NNLM), https://nnlm.gov/, can serve as a starting point.

In addition, sharing results with trade groups that serve such populations (through journal articles, posters at educational meetings, etc.) can help disseminate results. In addition, patient activists and support groups are a very good source of data sharing. Study groups among students and practitioners are yet another avenue for sharing and dissemination. Academicians at these facilities can encourage such collaborations, especially in the context of extracurricular activities and internships.

6. Challenges and Future Direction

Numerous barriers exist to creating an ideal, iterative cycle between research and practice. Strategies for embedding collaboration may take a variety of forms. Inclusion of proposed dissemination tactics into research grant proposals, utilizing collaborative models as directions for further study, and incorporating rigorous evaluation methodologies in program implementations are a just a few examples of how to enmesh research and practice.

7. Solutions

From a health literacy perspective, one of the more natural, intrinsic approaches to address the needs of effective chronic disease management is to insert a team of health literacy specialists, charged with infusing health literacy principles throughout an organization. Many models of such integration exist. Many tools, and successful case studies, exist to ease implementation of this process. Tools include:

- Ten Attributes of a Health Literate Health Care Organization [40] (and accompanying guidebook [41])
- Health Literacy Universal Precautions Toolkit Assessment Tool [42]
- Consumer Assessment of Healthcare Providers and Systems (CAHPS) [43]
- Hospital Consumer Assessment of Healthcare Providers and Systems (HCAHPS) [44]
- Health Literacy Tool Shed [45]
- Toolkit for Implementing the Chronic Care Model in an Academic Environment [46]

Additionally, at the 2016 IHA Health Literacy Conference, a panel including representatives from The Health Care Improvement Foundation (Philadelphia, PA), Carolinas HealthCare System (Charlotte, NC), and Children's Hospital Colorado (Aurora, CO) shared tips and tools used to effectively and successfully integrate health literacy policies, procedures, teams, accountabilities, and metrics into their respective organizations.

It stands to reason that success will follow when engaged teams of providers and administrators implement health literacy principles and practices into their efforts to improve specific metrics, such as chronic disease management for their patient populations.

8. Conclusion

Efforts to move the needle on integrating health literacy strategies into chronic disease management must include the international healthcare community. Existing collaborations at conferences such as the annual Health Literacy Research Conference (HARC) and IHA's annual Health Literacy Conference, in addition to robust discussions on the Health Literacy Discussion Listserv, are good starts. The nascent International Health Literacy Association (http://www.ihla.org) is another vehicle to stimulate discussion and collaboration, as is the new health literacy journal, Health Literacy Research and Practice.

Leaders, in health literacy and in healthcare, who understand the value of health literacy must work collaboratively and strategically to generate awareness, and ultimately initiate innovative collaborations to eliminate health disparities and promote health equity. Increasing the knowledge base, while sharing programs, testing approaches, and disseminating results are critical to achieving these goals.

References

[1] https://meps.ahrq.gov/data_stats/tables_compendia_hh_interactive.jsp?_SERVICE=MEPSSocket0&_PROGRAM=MEPSPGM.TC.SAS&File=HCFY2014&Table=HCFY2014_CNDXP_D&_Debug=. Retrieved December 7, 2016.
[2] http://nam.edu/wp-content/uploads/2015/07/NecessaryElement.pdf. Retrieved December 7, 2016.
[3] Berkman ND, Sheridan SL, Donahue KE, Halpern DJ, Crotty K. Low health literacy and health outcomes: an updated systematic review. Ann Intern Med. 2011;155(2):97-107. DOI: 10.7326/0003-4819-155-2-201107190-00005.
[4] Heijmans M, Waverijn G, Rademakers J, van der Vaart R, Rijken M. Functional communicative and critical health literacy of chronic disease patients and their importance for self-management. Patient Educ Couns. 2015;98(1):41-8. DOI: 10.1016/j.pec.2014.10.006.
[5] Wang RH, Hsu HC, Lee YJ, Shin SJ, Lin KD, An LW. Patient empowerment interacts with health literacy to associate with subsequent self-management behaviors in patients with type 2 diabetes: a prospective study in Taiwan. Patient Educ Couns. 2016;99(10):1626-31. DOI: 10.1016/j.pec.2016.04.001.
[6] Shaw SJ, Armin J, Torres CH, Orzech KM, Vivian J. Chronic disease self-management and health literacy in four ethnic groups. J Health Commun. 2012;17(3):67-81. DOI: 10.1080/10810730.2012.712623.
[7] Friis K, Lasgaard M, Rowlands G, Osborne RH, Maindal HT. Health literacy mediates the relationship between educational attainment and health behavior: a Danish population-based study. J Health Comm. 2016;21(2):54-60. DOI: 10.1080/10810730.2016.1201175.

[8] Taggart J, Williams A, Dennis S, Newall A, Shortus T, Zwar N, et al. A systematic review of interventions in primary care to improve health literacy for chronic disease behavioral risk factors. BMC Fam Pract. 2012;13:49. DOI: 10.1186/1471-2296-13-49

[9] http://www.who.int/gho/ncd/mortality_morbidity/en/. Retrieved December 15, 2016.

[10] http://www.ahrq.gov/sites/default/files/wysiwyg/professionals/prevention-chronic-care/decision/mcc/mccchartbook.pdf. Retrieved December 7, 2016.

[11] https://www.cms.gov/research-statistics-data-and-systems/statistics-trends-and-reports/nationalhealthexpenddata/downloads/highlights.pdf. Retrieved December 11, 2016.

[12] Vernon J, Trujillo A, Rosenbaum S, DeBuono B. Low health literacy: implications for national health policy. Storrs (CT): National Bureau of Economic Research; 2007.

[13] https://nces.ed.gov/pubs2006/2006483.pdf. Retrieved December 7, 2016.

[14] Paasche-Orlow MK, Wolf MS. The causal pathways linking health literacy to health outcomes. Am J Health Behav. 2007;31(1):S19-26. DOI: 10.5555/ajhb.2007.31.supp.S19

[15] Baker DW, Gazmararian JA, Williams MV, Scott T, Parker RM, Green D, et al. Functional health literacy and the risk of hospital admission among Medicare managed care enrollees. Am J Public Health. 2002;92(8):1278-83. DOI: 10.2105/AJPH.92.8.1278.

[16] Baker DW, Gazmararian JA, Williams MV, Scott T, Parker RM, Green D, et al. Health literacy and use of outpatient physician services by Medicare managed care enrollees. J Gen Intern Med. 2004;19(3):215-220. DOI: 10.1111/j.1525-1497.2004.21130.x.

[17] Williams MV, Parker RM, Baker DW, Parikh NS, Pitkin K, Coates WC, Nurss JR. Inadequate functional health literacy among patients at two public hospitals. JAMA. 1995;274(21):1677-1628. DOI: 10.1001/jama.1995.03530210031026.

[18] Scott TL, Gazmararian JA, Williams MV, Baker DW. Health literacy and preventive health care use among Medicare enrollees in a managed care organization. Med Care. 2002;40(5):395-404.

[19] Bennet CL, Ferreira MR, Davis TC, Kaplan J, Weinberger M, Kuzel T, et al. Relation between literacy, race, and stage of presentation among low-income patients with prostate cancer. J Clin Oncol. 1998;16(9):3101-4. DOI: 10.1200/jco.1998.16.9.3101.

[20] Williams MV, Baker DW, Honig EG, Lee TM, Nowlan A. Inadequate literacy is a barrier to asthma knowledge and self-care. Chest. 1998;114(4):1008-15. DOI: 10.1378/chest.114.4.1008.

[21] Mathers C, Loncar D. Projections of global mortality and burden of disease from 2002 to 2030. PLoS Med. 2006;3(11):e442. DOI: 10.1371/journal.pmed.0030442.

[22] http://www.cdc.gov/nchs/data/nvsr/nvsr65/nvsr65_04.pdf. Retrieved December 7, 2016.

[23] EJ Emanuel. How can the United States spend its health care dollars better. JAMA. 2016;316(24):2604-2606. DOI: 10.1001/jama.2016.16739

[24] Ferguson MO, Long JA, Zhu J, Small DS, Lawson B, Glick HA, Schapira MM. Low health literacy predicts misperceptions of diabetes control in patients with persistently elevated A1C. Diabetes Educ. 2015;41(3):309-19. DOI: 10.1177/0145721715572446.

[25] Zikmund-Fisher BJ, Exe NL, Witteman HO. Numeracy and literacy independently predict patients' ability to identify out-of-range test results. J Med Internet Res. 2014;16(8):e187. DOI: 10.2196/jmir.3241.

[26] https://www.iha4health.org/wp-content/uploads/2015/03/Improving-Health-Literacy-5-Minutes-at-a-Time-Brief-teaching-intervention-improves-mother.pdf. Retrieved December 12, 2016.

[27] Peek ME, Harmon SA, Scott SJ, Roberson TS, Tang H, Chin MH. Culturally tailoring patient education and communication skills training to empower African-Americans with diabetes. Transl Behav Med. 2012;2(3):296-308. DOI: 10.1007/s13142-012-0125-8

[28] https://www.iha4health.org/wp-content/uploads/2015/03/Diabetes-Conversation-Maps-Journey-to-Better-Diabetes-Education.pdf. Retrieved December 12, 2016.

[29] Rosal MC, Ockene IS, Restrepo A, White MJ, Borg A, Olendzki B, et al. Randomized trial of a literacy-sensitive, culturally tailored diabetes self-management intervention for low-income Latinos: Latinos en control. Diabetes Care. 2011;34(4):838-44. DOI: 10.2337/dc10-1981.

[30] Matsuoka S, Tsuchihashi-Makaya M, Kayane T, Yamada M, Wakabayashi R, Kato NP, Yazawa M. Health literacy is independently associated with self-care behavior in patients with heart failure. Patient Educ Couns. 2016;99(6):1026-32. DOI: 10.1016/j.pec.2016.01.003.

[31] http://www.who.int/mediacentre/factsheets/fs315/en/. Retrieved December 10, 2016.

[32] Ford ES, Murphy LB, Khavjou O, Giles WH, Holt JB, Croft JB. Total and state-specific medical and absenteeism costs of chronic obstructive pulmonary disease among adults aged ≥18 years in the United States for 2010 and projections through 2020. Chest. 2015;147(1):31-45. DOI: 10.1378/chest.14-0972.

[33] https://www.iha4health.org/wp-content/uploads/2016/06/Improve-health-literacy-to-increase-knowledge-and-health-outcome-effects-for-Vietnamese-children-with-asthma-in-a-community-practice-setting.pdf. Retrieved December 12, 2016.

[34] Paige SR, Stellefson M, Chaney BH, Alber JM. Pinterest as a resource for health information on chronic obstructive pulmonary disease (COPD): a social media content analysis. Am J Health Educ. 2016;46(4):241-51. DOI: 10.1080/19325037.2015.1044586

[35] Mitchell B, Begoray DL. Electronic personal health records that promote self-management in chronic illness. OJIN. 2010;15(3). DOI: 10.3912/OJIN.Vol15No03PPT01

[36] Rycroft-Malone J, Wilkinson JE, Burton CR, Andrews G, Ariss S, Baker R, et al. Implementing health research through academic and clinical partnerships: a realistic evaluation of the Collaborations for Leadership in Applied Health Research and Care (CLAHRC). Implement Sci. 2011;6:74. DOI: 10.1186/1748-5908-6-74.

[37] Walshe K, Rundall TG. Evidence-based management: from theory to practice in health care. Milbank Q. 2001;79(3):429–57.

[38] Lomas J. The in-between world of knowledge brokering. BMJ. 2007;334:129–32. DOI: 10.1136/bmj.39038.593380.AE.

[39] Marshall M, Pagel C, French C, Utley M, Allwood D, Fulop N, et al. Moving improvement research closer to practice: the Researcher-in-Residence model. BMJ Qual Saf. 2014;23:801–5. DOI: 10.1136/bmjqs-2013-002779.

[40] https://nam.edu/wp-content/uploads/2015/06/BPH_Ten_HLit_Attributes.pdf. Retrieved December 8, 2016.

[41] http://www.unitypoint.org/filesimages/Literacy/Health%20Literacy%20Guidebook.pdf. Retrieved December 8, 2016.

[42] http://www.ahrq.gov/sites/default/files/publications/files/healthlittoolkit2_4.pdf. Retrieved December 8, 2016.

[43] http://www.ahrq.gov/cahps/surveys-guidance/index.html. Retrieved December 9, 2016.

[44] http://www.hcahpsonline.org/surveyinstrument.aspx. Retrieved December 9, 2016.

[45] http://healthliteracy.bu.edu. Retrieved December 9, 2016.

[46] http://www.ahrq.gov/professionals/education/curriculum-tools/chroniccaremodel/index.html. Retrieved December 9, 2016.

Health Literacy
R.A. Logan and E.R. Siegel (Eds.)
IOS Press, 2017
© 2017 The authors and IOS Press. All rights reserved.
doi:10.3233/978-1-61499-790-0-444

Learning from the Field and Its Listserv: Issues That Concern Health Literacy Practitioners

Sabrina KURTZ-ROSSI[a,1], R.V. RIKARD[b], and Julie McKINNEY[c]
[a] *Department of Public Health & Community Medicine,*
Tufts University School of Medicine
[b] *Department of Media and Information, Michigan State University*
[c] *Health Literacy Discussion List Moderator & Health Literacy Consultant*

Abstract. This study assesses the content of email messages posted to the Health Literacy Discussion List (HLDL) during a two-year period. The study identifies issues of concern to list subscribers, describes the purposes the list serves for health professionals, and contributes to the health literacy literature by providing an email listserv as a research corpus. The authors conducted an inductive qualitative analysis of email posts to the HLDL from October 2013 to October 2015. Using an iterative process, the authors identified descriptive categories for types of posts and topics of posts. The first (SKR) and second (JM) authors reviewed subject lines of all 2,036 posts and brainstormed type and topic categories, independently read and sorted a random sample of 200 posts into those categories, and then discussed discrepancies. Based on the latter experience, the authors combined, added, or excluded certain categories and jointly created a detailed description for each type and topic category. We then sorted another random sample of 200 posts and generated a list of key words relating emails to topic categories. A Cohen's kappa reliability coefficient was calculated to establish intercoder reliability. The third author (RVR) then conducted key word searches for sorting the remaining 1,836 email posts. The existence and frequency of email clusters and the content of emails in these clusters were used to identify and explore in greater detail the "hot topics" of interest to the field. Our analysis suggests the utility of the HLDL as a platform for sharing information and resources, announcements and calls for action, technical assistance and professional discourse.

Keywords. Health literacy, email listserv, professional development, community of practice, content analysis

1. Introduction

This study assesses the content of email messages posted to the Health Literacy Discussion List (HLDL) during a two-year period. The study identifies issues of concern to list subscribers, describes the purposes the list serves for health professionals, and contributes to the health literacy literature by providing an email listserv as a research corpus.

---

[1] Sabrina Kurtz-Rossi, MEd, Department of Public Health and Community Medicine, Tufts University School of Medicine, 136 Harrison Avenue, Boston, MA 02155; E-mail: sabrina.kurtz_rossi@tufts.edu.

Listservs are computer-mediated discussion groups by which subscribers can send and receive electronic mail (email) messages. Listservs provide professionals with similar interests the opportunity to ask questions and make requests, share resources and information, and discuss issues of common concern. Subscribers send and receive messages (posts) to all members of the list. Members can either respond to the email messages they receive from the list or simply read the posts and not respond. A key question is what purposes do lists serve for professional communities of practice.

To understand how the HLDL serves the health literacy community of practice, the authors identified categories for types and topics of posts made to the list. We sorted emails into types of posts categories to better understand the utility of the list for members. We sorted emails into topical categories to assess the substantive areas of concern to listserv members.

This paper reviews studies of lists serving professionals and presents background information on the evolution of Health Literacy Discussion List (HLDL). The authors detail the inductive methodology used to identifying types and topics of posts made to the list. We report common themes discussed and suggest the ways in which the list supports subscribers and the health literacy field of research and practice. Finally, we discuss how this work may serve as a model for future research.

2. Background

Electronic discussion lists, also known as Listservs, are used within many professional disciplines to facilitate communication. Professionals with similar interests use listservs to exchange email messages, share information, ask questions, learn from others, and discuss relevant issues.

Professional organizations and associations often maintain listservs as a service to their field. For example, the American Evaluation Association maintains a listserv for members to exchange information and ideas related to evaluation. As new professionals enter the field, the list serves as a forum for offering feedback and soliciting advice [1].

Some discussion lists are unmoderated and allow all messages to go automatically to all list members. Other lists are moderated, meaning all email messages are read by a moderator, before they are allowed through to the group. A moderated format screens for inappropriate posts and may help promote and facilitate interaction.

Listservs are increasingly valued as a setting for investigation. There is a growing body of research looking at how and why groups of professionals such as teachers, nurses, and librarians use listservs and the topics they discuss [1, 2, 3, 4, 5, 6]. Investigators have developed methodologies for content analysis of emails posted from listservs and demonstrated these methods as reliable and valid ways of conducting research.

In one example, investigators conducted content analysis of emails posted to a discussion list for councilor educators and practitioners [4]. Neukrug and colleagues examined 9,197 emails posted to the list over a three-year period [4]. They identified 20 superordinate and 17 subordinate categories using an inductive approach. The majority of posts represented resource requests (29%) and personal communication (21%). Fifteen percent were categorized as program development, and 7% were jobs related.

Another study identified types of posts and types of knowledge shared by nurses through an online community of practice discussion list [3]. Ten types of posts were identified with 56% categorized as knowledge sharing and 33% as solicitation. The next most common type of post was job postings (6%). Through interviews with list members, Hara, Noriko Hew, Khe Foon [3] found that the moderator was pivotal to facilitating knowledge sharing.

2.1. The Health Literacy Discussion List

Adult educators and health professionals began to identify a link between health and literacy in the early 1990s. The National Adult Literacy Assessment (NALS) reported half of American adults had marginal literacy skills [7]. The findings led to concerns about the complexity of health information and people's ability to take medicine correctly, self-manage chronic diseases, and fill out medical forms. Numerous studies document the mismatch between the reading level at which health education material are written and the reading skills of the intended audience [8]. Growing evidence points to health literacy as a strong predictor of health status and health outcomes [8].

Health professionals from many disciplines began efforts to reduce the complexity of health information and increase ease of access to services. In this way, health literacy emerged as a professional subspecialty for some and a primary professional identity for others [9]. Further exploration of the link between literacy and health outcomes by researchers created a growing evidence base. As an emerging field, interaction among professionals from health, education and many other backgrounds and training generated health literacy knowledge, intervention tools, and best practices.

In 1996, the Literacy Information and Communication System (LINCS) established the LINCS Health Literacy Discussion List as an ongoing professional development forum for literacy practitioners, healthcare providers, health educators, researchers, policy makers and others to discuss health literacy needs and strategies. At its height, the list reported more than 1,500 subscribers from the United States, Canada, England, Ireland, Taiwan, Austria, New Zealand, The Netherlands, and Israel. List activity dropped when LINCS converted the email format to a web-based platform in 2011. From 2011 to early 2013, the moderator received personal emails from members saying they did not want to log into a web-based platform. Members expressed their preference to read and answer posts through email and voiced a clear dissatisfaction with the loss of professional discourse.

In response, the Institute for Healthcare Advancement (IHA) offered to host a listserv using the original email format. The Health Literacy Discussion List (HLDL) restarted in October 2013. The HLDL has more than 1,600 members and is an active online forum for discussion among a wide range of professionals. The list moderator screens all posts before releasing them to the group and deletes any that are spam. The moderator also monitors the subject lines to make sure they reflect the content of the post. This facilitates future searches through the archives. To encourage discussion, the moderator posts Wednesday Questions and periodically invites guests to facilitate discussion of current topics of interest.

Although studies have analyzed the content of professional listservs to identify utility and topics of interest, none have formally assessed the Health Literacy Discussion List (HLDL).

3. Methods

The authors analyzed 2,036 email posts to the Health Literacy Discussion List (HLDL) during a period of two years (October, 2013 – October 2015). Subscribers to the listserv agree to have their posts viewed by other subscribers and stored as a body of knowledge that can be searched and referenced for research. We applied a mixed methodological approach of inductive naturalistic inquiry and heuristic decision making to identify thematic codes that emerged from the data [10-12]. As such, this research is a descriptive evaluation of text and limited to the specific topics subscribers raise as well as the broader categories of subscriber posts. The authors developed descriptive categories for the types and topics of posts through an iterative process. Types of posts categories provided insight into the function of the listserv for members. Topics of posts categories highlighted the substantive areas of interest to listserv members.

The first (SKR) and third (JM) authors reviewed the subject lines of all 2,036 emails posts as the first step in the iterative process. Following that review we independently developed lists for the types and topics of posts. We combined the lists and placed them on a white board to review and discussion. The second author (RVR) facilitated a collaborative discussion to agree on a common understanding of the types and topics categories. Note: the third author (JM) was the HLDL moderator during the assessed time period, and the first (SKR) and second (RVR) authors were subscribers to the list during the assessed period. Figure 1 displays the preliminary list of eight types of posts categories and Figure 2 displays the preliminary list of 95 topics of posts categories.

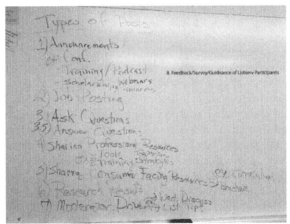

Figure 1. Preliminary List of Post Types

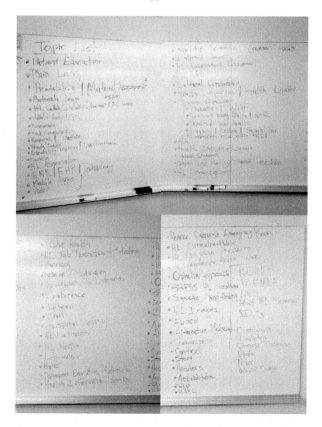

Figure 2. Preliminary List of Post Topics

The second iterative step involved creating a "tally sheet" to categorize a random sample of 200 listserv posts into the initial types and topics categories. The 200 posts were selected without replacement to the total 2,036 posts (i.e., 1,836 remaining posts). Each post received a unique post number (P) for identification purposes. SKR and JM independently read each of the 200 posts and categorized posts by type and topical area of interest. The tally sheets were returned to RVR to calculate intercoder reliability. Cohen's kappa reliability coefficient [13-14] estimates the level of intercoder reliability between raters analyzing qualitative data. Kappa values for the types of posts ranged from 0.42 (a "moderate" level of agreement) to 1.00 (an "almost perfect" level of agreement) [15]. Kappa values for the topical areas ranged from 0.09 (a "slight" level of agreement) to 1.00. The preliminary analyses suggested the need for further refinement as part of the heuristic decision making process [13]. During a weekly research meeting, SKR and JM each described their decision-making process to categorize posts by types and topical areas. RVR facilitated discussions and resolved disagreements on type and topics categorizing through consensus. Discussions lead to the development of a codebook containing the final list of six types of posts in Table 1 and 48 post topics in Table 2. The agreed upon list of types and topics guided the next iterative step.

Table 1. Types of Posts

Categories	Description of Categories
1. Announcements	This category primarily includes conference announcements and announcements for professional in-person trainings, podcasts, and webinars.
2. Job Postings	Included in this category are job postings from organizations hiring a health literacy position, and also questions about job descriptions.
3. Asking/Answering Questions	Posts placed in this category include questions from list members; answers to questions; requests for clarification; and thank you posts to those responding to questions.
4. Resources	This category includes asking for and sharing professional resources and materials (i.e. teaching tools, trainings, curricula, guidelines, print resources, websites, research articles, and other); and consumer facing resources and materials (i.e. brochures, booklets, curricula, consumer websites and other)
5. Service	Included in this category are requests for list members to provide feedback or guidance on policy or other issues, complete a questionnaire or survey, and calls for action affecting the field as a whole.
6. Discussion	Posts in this category were discussions of a theme, new idea or conceptual view of some aspect of health literacy, initiated by a list member or by the moderator. The two types of moderator-initiated posts are Wednesday Questions, posted most weeks and intended to stimulate discussion, and Guest Discussions, events scheduled for a few days to a week, where a guest moderator leads a focused discussion of a topic.

Table 2. Topics of Posts

Categories	Description of Categories | Key Words
1. Affordable Care Act (ACA)	Any post that refers to or is part of a discussion related to the U.S. Affordable Care Act (ACA).
2. Adult basic education (ABE)	Any post that refers to or is part of a discussion related to adult education, adult basic education (ABE), English language learning (ELL), ESL, ESOL, learner(s), teacher(s), tutoring
3. Alternative medicine(s)	Any post that refers to or is part of a discussion related to the alternative medicine(s) or home remedy(ies).
4. Assessment / measurement: individual	Any post that refers to or is part of a discussion related to health literacy measurement of individuals: screening tool(s), TOFLA, REALM, Newest Vital Signs, single question screen, health literacy assessment of patients, assessment in hospitals.
5. Assessment / measurement: population	Any post that refers to or is part of a discussion related to health literacy assessment of population(s): HLS-EU-Q, Ophelia, National Assessment of Adult Literacy (NAAL), BRFSS, PIACC.
6. Association, membership organization	Any post that refers to or is part of a discussion related to a health literacy association, membership organization, HLA, IHLA, AHL, I-HLA.
7. Award(s), funding	Any post that refers to or is part of a discussion related to health literacy award(s), grant(s), funding, scholarship(s).

8. Certification, accreditation

Any post that refers to or is part of a discussion related to a health literacy certification, accreditation.

9. Collaboration, coalition(s), partnership(s)

Any post that refers to or is part of a discussion related to collaboration(s), partnership(s), alliance(s) including all references to health literacy coalition(s), collaborate, collaboratively.

10. Conference(s), meeting(s),

Any post that refers to or is part of a discussion related to a health literacy conference(s), meeting(s), IOM meeting(s), summit, institute.

11. Consumer education, health education material(s)

Any post that refers to or is part of a discussion related to consumer education, health education materials (i.e., print, radio, websites, and other multi-media). Not social media or new technologies. NOT patient education.

12. Cultural competency

Any post that uses the term cultural competency, culture, cross-cultural, culturally and linguistically appropriate (CLAS)

13. Curriculum in the community or health setting for patients or the public

Any post that refers to or is part of a discussion related to a curriculum for teaching consumers or patients, community education, HLLI, workshop, k-12 school(s)

14. Curriculum for training health professionals

Any post that refers to or is part of a discussion related to training health professionals, continuing education, medical school(s), competencies, health professions educator(s), session(s), course(s), HLLI, syllabus, syllabi, webinar(s), professional development.

15. Disparities, health equity

Any post that refers to or is part of a discussion related to health disparities, health equity, unequal provision of quality health care. NOT social justice, privilege, power.

16. Definition of health literacy

Any post that refers to or is part of a discussion related to the definition of health literacy or a conceptualization of health literacy (i.e., two-way street concept).

17. Global, international health literacy

Any post that refers to or is part of a discussion related to global, international, or names a specific country.

18. Health communication

Any post that uses the term health communication.

19. Health literacy month

Any post that refers to or is part of a discussion related to health literacy month (HLM).

20. Health insurance, health insurance literacy

Any post that refers to or is part of a discussion related to health insurance, health insurance literacy.

21. History (how the field got started)

Any post that refers to or is part of a discussion related to the history of the field or how health literacy as a field of study and practice began.

22. Job announcement(s)

Any post that refers to or is part of a discussion related to a health literacy job announcement(s), job description, open position, employment, staff position, consulting.

23. Health literate organization(s)

Any post that refers to or is part of a discussion related to a health literate organization(s), Ten Attributes, assessment of organizational health literacy, health literacy environment(s), measure(s) to assess organizations

24.	Hospital, clinical setting(s)	Any post that refers to or is part of a discussion related to health literacy in hospitals setting(s), clinical setting(s), health care setting(s), doctor's office, medical center, including subcategories with references to emergency department (ED), emergency room (ER), healthcare system(s), hospital system(s), healthcare system(s), advanced directive(s), nurses, lab results, signage, wayfinding, navigation, navigator, universal precautions, patient safety, patient satisfaction.
25.	Humor	Any post that refers to or is part of a discussion related to humor.
26.	Informed consent	Any post that refers to or is part of a discussion related to informed consent in a hospital or health care setting for surgery or a procedure, or related to research.
27.	Language(s) other than English, interpreter, translation	Any post that refers to or is part of a discussion related to language(s) other than English, interpreter, interpreting, translation, multilingual, multi-lingual, other languages, non-English, Spanish.
28.	Legal	Any post that refers to or is part of a discussion related to legal issues.
29.	Librarian(s), health information literacy	Any post that refers to or is part of a discussion related to librarian(s), library(ies), health information literacy.
30.	Listserv related	Any post that is specifically listserv related such as etiquette and other guidelines from the moderator.
31.	Materials assessment	Any post that refers to or is part of a discussion related to materials assessment, readability, formulas, SMOG, Fry, SAM, CDC Index, PEMAT, check list, user feedback, user testing.
32.	Materials development, plain language materials or websites	Any post that refers to, requests for, or is part of a discussion related to developing plain language, easy-to-read, easy to use materials, website design, website guidelines, writing guidelines, design guidelines, guidelines for forms, survey(s) questionnaire(s), visual(s), image(s), headers, subheaders.
33.	Medicine(s), medication(s)	Any post that refers to or is part of a discussion related to medicine(s), medication(s), prescription (RX), labels, inserts, over-the-counter (OTC), pharmacy(ies).
34.	Numeracy	Any post that refers to or is part of a discussion related to numeracy, numerical.
35.	Patient education, patient education material(s)	Any post that refers to or is part of a discussion related to patient education, patient education materials (i.e., print, radio, websites, and other multi-media). Not social media or new technologies. NOT patient education.
36.	Patient engagement	Any post that uses the term patient engagement.
37.	Patient-provider communication	Any post that refers to or is part of a discussion related to patient-provider communication, oral communication, jargon.
38.	Public health, health promotion, social determinants of health	Any post that uses one of these terms public health, health promotion, social determinants of health.

39.	Research	Any post that refers to or is part of a discussion related to research finding(s), method(s), result(s), data, sampling, statistics, article(s), journal, participatory design, participatory research, research questions. NOT related to health literacy measurement or assessment.
40.	Practice, practitioner(s)	Any post that uses the term health literacy practice or practitioner.
41.	Risk communication	Any post that uses the term risk communication.
42.	Shared decision making	Any post that uses the term shared decision making or shared decision making aides.
43.	Social justice	Any post that refers to or is part of a discussion related to social justices, identity, bias, power, privilege, sexual orientation.
44.	Special populations / health topics	Any post that refers to or is part of a discussion relating to a specific population group or health topics of concern. Subcategories include pediatric(s), children, child, kids; teens, young adults, adolescent, youth; seniors, older adults, aging; pregnancy, prenatal, mother(s), maternal, maternity; disability(ies), accessibility, accessible; caregiver(s), parent(s); HIV/AIDS; cancer; women; flu; LEP, Immigrant(s), refugee(s), non-English speaking; diabetes; VA, veteran(s); incarcerated, prison, jails, criminal justice; mental health, behavioral health; nutrition; asthma; chronic disease(s); homeless.
45.	Story, narrative	Any post that is a personal story or talks about story as an effective form of communication.
46.	Teach-back	Any post that refers to or is part of a discussion related to teach-back, teachback, teach back.
47.	Technology	Any post that refers to or is part of a discussion related to technology. NOT including websites. Subcategories include chat, electronic medical record (EMR), electronic health records, smartphones, social media, mobile apps.
48.	Terminology, vocabulary, glossary of terms	Any post that refers to or is part of a discussion related to plain language vocabulary, glossary of terms, glossaries, terminology, common term(s).

A second random sample of 200 email posts were selected from the 1,836 remaining listserv posts. Using a revised "tally sheet" of type and topical areas, SKR and JM independently read and categorized the second sample of posts. The tally sheets were returned to RVR to calculate intercoder reliability. The kappa values for types of posts improved and ranged from 0.90 to 1.00 (an "almost perfect" level of agreement)[16] and kappa values for the topical categories ranged from 0.89 to 1.00 (a "substantial" to "almost perfect" level). To ensure and further validate the reliability for the topical categories of interest, RVR independently categorized the second random sample of 200 posts using the key word search function in Atlis.ti 7 [16]. Atlis.ti 7 key word search function includes the option to search and systematically analyze text using Boolean logic operators (e.g., AND, NOT, OR). Including the key word search results slightly increased the estimated kappa values for topical areas and ranged from 0.91 to 1.00 (an "almost perfect" level). The authors also identified clusters of "hot topics" most frequently discussed by listserv members from the total 2,036 posts. We elaborate further on the identified "hot topics" within the Results section.

4. Results

The authors extracted contributors' signature lines to examine the characteristics (i.e., location, degree(s) earned, and position title) of listserv members and identified 322. Of the 322 unique contributors to the list during the two-year period, 289 included a physical address within the signature. Nine countries were represented including Australia, Canada, Israel, Italy, New Zealand, Pakistan, The Netherland, United Kingdom, and the United States. The majority (89%) of addresses were located within the United States. We did not observe contributions to the listserv from South America and Africa. In terms of formal training, 22% of members listed a degree in Public Health, 17% in Nursing/Allied Health Science, and 11% in Library Sciences. In addition, 20 members listed a health literacy specific title in their signature line. Examples include, Health Literacy: Manger, Consultant, Director, Specialist and Coordinator.

4.1. Understanding the Function of the List for Members: Types of Posts

Categorizing types of posts provided insight into the function of the listserv for members. The results are displayed in Table 3.

Table 3. Types of Posts

Type of Post	Number of Posts	Percent of Posts
Announcements	170	8.3%
Job Postings	36	1.8%
Asking/Answering Questions	552	26.8%
Resources	382	18.5%
Service	21	1.0%
Discussion	799	38.8%

4.2. Identifying Issues of Importance to List Members: Topics of Posts

The authors identified eight "hot topic" areas of substantive importance to list members through our inductive approach. The eight topics of interest described here are: health literacy measurement and assessment, health literacy for public health, health literacy for health professionals, the U.S. Affordable Care Act (ACA) and health insurance, health literacy and equity, and health literacy collaborations. We selected example posts from HLDL to illustrate the diverse points of view associated with each of the topics. These examples were written by subscribers and taken verbatim from the HLDL, they were not edited or written by the authors.

4.2.1. Health Literacy Measurement and Assessment

Health literacy measurement is a recurring topic of interest to members of the listserv. For example, listserv members discussed the use of individual level health literacy measures in clinical settings:

> *Question:* I am reaching out to see if you might recommend a good instrument for assessing health literacy with older adults? We decided against REALM, but are using eHEALS and NVS. We are considering adding the brief health literacy screen. Do you have experience with this measure or alternatives that might work well face-to-face with this population? Thanks so much for any suggestions you can offer.

> *Response:* Most of my research is in underserved rural communities in South Carolina and I have found that most of the research participants cannot use the NVS. Thus, I have found the Single Item screen to provide some measure of health literacy. I am also interested in learning from the experiences others have with the various instruments.

> *Question:* The Joint Commission requires organizations to "perform a learning needs assessment that includes the patient's cultural and religious beliefs, emotional barriers, desire and motivation to learn, physical or cognitive limitations, and barriers to communication." Right now my organization includes a box to check for "literacy" in the learning needs assessment but we don't have a standardized way of determining when a patient/family has literacy barriers. I'm curious to learn if and how other organizations are using the learning needs assessment for health literacy.

> *Response:* My feeling is that time spent on getting valid patient feedback would benefit patients so much more than spending time on trying to figure out which patient goes in which category.

Listserv members also expressed interest in population based health literacy tools:

> Having coordinated the work on the HLS-EU-Q we are keen to use this instrument, but others may have good experiences, we can learn from. Thanks in advance....

> I am at the HARC conference now, and the folks who just released the data from the PIAAC study are about to share some findings with us. See piaacgateway.org. I believe this is going to be the next version of the NAAL.

Assessing the skills of health professionals appears to be an emerging topic of interest as one listserv member asked:

I am a research intern .... I am writing my Master's Thesis ... about Health Literacy among Primary Health Care Personnel and therefore I would like to request from you if you know already existing questionnaire that has been piloted and is available for using?

4.2.2. Health Literacy for the Public

Health literacy interventions outside clinical settings was another prevalent topic of discussion. The listserv moderator initiated an extensive discussion about health education efforts in K-12:

There currently exists a unique opportunity for health literacy advancement in K-12 education. Health literacy instruction in schools has historically been relegated to ancillary programs that are subject to budget cuts. Today, however, schools across the country are adopting the new Common Core State Standards (CCSS) in Math, English and Science. By aligning Health Literacy with CCSS it can become part of CCSS lessons and, as a result, an element of core instruction. We believe firmly that it is much easier to educate children in the concept of Health Literacy than it is to educate adults who typically already have some compromising health issue. Thanks for your interest. I hope others will join us in helping to insure that Health Literacy becomes a key element in CCSS instruction.

Other community oriented discussions focused on incorporating health literacy in adult and family literacy programs as well as English for speakers of other languages programs:

Question: I'm working on a developing a family literacy program for English language learners at my library, with a strong health literacy component. As a fan of the IHA's easy to read health books, I was looking into the IHA's HELP curriculum: https://www.iha4health.org/our-products/free-materials. I was curious if anyone on the list had experience implementing this curriculum. If so, I would be very interested in hearing how your program operated and any other details you would like to share!

Response: This page is rich in links to information on that may be helpful: http://www.ncsall.net/index.php@id=25.html. The sample lesson plans are very helpful. Also, there was some great work done in University of Illinois at Chicago, I think, on ABE and health literacy, but I can never find the curricula on the web. If anyone has a link, post it!!!! The lesson plans were great. A possible handout for you: http://say-ah.org/wp-content/uploads/SAY-AH-ENGLISH.pdf

Response: I would be interested in reading the answers to this inquiry. I remember attending an IHA Health Literacy Conference workshop a few years ago, where the speakers shared their experiences and outcomes with using the "What to Do When Your Child Gets Sick" books. Are there published reports on this matter?

Response: KidsHealth.org has a huge amount of content for kids, as well as for teens and for adults on a wide range of medical and behavioral issues - including very basic concepts. It's in English and in Spanish. There are a number of features that focus on helping family members talk to each other about important health topics.

4.2.3. Health Literacy for Health Professionals

Teaching and training future health professionals was a frequent topic of discussion as members shared materials to create clearly articulated learning objectives as well as tools and techniques to achieve competencies:

We have an undergraduate pre health class for our Interdisciplinary Health Services program. This program is a pre-program for a variety of clinical and non- clinical graduate programs (different elective tracks for each program) but they all take our health literacy class. I am uploading my syllabus as well. We also have an on campus and hybrid version of the class.

This summer I taught 'fundamentals of health literacy' to undergraduate pre-health students at the university. I am still working out some of the 'bugs' but found that the course was well received. The plan is to offer it annually as an elective. If you have suggestions for improvement, please share them with me.

Please share what anyone is doing for skill development or formal staff education. If you have any data of pre- and post-education that demonstrates results of your efforts in the way of improved patient satisfaction scores or fewer patient complaints centered around communication/education issues, etc. please share.

4.2.4. Affordable Care Act (ACA) and Health Insurance Literacy

Listserv members exchanged information and ideas related to the U.S. Affordable Care Act (ACA) and how to improve health insurance literacy. Given the introduction of the ACA in 2010, it is not surprising we found extensive discussion related to implementation strategies and materials:

Question: We're putting on our homepage a graphic about the ACA and how time is running out. I'm … concerned about the graphic and the wording. I think we should use the word "fine" or something less harsh than "penalty." A couple of other individuals who are doing this work, shy away from the word "penalty" because it is so negative – and I want people to make an informed decision, so if they are willing to pay the fine, that is well within their right. Thank you all in advance for your help! We're going to try to get this up tomorrow.

Response: Some people are calling the penalty a "shared responsibility payment" and some call it a fee. We are calling it a penalty and we give out a worksheet so people can figure what their penalty will be. Do you have a list of assisters & navigators? Telling people where to get that kind of help is good information to be giving out.

Response: You could call it a tax....that what the supreme court called it.

4.2.5. Health Literacy and Equity

Discussion of health literacy and cultural competency among list members appears to be an evolving topic. A listserv member requested clarification around integrating health literacy and cultural competency in healthcare delivery and training:

Question: We know that health literacy and cultural competence--or cultural sensitivity--are distinct, yet have many overlapping parts. If an organization wants to improve its capacity in both of these areas, how much is the effort integrated and how much is separate? How would you approach this dual challenge and why?

Response: I think cultural competence and health literacy are linked and that they need to be integrated systematically and integrated within all communications and interactions.

Response: I always include culture and language in my health literacy courses and professional development trainings. I used the Primer on Cultural Competency and Health Literacy (2013) to help me identify overlapping competencies and relevant teaching tools. I am really looking forward to teaching this new course... and learning from my students how well the approach works and what changes I will need to make.

Discussions among listserv members shifted from exploring equity in healthcare delivery to the topic of social justice, power and privilege in the healthcare system:

... last week our keynote speaker ... spoke of the social determinants of health. One of things she was adamant about is that it isn't "health equality" we should be striving for, but "health equity" – the subtle differences of which I had not truly understood until she explained it during her address...

… I have argued that our health literacy challenge is partially a result of the power and privilege of health industrial complex and how this leads to the oppression of patients. What I would like to see in future months is some discussion around power and privilege in medicine and any research that has examined it and how it impacts the communication flow between the system and patients.

4.2.6. Health Literacy Collaboration

Health literacy coalitions exist in a number of regions and states in the United States. Members of newly established coalitions post questions asking for support and advice. In response, leaders of established coalitions provide guidance and advice based on their own experience:

> I think that a coalition needs to start with a vision, a mission, goals and objectives decided by the members of the coalition. A vision is the big picture of what the ideal world would look like. The mission is a piece of the vision that the coalition wants to address, the goals are the focus of the coalition for a given period of time, and the objectives are the steps or processes to accomplish a goal. Ideally a coalition wants to start focusing on small, concrete goals that can be accomplished and used as models. Once those are accomplished, the coalition can serve more people with the same goal or decide on new goals.

> We begin each quarterly membership meeting by going around the room so that all of the 40+ participants we typically draw can introduce themselves and tell a little about their current health literacy projects. At the end of that exercise I always have the same reaction: the diversity of professions and organizations that seek a community of interest under the health literacy tent is awesome. I'm not the first to observe that health literacy is the common ground where public health, clinical care, and health services policy nourish each other. [The state coalition] deliberately cultivates that sense of health literacy as a commodious space for cross-disciplinary conversations.

4.2.7. Health Literate Organizations and Interventions in Healthcare

Numerous discussions centered on health literacy interventions in healthcare and clinical settings, and the concept of a health literate organization. Listserv members requested and exchanged information as well as offered to discuss interventions and available resources offline with others:

> *Request:* I am brainstorming for Health Literacy Month at my organization, and I would love to hear about the successes that you have had in the past especially when it comes to events/programs geared towards clinical staff. We are planning to do some tabling and set up some passive displays but it would be great to engage

staff in other ways. If you have ideas or experiences around this I (and presumably others!) would love to hear them.

Response: I just completed a project on this [signage] in primary care clinics. You can contact me directly if you would like to discuss. I used photography as a tool to explain to stakeholders and leaders what makes good signage, and what doesn't, after an in-depth assessment.

Response: Building Health Literate Organizations: A Guidebook to Achieving Organizational Change describes how organizations can move forward in achieving the attributes described in the Institute of Medicine discussion paper, "Ten Attributes of Health Literate Health Care Organizations". The guidebook offers an approach that enables organizations to start where they can begin to build a pattern of success, expanding to more than one area, eventually working in all key areas for results that can be sustained.

Response: We do not include it [teach back] in our policy as making policies too prescriptive opens brings the potential for liability and Joint Commission penalty if the policy is not followed 100% of the time. Teach back is taught and its use encouraged. It is documented in the patient education section of the EHR.

4.2.8. Plain Language Health Information

Listserv members frequently requested guidelines and information to develop materials in plain language and received invaluable expertise and exchange of resources:

Question: Does anyone know of any reasons why questions should or should not be used as headers/subheads in communications to the member/lay audience? I'm specifically looking for any guidelines, studies, or other evidence (e.g., expert opinions) that provide reasons either for or against this practice.

Response: Here is an article she wrote for PLAIN (Federal). It doesn't address headings as questions specifically but does say people like headings.

Question: The persons at the facilities with whom we are working have asked us to use very basic patient education materials due to the many factors that we know this population faces. Although we have education on all these topics, even 6-8th grade level literacy seems too high. Any suggestion of where to look for materials?

Response: Some of the sources I go to for some of the best clear, basic descriptions of medical conditions are through sources that have information in multiple languages. Some of these can be most easily found on MedlinePlus on their "Health Information in Multiple Languages" link. You can see they also have an "Easy-to-Read Materials" link, but those are not always 6th-8th grade.

Question: What are your thoughts on the best readability tool? Is there a HL industry standard? I have been trained in many of them and can't figure out which one is best.

Response: I suggest you look at CMS' Toolkit on Making Written Material Clear and Effective, Part 7: Using readability formulas: A cautionary note (https://www.cms.gov/Outreach-and-Education/Outreach/WrittenMaterials Toolkit/ToolkitPart07.html). Also look at tools that measure understandability and actionability, e.g., AHRQ's Patient Education Materials Assessment Tool (PEMAT - www.ahrq.gov/pemat) and CDC's Clear Communication Index (www.cdc.gov/ccindex/).

5. Discussion

This study describes how subscribers to the Health Literacy Discussion List (HLDL) use the service and what topics of discussion are of interest. The findings add to a growing body of literature that uses electronic discussion lists as a setting and corpus for research.

Among the study's limitations, the study's findings reflect only the assessed two-year time frame - from October 2013 to October 2015. The findings are limited to the activities of involved HLDL subscribers. The findings may or may not apply to subscribers who receive but do not interact with the listserv. The authors acknowledge a potential for selection bias since we are health literacy practitioners and were involved in HLDL activities during the study's assessed time period. Conversely, the authors' knowledge, experience, and involvement in HLDL and health literacy practice may have helped detect patterns in subscriber use.

In terms of basic use, the results suggest HLDL supports health literacy professionals by raising diverse topics and providing peer-generated feedback. Among its peer services, the HLDL: asks and answers questions; shares information and resources; provides technical assistance; and is a platform for professional discourse. The authors found subscribers use the list for: announcements; asking and answering questions; sharing resources; and discussion.

The majority of announcements are to promote professional development opportunities including conferences and online trainings. Subscribers also seek feedback, such as technical assistance regarding intervention approaches as well as sharing professional and consumer resources. Subscribers who are most inclined to use the list as a feedback resource, seem to be students or practitioners who are in the nascent stage of a health literacy job or career. These findings are consistent with other studies of how health and non-health professionals use a peer, subscriber listserv 1-6, 17, 18].

In terms of subscriber background, while some email lists serve subscribers with similar professional training, HLDL's members are professionally diverse. Nurses, librarians, and public health professionals all subscribe and use the HLDL.

By analyzing the listserv's signature lines, the authors found subscribers also represent an array of 20 job titles that include the words 'health literacy,' including Health Literacy Manager and Health Literacy Coordinator.

Interestingly, some subscribers described that professional isolation is an operant challenge for some health literacy practitioners around the world. For example, one subscriber posted: "I'm the only one in my workplace who is advocating for health literacy." Apparently for these and other subscribers, the HLDL is a place where health literacy practitioners create a sense of community and peer support. Some other specific health literacy issues discussed within the HLDL include: health literacy research and assessment; how the U.S. Affordable Care Act and health insurance impact health literacy; health literacy interventions in healthcare settings; peer coalition building; providing or finding plain language health information; and the training of health literacy and other health professionals [1].

In contrast, with one exception there was little interaction among HLDL subscribers regarding contemporary health information technological (HIT) issues, such as the use of social media to improve public access to health information and services as well as HIT interventions to improve health outcomes. Yet, HLDL subscribers discussed their experiences with electronic medical records (EMRs). Subscribers asked questions, shared resources, and discussed the implications of integrating a health literacy measure within patient EMRs.

In addition, some subscribers used the HLDL for what the authors term 'service to the field.' In these cases, subscribers would ask peers to take action in some way, or formally share their expertise in a survey. In one case, subscribers were asked to review the new design of a U.S. government website and provide feedback. In another case, subscribers were asked to advocate for the inclusion of health literacy questions in the U.S. Behavioral Risk Factor Surveillance System (BRFSS) survey and to give feedback on a set of draft questions. Another small, but noteworthy, use of the list is to post health literacy job announcements.

The findings additionally suggest subscribers appreciated the role and presence of HLDL's moderator. The study suggests subscribers value the ability of a moderator to facilitate peer discussion. The positive influence of the list moderator to generate discussion and engage subscribers is consistent with previous research [6].

The current research contributes to the growing literature on electronic discussion lists (listservs) as a setting for research. The study's methods include the use of an independent coding tool to assess the face validity of researcher-derived findings.

Finally, the study suggests electronic data can be a data corpus for researchers who wish to assess the content of electronic mediated communication. The current research describes the specific listserv use of some health literacy practitioners and suggests the importance of online discussions about research and practice within a professional community.

6. Implications

The authors suggest three broader implications of the HLDL for health literacy knowledge and practice: as an information repository, as a site for professional development, and as a forum for identifying needs and solutions prior to discourse at professional meetings and in publications.

First, the HLDL serves as an information repository for the field of health literacy. As pointed out, listserv members did not use the web-based version of the list for approximately two years. The change from an email listserv to a web-based system from 2011 to early 2013 resulted in a loss of professional discourse. To develop and maintain a corpus of professional thought, it is critical to have a communication system such as the HLDL the health literacy community of practice will use.

Second, the list serves the field as a site for peer to peer professional development and support. Similar to other professional listservs, the HLDL serves as a means to request information and share best practices. The HLDL is especially important to the development and socialization of new professionals and students. Long term subscribers share institutional knowledge of the field, while new subscribers ask for insights about ideas and practices.

Third, the HLDL is a forum where new topics and challenges (such as the adoption of electronic medical records) are discussed before they appear at conferences or in professional papers. During the early iterations of analysis, the authors also identified information communication technologies (ICTs) such as mobile app, webinars, chat, and social media as topics of discussion. The proliferation of ICTs highlight a need and opportunity not fully realized to utilize new technologies and ICTs to leverage and enhance health literacy practice.

7. Conclusions

Electronic discussion lists are a valuable mechanism for professional discourse and development. Content analysis of the HLDL suggests that a diverse group of professionals interested in health literacy use the list to make announcements, ask and answer questions, share information and resources, and discuss practical and conceptual issues.

Topics of discussion largely mirror those reflective of the time period and include "hot topics" such as assessment and measurement, the U.S. Affordable Care Act, and creating health literate organizations. List members also addressed topics that are not yet being addressed in research or publications but warrant more immediate outlets for discussion because they are already confronted in practice. Examples include electronic medical records and a growing interest in exploring the relationship between health literacy, equity, and social justice. The list and its members serve as a source for expertise and input on issues that affect the field as a whole, and a corpus for research and tracking emerging concepts that will shape development of health literacy study and practice.

References

[1] Christie CA, Azzam T. What's all the talk about? Examining EVALTALK, an evaluation listserv. Am J Eval. 2004; 25(2): 219-234. DOI 10.1177/109821400402500206.
[2] Bar-Ilan J, Assouline B. A content analysis of PUBYAC-- a preliminary study. ITAL. 1997; 16(4): 165-174.
[3] Hara N, Hew KF. Knowledge - sharing in an online community of healthcare professionals. Info Technology & People. 2007; 20(3): 235-261. DOI: 10.1108/09593840710822859.

[4] Neukrug E, Cicchetti R, Forman J, Kyser N, McBride R, Wisinger S. A content analysis of CESNET-L e-mail messages: directions for information delivery in higher education. J Comput High Educ. 2010; 22(1): 60-72. DOI: 10.1007/s12528-010-9029-0.

[5] Pennington T, Wilkinson C, Vance J. Physical educators online: what is on the minds of teachers in the trenches? Physical Educator. 2004; 61(1): 45.

[6] Wildemuth BM, Crenshaw L, Jenniches W, Harmes JC. What's everybody talking about?: Message functions and topics on electronic lists and newsgroups in information and library science. JELIS. 1997; 38(2): 137-156. DOI: 10.2307/40324217.

[7] Rudd R, Kirsch I, Yamamoto K. Literacy and health in America. In: Educational Testing Service. Princeton, NJ, 2004.

[8] Nielsen-Bohlman L, Panzer AM, Kindig DA. Health literacy: a prescription to end confusion. Washington, DC: The National Academies Press, 2004.

[9] World Education. Health literacy: new field, new opportunities. 2004; Boston, MA· http://www.healthliteracy.worlded.org/docs/tutorial/SWF/flashcheck/main.htm.

[10] Glaser B, Strauss A. The discovery grounded theory: strategies for qualitative inquiry, Chicago, IL: Aldin, 1967.

[11] Lincoln YS, Guba EG. Naturalistic inquiry. Sage, 1985.

[12] Vaast E, Walsham G. Grounded theorizing for electronically mediated social contexts, Eur. J. Inf. Syst. 2013; 22(1): 9-25. DOI: 10.1057/ejis.2011.26.

[13] Cohen J. Weighted Kappa: nominal scale agreement provision for scaled disagreement or partial credit, Psychol. Bull. 1968; 70(4): 213.

[14] Fleiss JL, Cohen J. The equivalence of weighted kappa and the intraclass correlation coefficient as measures of reliability. Educ. Psychol. Meas. 1973.

[15] Landis JR, Koch GG. The measurement of observer agreement for categorical data. Biometrics. 1977; 33(1): 159-174. DOI: 10.2307/2529310.

[16] Scientific Software Development GmbH, ATLAS.ti Version 7. In: Berlin, 2015.

[17] Irvine-Smith S. A series of encounters: The information behaviour of participants in a subject-based electronic discussion list. J. Info. Know. Mgmt. 2010; 09(03): 183-201. DOI: 10.1142/S0219649210002619 10.1142/S0219649210002619</p>.

[18] Marty PF, Alemanne ND. Engaging the experts in museum computing: seven years of queries on MCN-L. Curator 2013; 56(4): 421-433. DOI: 10.1111/cura.12042.

Health Literacy
R.A. Logan and E.R. Siegel (Eds.)
IOS Press, 2017
doi:10.3233/978-1-61499-790-0-464

Social Media: A Path to Health Literacy

Michelle ROBERTS[a],[1] Lizz CALLAHAN[b] and Catina O'LEARY[c]

[a] Health Literacy Media, Creative Director
[b] Health Literacy Media, Health Literacy Projects Manager
[c] Health Literacy Media, President and CEO

Abstract. Social media – websites and other online tools called social networks – serve as a tool to connect people and organizations around topics of common interest. Social media platforms offer tremendous opportunity to engage quickly and sometimes in depth with many and diverse stakeholders as people have the ability to communicate back-and-forth from anywhere in the world. As increasing numbers of people receive their news and health information online, it is important to ensure content delivered through online resources is accessible to diverse target audiences. This chapter discusses a mid-sized health literacy nonprofit organizations' social media philosophy and tactics during the past 10 years, as both social media and health literacy strategies evolved continuously. The integration of social media in health literacy program content depends on the use with best evidence health literacy strategies, such as the use of plain language techniques. Strategy and technical considerations for the implementation and integration of social media within a health literate health communications model are discussed.

Keywords. Health literacy, social media, communication

1. Introduction

Social media include websites and other online tools (called social networks) that enable people and organizations to get, create, and share content by interacting with others about topics of common interest. Examples of social networks include Facebook, Twitter, Instagram, LinkedIn, YouTube, and more.

Social media are a powerful mode of communication because they enable adults and adolescents to align around interpersonal relationships and common interests. Social networks also make it easier for users to remain in touch through the sharing of content and updates. Social media quickly mobilize people around issues that matter to them, and help to keep them informed. In fact, almost one-in-three Americans now get their news online, often through social media.

Social media and health literacy are interconnected, especially in the field of health promotion. A meta-analysis from O'Mara suggests that broad, generic health promotion programs and campaigns often fail to engage diverse communities because their health communication strategies overlook the unique culture and language of segmented populations as well as health literacy principles [1]. O'Mara suggests some important health literacy principles that could be more applied to improve health promotion and communication include: knowing the audience, understanding the

---

[1] Corresponding author: Michelle D. Roberts, MEd, MSJ, Creative Director, Health Literacy Missouri, 911 Washington Ave., Suite 625, St. Louis, MO 63101; E-mail: mroberts@healthliteracy.media

purpose of health messages, and creating social media messages to tailor to diverse populations.

Never before has it been more important to reach out to healthcare consumers online. The Pew Research Internet Project reports health information is one of the primary topics that people search on the Internet [2]. The use of digital media also has surpassed the amount of time most consumers spend with television, or other traditional media [2]. More than 60 percent of smartphone owners have used their phone to obtain information about a health condition, which makes social media a compelling platform for health promotion, health communication, and health literacy interventions [2].

Social media additionally are becoming a way to reach vulnerable populations and persons who are most impacted by health literacy barriers. For example, low-income and rural Americans rely on smartphones to access the internet and are more likely to use a smartphone to look for information about life decisions, such as individual and population health conditions [3]. Forty percent of adults in rural communities use at least one social media site [3]. Fifteen percent of Americans ages 18-29 rely on a smartphone for online access, as do 13 percent of persons with a yearly household income less than $30,000 [3].

The use of smartphone-friendly social media additionally provides a means to reach minority audiences. Twelve percent of U.S; African Americans and 13 percent of Latinos rely on a smartphone, compared with 4 percent of whites [3].

Social media are a powerful tool when they are used to widely disseminate clear and timely health information. According to a 2016 Pew Research Center survey, there are 1.86 billion monthly active Facebook users, 600 million monthly active Instagram users, and 317 million monthly active Twitter users [4].

No other mass medium provides similar direct-to-consumer interactive opportunities. No other mass medium provides real-time access where communicators can tell stories, release news, provide live-stream events, interviews, create original content, share and promote events, and pay to place customized content with the audience you seek to reach.

To optimize social media use, Korda suggests clear health information should be tailored to the demographic profile of the intended audience and users should be encouraged to participate and share content [5]. Korda adds that health promotion, health communication, and health literacy interventions can be based on theories of social and behavioral change [5].

Social media also are a powerful tool to spread clear health information, along with advancing partnerships among organizations that serve low-income populations, as well as face-to-face outreach, messages and messengers, and efforts to meet basic needs such as food and shelter [6].

With this background in mind, this chapter reviews the social media efforts of one organization that has tried to embed social media initiatives within health literacy principles. The chapter is divided into five sections. Section two outlines the history of Health Literacy Media, formerly Health Literacy Missouri, a nonprofit health literacy center located in the Midwestern region of the U.S. Section three addresses how HLM utilizes social media to establish its credibility and prominence as a health literacy expert and service provider. Section four focuses on how HLM uses its social media and digital expertise as a health literacy tool for its customers. The concluding section provides suggestions about how to use social media to improve health literacy for diverse populations.

2. The History of Health Literacy Media (HLM)

Health Literacy Media, established in December 2009 as Health Literacy Missouri, is one of the U.S.' largest health literacy, nonprofit organizations. Since its inception, Health Literacy Media's (HLM's) staff has created and implemented an in-depth menu of evidence-based health literacy services, and trained more than 16,000 health-related professionals who work with persons impacted by low health literacy. Integral to its activities, HLM seeks to create and disseminate social media messages customized for private and public health organizations that seek to communicate information to diverse audiences. By harnessing health literacy best practices (such as summarizing information, encouraging reflection, and creating a more personal tone), HLM helps its healthcare clients engage in conversations through social media.

HLM's social media programs are grounded in the idea that social media and health literacy center on relationships – both on and offline. An individual's peers are an important source of information when it comes to making health decisions. To that end, social media helps to facilitate conversations between like-minded peers and healthcare professionals about pertinent health topics [7].

The idea for the organization was born in October 2003, when the Regional Health Commission (RHC) in St. Louis approved a plan for primary and specialty care health services for the region, which was submitted to the U.S. Centers for Medicare and Medicaid Services as part of an agreement with the U.S. federal government. A key component of the plan was to reduce cultural barriers to health care and improve health literacy.

In early 2004, RHC formed a Regional Health Literacy Task Force, co-chaired by Will Ross M.D., Washington University School of Medicine, and Mark Mengle M.D., St. Louis University School of Medicine. The task force was charged to develop recommendations that supported the RHC's mission to: improve access to health care services; reduce health disparities; and improve health outcomes for the residents of the St. Louis region.

To backup, the partial impetus for these efforts stemmed from an array of individual and population health challenges partially indigenous to the St. Louis metropolitan area. For example, St. Louis' diabetes and cancer rates are higher than in some other areas within the state of Missouri as well as in the U.S.

The task force was asked to develop recommendations to strengthen communication between providers and patients, improve patient access and their ability to navigate the healthcare system, as well as build an infrastructure to sustain health literacy efforts.

After an assessment of existing literature and programs, the task force completed an action plan that was approved by the Regional Health Commission in 2004. Throughout 2005, the task force worked to prioritize and further develop its recommendations and solicit feedback from its advisory boards and the broader community. In April 2006, the RHC hosted "Building a Healthier St. Louis," a community-wide health summit, which convened more than 500 participants to provide input about the next steps to build health literacy and community health.

Concurrently, in 2005, the Missouri Foundation for Health (MFH), an independent philanthropic foundation dedicated to improving the health of the uninsured and underserved, also turned its attention to health literacy. MFH convened a Strategic Planning Committee to discuss efforts to incorporate health literacy into grant-capacity. The committee identified underlying health literacy concerns within previous proposals from 2002-2005, examined research recommendations from by the Institute of Medicine and the CDC's Community Preventive Services Task Force, and reviewed the literature about the human and financial impact of low health literacy.

In response, MFH created the Missouri Health Literacy Enhancement Committee (MHLE) in 2006, chaired by MFH board member Will Ross M.D. MHLE subsequently convened state partners in health literacy to form the Missouri Health Literacy Coordinating Council, chaired by Dr. Ross. With funding infrastructure from MFH, the coordinating council voted to create Health Literacy Missouri (HLM) as a free-standing non-profit agency. Within its first year, HLM became one of the most active health literacy centers in the U.S. Immediately, HLM implemented provider-training programs, hosted a state-wide health literacy summit, developed community-wide health literacy initiatives, and established an online library with more than 10,000 health literacy resources. Since 2009, HLM has continued to grow and build partnerships in the region, across the U.S., and around the world.

3. Social Media's Role in Helping to Build a Health Literacy Non-profit

Since 2009, HLM has built a robust social media presence with more than 7,000 followers across six platforms. While the initial followers were mostly other health literacy professionals, HLM's social media's current users includes: health journalists; international health information companies; hospital systems; global pharmaceutical companies; and consumers of health care (the general public).

HLM's social media presence quickly became a linchpin of the agency's health communications efforts. In early 2010, a health communications team launched HLM's first social media platforms in Twitter, Facebook, and LinkedIn. Initially, HLM's social media efforts were to create awareness about the concept of health literacy among the general public. Although the health literacy field was well established among researchers, HLM sought to boost the public understanding of the concept of health literacy and its social impact through the use of social media.

Hence, a primary strategy tried to help social media users increase their understanding of health literacy and to normalize and reduce communication chasms between health care professionals and the general public. HLM also intentionally decided to use social media to build public recognition and foster the organization's reputation as a trusted media source for healthcare issues. HLM's dual strategy was to provide information about health literacy into health related stories often covered by other news media outlets to potentially reach a larger audience. HLM additionally set a goal to involve stakeholders via the creation and maintenance of social media spaces to discuss health literacy issues. Finally, HLM sought to promote social media networking as a tactic to encourage potential stakeholders and partners to watch HLM's health information videos.

3.1. HealthLit Chats

The first major opportunity to use social media to discuss health literacy occurred just six months after HLM opened and the 2010 U.S. National Action Plan to Improve Health Literacy was released. The latter document identified key stakeholders, suggested activities and contributions, and set forth seven goals to improve health literacy with a focus on information, communication, and informed decision-making, access to services, research, and practice.

Using the National Action Plan as a focal point, HLM hosted more than a dozen Twitter Chats meetings on topics related to health literacy during the next 1.5 years. Much like an in-person meeting, Twitter Chats are the virtual equivalent of bringing an audience together in a conversation. Hence, HLM's Twitter Chats encouraged participants to ask questions of one or more experts, read other people's questions, and ask follow-up questions. On the first Thursday of each month, HLM hosted monthly discussions on Twitter that focused on a timely topic in health literacy. Participants were encouraged to respond to questions, post messages, and interact with other participants about a given topic during the scheduled discussion using the hashtag #healthlit.

Some specific topics included: Healthy People 2020; health literacy's role in health care reform; health literacy curriculum in schools of health professionals; and the aforementioned National Action Plan to Improve Health Literacy. HLM's first HealthLitChat in October 2010 attracted 92 people who posted 553 tweets during the 1.5-hour period.

Other participants included: representatives from healthfinder.gov, an information site operated by the U.S. Department of Health and Human Services; and spokespersons from the United States Health Resources & Services Administration and the Agency for Healthcare Research and Quality; as well as other health and health literacy organizations.

The success of the initial discussion encouraged the HLM staff to continue to engage a growing health literacy following on Twitter in additional productive conversations about important issues within the field.

The Twitter Chat program met HLM's early social media goals to raise awareness on a local and national level about the organization as well the importance of health literacy. The Twitter Chat program also advanced HLM's initial social media goals to: provide ideas; encourage others to share ideas for how to better communicate and distribute health literacy messages; generate discussion around health literacy; develop relationships with key health literacy experts and practitioners; encourage collaboration among other participants, boost Twitter followers; and increase overall social media reach.

3.2. Engaging with Legacy Broadcast Media

A key component of HLM's social media strategy has been to engage followers with original messages using video. In 2011, HLM partnered with the Higher Education Channel, HEC-TV, which is St. Louis' non-profit producer of education and arts television programming, to produce a 30-minute documentary about Missouri's health literacy challenges. Four different versions were produced (for health care professionals, policy makers, healthcare administrators and the general public). The latter approach was based on health literacy principles to provide materials tailored for specific audiences.

The documentary outlined the problem of health literacy as well as strategies to enhance health outcomes through improved communication strategies. The programs aired on public television and were promoted heavily through HLM's social media channels. The documentary won the 2012 Silver Telly Award and was nominated for a 2012 Mid-America Emmy by the National Academy of Television Arts & Sciences.

This early project established one of HLM's core and unique services: health literate video scripting and production.

4. Social Media and Video: A Service Line

In mid-2012, the founding HLM Board staff, with the Missouri Foundation for Health leadership, began a process to transition HLM from a Missouri based nonprofit heavily subsidized by the Foundation, to a self-sufficient, sustaining nonprofit organization. A multi-year exit strategy from Foundation grant supports was developed, which included a business plan to ensure stabilization and success. HLM's early success in social media and video content services suggested these strategies should be prioritized as key services in the future.

While the goal continued to create health literacy awareness via HLM's media activities, these efforts were supplemented by new initiatives to use social media to improve health outcomes. The expansion of HLM's social media mission was partially based on recent research that suggested the use of social and digital media was tied to health promotional/educational outcomes within some settings. For example, a multi-media based curriculum that encouraged 9th grade students to evaluate media messages was found to reduce their intentions to smoke more than a standard educational program (that was provided for the same age group) [8]. The study also suggested attitudes and intentions among youth are more likely to change if social media platforms were integrated within health educational interventions [8].

4.1. Health Insurance Literacy Social Media

HLM created social media initiatives to help Americans understand how to obtain and understand insurance following the 2011 introduction of the U.S. Affordable Care Act. The challenge to obtain and understanding health insurance became a barrier for some Americans who sought to use the Affordable Care Act (ACA) to obtain more affordable, accessible coverage. For example, ACA enrollment initially was adversely effected because 60 percent of those eligible to enroll in ACA's health insurance marketplaces did not understand key health insurance concepts [9]. The wise use of the ACA also required consumers to navigate corporate and government health insurance websites, as well as be more mindful of insurance-related details, such as varying premiums, deductibles, and copays.

In response, the Missouri Foundation for Health led a charge in Missouri to infuse necessary health and health insurance information into public conversation and support policy implementation through the creation and support of the Cover Missouri Coalition. Currently, the Cover Missouri Coalition includes about 800 health related partner organizations in Missouri, many of whom employ the navigators and assisters charged with directly communicating with the public on how to find, keep and use health insurance.

Early on, Cover Missouri Coalition leaders identified health literacy and, specifically, health insurance literacy, as a key component of strategy toward the overall goal of reducing the rate of insured in Missouri to 5% by 2017. While the coalition has not yet met that goal, primarily as a result of the complexity of the policy issues surrounding Medicaid's failed expansion in Missouri, by the end of the 2015 open enrollment period the rate of uninsured in Missouri was reduced to 9.8% [10].

HLM provides health literacy technical support for the Cover Missouri Coalition. In this role, HLM extended its social media experience to the larger group and was responsible for the conceptualization, creation and coordination of social media messages that support health insurance literacy (HIL) topics.

Cover Missouri contractors provided scheduled messages through social media (Tweets, Facebook posts, and YouTube videos) that focused on health insurance awareness and enrollment. HLM supplemented these efforts with messages focused on topics that boosted consumer understanding of health insurance. Some of the topics for messages were informed by HLM's interactions with Cover Missouri Coalition members.

Since 2014, HLM has created weekly social media messages (two to five messages per week) and distributed them to Cover Missouri coalition members. To date, HLM has written and distributed approximately 550 social media messages, including graphics and videos. HLM has developed three health literacy insurance social media campaigns: #healthinsurancelit Word of the Week, which defines a new health insurance term each week to help consumers understand their coverage; #ImCovered...now what? The latter helps consumers understand and use free preventive care benefits; and #healthcarehacks, which provides tips on how to optimize health care and health insurance services within a general health and health literacy framework.

HLM and its project partners – the Missouri Foundation for Health and the 800 Cover Missouri Coalition member organizations -- posted the messages on their social media platforms. While analytics are not associated with each of the partner groups' social media activities, within HLM's channels the messages were seen by an average of 257 people per Twitter message and 42 persons per Facebook message.

4.2. State of Oklahoma Thrive Social Media

HLM provided social media technical assistance to the U.S. State of Oklahoma Thrive Employee Wellness Program, which supports a health literacy and consumer engagement program for state employees, teachers and support staff, dependents, and state governmental retirees. This program potentially has an audience reach of more than 150,000 Oklahomans.

The goal of this program is to increase health literacy so state employees might better understand their health insurance coverage and make better decisions around seeking care. The program also empowers employees to become better advocates for their care and to leverage available financial resources.

HLM developed 53 messages and graphics for Facebook and Twitter. These messages highlighted and promoted a Health Literacy Webinar Series and supported health literacy and health insurance literacy topics. Some topics included: the importance of preventive care; ways to save money with health insurance; dates of open enrollment; and tips for seeing a physician. Since the internet site Thrive recently rebranded and created Facebook and Twitter accounts, HLM also created messages to introduce Thrive. The State of Oklahoma Thrive Employee Wellness Program is now considered launched and is maintained entirely by State of Oklahoma staff.

4.3. Health Insurance Literacy Consumer Health Insurance Video Series

Health literacy and adult education practitioners suggest that offering health information in video formats may be especially effective for low literacy populations. Widespread and diversified consumer access to computers and cell phones also now enable Internet-based video to diffuse culturally representative messages to diverse audiences. The potential of mobile phones to convey video-based is especially promising among Hispanic Americans, who are younger, more mobile, and socially connected than older Americans with a Latino heritage.

To supplement written materials, HLM developed 10 short videos using evidence-based health literacy principles to present health information to younger adults. The Health Insurance Video Series is a consumer-facing video series that educates consumers about health insurance, how to enroll in U.S. health insurance marketplaces, and steps after enrollment. Six of the videos were produced in English and four were in Spanish.

HLM worked with Bad Dog pictures and partners at International Institute of St. Louis (IISTL) to produce 10 consumer videos. HLM's communications staff wrote scripts for all 10 videos, which were reviewed by project partners. Other project partners edited and translated videos into Spanish. Another partner provided cultural and linguistic expertise during the script review and filming of the Spanish language videos.

All 10 videos were made available online (e.g., Vimeo, YouTube, Cover Missouri's website) by September 30, 2014, months before the beginning of the second open enrollment period in the U.S. health insurance marketplace portion of the ACA.

HLM designed and ordered 500 flash drives preloaded with pertinent consumer videos. HLM promoted and distributed the videos on flash drives and DVDs at in-person Cover Missouri meetings. HLM also made announcements through email distribution lists and social media. To promote the Spanish videos, other project staff at partner organizations shared the videos with seven St. Louis-based agencies and two statewide agencies organizations that serve Spanish-first speakers, such as Missouri Immigrant & Refugee Advocates (MIRA), Red Latina, and Office of Hispanic Ministry, through email announcements.

HLM continues to promote and distribute the consumer Health Insurance Video Series through meetings and emails, newsletter articles, social media, other messages for healthcare professionals, as well as the aforementioned media formats.

To encourage the use of the videos, HLM shared tips with consumers (e.g., play in waiting rooms and during enrollment appointments), and with staff at organizations (e.g., during staff meetings, new staff training, and social media). HLM shared tips during monthly meetings and through written materials on ShareFile. The video series has been shared with assisters nationwide, as the videos were featured in the Families USA resource slideshow in January 2016.

To date, the videos have received almost 5,000 views online and been distributed on more than 800 flash drives. The video series received a 2015 Clear Mark Award of Distinction from the Center for Plain Language.

4.4. Health Insurance Literacy "Clayton & Candra Got You Covered" Video Series for Enrollment Assisters and Health Care Professionals

As an effective alternative to print materials, HLM created ten training videos for enrollment assisters and health care professionals to enroll persons in diverse ACA programs. The videos supported and promoted health insurance literacy by explaining and demonstrating how to best communicate health insurance information to consumers.

HLM created a timeline to produce the assister how-to videos in two waves. The first five videos were produced to be released prior to the start of ACA's open enrollment period in 2016. To generate a list of topics for the assister how-to videos, HLM gathered input from key stakeholders. The selected topics included: calculating a consumer's modified adjusted gross income (MAGI); using teach-back to help consumers understand preventive care; providing clear action steps to help consumers talk to their insurance company; resolving myths related to the ACA's insurance marketplace; and assisting consumers to select a primary care provider.

The first five videos and accompanying handouts were available online in mid-September 2016 via YouTube and Vimeo. In just one and a half months, the videos received nearly 900 views online; the MAGI video received the most views (n=253). HLM also added the videos to the Cover Missouri flash drives and distributed more than 350 flash drives at Cover Missouri regional summits, in-person meetings, and HLM's annual summit. HLM promoted the videos among assisters and healthcare professionals through email announcements and newsletter messages, Cover Missouri meetings and regional summits, as well as a health insurance literacy Google group.

To supplement the videos, HLM created a handout for two of the videos that provided: 1) a worksheet for assisters to use when calculating a consumer's MAGI; and 2) a handout for assisters that provides consumer tips to talk to an insurance company. A link to each of these handouts was provided in the video description, and the handouts were available to Cover Missouri members through ShareFile. To obtain input about the videos from Cover Missouri Coalition (CMC) members, HLM developed an online survey to assess assisters' increase in knowledge about the video topics, their intention to apply the information and skills to their work, and references to undergird the content of the next five videos.

Thirteen CMC members completed the online survey. The majority of the survey participants either strongly or somewhat agreed that the furnished videos helped them reached a better understanding of each video topic. The majority of participants reported they were 'very likely' to apply the knowledge and skills they learned from the video in their work.

Following feedback from CMC members and others, HLM developed the remaining five videos in early November and made the videos available online via YouTube and Vimeo. The videos have been viewed online more than 7,000 times and have received nationwide recognition.

Three of the "Clayton & Candra Got You Covered" videos were picked up by AccentHealth as part of their patient educational programming in up to 30,000 outpatient waiting rooms across the U.S. AccentHealth provides TVs in qualified outpatient waiting room environments for health providers of all sizes across the U.S.. AccentHealth's educational programming is customized by specialty and patient population and is produced by CNN's Medical Unit.

HLM's videos also received a 2016 ClearMark Award of Distinction and a 2015 Digital Health Award. Enroll America showcased the videos on its Health Insurance Literacy Resource Hub.

5. Conclusion: Recommendations for Designing a Social Media Strategy

This chapter details the experience of Health Literacy Media – a mid-sized health literacy nonprofit communications group – in digital and social media during the past 10 years. HLM's overall experience suggests an underlying preference to utilize social media as a health communications medium to advance health literacy practices.

However, the latter is a challenge because social and digital media platforms continue to evolve -- often independently of the advances in theory and practice that occur within the field of health literacy. Nevertheless, HLM has found the integration of social and digital media with health literacy program content is fostered by the use of evidence-based health literacy principles, such as the use of plain language and communication strategies that are tailored for specific audiences.

In HLM's experience, the use of social media is enhanced by defined goals, such as helping uninsured consumers understand how to sign up for Marketplace coverage, educating people at risk for heart disease that they are at risk and specific strategies to lower that risk, and building an expert voice in the field to increase brand awareness.

HLM suggests health organizations should use specific goals to develop a plan of action to address the topics they want covered and build the conversation they seek to have, which positions their institutional voice within that conversation. For example, when HLM wanted to develop its presence as an important voice in the health literacy conversation, the organization used the Twitter-based HealthLitChat to make HLM visible in the field and to draw in and develop the voices already in the conversation. This combination of promoting both external and internal voices built good will, elevated a pluralistic conversation, and solidified HLM's place as an expert in the field. Overall, the equalizing influence of social media in building multi-level conversations fostered the aforementioned evolution.

5.1. Strategy Considerations

HLM's experience is there are diverse considerations to take into account when launching a social media plan. First, health care organizations should know with whom they are trying to build a relationship, what business goals they are trying to achieve, whether the initiatives are evidence-based, in addition to clarifying potentially diverse leadership responsibilities. Second, health care organizations need to consider the tone/manner used with an intended audience, how to assess interventions, how to operationalize success, and how to create culturally appropriate content for an intended audience.

To avoid potential embarrassment, the social media information provided by health care organizations also should be consistent with (or at least not contradict) the available evidence about the health care status of different populations within a region. For example, Jha, Lin and Savoia found most U.S. state health departments social media messages, frequently on Facebook, are inconsistent with the BRFSS (Behavioral Risk Factor Surveillance System) data about their region's health status [11]. Overall, it is difficult to envision how a social media intervention can generate long-range therapeutic health outcomes if it is not based on and directly addresses evidence-based public health needs.

Conceptually, HLM's experience is the judicious use of social media is associated with improvements in health behaviors and boosting the public's health literacy. HLM's experience also suggests improvements in health behaviors and boosting the public's health literacy are accelerated by the use of social media -- especially to communicate with vulnerable populations. However, the selection of social media platforms, the messages used, and the frequency of posts often are a byproduct of the specific health behavioral goals and health literacy enhancements established by an intervention's stakeholders, which includes the intended audience.

HLM emphasizes that getting to know your audience is both a strategy as well as a health literacy principle. Organizations need to define who they want to "talk to" through social media, and then make sure their content strategy and tone appeals to their desired audience.

Further, it is important to remember that in the world of social media the number of followers within organizations is relative. The number of followers on a social media page does not always suggest the engagement and relevance that resulted from a social media-based health intervention. Overall, HLM suggests that quality beats quantity and assessments (and goals) should be targeted to emphasize specific health outcomes more than broad ratings based on media use.

5.2. Technical Considerations

HLM suggests the attraction and engagement of intended followers depend on the relevance of social media posts. HLM suggests when an organization is telling its story, the narrative should be authentic as well as reflect a therapeutic, evidence-based perspective about individual and population health.

Organizations also should pay attention to their audience's concerns, watch how posts perform, adjust accordingly, and develop imagery and language that attract more followers.

The determination of the latter mandates the use of metrics. Social media health communication/promotion efforts should base metrics on what they hope to get from social media (sharing, click-throughs, sign-ups, office visits, etc) as well as the health care objectives they seek to advance. While metrics help keep track of which content gets the best response (to create more of it), the assessment of the association between social media and health outcomes also is vital to the future of the fields of health communication, health promotion, health literacy and demonstrates the value of social media-based intervention efforts by smaller organizations.

For the best results, HLM also suggests the use of plain language principles. Keep social media posts simple and easy to read by checking for spelling and grammar errors. Also, avoid writing in ALL CAPS, using jargon and insider buzzwords, and making every word a #hashtag. For organizations that work directly with consumers, it is best to be as personable as possible. A friendly, conversational tone often is helpful and is a proven health literacy tactic to work with vulnerable populations.

Timing is also important. A few strategically timed posts are better than a constant delivery of content to most followers. Fortunately, there are available tools to help organizations ascertain the best time to post, such as Facebook's analytic tools.

In addition, it is important to follow social media etiquette and recognize that different social networks have different "rules." For example, it is considered excessive to post more than once a day on platforms such as Facebook and LinkedIn. However, posting multiple times a day on Twitter currently is standard operating practice.

Social media managers need to be responsive when users or peers reach out via their social media links. Social media is an instant world; a line directly that connects a person or organization directly to their audience. Consequently, it is important to share content from like-minded organizations. This helps build a social media presence and is a productive tactic to post compelling content, increase the reach for trusted sources, and enhance connectivity to other organizations and individuals.

Although developing an effective and health literate social media strategy is a complex undertaking, it helped HIM grow from a regional health commission to one of the largest nonprofits in the U.S. With a set of defined goals, a clear action plan, and a well-developed understanding of the platforms, social media can help organizations be the voice in the field that many want to hear.

References

[1] O'Mara B. Social media, digital video and health promotion in a culturally and linguistically diverse Australia. Health Promot Int. 2013;28(3):466-476. DOI: 10.1093/heapro/das014.

[2] http://www.pewinternet.org/2015/04/01/us-smartphone-use-in-2015/. Retrieved May 19, 2017.

[3] http://www.pewinternet.org/fact-sheet-mobile. Retrieved May 19, 2017. Retrieved May 19, 2017.

[4] http://www.pewinternet.org/2016/11/11/social-media-update-2016/. Retrieved May 19, 2017.

[5] Korda ZI. Harnessing Social Media for Health Promotion and Behavior Change. Health Promot Pract. 2013;14(1):15-23. DOI: 10.1177/1524839911405850.

[6] Kreuter MW, McBride TD, Caburnay CA, Poor T, Thompson VLS, Alcaraz KI, Eddens KS, Rath S, Perkins H, Casey C. What can health communication science offer for ACA implementation? Five evidence-informed strategies for expanding Medicaid eEnrollment. Milbank Q. 2014;92(1):40-62. DOI: 10.1111/1468-0009.12040.

[7] Lau AY, Siek KA, Fernandez-Luque L, Tange H, Chhanabhai P, Li SY, Elkin PL, Arjabi A, Walczowski AA, Ang CS, Eysenbach, G. The role of social media for patients and consumer health. Yearb Med Inform. 2011; 6(1):131-138.

[8] Primack BA, Douglas EL, Land SR, Miller E, Fine MJ. Comparison of media literacy and usual education to prevent tobacco use: a cluster-randomized trial. J Sch Health. 2014;84(2):106-115. DOI: 10.1111/josh.12130.

[9] http://content.healthaffairs.org/content/33/1/161.full.pdf+html. Retrieved May 19,2017.

[10] United States Census Bureau. (2016). "Health insurance coverage in the United States: 2015." Report Number: P60-257. Retrieved from http://www.census.gov/library/publications/2016/demo/p60-257.html

[11] Jha A Lin L, Savoia EJ. The use of social media by state health departments in the US: Analyzing health communication through Facebook. J Community Health. 2016;41(1):174-179. DOI: 10.1007/s10900-015-0083-4.

Health Literacy
R.A. Logan and E.R. Siegel (Eds.)
IOS Press, 2017

477

Subject Index

478